Hartman's Nursing Assistant Care

Long-Term Care and Home Health

Susan Alvare
Jetta Fuzy, RN, MS
and Suzanne Rymer, MSTE, RN, C, LSW

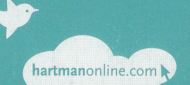

hartmanonline.com

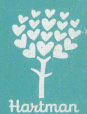

Hartman

ii

Credits

Managing Editor
Susan Alvare Hedman

Designer
Kirsten Browne

Illustrator
Thaddeus Castillo

Cover Illustrator
Jo Tronc

Page Layout
Thaddeus Castillo

Photography
Art Clifton/Dick Ruddy

Proofreaders
Kristin Calderon/Angela Storey/Michele Wiedemer

Sales/Marketing
Debbie Rinker/Caroyl Scott
Kendra Robertson/Erika Walker

Customer Service
Fran Desmond/Tom Noble
Angela Storey/Cheryl Garcia/Eliza Martin

Warehouse Coordinator
Chris Beck

Copyright Information

© 2009 by Hartman Publishing, Inc.
8529 Indian School Road, NE
Albuquerque, New Mexico 87112
(505) 291-1274
web: hartmanonline.com
e-mail: orders@hartmanonline.com

ISBN 978-1-60425-010-7
ISBN 978-1-60425-013-8 (Hardcover)

PRINTED IN CANADA

Notice to Readers

Though the guidelines and procedures contained in this text are based on consultations with healthcare professionals, they should not be considered absolute recommendations. The instructor and readers should follow employer, local, state, and federal guidelines concerning healthcare practices. These guidelines change, and it is the reader's responsibility to be aware of these changes and of the policies and procedures of her or his healthcare facility.

The publisher, author, editors, and reviewers cannot accept any responsibility for errors or omissions or for any consequences from application of the information in this book and make no warranty, expressed or implied, with respect to the contents of the book. The Publisher does not warrant or guarantee any of the products described herein or perform any analysis in connection with any of the product information contained herein.

Gender Usage

This textbook utilizes the pronouns "he," "his," "she," and "hers" interchangeably to denote healthcare team members and residents and clients.

Special Thanks

A special thank you goes to Beverly Cobb, RN, in Anthem, AZ for her invaluable assistance with our special care skills chapter.

Another warm thank you goes to Charles Illian, RN, BSN, CIC, our infection control expert in Orlando, FL for helping us with the infection prevention chapter. Charles, we couldn't have done it without you!

Thank you to Jill Holmes Long, MA, BSN, BS, RN, our go-to reviewer and author in Hayesville, NC for her important contributions to our mothers and newborns chapter and conflict resolution section.

A heartfelt thank you also goes to our insightful and wonderful reviewers, listed in alphabetical order:

Larry Bailey, RN, BA, BSN, HSTE
Mansfield, TX

Tracie L. Carter, LPN
Brunswick, GA

Regina G. Cottrell, MN-Ed, BS, RN
Chandler, AZ

Margaret J. Denault, M.Ed., RN-BC, SDS
Becket, MA

Mandy Farmer, LPN, HCC Instructor
Fort Cobb, OK

Pamela Hatchett, LPN
Brunswick, GA

Elizabeth A. Huss, RN, BSN
Austin, TX

Janice M. Joyce, RN, BSN
Springfield, IL

Vivian Luzar, RNC
Niles, OH

Aretha D. Meggett, LPN/SNRN
Pittsburgh, PA

Gloria Stafford, RN
Austin, TX

Beverly Vespico, MHA, RN, C
Harveys Lake, PA

Nancy Whatley, RN
William J. Whatley, Administrator
Colorado Springs, CO

Betty Wolfe, RN
Tulsa, OK

Contents

24 Introduction to Home Care

25 Infection Prevention and Safety in the Home

26 Medications in Home Care

27 New Mothers, Infants, and Children

Procedures

Using a Hartman Textbook

Understanding how your book is organized and what its special features are will help you make the most of this resource!

We have assigned each chapter its own colored tab. Each colored tab contains the chapter number and title, and you'll see them on the side of every page.

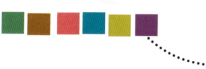

1. List examples of legal and ethical behavior

Everything in this book, the student workbook, and your instructor's teaching material is organized around learning objectives. A learning objective is a very specific piece of knowledge or a very specific skill. After reading the text, if you can do what the learning objective says, you know you have mastered the material.

bloodborne pathogens

You'll find bold key terms throughout the text followed by their definition. They are also listed in the glossary at the back of this book.

Giving a back rub

All care procedures are highlighted by the same black bar for easy recognition.

Guidelines:
Handwashing

Care Guidelines and Observing and Reporting are colored green for easy reference.

Residents' Rights
Cuts, Scrapes, and Rashes

These boxes teach important information on how to support and promote Resident's Rights, as well as providing other types of important information.

Chapter Review

Chapter-ending questions test your knowledge of the information found in the chapter. If you have trouble answering a question, you can return to the text and reread the material.

1

Understanding Healthcare Settings

1. Discuss the structure of the healthcare system and describe ways it is changing

Welcome to the world of health care. Health care is a growing field. The healthcare system refers to all the different kinds of providers, facilities, and payers involved in delivering medical care. **Providers** are people or organizations that provide health care, including doctors, nurses, clinics, and agencies. **Facilities** are places where care is delivered or administered, including hospitals, long-term care facilities or nursing homes, and treatment centers. **Payers** are people or organizations paying for healthcare services. These include insurance companies, government programs like Medicare and Medicaid, and the individual person needing care. Together, all these people, places, and organizations make up our healthcare system.

This textbook will focus on two types of care: long-term care and home health care. **Long-term care (LTC)** is given in long-term care facilities (LTCF) for people who need 24-hour, supervised nursing care. This type of care is given to people who need a high level of care for ongoing conditions. The term "nursing homes" was once widely used to refer to these facilities; Now, however, they are often called long-term care facilities, skilled nursing facilities, residential facilities, rehabilitation centers, or extended care facilities.

People who live in long-term care facilities may be disabled and/or elderly. They may arrive from hospitals or other healthcare settings. Their **length of stay** (the number of days a person stays in a healthcare facility) may be short, such as a few days or a few months, or longer than six months. Some of these people will have a **terminal illness**, which means that the person is expected to die from the illness. Other people may recover and return to their homes or to other living facilities or situations.

Most conditions seen in LTC are **chronic**. This means they last a long period of time, even a lifetime. Chronic conditions include physical disabilities, heart disease, stroke, and dementia. (You will learn more about these disorders and diseases in Chapter 18.)

People who live in long-term care facilities are usually called "residents" because it is where they reside or live. These places are their homes for the duration of their stay (Fig. 1-1).

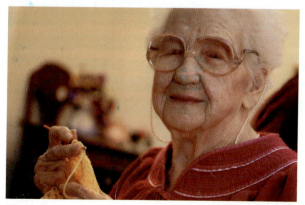

Fig. 1-1. *Long-term care is given to people who need a high level of care for ongoing conditions. People who live in long-term care facilities are called "residents" because they reside in the facility and it is their home.*

Home health care takes place in a person's home (Fig. 1-2). This type of care is also generally given to people who are older and are chronically ill but who are able to and wish to remain at home. Home care may also be needed when a person is weak after a recent hospital stay. Skilled assistance or monitoring may be required. People who receive home care are usually referred to as "clients."

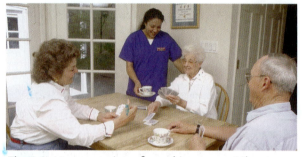

Fig. 1-2. Home care is performed in a person's home. People receiving home care are generally referred to as "clients."

In some ways, working as a home health aide is similar to working as a nursing assistant. Almost all care described in this textbook for nursing assistants applies to home health aides. Most of the personal care and basic nursing procedures are the same. Home health aides may also clean, shop for groceries, do laundry, and cook. There is information on home care throughout the textbook, but Chapters 24 through 30 deal solely with home care.

Home health aides may have more contact with the client's family. They also will work more independently, although a supervisor monitors their work. The advantage of home health care is that clients do not have to leave home. They may have lived there for many years, and staying at home can be comforting.

People who need long-term care or home care will have different **diagnoses**, or medical conditions determined by a doctor. The stages of illnesses or diseases affect how sick people are and how much care they will need. The job of nursing assistants and home health aides will also vary. This is due to each person's different symptoms, abilities, and needs.

Other healthcare settings include the following:

- **Assisted living** facilities provide some help with daily care, such as showers, meals, and dressing. Help with medications may also be given. People who live in these facilities do not need skilled, 24-hour care, and they are relatively independent. Assisted living facilities allow more independent living in a home-like environment. A resident can live in a single room or an apartment; however, some residents have roommates. An assisted living facility may be attached to a long-term care facility, or it may stand alone. "Boarding home" is another term that may be used to refer to assisted living facilities.

- **Adult daycare** is care given at a facility during daytime working hours. Generally, adult daycare is for people who need some help but are not seriously ill or disabled. Adult daycare centers give different levels of care. Adult daycare can also provide a break for spouses, family members, and friends.

- **Acute care** is given in hospitals and ambulatory surgical centers. It is for people who have an immediate illness. People are admitted for short stays for surgery or diseases. Acute care is 24-hour skilled care for temporary, but serious, illnesses or injuries (Fig. 1-3). **Skilled care** is medically necessary care given by a skilled nurse or therapist. This care is available 24 hours a day. It is ordered by a doctor, and involves a treatment plan.

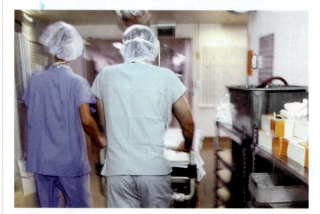

Fig. 1-3. Acute care is performed in hospitals for illnesses or injuries that require immediate care.

- **Subacute care** can be given in a hospital or in a long-term care facility. Subacute care is given to people who have had an acute injury or illness or problem resulting from a disease. These patients need treatment that requires more care and observation than some long-term care facilities can give and less care than acute illnesses require. Treatment usually ends when the condition has stabilized and/or after the predetermined time period for treatment has been completed. The cost is usually less than a hospital but more than long-term care. You will learn more about subacute care in Chapter 22.

- **Outpatient care** is usually given for less than 24 hours. It is for people who have had treatments or surgery and need short-term skilled care.

- **Rehabilitation** is care given in facilities or homes by a specialist. Physical, occupational, and speech therapists restore or improve function after an illness or injury. You will learn more about rehabilitation and related care in Chapter 21.

- **Hospice care** is given in facilities or homes for people who have six months or less to live. Hospice workers give physical and emotional care and comfort, while also supporting families. You will learn more about hospice care in Chapter 23.

Who will pay for medical care may determine what kind of care a person receives and where he receives it. Often payers control the amount and types of healthcare services people receive. Traditional insurance companies offer plans that pay for the health care of plan members. Most people covered by traditional insurance are part of a plan at their place of work. The costs are paid for by the employer, the employee, or shared by both. The costs have risen greatly, however, and many employers and employees can no longer afford to pay for traditional insurance plans.

As a reaction to the increased costs of traditional insurance plans, many employers and employees belong to **health maintenance organizations (HMOs)**. HMOs require that you use a particular doctor or group of doctors except in case of emergency. The doctors working for HMOs are paid to provide care while keeping costs down. Thus they may see more patients, order fewer tests, or cut costs in other ways.

Preferred provider organizations (PPOs) are another healthcare option used to reduce costs. A PPO is a network of providers that contract to provide health services to a group of people. Employees are given incentives to use network providers. Employers are given reduced, fee-for-service rates for getting employees to participate in the network. A person in a PPO may still get health care outside the network of providers, but must pay a higher portion of the cost.

If you become seriously ill, you may be admitted to a hospital. The costs of hospital care have risen greatly. To make up for it, healthcare payers are controlling who can be admitted to a hospital and for how long. After release from the hospital, many people need continuing care. This is particularly true as people are released after shorter hospital stays. Continuing care may be provided in a long-term care facility, a rehabilitation hospital, or by a home health agency. The type of care depends on the medical condition and needs of the patient or client.

Our healthcare system is constantly changing. As we develop new and better ways of caring for people, care becomes more expensive. Better health care helps people live longer, which leads to a larger elderly population that may need additional health care. New discoveries and expensive equipment have also driven healthcare costs higher (Fig. 1-4).

HMOs and PPOs continue to replace traditional insurance plans. This affects the amount and quality of health care provided. These cost control strategies are often called **managed care**. In the past, the goal of health care was to make sick people well. Today it is to get sick people well in the most efficient (least expensive) way possible.

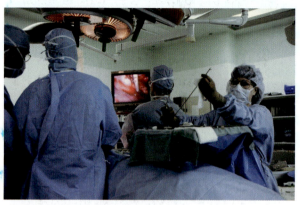

Fig. 1-4. Technology makes it possible to offer better health care, but equipment can be expensive.

2. Describe a typical long-term care facility

Long-term care facilities (LTCF) are businesses that provide skilled nursing care 24 hours a day. These facilities may offer assisted living housing, dementia care, or subacute care. Some facilities offer specialized care, while others care for all types of residents. The typical long-term care facility offers personal care for all residents and focused care for residents with special needs. Personal care includes bathing, skin, nail and hair care, and assistance with walking, eating, dressing, transferring, and toileting. All of these daily personal care tasks are called "activities of daily living," or ADLs.

Other common services offered at LTCFs include the following:

- Physical, occupational, and speech therapy

- Wound care

- Care of different types of tubes and **catheters** (a thin tube inserted into the body that is used to drain fluids or inject fluids)

- Nutrition therapy

- Management of chronic diseases, such as AIDS, diabetes, chronic obstructive pulmo-

nary disease (COPD), cancer, and congestive heart failure (CHF)

When specialized care is offered at long-term care facilities, the employees must have special training. Residents with similar needs may be placed in units together. Non-profit companies or for-profit companies can own long-term care facilities.

3. Describe residents who live in long-term care facilities

There are some general statements that can be made about residents in nursing homes. However, more important than understanding the entire population is understanding the individuals for whom you will care. Make sure you know how to care for residents based on their needs, illnesses, and preferences.

According to the National Center for Health Statistics, almost 91 percent of long-term care residents in the U.S. are over age 65. Only nine percent are younger than 65. Almost 72 percent of residents are female (Fig. 1-5). More than 85 percent are Caucasian. This is a much larger percentage than the U.S. population as a whole. About one-third of residents come from a private residence; over 50 percent come from a hospital or other facility.

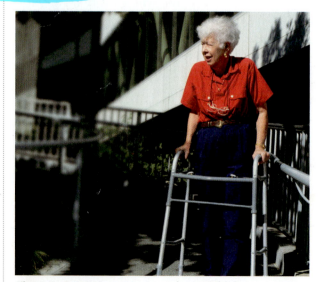

Fig. 1-5. Caucasian women make up a high percentage of residents in long-term care facilities.

The length of stay of almost one-half of residents is six months or more. These residents need enough help with their activities of daily living that 24-hour care is needed. Often, they did not have caregivers available to give enough care for them to live in the community. The groups with the longest average stay are the developmentally disabled. They are often younger than 65. You will learn more about these groups in Chapter 8.

The other half of residents stay for less than six months. This group generally falls into two categories. The first category is residents admitted for terminal care. They will die in the facility. The second category is residents admitted for rehabilitation or temporary illness. They will recover and return to the community. As you can imagine, care of these residents may be very different.

Dementia is defined as the loss of mental abilities, such as thinking, remembering, reasoning, and communicating. Various studies place the number of nursing home residents with dementia between 50 and 90 percent. Dementia and other mental disorders are major causes of nursing home admissions. Many residents are admitted with other disorders as well. However, the disorders themselves are often not the main reason for admission. It is most often the lack of ability to care for oneself and the lack of a support system that leads people into a facility.

A support system is vital in allowing the elderly to live outside a facility. For every elderly person living in a long-term care facility, at least two with similar disorders and disabilities live in the community.

You may notice the lack of outside support given to your residents. It is one reason you will care for the "whole person" instead of only the illness or disease. Residents have many needs besides bathing, eating, drinking, and toileting. These needs will go unmet if staff do not work to meet them.

4. Explain policies and procedures

You will be told where to locate a list of policies and procedures that all staff members are expected to follow. A **policy** is a course of action that should be taken every time a certain situation occurs. For example, a very basic policy is that healthcare information must remain confidential. A **procedure** is a method, or way, of doing something. For example, your facility will have a procedure for reporting information about residents. The procedure explains what form to complete, when and how often to fill it out, and to whom it is given. You will be told where to find a list of policies and procedures that all staff are expected to follow.

Common policies at long-term care facilities include the following:

- All resident information must remain confidential. This is not only a facility rule, it is also the law. See Chapter 3 for more information on confidentiality, including the Health Insurance Portability and Accountability Act (HIPAA).

- The plan of care must always be followed. Nursing assistants should perform tasks assigned by the care plan. They should not do any tasks that are not included or approved by the nurse.

- Nursing assistants should not do tasks not included in the job description.

- Nursing assistants must report important events or changes in residents to a nurse.

- Personal problems must not be discussed with the resident or the resident's family.

- Nursing assistants should not take money or gifts from residents or their families (Fig. 1-6).

- Nursing assistants must be on time for work. They must be dependable.

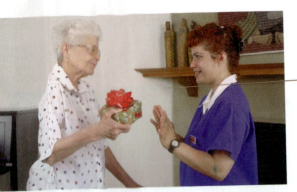

Fig. 1-6. *Nursing assistants should not accept money or gifts because it is unprofessional and may lead to conflict.*

Your employer will have policies and procedures for every resident care situation. Written procedures may seem long and complicated, but each step is important. Become familiar with your facility's policies and procedures.

5. Describe the long-term care survey process

Inspections are done to make sure long-term care facilities (and home health agencies) follow state and federal regulations. Inspections are done every 9 to 15 months by the state agency that licenses facilities. These inspections are called surveys. They may be done more often if a facility has been cited. To **cite** means to find a problem through a survey. Inspections may be done less often if the facility has a good record. Inspection teams include a variety of trained healthcare professionals.

Surveyors study how well staff care for residents. They focus on how residents' nutritional, physical, social, emotional, and spiritual needs are being met. They interview residents and family and observe staff's interactions with residents and the care given. They review resident charts and observe meals. Surveys are one reason the "paperwork" part of a nursing assistant's job is so important.

If a facility is cited for not following a federal or state regulation, surveyors use tags (F-Tags or N-Tags) to note these problems.

When surveyors are in your facility, try not to be nervous. Give the same great care you do every day. Answer any questions to the best of your ability. If you do not know the answer, be honest. Never guess. Tell the surveyor that you do not know the answer but will find out as quickly as possible, then do just that. Do not offer any information unless asked.

The **Joint Commission**, formerly the Joint Commission on Accreditation of Healthcare Organizations (JCAHO), is an independent, not-for-profit organization that evaluates and accredits healthcare organizations. Its goal is to improve the safety and quality of care given to patients, clients, and residents. For an organization to receive accreditation from the Joint Commission, it must undergo a comprehensive survey process at least every three years. The survey process includes carefully checking performance in specific areas, such as patient rights, treatment, and infection prevention.

The surveys that the Joint Commission performs are not affiliated with state inspections. Healthcare organizations are not required to participate in the Joint Commission's survey process; this is done on a volunteer basis. Organizations that are accredited by the Joint Commission include hospitals, long-term care facilities, rehabilitation centers, hospice services, home care agencies, laboratories, and other organizations.

6. Explain Medicare and Medicaid

The **Centers for Medicare & Medicaid Services (CMS),** formerly known as the Health Care Finance Administration (HCFA), is a federal agency within the U.S. Department of Health and Human Services (Fig. 1-7). CMS runs two national healthcare programs—Medicare and Medicaid. They both help pay for health care and health insurance for millions of Americans. CMS has many other responsibilities as well.

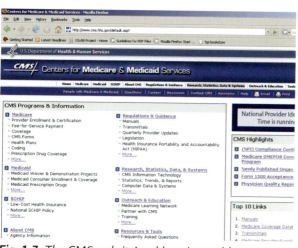

Fig. 1-7. *The CMS website's address is cms.hhs.gov.*

Medicare is a health insurance program that was established in 1965 for people aged 65 or older. It also covers people of any age with permanent kidney failure or certain disabilities. Medicare has four parts. Part A helps pay for care in a hospital or skilled nursing facility or for care from a home health agency or hospice. Part B helps pay for doctor services and other medical services and equipment. Part C allows private health insurance companies to provide Medicare benefits. Part D helps pay for medications prescribed for treatment. Medicare will only pay for care it determines to be medically necessary.

Medicaid is a medical assistance program for low-income people. It is funded by both the federal government and each state. Eligibility is determined by income and special circumstances. People must qualify for this program.

Medicare and Medicaid pay long-term care facilities a fixed amount for services. This is based on the resident's need upon admission.

Home Care Focus

For home care, Medicare pays for intermittent, not continuous, services provided by a certified home health agency. The agency must meet specific guidelines established by Medicare. To qualify for home health care, Medicare recipients must usually be unable to leave home, and their doctors must determine that they need home health care. Medicare will

pay the full cost of most covered home healthcare services. However, Medicare will not pay for round-the-clock home health care. Home health care plays an important role when skilled care is needed on a part-time basis.

7. Discuss the term "culture change" and describe Pioneer Network and The Eden Alternative

Culture change is a term given to the process of transforming services for elders so that they are based on the values and practices of the person receiving care. Culture change involves respecting both elders and those working with them. Core values are choice, dignity, respect, self-determination, and purposeful living. To honor culture change, healthcare settings may need to change organization practices, physical environments, and relationships at all levels.

Pioneer Network was formed in 1997 by a small group of professionals in long-term care to advocate for person-directed care. This group called for a change in how elders are treated wherever they live—whether in care facilities or at home. Pioneer Network promotes a movement away from institutions and promotes caring environments in which a person's individual voice is heard and his or her choices are respected. For more information about this organization, visit pioneernetwork.net.

The Eden Alternative is a not-for-profit organization founded in the mid 1990s by Dr. William Thomas. Its ongoing focus is to improve the lives of elders and their caregivers by creating environments that support growth and development, while trying to eliminate problems of loneliness, helplessness, and boredom that many elderly people suffer.

The Eden Alternative offers education, resources and consulting services to help make environments for the elderly meaningful. Places that have adopted the Eden Alternative's philosophy are typically filled with plants and animals, and are regularly visited by children. The Eden Alternative strives to improve the quality of life and quality of care for the elderly (Fig. 1-8). For more information about this organization, visit their website at edenalt.org.

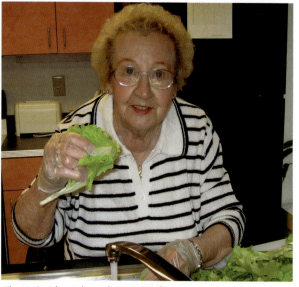

Fig. 1-8. *The Eden Alternative focuses on eliminating boredom, loneliness, and helplessness by promoting meaningful elder care.* (PHOTO COURTESY OF THE EDEN ALTERNATIVE)

Chapter Review

1. What is long-term care?

2. What is home health care?

3. List one fact about each of the following healthcare settings: assisted living facilities, adult daycare, acute care, subacute care, outpatient care, rehabilitation, and hospice care.

4. List five services commonly offered at long-term care facilities.

5. Who makes up the majority of nursing home residents—men or women?

6. What are two general categories of residents who stay in a care facility for less than six months?

7. List five common policies at long-term care facilities.

8. List two ways that surveyors study how well staff care for residents in a facility.

9. Briefly describe what the Medicare and Medicaid programs do.

10. List three problems that elderly people may face that The Eden Alternative tries to eliminate.

2

The Nursing Assistant and the Care Team

1. Identify the members of the care team and describe how the care team works together to provide care

Residents will have different needs and problems. Healthcare professionals with different kinds of education and experience will help care for them. This group is known as the "care team." Members of the care team include the following:

Nursing Assistant (NA) or Certified Nursing Assistant (CNA). The nursing assistant (NA) performs delegated tasks, such as taking vital signs, and provides routine personal care, such as bathing residents and helping with toileting. Nursing assistants must have at least 75 hours of training, and in many states, training exceeds 100 hours. Nursing assistants spend more time with residents than other members of the care team. That is why they act as the "eyes and ears" of the team. Observing and reporting changes in the resident's condition or abilities is a very important role of the NA (Fig. 2-1).

Registered Nurse (RN). A registered nurse is a licensed professional who has completed two to four years of education. RNs have diplomas or college degrees and have passed a licensing exam administered by the state board of nursing. Registered nurses may have additional academic degrees or education in specialty areas. In long-term care, a registered nurse coordinates, manages, and provides skilled nursing care.

This includes administering special treatments and giving medication as prescribed by a physician. A registered nurse also assigns tasks and supervises daily care of residents by nursing assistants.

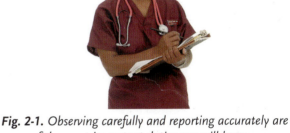

Fig. 2-1. *Observing carefully and reporting accurately are some of the most important duties you will have.*

Licensed Practical Nurse (LPN) or Licensed Vocational Nurse (LVN). A licensed practical nurse or licensed vocational nurse is a licensed professional who has completed one to two years of education. A LPN/LVN administers medications and gives treatments. LPNs may also supervise nursing assistants' daily care of residents.

Physician or Doctor (MD or DO). A doctor's job is to diagnose disease or disability and prescribe treatment. Doctors have graduated from four-year medical schools, which they attended after receiving bachelor's degrees. Many doctors also take specialized training programs after medical school (Fig. 2-2).

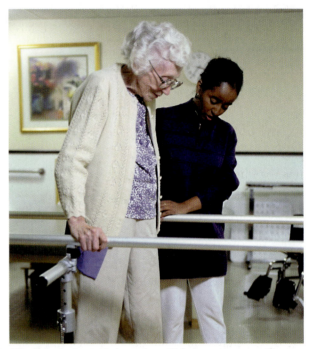

Fig. 2-2. Doctors diagnose disease and prescribe treatment.

Physical Therapist (PT). A physical therapist evaluates a person and develops a treatment plan to increase movement, improve circulation, promote healing, reduce pain, prevent disability, and help the resident regain or maintain mobility (Fig. 2-3). A PT administers therapy in the form of heat, cold, massage, ultrasound, electricity, and exercise to muscles, bones, and joints. For example, a PT helps a person to safely use a walker, cane, or wheelchair. Physical therapist education programs are offered at two degree levels: doctoral and master's. Entrance into these programs usually requires an undergraduate degree. Master's degree programs usually last two years, and doctoral degree programs last three years. PTs have to pass national and state licensure exams before they can practice.

Occupational Therapist (OT). An occupational therapist helps residents learn to compensate for disabilities. An OT helps residents perform **activities of daily living (ADLs)**. ADLs are personal daily care tasks. They include bathing, dressing, caring for teeth and hair, toileting, and eating and drinking. This often involves equipment called **assistive** or **adaptive devices** (Fig. 2-4). (See Chapter 21 for more information.) For example, an OT can teach a person to use a special fork to feed himself. The OT observes a resident's needs and plans a treatment program. Occupational therapists generally have an

undergraduate degree before being admitted to either a doctoral or master's program, but some students are admitted without a bachelor's degree. OTs have to pass a national certification examination and most must be licensed within their state.

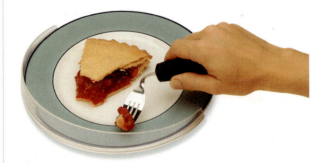

Fig. 2-3. A physical therapist will help restore specific abilities.

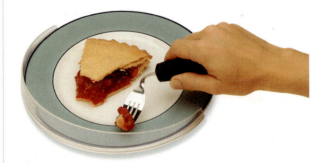

Fig. 2-4. An occupational therapist will help residents learn to use adaptive devices, such as this one for eating. (PHOTO COURTESY OF NORTH COAST MEDICAL, INC. 800-821-9319)

Speech-Language Pathologist (SLP). A speech-language pathologist helps with speech and swallowing problems. An SLP identifies communication disorders, addresses factors involved in recovery, and develops a plan of care to meet short- and long-term recovery goals. An SLP teaches exercises to help the resident improve or overcome speech problems. For example, after a stroke, a person may not be able to speak or speak clearly. An SLP may use a picture board to help the person communicate thirst or pain. An SLP also evaluates a person's ability to swallow food and drink. Speech-language pathologists (SLPs) are generally required to have a master's degree in speech-language pathology. Most states require that SLPs be licensed or certified to work.

Registered Dietitian (RD). A registered dietitian creates diets for residents with special needs. Special diets can improve health and help manage illness. RDs may supervise the preparation and service of food and educate others on healthy nutritional habits. Registered dietitians have completed a bachelor's degree and may also have a master's degree or have completed postgraduate work. Most states require that RDs be licensed or certified.

Medical Social Worker (MSW). A medical social worker determines residents' needs and helps get them support services, such as counseling. He or she may help residents obtain clothing and personal items if the family is not involved or does not visit often. A medical social worker may book appointments and transportation. Generally, MSWs hold a master's degree in social work.

Activities Director. The activities director plans activities for residents to help them socialize and stay physically and mentally active. These activities are meant to improve and maintain residents' well-being and to prevent further complications from illness or disability. An activities director may have a bachelor's degree, associate degree, or qualifying work experience. An activities director may be called a "recreational therapist" depending upon education and experience.

Resident and Resident's Family. The resident is an important member of the care team. The resident has the right to make decisions and choices about his or her own care. The resident's family may also be involved in these decisions. The care team revolves around the resident and his or her condition, treatment, and progress. Without the resident, there is no care team.

Information on home health aides as members of the care team is found in Chapter 24.

2. Explain the nursing assistant's role

Nursing assistants can have many different titles. "Nurse aide," "certified nurse aide," "unlicensed assistive personnel," and "certified nursing assistant" are some examples. This textbook will use the term "nursing assistant."

Nursing assistants (NAs) perform assigned nursing tasks, such as taking a resident's temperature. Nursing assistants also provide personal care, such as bathing residents, helping them eat and drink, and helping with hair care (Fig. 2-5). Promoting independence and self-care are other very important tasks that nursing assistants do. Other nursing assistant duties include the following:

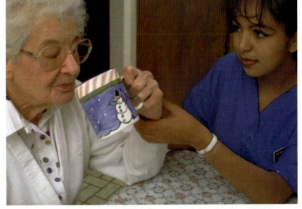

Fig. 2-5. Encouraging residents to drink often will be an important part of your job.

- Feeding residents

- Helping residents with toileting needs

- Assisting residents to move around safely

- Keeping residents' living areas neat and clean

- Encouraging residents to eat and drink
- Caring for supplies and equipment
- Helping dress residents
- Making beds
- Giving backrubs
- Helping residents with mouth care

Nursing assistants are generally not allowed to give medications; nurses are responsible for giving medications. Some states allow nursing assistants to work with medications after receiving special training. Examples of other tasks that nursing assistants are generally not allowed to do are inserting/removing tubes, changing sterile dressings, and giving tube feedings.

Nursing assistants spend more time with residents than other care team members do. They act as the "eyes and ears" of the care team. Observing changes in a resident's condition and reporting them is a very important role of the NA. Another is writing down important information about the resident; this is called **charting**.

Nursing assistants are part of a team of health professionals. Everyone, including the resident, works closely together to meet goals. Goals include helping residents to recover from illnesses or to do as much as possible for themselves.

Residents' Rights

Responsibility for Residents

All residents are the responsibility of each nursing assistant. You will receive assignments to do tasks, care, and paperwork for specific residents. If you see a resident who needs help, even if he or she is not on your assignment sheet, provide the needed care.

3. Explain professionalism and list examples of professional behavior

Professional means having to do with work or a job. The opposite of professional is **personal**, which refers to your life outside your job, such as your family, friends, and home life. **Profes-**

sionalism is how you behave when you are on the job. It includes how you dress, the words you use, and the things you talk about. It also includes being on time, completing tasks, and reporting to the nurse. For an NA, professionalism means following the care plan, making careful observations, and reporting accurately. Following policies and procedures is an important part of professionalism. Residents, coworkers, and supervisors respect employees who behave in a professional way. Professionalism will help you keep your job and may help you earn promotions and raises.

A professional relationship with residents includes the following:

- Keeping a positive attitude
- Doing only the assigned tasks you are trained to do and that are listed in the care plan
- Keeping all residents' information confidential
- Being polite and cheerful, even if you are not in a good mood (Fig. 2-6)

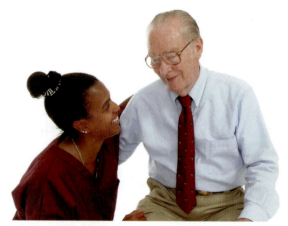

Fig. 2-6. *Being polite and cheerful is something that will be expected of you.*

- Not discussing your personal problems
- Not using profanity, even if a resident does
- Listening to the resident
- Calling a resident "Mr.," "Mrs.," "Ms.," or "Miss," or by the name he or she prefers

- Never giving or accepting gifts
- Always explaining the care you will provide before providing it
- Following practices, such as handwashing, to protect yourself and residents

A professional relationship with an employer includes the following:

- Completing tasks efficiently
- Always following all policies and procedures
- Always documenting and reporting carefully and correctly
- Communicating problems with residents or tasks
- Reporting anything that keeps you from completing duties
- Asking questions when you do not know or understand something
- Taking directions or criticism without getting upset
- Being clean and neatly dressed and groomed
- Always being on time
- Telling your employer if you cannot report for work
- Following the chain of command
- Participating in education programs
- Being a positive role model for your facility

Nursing assistants must be

Compassionate: Being **compassionate** is being caring, concerned, considerate, empathetic, and understanding. Demonstrating **empathy** means entering into the feelings of others. Compassionate people understand others' problems. They care about them. Compassionate people are also sympathetic. Showing **sympathy** means sharing in the feelings and difficulties of others.

Honest: A person who is honest tells the truth and can be trusted. Residents need to feel that they can trust those who care for them. The care team depends on your honesty in planning care. Employers count on truthful records of your care and observations.

Tactful: **Tact** is the ability to understand what is proper and appropriate when dealing with others. It is the ability to speak and act without offending others.

Conscientious: People who are **conscientious** always try to do their best. They are guided by a sense of right and wrong and have principles. They are always alert, observant, accurate, and responsible. Conscientious care means making accurate observations and reports, following assignments and the care plan, and taking responsibility for actions (Fig. 2-7). For example, taking accurate measurements of vital signs, such as temperature or pulse, is important. Other members of the care team will make treatment decisions based on your measurements. Without conscientious care, a resident's health and well-being are in danger.

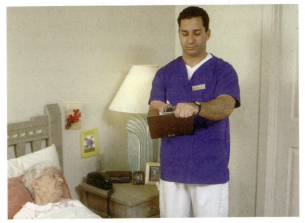

Fig. 2-7. Nursing assistants must be conscientious about documenting observations and procedures.

Dependable: Nursing assistants must make and keep commitments. You must report to work on time. You must skillfully do assigned tasks, avoid too many absences, and help your peers when they need it.

Respectful: Being respectful means valuing other people's individuality. This includes their age, religion, culture, feelings, and beliefs. People who are respectful treat others politely and kindly. You should care about people's self-esteem. Do not do or say anything that will harm it. You must not disrespect others by gossiping about them. Respect the various cultures and practices of your residents and others.

Unprejudiced: You will work with many different people from different backgrounds. You must give each resident the same quality care regardless of age, gender, sexual orientation, religion, race, ethnicity, or condition.

Tolerant: You may not like or agree with things that your residents or their families do or have done. However, your job is to care for each resident as assigned, not to judge him or her. Put aside your opinions, and see each resident as an individual who needs your care.

4. Describe proper personal grooming habits

Regular grooming makes you feel good about yourself, and it makes others feel good about you (Fig. 2-8). Grooming affects how confident residents feel about the care you give. Good nursing assistants have the following personal grooming habits:

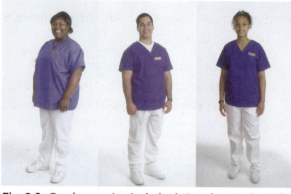

Fig. 2-8. Good grooming includes being clean and neatly dressed. Keep long hair tied back, and apply makeup lightly. Wear clean clothes and comfortable, clean shoes.

- Bathing or showering daily and using deodorant or anti-perspirant (do not use perfume or cologne, as some residents may be intolerant of some odors)

- Brushing teeth frequently and using mouthwash when necessary

- Keeping hair clean and neatly brushed or combed, tying long hair back in a bun or ponytail

- Keeping facial hair short, clean, and neat (men)

- Dressing neatly in a uniform that is washed and ironed

- Not wearing clothes that are too tight or too baggy, torn or stained, or too revealing (short skirts, low-cut blouses, see-through fabrics)

- Not wearing large jewelry (the main exception to this rule is to wear a simple, waterproof watch that is used to take vital signs and record events)

- Not having visible tattoos and body piercings, except for the ear lobes

- Wearing comfortable, clean, and high quality shoes.

- Keeping fingernails short, smooth, and clean

- Not wearing artificial nails, extenders, overlays, etc. because they harbor bacteria

- Wearing little or no makeup

Your facility will have rules about your appearance. Know these rules and always follow them.

5. Explain the chain of command and scope of practice

As a nursing assistant, you will be carrying out instructions given to you by a nurse. The nurse is acting on the instructions of a physician or other member of the care team. This is called the chain of command. It describes the line of authority and helps to make sure that your residents get proper health care. The chain of command also protects you and your employer from liability. **Liability** is a legal term that means someone can be held responsible for harming someone else. For example, imagine that something you do for a resident harms him. However, what you did was in the care plan and was done according to policy and procedure. Then you may not be liable, or responsible, for hurting the resident. However, if you do something not in the care plan that harms a resident, you could be held responsible. That is why it is important to follow instructions in the care plan and know the chain of command (Fig. 2-9).

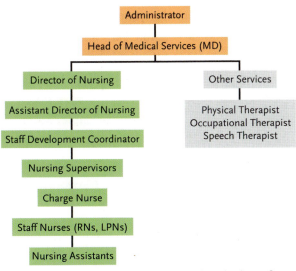

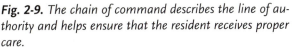

Fig. 2-9. *The chain of command describes the line of authority and helps ensure that the resident receives proper care.*

Nursing assistants must understand what they can and cannot do. This is important so that you do not harm a resident or involve yourself or your employer in a lawsuit. Some states certify that a nursing assistant is qualified to work. However, nursing assistants are not licensed healthcare providers. Everything in your job is assigned to you by a licensed healthcare professional. You work under the authority of another person's license. That is why these professionals will show great interest in what you do and how you do it.

Every state grants the right to practice various jobs in health care through licensure. Examples include a license to practice nursing, medicine, or physical therapy. All members of the care team work under each professional's "scope of practice." (A **scope of practice** defines the

things you are allowed to do and how to do them correctly.

Laws and regulations on what NAs can and cannot do vary from state to state. However, some procedures are not performed by nursing assistants under any circumstances. Tasks that are said to be outside the scope of practice of a nursing assistant include the following:

- NAs do not administer medications unless trained and assigned to do so.

- NAs do not honor a request to do something outside the scope of practice, not listed in the care plan, or not on the assignment sheet. In this situation an NA should explain that he or she cannot do the task requested. The request should then be reported to a nurse. This is true even if a nurse or doctor asks the NA to perform the task. The NA should refuse to perform the task and explain why. Refusing to do something that the NA cannot legally do is the NA's right and responsibility.

- NAs do not usually perform procedures that require sterile technique. For example, changing a sterile dressing on a deep, open wound requires sterile technique.

- NAs do not diagnose or prescribe treatments or medications.

- NAs do not tell the resident or the family the diagnosis or the medical treatment plan. This is the responsibility of the doctor or nurse.

Your instructor or employer may provide a list of other tasks outside your scope of practice. In some cases, you may be trained to do a particular task that your employer does not want nursing assistants to perform. Know which tasks these are and do not perform them. Many of these specialized tasks require more training. It is important to learn how to refuse a task for which you have not been trained, or which is outside your scope of practice.

6. Define "care plan" and explain its purpose

A care plan is created for each resident by the nurse or doctor. It is individualized for each resident to help achieve the goals of care. The resident assists with developing the care plan. The care plan lists the steps and tasks the care team, including nursing assistants, must perform (Fig. 2-10). It states how often these tasks should be performed and specifies how they should be carried out.

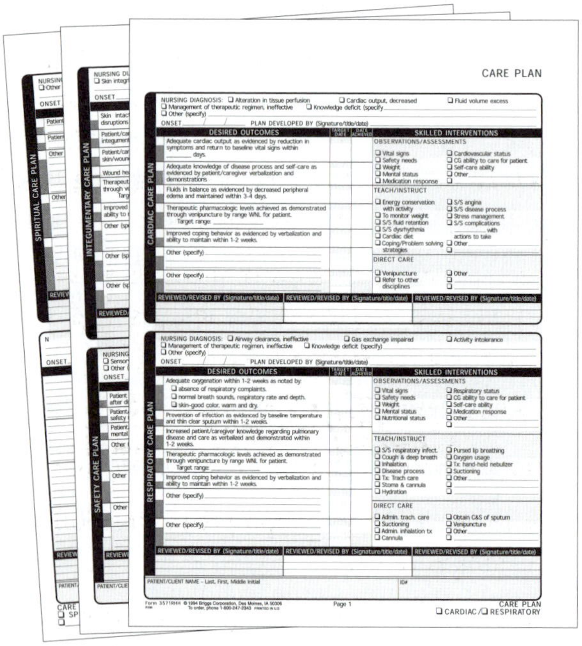

Fig. 2-10. *Sample resident care plans.* (REPRINTED WITH PERMISSION OF BRIGGS CORPORATION, DES MOINES, IOWA, 800-247-2343, WWW.BRIGGSCORP.COM)

The care plan is a guide to help the resident reach and maintain the best level of health possible. **Activities not listed on the care plan should not be performed.** The care plan must be followed very carefully.

Care planning should involve input from the resident and/or the family, as well as healthcare professionals. Healthcare professionals will assess the resident's physical, financial, social, and psychological needs. After the doctor prescribes treatment, the supervisor, nurses, and other care team members formulate the care plan.

Many factors are considered when formulating a care plan. These include the following:

- The resident's health and physical condition

- The resident's diagnosis and treatment

- The resident's goals or expectations

Multiple care plans may be necessary for some residents. In these situations, the nurse will coordinate the resident's overall care. There may be one care plan for the nursing assistant to follow. There may be separate care plans for other providers, such as the physical therapist.

Throughout this text you will read how important it is to make observations and report them to the nurse. Sometimes even simple observations are very important. The information you collect, such as vital signs, and the changes you observe are both important in determining how care plans may need to change. Because you spend so much of your time with residents, you may have a lot of valuable information about them that will help in care planning. You may be asked to attend care planning meetings. If you attend these meetings, do not be afraid to speak up. Share your observations of your residents. If you are not sure what is important to say, speak to a nurse before the meeting to find out.

7. Describe the nursing process

Care plans must be updated as the resident's condition changes. Reporting changes and problems to the nurse is a very important role of the nursing assistant. That is how the care team revises care plans to meet the resident's changing needs.

To communicate with other care team members, nurses use the nursing process (Fig. 2-11). The process has five steps:

- **Assessment**: getting information about the resident's status from different sources, including medical history, physical assessment, and environment, and reviewing this information

- **Diagnosis**: identifying the health problems after looking at all the resident's needs

- **Planning**: setting goals and creating a care plan to meet the resident's needs

- **Implementation**: putting the care plan into action; giving care

- **Evaluation**: a careful examination to see if the goals are being met

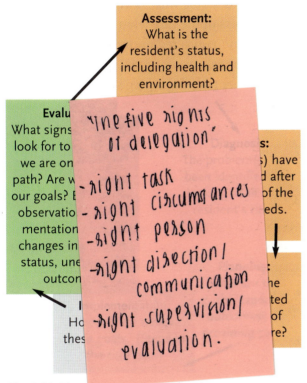

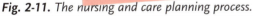

Fig. 2-11. The nursing and care planning process.

The goal of the nursing process is to meet the resident's nursing needs. Good communication between all care team members and the resident is vital. It helps ensure the success of the nursing process. This process constantly changes as new information is collected and reported. Nursing assistants are an important part of this process; their observations and reports may trigger changes in the process.

8. Describe "The Five Rights of Delegation"

While care planning, nurses decide which tasks to delegate to other team members, such as nursing assistants. Everything you do in your job is delegated to you by a licensed healthcare professional, and licensed nurses are accountable for care. This includes all delegated tasks. The National Council of State Boards of Nursing has identified "The Five Rights of Delegation." This can be used as a mental checklist to help nurses in the decision-making process.

"The Five Rights of Delegation" are the "Right Task," "Right Circumstance," "Right Person," "Right Direction/Communication," and "Right Supervision/Evaluation." Before delegating tasks, nurses may consider these questions:

- Is there a match between the resident's needs and the NA's skills, abilities, and experience?

- What is the level of resident stability?

- Is the NA the right person to do the job?

- Can the nurse give appropriate direction and communication?

- Is the nurse available to give the supervision, support, and help that the NA needs?

There are questions you may want to ask yourself before accepting a task. Consider these questions:

- Do I have all the information I need to do this job? Are there questions I should ask?

- Do I believe that I can do this task? Do I have the necessary skills?

- Do I have the needed supplies, equipment, and other support?

- Do I know who my supervisor is, and how to reach him/her?

- Do we both understand who is doing what?

Do not be afraid to ask for help. If you need any more information or are unsure about something, communicate this to the nurse. If you feel that you do not have the skills for a task, or the task is not within your scope of practice, discuss this with the nurse.

9. Demonstrate how to manage time and assignments

When you take care of residents, it is important to manage your time well every day. You will have a variety of tasks to do during your shift. Managing time properly will help you to complete these tasks. Many of the ideas for managing time on the job can be used to manage your personal time as well. The following ideas are basic ways to manage time:

Plan ahead. Planning is the single best way to help you manage your time better. Sometimes you may feel you do not even have the time to plan. Take the time to sit down and list everything you have to do. Take time to check to see if you have all the supplies needed for a procedure. Often just making the list and taking the time to recheck will help you feel better. This will get you focused.

The nurse will make your work assignments. He or she bases this on needs of residents and availability of staff. The assignments will allow staff to work as team. Your responsibilities in completing assignments include the following:

- Helping others when needed

- Never ignoring a resident who needs help

- Answering all call lights even if you are not assigned to a particular resident

- Notifying the nurse if you cannot complete an assignment

Prioritize. Identify the most important things to get done. Do these first.

Make a schedule. Write out the hours of the day and fill in when you will do what. This will help you be realistic.

Combine activities. Can you visit with residents while providing care? Work more efficiently when you can.

Get help. It is not reasonable for you to do everything. Sometimes you will need help to ensure a resident's safety. Do not be afraid to ask for help.

Chapter Review

1. Briefly describe what each of the following members of the care team does: nursing assistant; registered nurse; physician; physical therapist; occupational therapist; speech language pathologist; registered dietitian; medical social worker; activities director; and resident and resident's family.

2. List six examples of duties that nursing assistants perform.

3. List two duties that nursing assistants do not usually perform.

4. Describe professionalism. List five examples of professional behavior with residents.

5. List seven examples of professional behavior with an employer.

6. List eight personal qualities that are important for nursing assistants to have.

7. Why do you think it is important for nursing assistants to keep their hair tied back if they have long hair?

8. Why would wearing comfortable shoes be important to nursing assistants?

9. Give one reason why the chain of command is important.

10. List three tasks that are said to be outside the scope of practice of a nursing assistant.

11. Why are observing and reporting even simple observations about a resident important?

12. What are three factors considered when forming a care plan?

13. List five steps in the nursing process.

14. List the "Five Rights of Delegation."

15. What should a nursing assistant do if he feels he does not have the skills necessary to perform a task?

16. List five steps in managing time and assignments.

3
Legal and Ethical Issues

1. Define the terms "law" and "ethics" and list examples of legal and ethical behavior

Ethics and laws guide our behavior. **Ethics** are the knowledge of right and wrong. An ethical person has a sense of duty and responsibility toward others. He or she always tries to do what is right. If ethics tell us what we should do, laws tell us what we must do. **Laws** are usually based on ethics. Governments establish laws to help people live peacefully together and to ensure order and safety. When someone breaks the law, he or she may be punished by having to pay a fine or spend time in prison.

Ethics and laws are extremely important in health care (Fig. 3-1). They protect people receiving care and guide people giving care. Nursing assistants, home health aides, and other health-care providers should be guided by a code of ethics. They must know the laws that apply to their jobs.

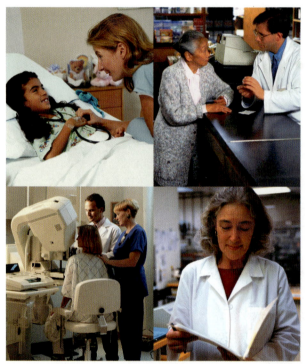

Fig. 3-1. Behaving ethically and following the law applies to all healthcare providers.

Guidelines:
Legal and Ethical Behavior

G   Be honest at all times. Stealing from a resident and lying about care you provided are examples of dishonesty. Communicate honestly with all team members.

G   Protect residents' privacy. Do not discuss their cases except with other members of the care team. Keeping resident information confidential is one of the residents' rights, which are covered later in this chapter. All team members must keep resident information confidential.

G   Keep staff information confidential. You should not share information about your coworkers at home or anywhere else.

G Report abuse or suspected abuse of residents, and assist residents in reporting abuse if they wish to make a complaint of abuse. You will learn more about this later in this chapter.

G Follow the care plan and your assignments. If you make a mistake, report it promptly. This helps prevent any further problems. Reporting mistakes promotes the safety and well-being of all residents.

G Do not perform any task outside your scope of practice.

G Report all resident observations and incidents to the nurse.

G Document accurately and promptly.

G Follow rules on safety and infection control. You will learn more about these rules in Chapters 5 and 6.

G Do not accept gifts or tips.

G Do not get personally or sexually involved with residents or their family members or friends.

Many associations, organizations, and companies have created their own "Code of Ethics" for their members or employees to follow. These vary, but generally they focus on promoting proper conduct and high standards of practice. If your facility has its own "Code of Ethics," you will be given a copy and expected to follow it.

Tip

Crimes in Healthcare Settings

Most of the crimes that occur in the community can also occur in healthcare settings. Theft is frequently reported. Physical abuse, including hitting, punching, shoving, and rough handling, and many other types of abuse can occur. Violations of residents' rights are reported and can be prosecuted as a crime. As you read through this chapter, pay close attention to the many legal issues. Know what to observe and how to report any illegal activity. Your vigilance can help prevent crimes and promote legal and ethical behavior in the workplace.

2. Explain the Omnibus Budget Reconciliation Act (OBRA)

Due to reports of poor care and abuse in long-term care facilities, the U.S. government passed the **Omnibus Budget Reconciliation Act (OBRA)** in 1987. It has been updated several times since. OBRA set minimum standards for nursing assistant training. Nursing assistants must complete at least 75 hours of training and must pass a competency evaluation (testing program) before they can be employed. They must attend regular in-service education to keep their skills updated.

OBRA requires that states keep a current list of nursing assistants in a state registry.

OBRA sets guidelines for minimum staff requirements. It specifies the minimum services that long-term care facilities must provide. Another important part of OBRA is the resident assessment requirements. OBRA requires complete assessments on every resident. The assessment forms are the same for every facility.

A resident assessment system was developed in 1990 and is revised periodically. It is called the **Minimum Data Set (MDS)** (Fig. 3-2). The MDS is a detailed form with guidelines for assessing residents. It also lists what to do if resident problems are identified. Facilities must complete the MDS for each resident within 14 days of admission and again each year. In addition, the MDS for each resident must be reviewed every three months. A new MDS must be done when there is any major change in the resident's condition.

OBRA made major changes in the survey process. You first learned about the survey process in Chapter 1. The results from surveys are available to the public and posted in the facility.

OBRA also identifies important rights for residents in long-term care facilities. You will learn more about them in the next learning objective.

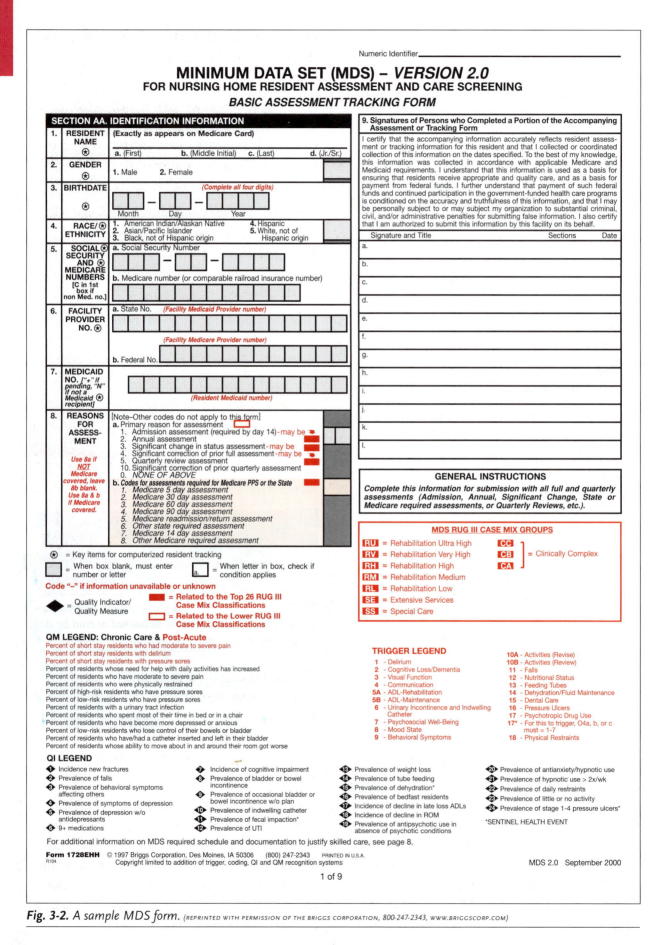

Fig. 3-2. *A sample MDS form.* (REPRINTED WITH PERMISSION OF THE BRIGGS CORPORATION, 800-247-2343, WWW.BRIGGSCORP.COM)

3. Explain residents' rights and discuss why they are important

Residents' rights relate to how residents must be treated while living in a facility. They provide an ethical code of conduct for healthcare workers. Facilities give residents a list of these rights and review each right with them. You need to be familiar with residents' rights, which are very detailed. They include the following:

Quality of life: Residents have the right to the best care available. Dignity, choice, and independence are important parts of quality of life.

Services and activities to maintain a high level of wellness: Residents must receive the correct care. Their care should keep them as healthy as possible every day. Health should not decline as a direct result of the facility's care.

The right to be fully informed about rights and services: Residents must be told what care and services are available. They must be told the fees for each service. They must be made aware of all their legal rights. Legal rights must be explained in a language they can understand. This includes being given a written copy of their rights. They have the right to be notified in advance of any change of room or roommate. They have the right to communicate with someone who speaks their language. They have the right to assistance for any sensory impairment. Blindness is one type of sensory impairment.

The right to participate in their own care: Residents have the right to participate in planning their treatment, care, and discharge. Residents have the right to refuse medication, treatment, care, and restraints. They have the right to be told of changes in their condition. They have the right to review their medical record. Informed consent is a concept that is part of participating in one's own care. A person has the legal and ethical right to direct what happens to his or her body. Doctors also have an ethical duty to involve the person in his or her health care. **Informed consent** is the process by which a person, with the help of a doctor, makes informed decisions about his or her health care.

The right to make independent choices: Residents can make choices about their doctors, care, and treatments. They can make personal decisions, such as what to wear and how to spend their time. They can join in community activities, both inside and outside the care facility.

The right to privacy and confidentiality: Residents can expect privacy when care is given. Their medical and personal information cannot be shared with anyone but the healthcare team. Residents have the right to private, unrestricted communication with anyone they choose (Fig. 3-3).

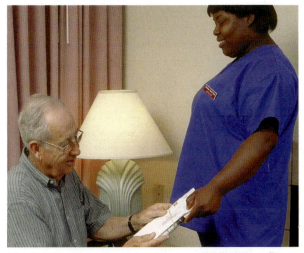

Fig. 3-3. Residents have the right to private communication with anyone; mail cannot be opened or read by staff, unless someone is directed to do so by the resident.

The right to dignity, respect, and freedom: Residents must be respected and treated with dignity by caregivers. They cannot be abused, mistreated, or neglected in any way. You will learn more about abuse and neglect in the next learning objective.

The right to security of possessions: Residents' personal possessions must be safe at all times. They cannot be taken or used by anyone without a resident's permission. Residents have the right to manage their own finances or choose someone to do it for them. Residents can ask the care facility to handle their money and in this case, the resident must sign a written statement. If the care facility handles residents' financial affairs, residents must have access to their accounts and financial records, and they must receive quarterly statements, among other things.

Rights during transfers and discharges: Location changes must be made safely and with the resident's knowledge and consent. Residents have the right to stay in a facility unless a transfer or discharge is needed.

The right to complain: Residents have the right to make complaints and voice grievances without fear of punishment. Facilities must work quickly try to resolve complaints.

The right to visits: Residents have the right to visits from family, friends, doctors, clergy members, groups, and others (Fig. 3-4).

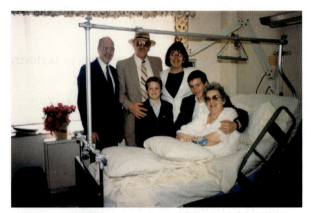

Fig. 3-4. Residents have the right to visitors.

Rights with social services: The care facility must provide residents with access to social services, including counseling, assistance in solving problems with others, and help contacting legal and financial professionals.

The Americans with Disabilities Act (ADA)

The Americans with Disabilities Act (ADA) became a law in 1990. It was passed to help people with disabilities gain skills, do jobs they want to do, and take part in desired activities. The ADA prohibits discrimination because of a disability. The law requires that employers, schools, and businesses offer equal opportunities to individuals with disabilities to use the services in our society and improve their quality of life.

Persons with disabilities need to be able to get into and around in buildings and use the bathrooms, drinking fountains, and other areas. The law requires new buildings to be accessible and for older buildings to be updated when they are renovated.

Americans with disabilities have the right to education, employment, and all the services offered to the public. Schools, colleges, and many employers are not allowed to discriminate and must make reasonable accommodations, or changes, to make their services available. Examples of accommodations are providing a large screen for a computer, or allowing a service dog. Providers of health care, social services, transportation, restaurants, hotels, and recreation are also not allowed to discriminate against persons with disabilities. They must provide equal opportunities, which may include making some changes to their services.

4. Discuss abuse and neglect and explain how to report abuse and neglect

The healthcare community has become aware of the growing problem of elder abuse and neglect. In their "National Elder Abuse Incidence Study" published in 1998, The National Center on Elder Abuse estimated that more than a million elders suffered abuse or neglect in a single year, many of them in nursing homes. This study also found that for every reported incident of elder abuse or neglect, approximately five go unreported.

The National Citizens' Coalition for Nursing Home Reform (NCCNHR) is a national nonprofit organization founded in 1975 to protect the rights, safety, and dignity of long-term care residents. In a fact sheet compiled by the NCCNHR (nccnhr.org), they list this statistic: "in 2000, states reported 472,813 reported incidents of abuse." They also mention that "The National Academies estimate between 1 and 2 million Americans age 65 or older have been injured, exploited, or otherwise mistreated by someone on whom they depended for care."

As the elderly population grows, this problem may become worse. Elderly people may be abused intentionally or unintentionally, through ignorance, inexperience, or inability to care for them. People who abuse elders may mistreat them physically, psychologically, sexually, verbally, financially, and/or materially. They may deprive them of their rights or they may neglect them by failing to provide food, clothing, shelter, or medical care. Some older adults may also become self-abusive or neglect their own needs. In order to help prevent abuse and neglect, it helps if you understand more about the different types of each.

Neglect means harming a person physically, mentally, or emotionally by failing to provide needed care. Neglect can be divided into two categories: active neglect and passive neglect. **Active neglect** is purposely harming a person by failing to provide needed care. Examples of active neglect are leaving a bedridden resident alone for lengthy periods or willfully denying the resident food, dentures, or eyeglasses. **Passive neglect** is unintentionally harming a person physically, mentally, or emotionally by failing to provide needed care. The caregiver may not know how to properly care for the resident, or may not understand the resident's needs.

Negligence means actions, or the failure to act or provide the proper care for a resident, that result in unintended injury. An example of negligence is an NA forgetting to lock a resident's wheelchair before transferring her. The resident falls and is injured. **Malpractice** occurs when a person is injured due to professional misconduct through negligence, carelessness, or lack of skill.

Abuse means purposely causing physical, mental, or emotional pain or injury to someone. There are many forms of abuse, including the following:

- **Physical abuse** refers to any treatment, intentional or not, that causes harm to a person's body. This includes slapping, bruising, cutting, burning, physically restraining, pushing, shoving, or even rough handling.

- **Psychological abuse** is emotionally harming a person by threatening, scaring, humiliating, intimidating, isolating, insulting, or treating him or her as a child.

- **Verbal abuse** involves the use of language—spoken or written—that threatens, embarrasses, or insults a person.

- **Assault** is threatening to touch a person without his or her permission. The person feels fearful that he or she will be harmed. Telling a resident that she will be slapped if she does not stop yelling is an example of assault.

- **Battery** means a person is actually touched without his or her permission. An example is an NA hitting or pushing a resident, which is also physical abuse. Forcing a resident to eat a meal is another example of battery.

- **Sexual abuse** is forcing a person to perform or participate in sexual acts against his or her will. This includes unwanted touching and exposing oneself to a person. It also includes sharing pornographic material.

- **Financial abuse** is stealing, taking advantage of, or improperly using the money, property, or other assets of another.

- **Domestic violence** is abuse by spouses, intimate partners, or family members. It can be physical, sexual, or emotional. The victim can be a man or woman of any age or a child.

- **Workplace violence** is abuse of staff by residents or other staff members. It can be verbal, physical, or sexual. This includes improper touching and discussion about sexual subjects.

- **Involuntary seclusion** is separating a person from others against the person's will. For example, an NA confines a resident to his room without his consent.

- **Sexual harassment** is any unwelcome sexual advance or behavior that creates an intimidating, hostile, or offensive working environment. Requests for sexual favors, unwanted touching, and other acts of a sexual nature are examples of sexual harassment.

- **Substance abuse** is the use of legal or illegal drugs, cigarettes, or alcohol in a way that harms oneself or others. You will learn more about this in Chapter 20.

Nursing assistants must never abuse residents in any way. They must also try to protect residents from others who abuse them. If you ever see or suspect that another caregiver, family member, or resident is abusing a resident, report this immediately to the nurse in charge. **Reporting abuse is not an option—it is the law.**

If action is not taken, keep reporting up the chain of command, and do this until action is taken. If no appropriate action is taken at the facility level, call the state abuse hotline, which is an anonymous call.

Nursing assistants must follow the chain of command when reporting abuse. They do not report directly to the authorities. If a life-or-death situation is witnessed, remove the resident to a safe place, if possible. Get help immediately or have someone go for help. Do not leave the resident alone.

Observing and Reporting:
Abuse and Neglect

These are "suspicious" injuries. They should be reported:

- %ᴿ Poisoning or traumatic injury
- %ᴿ Teeth marks
- %ᴿ Belt buckle or strap marks
- %ᴿ Old and new bruises, contusions and welts
- %ᴿ Scars
- %ᴿ Fractures, dislocation

- %ᴿ Burns of unusual shape and in unusual locations; cigarette burns
- %ᴿ Scalding burns
- %ᴿ Scratches and puncture wounds
- %ᴿ Scalp tenderness and patches of missing hair
- %ᴿ Swelling in the face, broken teeth, nasal discharge
- %ᴿ Bruises, bleeding, or discharge from the vaginal area

Signs that could indicate abuse include the following:

- %ᴿ Yelling obscenities
- %ᴿ Fear, apprehension, fear of being alone
- %ᴿ Poor self-control
- %ᴿ Constant pain
- %ᴿ Threatening to hurt others
- %ᴿ Withdrawal or apathy (Fig. 3-5)

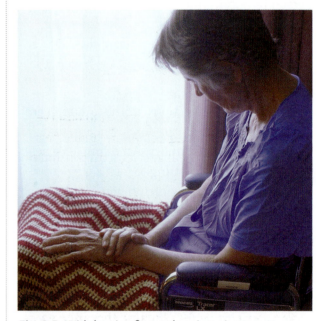

Fig. 3-5. *Withdrawing from others is an important change to report.*

- %ᴿ Alcohol or drug abuse
- %ᴿ Agitation or anxiety, signs of stress
- %ᴿ Low self-esteem
- %ᴿ Mood changes, confusion, disorientation

- **⁰/ʀ** Private conversations are not allowed, or the family member/caregiver is present during all conversations
- **⁰/ʀ** Resident or family reports of questionable care

Signs that could indicate neglect include the following:

- **⁰/ʀ** Pressure sores
- **⁰/ʀ** Body not clean
- **⁰/ʀ** Body lice
- **⁰/ʀ** Unanswered call lights
- **⁰/ʀ** Soiled bedding or incontinence briefs not being changed
- **⁰/ʀ** Poorly-fitting clothing
- **⁰/ʀ** Refusal of care
- **⁰/ʀ** Unmet needs relating to hearing aids, eyeglasses, etc.
- **⁰/ʀ** Weight loss, poor appetite
- **⁰/ʀ** Uneaten food
- **⁰/ʀ** Dehydration
- **⁰/ʀ** Fresh water or beverages not being passed each shift

You will be in an excellent position to observe and report abuse or neglect. As mentioned earlier NAs have an ethical and legal responsibility to observe for signs of abuse and report suspected cases to the charge nurse. In some states, nursing assistants are considered "mandated reporters" and can be convicted of a crime for not reporting knowledge of abuse or neglect of a resident. **Mandated reporters** are people who are legally required to report suspected or observed abuse or neglect because they have regular contact with vulnerable populations, such as the elderly in facilities.

If abuse is suspected or observed, give the nurse as much information as possible. If residents want to make a complaint of abuse, you must assist them in every way. This includes telling them of the process and their rights.

Never retaliate against (punish) residents complaining of abuse. If you see someone being cruel or abusive to a resident who made a complaint, you must report it. All care team members are responsible for residents' safety. Take this responsibility seriously. Help end the disturbing trend of elder abuse and neglect.

Residents' Rights

Vulnerable Adults

Some states have Vulnerable Adults Acts or Adult Protective Service (APS) laws. These laws are written by each state, and are not the same throughout the country. There are states that do not have any such laws.

In general, these Vulnerable Adults Acts or Adult Protective Service laws protect individuals who because of a physical or mental impairment need help from other people for their care. The residents of long-term care facilities, assisted living and other institutions fit into this category.

It is important to know the laws in your state. However, even if your state does not have a specific law like the ones above, residents of long-term care facilities are covered by the federal laws relating to residents' rights, which also forbid abuse and neglect and require reporting if these acts do occur.

5. List examples of behavior supporting and promoting residents' rights

You can help protect your residents' rights in the following ways:

- Never abuse a resident physically, emotionally, verbally, or sexually.
- Watch for and report any signs of abuse or neglect immediately.
- Call the resident by the name he or she prefers.
- Involve residents in your planning. Allow the residents to make as many choices as possible about when, where, and how care performed.
- Always explain a procedure to a resident before performing it.

- Do not unnecessarily expose a resident while giving care.

- Respect a resident's refusal of care. Residents have a legal right to refuse treatment and care. However, report the refusal to the nurse immediately.

- Inform the nurse if a resident voices concerns, complaints, or has questions about treatment or the goals of care.

- Be truthful when documenting care.

- Do not talk or gossip about residents. Keep all resident information confidential.

- Knock and ask for permission before entering a resident's room. (Fig. 3-6).

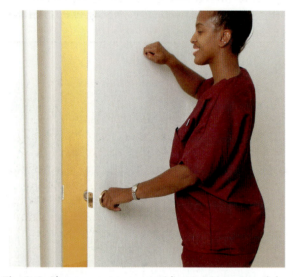

Fig. 3-6. Always respect your residents' privacy. Knock before entering their rooms, even if the door is open.

- Do not accept gifts or money.

- Do not open a resident's mail or look through his belongings.

- Respect residents' personal possessions. Handle them gently and carefully. Keep personal items labeled and stored, according to facility policy.

- Report observations about a resident's condition or care.

- Help resolve disputes by reporting them to the nurse.

6. Describe what happens when a complaint of abuse is made against a nursing assistant

The Nurse Aide Training Competency Evaluation Program (NATCEP) makes the rules about training and testing nursing assistants. The state programs make sure that federal rules are followed in nursing facilities that receive payment from Medicare or Medicaid. Setting up and running the nursing assistant registry is also a part of this program. This registry keeps track of each nursing assistant working in that state.

If a nursing assistant is accused of abusing a resident, the facility will investigate according to its policies and procedures. If they determine abuse has occurred, a report must be made to the Nurse Aide Training Competency Evaluation Program (NATCEP).

The nursing assistant will be notified of any complaint made about him or her to NATCEP. The nursing assistant can request a hearing. NATCEP will investigate and decide whether or not to mark in the nursing assistant's record that he or she was abusive. Some states have an abuse registry and will place the nursing assistant's name this list. Other states do not have a separate list but will add the information on the required registry of nursing assistants.

If NATCEP places the nursing assistant on the abuse registry and marks the record that he or she was abusive, the nursing assistant will not be allowed to work in a certified nursing facility. All nursing facilities must check the registry before hiring a nursing assistant. They will be told of the abuse when they inquire.

7. Explain how disputes may be resolved and identify the ombudsman's role

An **ombudsman** is assigned by law as the legal advocate for residents. The Older Americans Act (OAA) is a federal law that requires all states have an ombudsman program. The ombudsman visits facilities and listens to residents. He or she decides what action to take if there are problems. Ombudsmen can help resolve conflicts and settle disputes concerning residents' health, safety, welfare, and rights. The ombudsman will gather information and try to resolve the problem on the resident's behalf, and may suggest ways to solve the problem. Ombudsmen provide an ongoing presence in long-term care facilities. They monitor care and conditions.

An ombudsman typically does the following tasks:

- Advocates for residents' rights and quality care
- Educates consumers and care providers
- Investigates and resolves complaints
- Appears in court and/or in legal hearings
- Works with investigators from the police, adult protective services, and health departments to resolve complaints (Fig. 3-7)
- Gives information to the public

Each state has a department that performs surveys and is responsible for enforcing long-term care facility laws and rules. Generally, this is the responsibility of the state's department of health. Complaints may be made directly to the state agency. Each one has policies and procedures that are used to follow up on complaints.

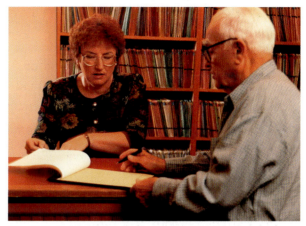

Fig. 3-7. *An ombudsman is a legal advocate for residents. He or she may work with other agencies to resolve complaints.*

Residents' Rights

Residents' Council

A Residents' Council is a group of residents who meet regularly to discuss issues related to the long-term care facility. This Council gives residents a voice in facility operations. Topics of discussion may include facility policies, decisions regarding activities, concerns, and problems. The Residents' Council offers residents a chance to provide suggestions on improving the quality of care. Council executives are elected by residents. Family members are invited to attend meetings with or on behalf of residents. Staff may participate in this process when invited by Council members.

8. Explain HIPAA and list ways to protect residents' privacy

To respect **confidentiality** means to keep private things private. You will learn confidential (private) information about your residents. You may learn about a resident's state of health, finances, and relationships. Ethically and legally, you must protect the confidentiality of this information. You should not tell anyone except members of the care team anything about your residents.

Congress passed the Health Insurance Portability and Accountability Act (HIPAA) in 1996. It was further defined and revised in 2001 and 2002. One of the reasons this law was passed is to help keep health information private and secure. All healthcare organizations must take special steps to protect health information. They and their employees can be fined and/or imprisoned if they break rules to protect patient privacy. This applies to all healthcare providers, including doctors, nurses, nursing assistants, and all care team members.

Under this law, a person's health information must be kept private. It is called **protected health information (PHI)**. Examples of PHI include the patient's name, address, telephone number, social security number, e-mail address, and medical record number. Only people who must have information to provide care or to process records should know this information (Fig. 3-8). They must make sure they protect the information so that it does not become known or used by anyone else. It must be kept confidential.

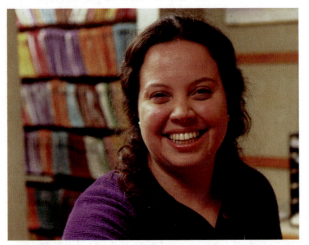

Fig. 3-8. Special care must be taken to keep medical records confidential. Only people who give care or process records should have access to this information.

NAs cannot give out any information about a resident to anyone not directly involved in the resident's care, unless the resident gives official consent or unless the law requires it. For ex-

ample, if a neighbor asks you how a resident is doing, you should reply, "I'm sorry, but I cannot share that information. It's confidential." That is the correct response to anyone who does not have a legal reason to know about the resident. Other ways to protect residents' privacy include the following guidelines:

Guidelines:
Protecting Privacy

G Make sure you are in a private area when you are listening to or reading your messages.

G Know with whom you are speaking on the phone. If you are not sure, get a name and number, and call back after you get approval.

G When talking to a care team member on the phone, use regular phones, not cell phones. Cell phones can be scanned.

G Do not talk about residents in public places (Fig. 3-9). Public areas include elevators, grocery stores, lounges, waiting rooms, parking garages, schools, restaurants, etc.

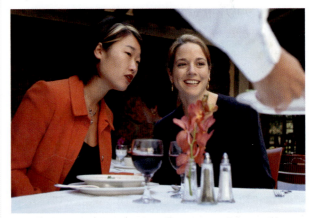

Fig. 3-9. Do not discuss any information about residents in any public place, such as grocery stores or restaurants. Only discuss residents' information with the care team.

G Use confidential rooms for reports to other care team members.

G If you see a resident's family member or a former resident in public, be careful in greeting him or her. He or she may not want others to know about the family member or that he or she has been a resident.

G Do not bring family or friends to the facility to meet residents.

G Make sure nobody can see health or personal information on your computer screen while you are working.

G Log off when not using your computer.

G Do not give confidential information in e-mails because you do not know who has access to your messages.

G Make sure fax numbers are correct before faxing any healthcare information. Use a cover sheet with a confidentiality statement.

G Do not leave papers or documents where others may see them.

G Store, file, or shred documents according to your facility's policy.

G If you find documents with a resident's information, give them to the nurse.

All healthcare workers must follow HIPAA regulations no matter where they are or what they are doing. There are serious penalties for violating these regulations. Penalties differ depending upon the violation and can include:

• Fines ranging from $100 to $250,000

• Prison sentences of up to ten years

Maintaining confidentiality is a legal and ethical obligation. It is part of respecting your residents and their rights. Discussing a resident's care or personal affairs with anyone other than members of the care team violates the law.

9. Explain the Patient Self-Determination Act (PSDA) and discuss advance directives

The Patient Self-Determination Act (PSDA) was passed in 1990 as an amendment to OBRA. The PSDA requires all healthcare agencies receiving Medicare and Medicaid money to give adults, during admission or enrollment, information about their rights relating to advance directives. **Advance directives** are legal documents that allow people to choose what medical care they wish to have if they cannot make those decisions themselves. Advance directives can also name someone to make decisions for a person if that person becomes ill or disabled. Living wills and durable power of attorney for health care are examples of advance directives.

A **living will** states the medical care a person wants, or does not want, in case he or she becomes unable to make those decisions him- or herself. It is called a "living will" because it takes effect while the person is still living. It may also be called a "directive to physicians," "health care declaration," or "medical directive." A living will is not the same thing as a will. A will is a legal declaration of how a person wishes his or her possessions to be disposed of after death.

A **durable power of attorney for health care** is a signed, dated, and witnessed paper that appoints someone else to make the medical decisions for a person in the event he or she becomes unable to do so. This can include instructions about medical treatment the person wants to avoid.

A **do-not-resuscitate (DNR)** order is another tool that helps medical providers honor wishes about care. A DNR order tells medical professionals not to perform CPR. CPR (cardiopulmonary resuscitation) refers to medical procedures to restart the heart and breathing. You will learn more about CPR in Chapter 7. A DNR order means that medical personnel will not attempt emergency CPR if breathing or the heartbeat stops. In general, DNR orders are appropriate for those in the final stages of a terminal illness or who suffer from a serious condition.

According to the Patient Self-Determination Act, rights relating to advance directives that must be given upon admission include the following:

- The right to participate in and direct health-care decisions

- The right to accept or refuse treatment

- The right to prepare an advance directive

- Information on the facility's policies that govern these rights

The act prohibits discriminating against a patient who does not have an advance directive. The PSDA requires documentation of patient information and ongoing community education on advance directives.

Advance Directives

Laws related to advance directives vary from state to state. Here are a few resources that may help you locate the proper forms for your state:

- The National Hospice and Palliative Care Organization (NHPCO) is a nonprofit organization that represents hospice and palliative care programs in the United States. NHPCO is involved with improving care for people who are dying and their loved ones. For more information visit their website at caringinfo.org, or call 800-658-8898.

- The U.S. Living Will Registry is a privately held organization that electronically stores advance directives, organ donor information and emergency contact information, and makes them available to healthcare providers across the country 24 hours a day. For more information about the U.S. Living Will Registry, call 800-LIV-WILL (800-548-9455) or visit their website at uslivingwillregistry.com.

Chapter Review

1. What is the difference between ethics and laws?

2. List eight examples of legal and ethical behavior for a nursing assistant.

3. What is the minimum number of hours of training that nursing assistants must complete as required by OBRA?

4. How soon must a Minimum Data Set (MDS) be completed on new residents after admission?

5. What is the purpose of residents' rights?

6. Pick five residents' rights in Learning Objective 3 that are most important to you and explain why you chose those particular rights.

7. If a nursing assistant sees abuse or suspects that a resident is being abused, what is her responsibility?

8. List five possible signs of abuse that should be reported by the nursing assistant. List five possible signs of neglect that should be reported by the nursing assistant.

9. If residents want to make a complaint of abuse, what is the role of the nursing assistant?

10. Pick three of the examples of behavior promoting residents' rights in Learning Objective 5. Describe how it supports or promotes residents' rights.

11. What happens if a nursing assistant is accused of abusing a resident?

12. What does an ombudsman do?

13. What is a Residents' Council?

14. What is one important reason that HIPAA was passed?

15. List five examples of a person's protected health information (PHI).

16. To whom is a nursing assistant allowed to give information about a resident?

17. To what members of the healthcare team does HIPAA apply?

18. Define "advance directives" and briefly describe two examples.

19. List three rights relating to advance directives that the PSDA requires be given to a resident at the time of admission.

4

Communication and Cultural Diversity

1. Define the term "communication"

Communication is the process of exchanging information with others. It is a process of sending and receiving messages. People communicate by using signs and symbols, such as words, drawings, and pictures. They also communicate by their behavior.

The simplest form of communication takes place between two people (Fig. 4-1). The person who communicates first is the "sender" who sends a message. The person who receives the message is called the "receiver." Receiver and sender constantly switch roles as they communicate.

The third step is providing feedback. The receiver repeats the message or responds to it in some way. This lets the sender know the mes-

sage was received and understood. Feedback is especially important when working with the elderly. Nursing assistants must take time to make sure residents understand messages.

All three steps must occur before the communication process is complete. During a conversation, this three-step process is repeated over and over.

Effective communication is a vital part of your job. Nursing assistants must communicate with supervisors, the care team, residents, and family members. A resident's health depends on how well you communicate your observations and concerns to the nurse. You must also be able to communicate clearly and respectfully in stressful or confusing situations.

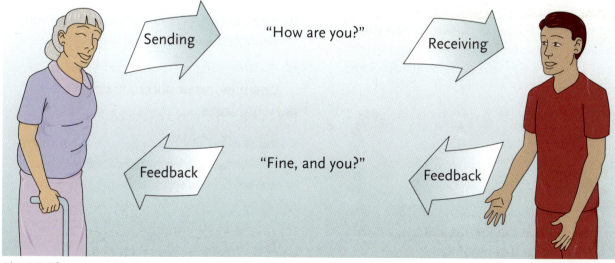

"How are you?"

Sending

Receiving

Feedback

"Fine, and you?"

Feedback

Fig. 4-1. *The communication process consists of sending a message, receiving a message, and providing feedback.*

2. Explain verbal and nonverbal communication

Communication is either verbal or nonverbal. **Verbal communication** involves the use of words or sounds, spoken or written. Oral reports are an example of verbal communication. It is important to use words that have the same meaning to both the sender and the receiver. Misunderstandings may occur if each person interprets the same words differently. For example, if you ask a resident to "turn on the light" when she needs help, she may not understand that you actually meant for her to push the call button.

Nonverbal communication is the way we communicate without using words. Examples include shaking your head or shrugging your shoulders. Nonverbal communication includes how a person says something. For example, you might say, "I'll be right there, Mrs. Gonzales." This communicates that you are ready and willing to help. But saying the same phrase in a different tone can communicate frustration and annoyance: "I'll be right there, Mrs. Gonzales!"

Body language is another form of nonverbal communication. Movements, facial expressions, and posture can express different attitudes or emotions. Just as with speaking, you send messages with your body language. Other people receive and interpret them. For example, slouching in a chair and sitting erect send two different messages (Fig. 4-2). Slouching says that you are bored, tired, or hostile. Sitting up straight sends the message that you are interested and respectful.

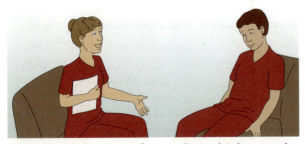

Fig. 4-2. *Body language often speaks as plainly as words. Which of these people seems more interested in the conversation they are having?*

Other examples of positive nonverbal communication include smiling, nodding your head, and looking at the person who is speaking.

Sometimes people send one message verbally and a very different message nonverbally. Nonverbal communication often tells us how someone is feeling. This message may be quite different from what he or she is saying. For example, a resident who tells you "I'm feeling fine today," but does not want to get out of bed and winces in pain, is sending two very different messages. Paying attention to nonverbal communication helps you give better care. Communicate to the nurse your observation that the resident is staying in bed and appears to be wincing in pain despite what he says.

You must also be aware of your own verbal and nonverbal messages. If you say "It's nice to see you today, Mr. Lee" but you do not smile or look him in the eye, he may feel that you are not really all that happy to see him.

When communication is confusing, try to clarify it. Ask for an explanation of the message. Say something like, "Mrs. Jones, you've just told me something that I don't understand. Would you explain it to me?" Or state what you have observed and ask if the observation is correct. For example, "Mrs. Jones, I see that you're smiling, but I hear by the sound of your voice that you may be sad. Are you sad?" Take the time to clarify communication. It can help you know your residents better and avoid misunderstandings.

3. Describe ways different cultures communicate

Cultural diversity has to do with the different groups of people with varied backgrounds and experiences living together in the world. Positive responses to cultural diversity include acceptance and knowledge, not **bias**, or prejudice. A **culture** is a system of learned behaviors by a group of people that are considered to be the tradition of that people and are passed on from one generation to the next. Each culture may have different knowledge, behaviors, beliefs, values, attitudes, religions, and customs.

Nonverbal communication may depend on personality or cultural background. Some people are more animated when they speak. They use lots of gestures and facial expressions. Other people speak quietly or calmly, regardless of their moods. Depending on their cultural background, people may make motions with their hands when they talk. They may stand close to the person to whom they are talking, or touch the other person.

People from some cultural groups stand further apart when talking than people from other groups. When one person moves closer, the other person may view it as a threat. Be sensitive to your residents' needs. Let them decide how close they want to be when talking to you.

The use of touch and eye contact also varies with cultural background and personality (Fig. 4-3). For some people, touching is welcome. It expresses caring and warmth. For others, it seems threatening or harassing. In the United States, we often talk about "looking someone straight in the eye" or speaking "eye to eye." We see eye contact as a sign of honesty. However, in some cultures, looking someone in the eye may seem overly bold or disrespectful.

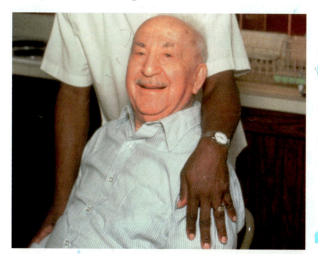

Fig. 4-3. How a person perceives your touch may depend on his cultural background.

Learning each resident's behavior can be a challenge. However, it is an important part of communication. It is especially vital in a multi-cultural society (a society made up of many cultures), such as the United States. Be aware of all the messages you send and receive. As you listen and observe carefully, you will learn to better understand your residents' needs and feelings.

4. Identify barriers to communication

Communication can be blocked or disrupted in many ways (Fig. 4-4). Following are some barriers and ways to avoid them:

Resident does not hear you, does not hear correctly, or does not understand. Face the resident. Speak more slowly than you do with family and friends. Speak clearly. Use a low, pleasant voice. Do not whisper or mumble. If the resident says he cannot hear you, speak more loudly. However, use a pleasant, professional tone. If the resident wears a hearing aid, check that it is on and is working properly.

Resident is difficult to understand. Be patient and take time to listen. Ask the resident to repeat or explain. State the message in your own words to make sure you have understood.

Message uses words receiver does not understand. Do not use medical terms with residents. Speak in simple, everyday words. Ask what a word means if you are not sure.

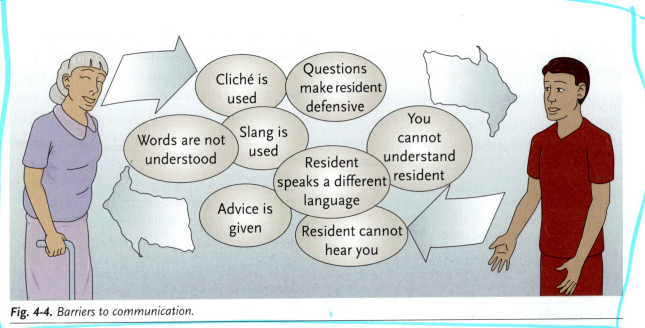

Fig. 4-4. *Barriers to communication.*

Using slang confuses the message. Avoid using slang words that are unprofessional or may not be understood. Do not curse or use profanity, even if the resident does.

Avoid using clichés. Clichés are phrases that are used over and over again and do not really mean anything. For example, "Everything will be fine" is a cliché. Instead of using a cliché, listen to what your resident is really saying. Respond with a meaningful message. For example, if a resident is afraid of having a bath, say "I understand that it seems scary to you. What can I do to make you more comfortable?" Do not say, "Oh, it'll be over before you know it."

Asking "why" makes the resident defensive. Avoid asking "why" when a resident makes a statement. "Why" questions make people feel defensive. For example, a resident may say she does not want to go for a walk today. If you ask "why not?" you may receive an angry response. Instead, ask, "Are you too tired to take a walk? Is there something else you want to do?" Your resident may then be willing to discuss the issue.

Giving advice is inappropriate. Do not offer your opinion or give advice. Giving medical advice is not within the scope of your practice. It could be dangerous.

Yes/no answers end a conversation. Ask open-ended questions that need more than a "yes" or "no" answer. Yes and no answers bring conversation to an end. For example, if you want to know what your resident likes to eat, do not ask "Do you like vegetables?" Instead, try, "Which vegetables do you like best?"

Resident speaks a different language. If a resident speaks a different language than you do, speak slowly and clearly. Keep your messages short and simple. Be alert for words the resident understands. Also be alert for signs the resident is only pretending to understand you. You may need to use pictures or gestures to communicate. Ask the resident's family, friends, or other staff members who speak the resident's language for help. Be patient and calm

Nonverbal communication changes the message. Be aware of your body language and gestures when you are speaking. Look for nonverbal messages from residents and clarify them. For example, "Mr. Feldman, you say you're feeling fine but you seem to be in pain. Can I help?"

5. List ways to make communication accurate and explain how to develop effective interpersonal relationships

In addition to avoiding the barriers to communication listed above, the following techniques will help ensure that you send and receive clear, complete messages.

Be a good listener. Allow the other person to express her ideas completely. Concentrate on what she is saying, and do not interrupt. Do not finish her sentences even if you know what she is going to say. When she is finished, restate the message in your own words to make sure you have understood.

Provide feedback as you listen. Active listening means focusing on the person sending the message and giving feedback. Feedback might be an acknowledgment, a question, or repeating the sender's message. Offer general but leading responses, such as "Oh?" or "Go on," or "Hmm." By doing this you are actively listening, providing feedback, and encouraging the sender to expand the message.

Bring up topics of concern. If you know of a topic that might concern a resident, raise the issue in a general, non-threatening way. This lets the resident decide whether or not to discuss it. For example, if you see that your resident is unusually quiet, you could say, "Mrs. Jones, you seem so quiet today." Or you may notice a certain emotion. You might say, "Mrs. Jones, you seemed upset earlier. Would you like to talk about it?"

Let some pauses happen. Use silence for a few moments at a time. This encourages the resident to gather his or her thoughts and compose messages.

Tune in to other cultures. Learn the words and phrases of your resident's culture. This shows that you respect the culture and are interested in what the resident has to say. It will help you understand your resident's messages more fully. Be careful about using new words and terms, though. Some may have a different meaning than what you thought. The important thing is to understand words and expressions when others use them. Do not be judgmental; accept people who are different from you.

Accept a resident's religion or lack of religion. Religious differences also affect communication. Religion can be very important in people's lives, particularly when they are ill or dying. Respect residents' religious beliefs, practices, or lack of beliefs, especially if they are different from yours. Never question your residents' beliefs. Do not discuss your beliefs with them.

Understand the importance of touch. Softly patting residents' hands or shoulders or holding their hands may communicate caring. Some people's backgrounds may make them less comfortable being touched. Ask permission before touching residents. Be sensitive to their feelings. You must touch residents in order to do your job. However, recognize that some residents feel more comfortable when there is little physical contact. Learn about your residents and adjust care to their needs.

Ask for more. When residents report symptoms, events, or feelings, have them repeat what they have said. Ask them for more information.

Make sure communication aids are clean and in good working order (Fig. 4-5). These include hearing aids, glasses, dentures, and wrist or hand braces. Tell the nurse if they do not work properly or are dirty or damaged.

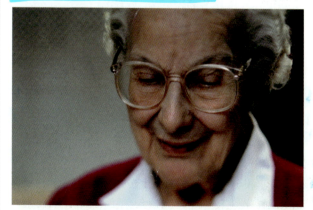

Fig. 4-5. *Glasses must fit well, be clean, and be in good condition. Tell the nurse if you think communication aids are not clean or not working properly.*

Proper Communication

When communicating with your residents, remember the following steps:

- Always greet the resident by his or her preferred name.
- Identify yourself.
- Focus on the proper topic to be discussed.
- Face the resident while speaking. Avoid talking into space.
- Talk with the resident while giving care.
- Listen and respond when the resident speaks. Praise the resident and smile often.
- Encourage the resident to interact with you and others.
- Be courteous.
- Tell the resident when you are leaving the room.

Residents' Rights

Names

Call residents by the names that they prefer you to use. Do not refer to them by their first names unless they have told you that it is OK to do so. Do not use disrespectful terms such as "sweetie," "honey," or "dearie."

Having good relationships with residents, their family members, and the care team will help you provide excellent care. You should not try to become friends with your residents. However, you should try to develop warm professional relationships with them based on trust. Good communication will help you get to know your residents. It will also help them learn to trust you. In addition to the strategies already discussed, the following tips can help you communicate well and develop good relationships:

Avoid changing the subject when your resident is discussing something. This is true even if the subject makes you feel uncomfortable or helpless. For example, a resident might say, "I'm having so much pain today." Do not try to avoid the topic by asking the resident if he wants to watch television. This makes the resident feel that you are not interested in him or what he is talking about.

Do not ignore a resident's request. Ignoring a request is considered negligent behavior. Honor the request if you can. Otherwise, explain why the request cannot be fulfilled. Always report such requests to the nurse.

Do not talk down to an elderly or disabled person or a child. Talk to your residents and their families as you would talk to any person. Make adjustments if someone is visually- or hearing-impaired. Guidelines for visually and hearing-impaired residents are found later in the chapter.

Sit near the person who has started the conversation. This shows you find what he or she is saying important and worth your time.

Lean forward in your chair when someone is speaking to you. Leaning forward communicates interest. Pay attention to your nonverbal communication. If you fold your arms in front of you, you send the negative message that you wish to distance yourself from the speaker.

Talk directly to the person whom you are assisting. Do not talk to other staff while helping residents (Fig. 4-6). Avoid gossip. Do not criticize other staff members.

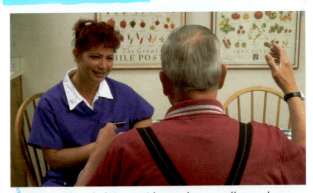

Fig. 4-6. *When helping residents, do not talk to other staff. Do not talk over residents' heads. Look and speak directly to the person you are helping.*

Approach the person who is talking. Even if you are in another area of the room, approach the person. This tells the person you are interested in what he or she has to say.

Put yourself in other people's shoes. Try to understand what they are going through. This is called empathy. Ask yourself how you would feel if you were confined to bed or needed help to go to the bathroom. Do not tell residents you know how they feel because you do not know exactly how they feel. Do say things like, "I can imagine this must be difficult for you."

Show residents' families and friends that you have time for them, too. Communicate with them. Do not discuss a resident's care with friends or family members, but listen if they want to talk. Be respectful and nice, and give privacy for visits. Do not interfere with private family business. Families are great sources of information for residents' personal preferences, history, diet, habits, and routines. Ask them questions. If you see any abusive behavior towards a resident during a visit, report it immediately to the nurse.

6. Explain the difference between facts and opinions

A fact is something that is definitely true. For example, "Mr. Ford has lost four pounds this month." You can back up this fact with evidence: weighing Mr. Ford and comparing his current weight to his weight last month. An opinion is something someone believes to be true, but is not definitely true. "I think Mr. Ford looks thinner," is an opinion. It might be true, but you cannot back it up with evidence. Separating facts from opinions will make you a better communicator.

Using facts instead of your opinion lets you communicate in a more professional way. When communicating with members of the healthcare team, separate facts and opinions. For example, "Mr. Morgan is acting like he had a stroke," is an opinion and could very well be wrong. Instead, report the facts: "Mr. Morgan has lost strength on his right side and his speech is slurred." When you need to report your opinion, begin it with "I think...." Then it is clear that you are giving your opinion and not a fact you have observed.

7. Explain objective and subjective information and describe how to observe and report accurately

When making any report, you must collect the right information before documenting it. Facts, not opinions, are most useful to the nurse and the care team. Two kinds of factual information are needed in your reporting. **Objective information** is based on what you see, hear, touch, or smell. Objective information is collected by using the senses. **Subjective information** is something you cannot or did not observe, but is based on something the resident reported to you that may or may not be true. An example of objective information is, "Mr. McClain is holding his head and rubbing his temples." A subjective report of the same situation might be, "Mr. McClain says he has a headache." The nurse needs factual information in order to make decisions about care and treatment. Both objective and subjective reports are valuable.

In any report, make sure what you observe (signs) and what the resident reports to you (symptoms) are clearly noted. For example, "Ms. Scott reports pain in left shoulder." You are not expected to make diagnoses based on signs and symptoms you observe. Your observations, however, can alert staff to possible problems. In order to report accurately, observe your residents accurately. To observe accurately, use as many senses as possible to gather information (Fig. 4-7). Some examples follow.

Sight. Look for changes in resident's appearance. These include rashes, redness, paleness, swelling, discharge, weakness, sunken eyes, and posture or gait (walking) changes.

Hearing. Listen to what the resident tells you about his condition, family, or needs. Is he speaking clearly and making sense? Does he show emotions, such as anger, frustration, or sadness? Is breathing normal? Does the resident wheeze, gasp, or cough? Is the area calm and quiet enough for him to rest as needed?

Touch. Does your resident's skin feel hot or cool, moist or dry? Is the pulse rate regular?

Smell. Do you notice odor from the resident's body? Odors could suggest poor bathing, infections, or incontinence. **Incontinence** is the inability to control the bladder or bowels. Breath odor could suggest use of alcohol or tobacco, indigestion, or poor oral care.

Using all your senses will help you make the most complete report of a resident's situation.

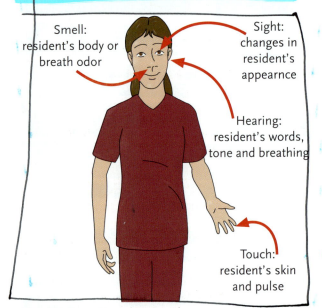

Smell: resident's body or breath odor

Sight: changes in resident's appearnce

Hearing: resident's words, tone and breathing

Touch: resident's skin and pulse

Fig. 4-7. Reporting what you observe means using more than one sense.

8. Explain how to communicate to other team members

Nursing assistants will communicate regularly with care team members, residents and their families and friends. NAs should communicate freely with the charge nurse regarding residents. Keep the nurse informed of all important issues during your shift. Share information with other staff members as needed for quality of care. You may need to share a resident's personal information with another nursing assistant to help her give care to a resident. However, the activities staff may have no need to know that same information. Refer any doctor's questions to the nurse.

Always respect your resident's privacy. When giving information to other members of the care team, be sure that other residents or staff cannot overhear. Be cautious when communicating with residents and their families and friends. Do not tell them any new information about the resident's condition or any new diagnoses. That is the nurse's or doctor's responsibility. When in doubt, ask the nurse what you can say. The resident may not want information shared with family members and that is his legal right.

Use the chain of command to voice any complaints you may have. Go to your charge nurse first. Refer to the facility's policies or procedures if your complaint is not resolved. If you feel that your charge nurse has abused a resident, communicate this to her supervisor.

9. Describe basic medical terminology and abbreviations

Throughout your training, you will learn medical terms for specific conditions. For example, the medical term for a runny nose is nasal discharge; a resident whose skin is pale or blue is called **cyanotic**. Medical terms are made up of roots, prefixes, and suffixes. A root is a part of a word that contains its basic meaning or definition. The prefix is the word part that precedes the root to help form a new word. The suffix is the word part added to the end of a root that helps form a new word. Prefixes and suffixes are called "affixes" because they are attached to a root. Here are some examples:

- The root "derm" or "derma" means skin. The suffix "itis" means inflammation. Dermatitis is an inflammation of the skin.

- The prefix "brady" means slow. The root "cardia" means heart. "Bradycardia" is slow heartbeat or pulse.

- The suffix "pathy" means disease. The root "neuro" means of the nerve or nervous system. Neuropathy is a nerve disease or disease of the nervous system.

When speaking with residents and their families, use simple, non-medical terms. Do not use medical terms, because they may not understand these terms. But when you speak with the care team, using medical terminology will help you give more complete information.

Abbreviations are a way to communicate more efficiently with other caregivers. For example, the abbreviation "p.r.n." means "as necessary." "BP" means "blood pressure." It is important to learn the standard medical abbreviations your facility uses. Use them to report information briefly and accurately. You may need to know these abbreviations to read assignments or care plans. Here is a brief list of abbreviations, and more are located at the end of this textbook. Check with your facility to see if there are terms you must know.

Common Abbreviations

$\bar{a}$	before
abd	abdomen
ac, AC	before meals
ad lib	as desired
am	morning
amb	ambulate
AP	apical pulse
b.i.d., bid	twice daily
BM, B.M.	bowel movement
BP	blood pressure
$\bar{c}$	with
C	Celsius degree
c/o	complains of
CHF	congestive heart failure
CPR	cardiopulmonary resuscitation
DNR	do not resuscitate
dx or DX	diagnosis
F	Fahrenheit degree
FBS	fasting blood sugar
ft	foot
FWB	full weight-bearing
GI	gastrointestinal
H_2O	water
hr.	hour
hs	hours sleep
I&O	intake and output
NKDA	no known drug allergies
NPO	nothing by mouth
NWB	no weight-bearing (absolutely no weight on leg)
O_2	oxygen
OOB	out of bed
P	pulse
$\bar{p}$	after
p.c., pc	after meals
po	by mouth
PRN	as necessary
PWB	partial weight-bearing
Q	every
R	respirations
ROM	range of motion
$\bar{s}$	without
SOB	shortness of breath
stat	at once
t.i.d., tid	three times a day
TPR	temperature, pulse, respiration
v.s., VS	vital signs
w/c, W/C	wheelchair

10. Explain how to give and receive an accurate report of a resident's status

Nursing assistants must make brief and accurate oral and written reports to residents and staff. Good communication skills are needed to collect information about residents. These skills will help you get information from residents and their families to report to the care team. This information may be written or given in oral reports from shift to shift. Remember that all resident information is confidential; only share information with members of the care team.

Your careful observations are very important to the health and well-being of all residents. Signs and symptoms that should be reported will be discussed throughout this textbook. Some of your observations will need to be reported immediately to the nurse. Deciding what to report immediately involves critical thinking. Anything that endangers residents should be reported at once, including the following:

- Falls
- Chest pain
- Severe headache
- Trouble breathing
- Abnormal pulse, respiration, or blood pressure
- Change in mental status
- Sudden weakness or loss of mobility
- High fever
- Loss of consciousness
- Change in level of consciousness
- Bleeding
- Change in resident's condition
- Bruises, abrasions, or other signs of possible abuse (Chapter 3)

Use oral reports to discuss your experiences with residents and your observations of residents' conditions. Use facts, not opinions. For an oral report, write notes so you do not forget to report any important details; do not rely on your memory alone. Following an oral report, document when, why, about what, and to whom an oral report was given.

Sometimes the nurse or another member of the care team will give you a brief oral report on one of your residents. Listen carefully and take notes (Fig. 4-8). Ask about anything you do not understand. At the end of the report, restate what you have been told to make sure you understand.

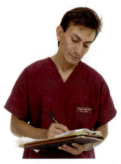

Fig. 4-8. *Take notes so you can remember facts and report accurately.*

11. Explain documentation and describe related terms and forms

Nursing assistants spend more time with residents than other members of the care team. You may observe things about your residents that nurses or doctors have not noticed. You will not make diagnoses or decide on treatment. However, you will have valuable information about residents that will help in care planning. Documenting accurately is the key to care planning. A thorough written record shows your observations to others. It helps you remember details about each resident.

Because you will see many residents during the day, you cannot remember everything that each resident did or said, or every observation you make. Documentation gives you an up-to-date record of each resident's care. You must learn to document accurately. Always take the time to observe and record carefully. Follow your facility's policies and procedures for documentation. Because documentation is so important, do not put it off until later.

A medical chart is a legal document. What is written in the chart is considered in court to be what actually happened. If you gave a resident a bath and took his temperature, but never documented it, you could not necessarily prove that you actually performed the care. In general, if something does not appear in a resident's chart, it did not legally happen. Failing to document your care could cause very serious legal problems for you and your employer. It could also cause harm to your resident. Remember: if you did not document it, you did not do it.

Information found in medical chart includes the following:

- Admission sheet (protected health information about the person, such as name, address, social security number, and date of birth, among other items)

- Medical history (illnesses, immunizations, medications, previous surgeries, family and social histories)

- Doctor's orders (instructions given to other members of the care team)

- Progress notes (updates from all care team members detailing changes or new information in the person's condition)

- Test results (blood tests, lab results, other tests)

- Graphic sheet (vital signs, intake and output, bladder and bowel elimination)

- Nurse's notes (the person's reported symptoms and actions taken to address them)

- Flow sheets (check-off sheets for documenting care; may also be called an ADL (activities of daily living) sheet (Fig. 4-9)

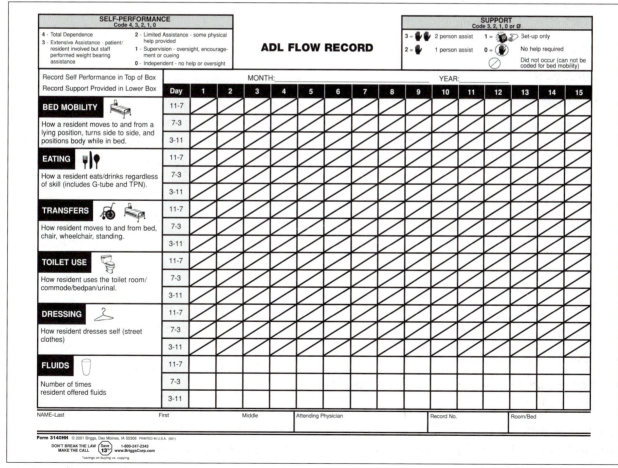

Fig. 4-9. *Some facilities use an ADL flow sheet for documenting care.* (REPRINTED WITH PERMISSION OF BRIGGS CORPORATION, 800-247-2343, WWW.BRIGGSCORP.COM)

If your facility's policies allow you to chart in a medical record, remember: there are legal aspects to your documentation. Careful charting is important for these reasons:

- It is the only way to guarantee clear and complete communication among all the members of the care team.

- It is a legal record of every resident's treatment. Medical charts are used in court as evidence.

- Documentation protects you and your employer from liability by proving what you did.

- Documentation gives an up-to-date record of the status and care of each resident.

Guidelines:
Careful Documentation

G Write your notes immediately after the care is given. This helps you to remember important details. Always wait to document until after you have completed care. Do not record any care before it has been done.

G Think about what you want to say before writing. Be as brief and as clear as possible.

G Write facts, not opinions.

G Write as neatly as you can. Use black ink.

G If you make a mistake, draw one line through it, and write the correct word or words. Put your initials and the date. Never erase what you have written. Do not use correction fluid (Fig. 4-10).

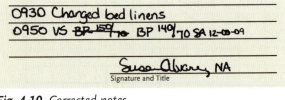
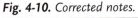

Fig. 4-10. Corrected notes.

G Sign your full name and title, and write the correct date.

G Document as specified in the care plan.

Nursing assistants may need to document using the 24-hour clock, or military time (Fig. 4-11). Regular time uses the numbers 1 to 12 to show each of the 24 hours in a day. In military time, the hours are numbered from 00 to 23: midnight is expressed as 00 (although it can also be written as 24), 1 a.m. is 01, 1 p.m. is 13, and so on.

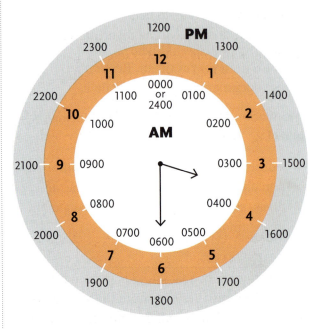

Fig. 4-11. Divisions in the 24-hour clock.

Both regular and military time list minutes and seconds the same way. The minutes and seconds do not change when converting from regular to military time. The abbreviations a.m. and p.m. are used in regular time to show what time of day it is. However, these are not used in military time, since specific numbers show each hour of the day.

To change the regular hours between 1:00 p.m. to 11:59 p.m. to military time, add 12 to the regular time. For example, to change 3:00 p.m. to military time, add 3 + 12. The time is expressed as 1500 (fifteen-hundred) hours. To change 4:22 p.m. to military time, add 4 + 12. The minutes do not change. The time is expressed as 1622 hours.

Midnight is the only time that differs. Midnight can be written as 0000, and it can also be written as 2400. This follows the rule of adding 12 to the regular time. Follow your facility's policy on whether to use 0000 or 2400 to express midnight.

You first learned about the Minimum Data Set (MDS) manual in Chapter 3. It is an assessment tool to give facilities a structured, standardized approach to care. The MDS manual offers a detailed guide to help nurses complete assessments accurately. The reporting you do on changes in your residents may "trigger" a needed assessment. Always report changes you notice to the nurse. They may be a sign of an illness or problem. By reporting them promptly, a new MDS assessment can be done if needed.

12. Describe incident reporting and recording

An **incident** is an accident or unexpected event during the course of care. It is not part of the normal routine in a facility. An error in care, such as feeding a resident from the wrong meal tray, is an incident. A fall or injury to a resident, employee, or visitor is another type of incident. An accusation from a resident or family member against staff is another example of an incident. Employee injuries also require reporting. In general, file a report when any of the following incidents occur:

* A resident falls

* You or a resident break or damage something

* You make a mistake in care

* A resident or a family member makes a request that is out of your scope of practice

* A resident or a family member makes sexual advances or remarks

* Anything happens that makes you feel uncomfortable, threatened, or unsafe

* You get injured on the job

* You are exposed to blood or body fluids

Reporting and documenting incidents is done to protect everyone involved. This includes the resident, your employer, and you. When documenting incidents, complete the report as soon as possible and give it to the charge nurse. This is important so that you do not forget any details.

State and federal guidelines require incidents to be recorded in an incident report (Fig. 4-12). The information in an incident report is confidential.

If a resident falls, and you did not see it, do not write "Mr. G fell." Instead write "found Mr. G on the floor," or "Mr. G states that he fell." For your protection, write a brief and accurate description of the events as they happened. Never place any blame or liability within the incident report.

Incident reports help demonstrate areas where changes can be made to avoid repeating the same incident. When completing an incident report, follow these guidelines:

Guidelines:
Incident Reporting

G Tell what happened. State the time, and the mental and physical condition of the person.

G Tell how the person tolerated the incident (his reaction).

G State the facts; do not give opinions.

G Do not write anything in the incident report on the medical record (incident reports are confidential).

G Describe the action taken to give care.

G Include suggestions for change.

13. Demonstrate effective communication on the telephone

You may be asked to make a call or answer the telephone at your facility. A home health aide working in the home may need to answer the phone for clients or call a supervisor.

Form 875/2 (if 2 part set) or
Form 875/3 (if 3 part set)

BRIGGS, Des Moines, IA 50306 (800) 247-2343

Printed in U.S.A.

INCIDENT REPORT

> "An incident is any happening which is not consistent with the routine operation of the hospital or the routine care of a particular patient. It may be an accident or a situation which might result in an accident."

PERSON INVOLVED	(Last Name)　　　(First Name)　　　(Middle Initial)　　Mr. ❑:　　Mrs. ❑:　　Child ❑:　　Male ❑:　　Female ❑:　　Age _____

PATIENT ❑	Room No.　　　　State Cause for Hospitalization

Patient's Condition Before Incident
Normal ❑:　　Senile ❑:　　Disoriented ❑:　　Sedated ❑:　　Other

Were Bed Rails Present? Yes ❑:　No ❑:　Up ❑:　Down ❑:　Ordered ❑:	Was Height of Bed Adjustable? Yes ❑:　No ❑:　Up ❑:　Down ❑:

EMPLOYEE ❑	Department	Job Title

VISITOR ❑	Home Address	Home Phone

OTHER ❑	Occupation	Reason for Presence at the Hospital

Exact Location of Incident	Date of Incident	Time of Incident　❑ A.M.　❑ P.M.

Property Involved ❑:　　Equipment Involved ❑:　　Describe

Description of Incident by Person Involved

_____

_____

Describe Exactly What Happened: Why It Happened: What Causes Were. If an injury, State Part of Body Injured. If Property or Equipment Damaged, Describe Damage.

_____

_____

_____

Name, Address & Phone No. of Witness(es)

Was It Necessary to Notify Physician?　　Yes ❑　No ❑	Time of Notification　　　　a.m./p.m.	Time Responded　　　　a.m./p.m.

Was Person Involved Seen by a Physician?　　Yes ❑　No ❑	Time Seen　❑ A.M.　❑ P.M.	Where

Physician's Name	T. _____　P. _____　R. _____　B.P. _____

Statement of Physician:

_____

_____

Date of Report	Title & Signature of Person Preparing Report

Additional Comments:

_____

Form 875 BRIGGS, Des Moines, IA 50306 (800) 247-2343
PRINTED IN U.S.A.

INCIDENT REPORT

Fig. 4-12. A sample incident report. (REPRINTED WITH PERMISSION OF BRIGGS CORPORATION, 800-247-2343, WWW.BRIGGSCORP.COM)

When making a call, follow these steps:

- Always identify yourself before asking to speak to someone. Never ask, "Who is this?" when someone answers your call.

- After you have identified yourself, ask for the person with whom you need to speak.

- If the person you are calling is available, identify yourself again. State why you are calling. Planning your call before you pick up the phone will help you be as efficient as possible.

- If the person is not available, ask if you can leave a message. Always leave a brief message, even if it is only to say you called. The message shows that you were trying to reach someone.

- Leave a brief and clear message. Do not give more information than necessary. A basic message includes your name, your facility's name, the phone number you are calling from, and a brief description of the reason for your call.

- Thank the person who takes the message for you. Always be polite over the telephone, as you would be in person.

When answering calls, follow these steps:

- Always identify your facility's name and your name. Be friendly and professional.

- If you need to find the person the caller wishes to speak with, place the caller on hold after asking if it is OK to do so.

- If the caller has to leave a message, write it down and repeat it to make sure you have the correct message. Ask for proper spellings of names. Do not ask for more information than the person needs to return the call: a name, short message, and phone number is enough. Do not give out any information about staff or residents.

- Thank the person for calling and say goodbye.

14. Understand guidelines for basic office machines and computers

There are many types of machines you will encounter in various healthcare settings, and you may already be familiar with most of them. Following is some brief information on office machines and computers. These machines or devices can make communication easier, faster, and more accurate.

Photocopier

A photocopier, commonly called a "copier," is a machine that makes paper copies of documents and other images quickly. To operate a copier, open the lid. Place the document to be copied face-down on the glass. There may be marks on the sides of the glass to show where to place different-sized documents. Select the options you want, such as how many copies you want. Other options may include enlarging or decreasing the image, making it lighter or darker, and collating the copies. Collate means to assemble or arrange in the proper order. Once you have selected the options you want, press the start button.

Fax Machine

A fax machine transfers copies of documents over a telephone network. Fax machines also function as photocopiers. To send a fax, place the piece of paper to be faxed in the document feeder. The machine should have instructions on whether the document must be placed face-down or face-up. Enter the phone number that you want to send the fax to, and press the send button. You may need to dial a special number to reach an outside line. After the fax has been transmitted, you may receive a printed confirmation from the paper tray below.

Calculator

A calculator performs mathematical calculations. Calculators have standard symbols for performing these calculations. They include a plus sign (+) for addition problems, a minus sign (-) for subtraction, a multiplication symbol (x or *), a division sign (÷), and an equal sign (=).

You must be able to understand basic math in order to use a calculator to perform these processes. Most calculators have numbers in the middle or bottom of the device. They begin with zero and work upwards in rows of three until you reach the number 9.

Computer

Computers are electronic devices that process and store information. They may be used in various ways in your facility. Some facilities and hospitals use computers to document information; this is faster and more accurate than writing information by hand. Doctors and nurses may carry computers from room to room to review medical records, document symptoms, tests, and treatments, manage medications, and perform other functions. Computers may be used to transmit records or other patient information to other facilities and healthcare professionals. They may be used for research. Employees may use computers to clock in and out when they work, so that their total hours worked are calculated for a specific time period for payment.

Computers are used to send and receive e-mail and access the Internet. E-mail, short for "electronic mail," is a system for sending and receiving messages electronically over a computer system or network. The Internet is a worldwide communications system that links a network of computers.

If your facility uses computers for documentation, research, tracking employee hours, or any other reason, you will be trained how to use them. HIPAA privacy guidelines apply to computer use. Make sure nobody can see private and protected health or personal information on your computer screen. Do not share confidential information with anyone except the care team.

15. Explain the resident call system

Long-term care facilities are required to have call systems—often called "call lights,"—so that residents can call for help whenever they need it. They are in resident rooms and bathrooms. Some have strings for residents to pull and others have buttons to be pushed. The signal is usually both a light outside the room and a sound that can be heard in the nurses' station. This is the primary way a resident can call for help. Always respond immediately when you see the light or hear the sound. Respond in a courteous and respectful manner. Check each time before you leave a room to make sure that the call light is within the resident's reach. Make sure that the resident knows how to use it.

16. List guidelines for communicating with residents with special needs

Due to illness or impairments, some residents will need special techniques to aid communication. An **impairment** is a loss of function or ability; it can be a partial or complete loss. Special techniques for different conditions are listed below. Information on communicating with residents who have dementia, such as Alzheimer's disease, is in Chapter 19. Guidelines for communicating with residents who are mentally ill are in Chapter 20.

Hearing Impairment or Deafness

Persons who have impaired hearing or are deaf may have lost their hearing gradually, or they may have been born deaf. If they have a gradual hearing loss, they may not be conscious of it. Signs of hearing loss include the following:

- Speaking loudly

- Leaning forward when someone is speaking

- Cupping the ear to hear better

- Responding inappropriately

- Asking the speaker to repeat what has been said

- Speaking in a monotone

- Avoiding social gatherings or acting irritable in the presence of people who are having a conversation

- Suspecting others of talking about them or of deliberately speaking softly

People who have hearing impairment may use a hearing aid, they may read lips, or use sign language. People with impaired hearing also closely observe the facial expressions and body language of others to add to their knowledge of what is being said. Hearing loss may affect how well residents can express their needs.

Guidelines:
Hearing Impairment

G If the person has a hearing aid, make sure he or she is wearing it and that it is working properly (Fig. 4-13). There are many types of hearing aids. Follow manufacturer's directions for cleaning. In general, the hearing aid needs to be cleaned daily. Wipe it with alcohol using a tissue or soft cloth. Do not put it in water. Handle the hearing aid carefully. Do not drop it. Always store it inside its case when it is not worn. Turn it off when it is not in use. Remove it before showers or when bathing resident and during the night. When storing it for an extended period of time, remove the battery.

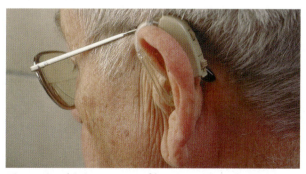

Fig. 4-13. This is one type of hearing aid. Make sure hearing aids are turned on.

G Reduce or remove noise, such as TVs, radios, and loud speech. Close doors if needed.

G Get residents' attention before speaking. Do not startle them by approaching from behind. Walk in front or touch them lightly on the arm to show you are near.

G Speak clearly and slowly. Directly face the person (Fig. 4-14). Make sure there is enough light in the room. The light should be on your face, rather than on the resident's. Ask if he or she can hear what you are saying.

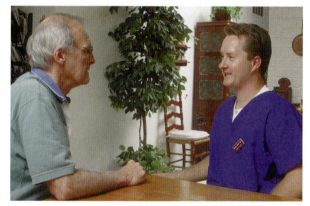

Fig. 4-14. Speak face-to-face in good light.

G Do not shout at the resident or mouth the words in an exaggerated way.

G Keep the pitch of your voice low.

G Residents may read lips, so keep hands away from your face while talking.

G Know which ear hears better. Try to speak to and stand on that side.

G Use short sentences and simple words. Avoid sudden topic changes.

G Repeat what you have said using different words, when needed. Some hearing-impaired people want you to repeat exactly what you said. This is because they miss only a few words.

G Use picture cards or a notepad as needed.

G Hearing impaired residents may hear less when they are tired or ill. This is true of everyone. Be patient and empathetic.

G Hearing decline can be a normal aspect of aging. Be matter-of-fact about this. Be understanding and supportive.

Vision Impairment

Like hearing impairment, vision impairment can affect people of all ages. It can exist at birth or develop gradually. It can occur in one eye or in both. It can also be the result of injury, illness, or aging. Some vision impairment causes people to wear corrective lenses. These can be contact lenses or eyeglasses. **Farsightedness** is the ability to see objects in the distance better than objects nearby. It develops in most people as they age. **Nearsightedness** is the ability to see things near but not far. It may occur in younger persons. Some people need to wear eyeglasses all the time. Others only need them to read or for activities, such as driving, that require seeing distant objects. There is more information on vision impairment in Chapter 18.

Guidelines:
Vision Impairment

G If the person has glasses, make sure they are clean and that he or she wears them. Clean glass lenses with water and soft tissue. Clean plastic lenses with cleaning fluid and a lens cloth. Also, make sure that glasses are in good condition and fit well. If they do not, inform the nurse.

G Knock on the door and identify yourself when you enter the room. Do this before touching the resident. Explain why you are there and what you would like to do. Let the resident know when you are leaving the room.

G Always tell the resident what you are doing while caring for him. Give specific directions, such as, "On your right" or, "In front of you." Talk directly to the resident whom you are assisting. Do not talk to other residents or staff members.

G Make sure there is proper lighting in the room. Face the resident when speaking.

G When you enter a new room with the resident, orient him or her to the area. Describe the things you see around you. Do not use words such as "see," "look," and "watch."

G Tell the resident where the call light is.

G Use the face of an imaginary clock as a guide to explain the position of objects that are in front of resident. For example,"There is a sofa at 7 o'clock" (Fig. 4-15).

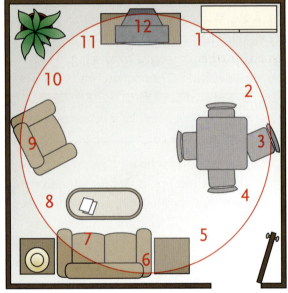

Fig. 4-15. The face of a clock can explain the position of objects.

G Do not move personal items or furniture without the resident's knowledge and permission.

G Put everything back where it was found.

G Leave the door completely open or completely closed.

G Encourage the use of the other senses, such as hearing, touch, and smell.

G Encourage the resident to feel and touch things, such as clothing, furniture, or items in the room.

G Offer large-print newspapers, magazines, and books.

G Use large clocks, clocks that chime, and radios to help keep track of time.

G Get books on tape and other aids from the local library or support organizations.

G If the resident has a guide dog, do not play with or distract it or feed it.

CVA or Stroke

The medical term for a stroke is a **cerebrovascular accident (CVA)**. CVA, or stroke, is caused when the blood supply to the brain is cut off suddenly by a clot or a ruptured blood vessel (Fig. 4-16). Without blood, part of the brain gets no oxygen. This causes brain cells to die. Brain tissue is further damaged by leaking blood, clots, and swelling. These cause pressure on surrounding areas of healthy tissue. Strokes can be mild or severe. Afterward, a resident may experience any of the following:

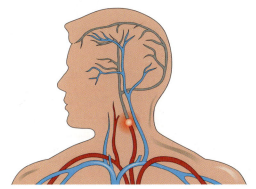

Fig. 4-16. A stroke is caused when the blood supply to the brain is cut off suddenly by a clot or ruptured blood vessel.

- Paralysis on one side of the body, called **hemiplegia**

- Weakness on one side of the body, called **hemiparesis**

- Inability to speak or speak clearly, called **expressive aphasia**

- Inability to understand spoken or written words, called **receptive aphasia**

- Loss of sensations such as temperature or touch

- Loss of bowel or bladder control

- Confusion

- Poor judgment

- Memory loss

- Loss of cognitive abilities

- Tendency to ignore one side of the body, called one-sided neglect

- Laughing or crying without any reason, or when it is inappropriate, called **emotional lability**

- Difficulty swallowing, called **dysphagia**

Depending on the severity of the stroke and speech loss or confusion, these guidelines may help:

Guidelines:
Communication and Stroke

G Keep questions and directions simple. Give directions one step at a time.

G Phrase questions so they can be answered with a "yes" or "no." For example, when helping a resident with eating, ask, "Would you like to start with a drink of milk?"

G Agree on signals, such as shaking or nodding the head or raising a hand or finger for "yes" or "no."

G Give residents time to respond. Listen attentively.

G Use a pencil and paper if the resident can write. A thick handle or tape around it may help the resident hold it more easily.

G Never call the weaker side the "bad side," or talk about the "bad" leg or arm. Use the term "weaker" or "involved" to refer to the side with paralysis or weakness.

G Keep the call signal within reach of residents. They can let you know when you are needed.

G Use pictures, gestures, or pointing. Use communication boards or special cards to aid communication (Fig. 4-17).

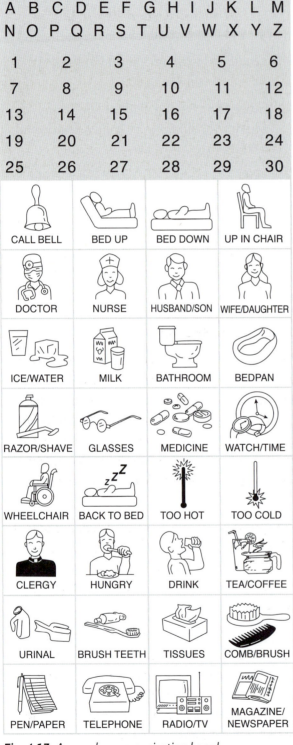

Fig. 4-17. A sample communication board.

You will learn more about caring for someone who has had a CVA in Chapter 18.

Combative Behavior

Residents may display **combative**, meaning violent or hostile, behavior. Such behavior includes hitting, pushing, kicking, or verbal attacks. It may be the result of disease affecting the brain. It may also be due to frustration. Or it may just be part of someone's personality. In general, combative behavior is not a reaction to you. Try not to take it personally.

Always report and document combative behavior. Even if you do not find the behavior upsetting, the care team needs to be aware of it. Use these guidelines when dealing with combative behavior:

Guidelines:
Combative Behavior

G Block physical blows or step out of the way, but never hit back (Fig. 4-18). No matter how much a resident hurts you, or how angry or afraid you are, never hit or threaten a resident.

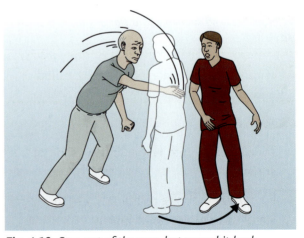

Fig. 4-18. Step out of the way, but never hit back.

G Remain calm. Lower the tone of your voice.

G Be flexible and patient.

G   Stay neutral.

G   Try not respond to verbal attacks. Do not argue. Do not accuse the resident of wrong-doing.

G   Do not use gestures that could frighten or startle the resident.

G   Be reassuring and supportive.

G   Consider what provoked the resident. Sometimes something as simple as a change in caregiver or routine can be very upsetting to a resident. Leave the resident alone if you can safely do so. Get help to take the resident to a quieter place.

Anger

Anger is a natural emotion that has many causes, such as disease, fear, pain, and loneliness. A loss of independence due to illness can cause anger. Anger may also just be a part of someone's personality. Some people get angry more easily than others.

People express anger in different ways. Some may shout, yell, threaten, throw things, or pace. Others express their anger by withdrawing, being silent, or sulking.

Always report angry behavior to the nurse. Use these guidelines when dealing with angry residents:

Guidelines:
Angry Behavior

G   Stay calm.

G   Try not respond to verbal attacks. Do not argue.

G   Empathize with the resident. Try to understand what he or she is feeling.

G   Try to find out what caused the resident's anger. Using silence may help the resident explain.

G   Treat the resident with dignity and respect. Explain what you are going to do and when you will do it.

G   Answer call lights promptly.

G   Stay at a safe distance if the resident becomes combative.

Assertive vs. Aggressive Behavior

A person is behaving assertively when he expresses thoughts, feelings, and beliefs in a direct and honest way. Being assertive involves respect for a person's own needs and feelings and for those of other people. It is not the same as being aggressive, combative, or angry.

A person is behaving aggressively when he expresses thoughts, feelings, and beliefs in ways that humiliate, disgrace, or overpower the other person. Little or no respect is shown for the needs or feelings of others. Report aggressive behavior when you witness it.

Inappropriate Behavior

Some residents will demonstrate inappropriate behavior. Inappropriate behavior from a resident includes trying to establish a personal, rather than a professional, relationship. Examples include asking personal questions, requesting visits on personal time, asking for or doing favors, giving tips or gifts, and loaning or borrowing money.

Inappropriate behavior includes making sexual advances and comments. Sexual advances include any sexual words, comments, or behavior that makes you feel uncomfortable. Report this behavior to the nurse immediately.

Inappropriate behavior also includes residents removing their clothes or touching themselves in public. Illness, dementia, confusion, and medication may cause this behavior. If you encounter any embarrassing situation, be matter-of-fact. Do not over-react, as it may actually reinforce the behavior. Try to distract the person. If that does not work, gently direct the resident to a private area, and notify the nurse.

Confused residents may have problems that mimic inappropriate sexual behavior. They may have an uncomfortable rash, clothes that are too tight, too hot, or too scratchy, or they may need to go to the bathroom. Consider and watch for these problems.

When residents behave inappropriately, report the behavior, even if you think it was harmless.

Residents' Rights

Never hit a resident.

Unfortunately, it is not uncommon to read or hear about physical abuse of the elderly by caregivers. These caregivers may be family, friends, or care team members. Often, physical abuse is due to stressful situations causing the caregiver to lash out quickly.

You can never hit a resident, no matter how a resident may have provoked you. Hitting a resident is considered abuse and is grounds for termination and legal action. If you feel that you need help handling stressful situations, talk with the charge nurse.

Chapter Review

1. Briefly describe three steps in the communication process.

2. Define nonverbal communication and give one example that is not listed in the textbook.

3. What does the word "culture" mean?

4. What is one positive response to cultural diversity?

5. Why should "why" questions be avoided when talking with residents?

6. If a resident speaks a different language than the nursing assistant does, what can the nursing assistant do?

7. What is one way to provide feedback while listening?

8. What can silence or pauses help a resident do?

9. What is one reason that a nursing assistant should not ignore a resident's request?

10. Why should a nursing assistant sit near a resident who has started a conversation?

11. For each statement, decide whether it is a fact or an opinion. Write "F" for fact and "O" for opinion.

    ___ Mr. Moore looked terrible today.

    ___ Mr. Gaston had a fever of 100.7° F.

    ___ Ms. Martino needs to make some friends.

    ___ Mr. Klein has not had a visitor since last Tuesday.

    ___ The doctor says Mrs. Storey has to walk once a day.

12. What is objective information? What is subjective information?

13. Why should nursing assistants use simple, non-medical terms when speaking with residents and their families?

14. What does the abbreviation "ROM" stand for?

15. What does the abbreviation "NPO" stand for?

16. What does the abbreviation "DNR" stand for?

17. List ten signs and symptoms that should be reported immediately to the nurse.

18. Describe four reasons why careful documentation is important.

19. When should care be documented—before or after it is done?

20. Convert 10:00 p.m. to military time.

21. Convert 1400 hours to regular time.

22. What is an incident at a facility?

23. List four guidelines for incident reporting.

24. Give an example of a proper greeting when answering the phone.

25. What are computers? Give two reasons why they may be used in a facility.

26. What is the purpose of the resident call light or call system?

27. When a resident has a hearing impairment, on whose face should the light be shining while communicating—the resident's or the nursing assistant's?

28. How can a nursing assistant explain the position of objects in front of a visually impaired resident?

29. How should questions be phrased to a resident who has had a stroke?

30. How should a nursing assistant refer to the weaker side of a resident who has had a stroke?

31. What should a nursing assistant always do after a resident behaves inappropriately?

5

Preventing Infection

1. Define "infection control" and related terms

Infection control is the term for measures practiced in healthcare facilities to prevent and control the spread of disease. Working to prevent the spread of disease is the responsibility of all care team members. Know your facility's infection control policies; they are there to help protect you, residents, and others from disease.

A **microorganism** is a living thing or organism that is so small that it can be seen only through a microscope. A **microbe** is another name for a microorganism. Microorganisms are always present in the environment (Fig. 5-1). **Infections** occur when harmful microorganisms, called **pathogens**, invade the body and multiply.

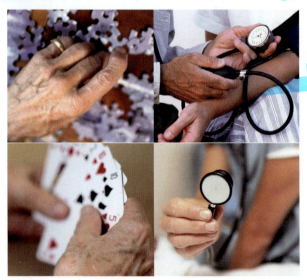

Fig. 5-1. Microorganisms are always present in the environment. They are on almost everything we touch.

Generally, there are two types of infections: systemic and localized. A **systemic infection** is in the bloodstream and is spread throughout the body. It causes general symptoms, such as fever, chills, or mental confusion. A **localized infection** is confined to a specific location in the body and has local symptoms. Its symptoms are near the site of infection. For example, if a wound becomes infected, the area around it may become red, hot, and painful.

Another type of infection is a healthcare-associated infection, or nosocomial infection. **Healthcare-associated infections (HAIs)** are infections that patients acquire within healthcare settings that result from treatment for other conditions.

Medical asepsis is the process of removing pathogens, or the state of being free of pathogens. It refers to the clean conditions you want to create in your facility and is used in all healthcare settings. In healthcare settings, the term **"clean"** means objects are not contaminated with pathogens. The term **"dirty"** means that objects have been contaminated with pathogens. **Surgical asepsis** is the state of being free of all microorganisms, not just pathogens. Surgical asepsis, also called "sterile technique," is used for many types of procedures, such as dressing wounds and changing catheters.

Preventing the spread of infection is very important. To understand how to prevent disease you must first understand how it is spread.

Tip

Infection Prevention

Many facilities now use the term "infection prevention," rather than "infection control." The reason for this is that infections should not be allowed to develop and then need to be controlled. Instead, they should be prevented.

2. Describe the chain of infection

The **chain of infection** is a way of describing how disease is transmitted from one living being to another (Fig. 5-2). Definitions and examples of each of the six links in the chain of infection follow.

1. Causative Agent
2. Reservoir
3. Portal of Exit
4. Mode of Transmission
5. Portal of Entry
6. Susceptible Host

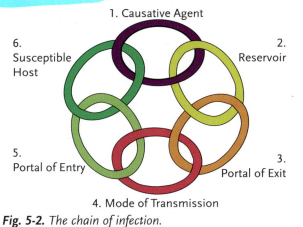

Fig. 5-2. The chain of infection.

Link 1: The **causative agent** is a pathogen or microorganism that causes disease. Normal flora are the microorganisms that live in and on the body and do not cause harm. When they enter a different part of the body, they may cause an infection. Causative agents include bacteria, viruses, fungi, and protozoa.

Link 2: A **reservoir** is a place where the pathogen lives and grows. It can be a person, animal, plant, soil, or substance. Microorganisms grow best in warm, dark, and moist places where food is present. Some microorganisms need oxygen to survive; others do not. Examples of reservoirs include the lungs, blood, and the large intestine.

Link 3: The **portal of exit** is any body opening on an infected person that allows pathogens to leave, such as the nose, mouth, eyes, or a cut in the skin (Fig. 5-3).

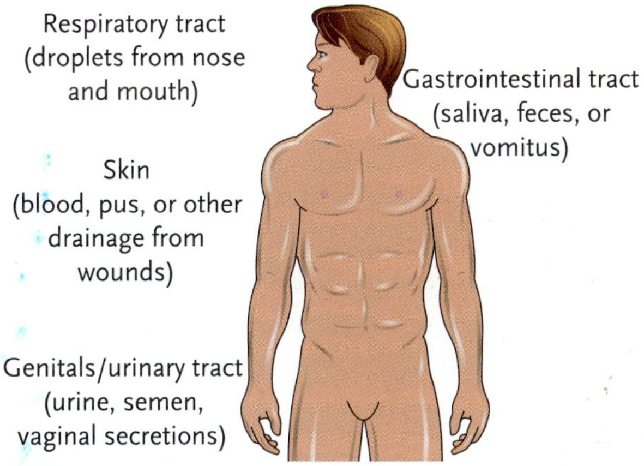

Respiratory tract (droplets from nose and mouth)
Gastrointestinal tract (saliva, feces, or vomitus)
Skin (blood, pus, or other drainage from wounds)
Genitals/urinary tract (urine, semen, vaginal secretions)

***Fig. 5-3.** Portals of exit.*

Link 4: The **mode of transmission** describes how the pathogen travels from one person to the next person. Transmission can happen through the air or through direct or indirect contact. **Direct contact** happens by touching the infected person or his secretions. **Indirect contact** results from touching something contaminated by the infected person, such as a tissue or clothes.

Link 5: The **portal of entry** is any body opening on an uninfected person that allows pathogens to enter. This can occur through the nose, mouth, eyes, other mucous membranes, a cut in the skin, or dry/cracked skin (Fig. 5-4). **Mucous membranes** are the membranes that line body cavities, such as the mouth, nose, eyes, rectum, and genitals.

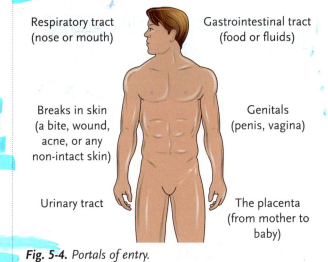

Respiratory tract (nose or mouth)
Gastrointestinal tract (food or fluids)
Breaks in skin (a bite, wound, acne, or any non-intact skin)
Genitals (penis, vagina)
Urinary tract
The placenta (from mother to baby)

***Fig. 5-4.** Portals of entry.*

Link 6: A **susceptible host** is an uninfected person who could get sick. Examples include all healthcare workers and anyone in their care who is not already infected with that particular disease.

If one of the links in the chain of infection is broken, then the spread of infection is stopped. By using infection prevention practices, you can help stop pathogens from traveling (Link 4) and getting on your hands, nose, eyes, mouth, skin, etc. (Link 5). You can also reduce your chances of getting sick by having immunizations (Link 6) for diseases such as hepatitis B and influenza.

Transmission (passage or transfer) of most **infectious**, or contagious, diseases can be prevented by always taking a few precautions. Washing your hands is the most important way to stop the spread of infection. All caregivers should wash their hands often.

3. Explain why the elderly are at a higher risk for infection and identify symptoms of an infection

The elderly are at a higher risk for infection. This is due, in part, to weakened immune systems as a result of aging. Weakened immune systems can also result from chronic illnesses. Other physical changes of aging, such as decreased circulation and slow wound healing, may also contribute to infections in the elderly.

Older adults are at risk for **malnutrition** and dehydration. A person who is malnourished is not getting the proper nutrition. **Dehydration** is a condition that results from inadequate fluid in the body. These conditions can result from difficulty chewing and/or swallowing, lack of appetite and thirst, illnesses, weakness, and medication. Both malnutrition and dehydration are serious conditions (see Chapter 15). When the body is not getting the nutrients and fluid it needs, the risk of infection greatly increases. Also, the elderly may have limited mobility, which is another risk factor for serious problems, such as pressure sores, skin infections, and pneumonia.

The elderly are hospitalized more often than younger people. This makes them more likely to get healthcare-associated infections. Difficulty swallowing and incontinence increase the risk of respiratory and urinary tract infections. Feeding tubes, oxygen tubes, and other types of tubing, such as catheters (see Chapter 16), increase the risk of infection.

Infection is more dangerous for the elderly because even a simple cold can turn into a life-threatening illness such as pneumonia. It also may take longer for older people to recover from an infection or illness. This is why preventing infection is so important. Nursing assistants play an important role in preventing infection.

You will need to recognize signs and symptoms of infections so that you can report them to the nurse.

Observing and reporting:
Localized and Systemic Infections

Signs and symptoms of a localized infection are:

O/R Pain

O/R Redness

O/R Pus

O/R Swelling

O/R Drainage (fluid from a wound or cavity)

O/R Heat to the site

Signs and symptoms of a systemic infection are:

O/R Fever

O/R Body aches

O/R Chills

O/R Nausea

O/R Vomiting

O/R Weakness

O/R Headache

O/R Mental confusion

O/R Drop in person's normal blood pressure

4. Describe the Centers for Disease Control and Prevention (CDC) and explain standard precautions

The **Centers for Disease Control and Prevention (CDC)** is a government agency under the Department of Health and Human Services (HHS) that issues information to protect the health of individuals and communities. It promotes public health and disease, injury, and disability prevention and control through education. In 1996, the CDC recommended a new infection control system to reduce the risk of contracting infectious diseases in healthcare settings. In 2007 some additions and changes were made to this system.

There are two tiers of precautions within the infection control system: standard precautions and transmission-based, or isolation, precautions. To **isolate** means to keep something separate, or by itself.

Following **standard precautions** means treating all blood, body fluids, non-intact skin (like abrasions, pimples, or open sores), and mucous membranes (lining of mouth, nose, eyes, rectum, or genitals) as if they were infected with an infectious disease. Following standard precautions is the only safe way of doing your job. You cannot tell by looking at your residents or their medical charts if they have a contagious disease such as HIV, hepatitis, or influenza.

Under standard precautions, "body fluids" include saliva, sputum (mucus coughed up), urine, feces, semen, vaginal secretions, and pus or other wound drainage. They do not include sweat.

Standard precautions and transmission-based precautions are a way to stop the spread of infection. They interrupt the mode of transmission. In other words, these guidelines do not stop an infected person from releasing pathogens. However, by following these guidelines you help prevent those pathogens from infecting you or those in your care:

- Always practice standard precautions with every single person in your care.
- Transmission-based precautions vary based on how an infection is transmitted. When indicated, they are used **in addition** to the standard precautions. You will learn more about these precautions later in the chapter.

Guidelines:
Standard Precautions

G **Wash your hands** before putting on gloves. Wash your hands immediately after removing your gloves. Be careful not to touch clean objects with your used gloves.

G **Wear gloves** if you may come into contact with: blood; body fluids or secretions; broken skin, such as abrasions, acne, cuts, stitches, or staples; or mucous membranes. Such situations include mouth care, toilet assistance, perineal care, helping with a bedpan or urinal, cleaning up spills, cleaning basins, urinals, bedpans, and other containers that have held body fluids, and disposing of wastes.

G **Remove gloves** immediately when finished with a procedure.

G **Immediately wash all skin surfaces that have been contaminated** with blood and body fluids.

G **Wear a disposable gown** that is resistant to body fluids if you may come into contact with blood or body fluids.

G **Wear a mask and protective goggles** if you may come into contact with splashing or spraying blood or body fluids (for example, emptying a bedpan).

G **Wear gloves and use caution when handling razor blades, needles, and other sharps.** **Sharps** are needles or other sharp objects. Discard these objects carefully in a puncture-resistant biohazard container.

G **Never attempt to put a cap on a needle or syringe**. Dispose of them in a biohazardous waste container. (Fig. 5-5).

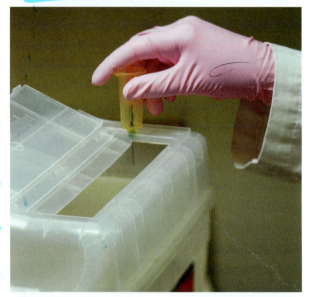

Fig. 5-5. One type of biohazardous waste container.

G **Avoid nicks and cuts** when shaving residents.

G **Carefully bag all contaminated supplies.** Dispose of them according to your facility's policy.

G **Clearly label body fluids that are saved for a specimen** with the resident's name and a bio-hazard label. Keep them in a container with a lid. Put in a biohazardous specimen bag for transportation, if required.

G **Dispose of contaminated wastes** according to your facility's policy. Waste containing blood or body fluids is considered biohazardous waste. Liquid waste can usually be disposed through the regular sewer system as long as there is no splashing, spraying, or aerosol-izing of the waste as it is being disposed. Appropriate PPE needs to be worn, followed by proper removal and handwashing. Follow instructions at your facility.

Again, standard precautions should ALWAYS be practiced on those in your care regardless of their infection status. You cannot tell by how someone looks or acts, or even by reading his or her chart, if he or she carries a bloodborne disease. If you practice standard precautions, you greatly reduce the risk of transmitting infection to yourself and others. You will learn more about following standard precautions in the next several learning objectives.

5. Explain the term "hand hygiene" and identify when to wash hands

In your work you will use your hands constantly. Microorganisms are on everything you touch. Washing your hands is the single most important thing you can do to prevent the spread of disease (Fig. 5-6).

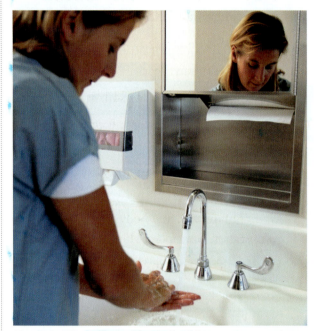

Fig. 5-6. All people working in health care must wash their hands often. Washing your hands is the most important thing you can do to prevent the spread of disease.

The CDC has defined **hand hygiene** as hand-washing with either plain or antiseptic soap and water and using alcohol-based hand rubs. Alcohol-based hand rubs include gels, rinses, and foams. They do not require the use of water. **Hand antisepsis** refers to washing hands with water and soap or other detergents that contain an antiseptic agent.

Alcohol-based hand rubs—often just called "hand rubs"—have proven effective in reducing bacteria on the skin. However, they are not a substitute for proper handwashing. Always use plain or antimicrobial soap and water for visibly soiled hands. An **antimicrobial** agent destroys or resists pathogens. Once hands are clean, hand rubs can be used in addition to handwashing any time your hands are not visibly soiled. When using a hand rub, the hands must be rubbed together until the product has completely dried. Use hand lotion to prevent dry, cracked skin.

If you wear rings, consider removing them while working. Rings may increase the risk of contamination. Keep your fingernails short, smooth, and clean. Do not wear artificial nails or extenders because they harbor bacteria and increase the risk of contamination.

You should wash your hands:

- When you arrive at work
- Whenever they are visibly soiled
- Before, between, and after all contact with residents
- Before putting on gloves and after removing gloves
- After contact with any body fluids, mucous membranes, non-intact skin, or dressings
- After handling contaminated items
- After contact with objects in the resident's room (care environment)
- Before and after touching meal trays and/or handling food
- Before and after feeding residents
- Before getting clean linen
- After touching garbage or trash
- After picking up anything from the floor
- After using the toilet
- After blowing your nose or coughing or sneezing into your hand
- Before and after you eat
- After smoking

- After touching areas on your body, such as your mouth, face, eyes, hair, ears, or nose
- Before and after applying makeup
- After any contact with pets and after contact with pet care items
- Before leaving the facility

Washing hands

Equipment: soap, paper towels

1. Turn on water at sink. Keep your clothes dry, because moisture breeds bacteria.

2. Angle your arms down, holding your hands lower than your elbows. This prevents water from running up your arm. Wet hands and wrists thoroughly (Fig. 5-7).

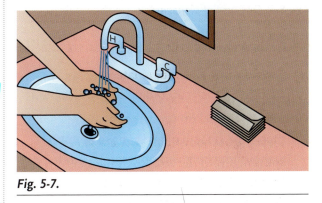

Fig. 5-7.

3. Apply skin cleanser or soap to your hands.

4. Rub hands together and fingers between each other to create a lather. Lather all surfaces of your fingers and hands, including your wrists (Fig. 5-8). Use friction for at least 20 seconds. Friction helps clean.

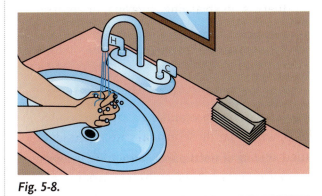

Fig. 5-8.

5. Clean your nails by rubbing them in palm of other hand.

6. Being careful not to touch the sink, rinse thoroughly under running water. Rinse all surfaces of your hands and wrists. Run water down from wrists to fingertips. Do not run water over unwashed arms down to clean hands (Fig. 5-9).

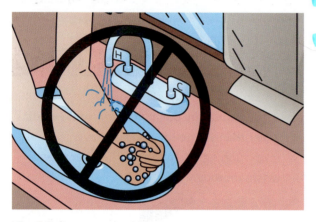

Fig. 5-9.

7. Use a clean, dry paper towel to dry all surfaces of your hands, wrists, and fingers. Do not wipe towel on unwashed forearms and then wipe clean hands. Dispose of towel without touching wastebasket. If your hands touch the sink or wastebasket, start over.

8. Use a clean, dry paper towel to turn off the faucet (Fig. 5-10). Do not contaminate your hands by touching the surface of the sink or faucet.

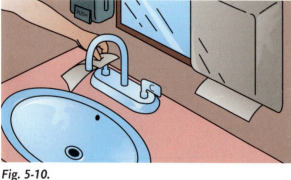

Fig. 5-10.

9. Dispose of used paper towel(s) in wastebasket immediately after shutting off faucet.

6. Discuss the use of personal protective equipment (PPE) in facilities

Personal protective equipment (PPE) is equipment that helps protect employees from serious workplace injuries or illnesses resulting from contact with workplace hazards. In long-term care facilities, PPE helps protect you from contact with potentially infectious material. Your employer is responsible for giving you the appropriate PPE to wear.

Personal protective equipment includes gloves, gowns, masks, goggles, and face shields. Gloves protect the hands. Gowns protect the skin and/or clothing. Masks protect the mouth and nose. Goggles protect the eyes. Face shields protect the entire face—the mouth, nose, and eyes.

Gloves

You must wear gloves when there is a chance you may come into contact with body fluids, open wounds, or mucous membranes. Your facility will have specific policies and procedures on when to wear, or don, gloves. Learn and follow these rules. Always wear gloves for the following tasks:

- Any time you might touch blood or any body fluid, including vomitus, urine, feces, or saliva

- Performing or helping with mouth care or care of any mucous membrane

- Performing or helping with **perineal care** (care of the genitals and anal area)

- Performing personal care on **non-intact skin**—skin that is broken by abrasions, cuts, rashes, acne, pimples, or boils

- Assisting with personal care when you have open sores or cuts on your hands

- Shaving a resident

- Disposing of soiled bed linens, gowns, dressings, and pads

Clean, non-sterile gloves are generally adequate. They may be vinyl, latex, or nitrile; however, some people are allergic to latex. If you are, let the nurse know. Alternative gloves will be provided. Tell the nurse if you have dry, cracked, or broken skin. Gloves should fit your hands comfortably. They should not be too loose or too tight.

If you have cuts or sores on your hands, first cover these areas with bandages or gauze, and then put on gloves. Disposable gloves are to be worn only once. They may not be washed or disinfected for reuse. Change gloves right before contact with mucous membranes or broken skin, or if gloves are soiled, torn, or damaged. Wash your hands before putting on fresh gloves.

Putting on gloves

1. Wash your hands.

2. If you are right-handed, slide one glove on your left hand (reverse if left-handed).

3. With gloved hand, slide the other hand into the second glove.

4. Interlace fingers. Smooth out folds and create a comfortable fit.

5. Carefully look for tears, holes, or discolored spots. Replace the glove if needed.

6. If wearing a gown, pull the cuff of the gloves over the sleeve of gown (Fig. 5-11).

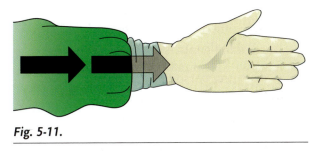

Fig. 5-11.

Remove, or doff, gloves promptly after use and wash your hands. Remove your gloves before touching non-contaminated items or surfaces. You are wearing gloves to protect your skin from becoming contaminated. After giving care, your gloves are contaminated. If you open a door with the gloved hand, the doorknob becomes contaminated. Later, when you open the door with an ungloved hand, you will be infected even though you wore gloves during the procedure. It is a common mistake to contaminate the room around you. Do not do this. Before touching surfaces, remove your gloves. Wash your hands. Afterward, put on new gloves if needed.

Taking off gloves

1. Touch only the outside of one glove. Pull the first glove off by pulling down from the cuff (Fig. 5-12).

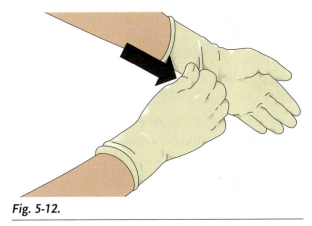

Fig. 5-12.

2. As the glove comes off your hand, it should be turned inside out.

3. With the fingertips of your gloved hand, hold the glove you just removed. With your ungloved hand, reach two fingers inside the remaining glove. Be careful not to touch any part of the outside of glove (Fig. 5-13).

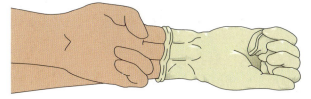

Fig. 5-13.

4. Pull down, turning this glove inside out and over the first glove as you remove it.

5. You should now be holding one glove from its clean inner side. The other glove should be inside it.

6. Drop both gloves into the proper container.

7. Wash your hands.

The guidelines for wearing other PPE are the same as for gloves. You should wear PPE if there is a chance you could come into contact with body fluids, mucous membranes, or open wounds. Gowns, masks, goggles, and face shields are worn when splashing or spraying of body fluids or blood could occur.

Gowns

Clean, non-sterile gowns protect your exposed skin. They also prevent soiling of your clothing. Gowns should fully cover your torso. They should fit comfortably over your body, and have long sleeves that fit snugly at the wrist. When finished with a procedure, remove the gown as soon as possible and wash your hands.

Putting on a gown

1. Wash your hands.

2. Open the gown. Hold out in front of you and allow gown to open. Do not shake it. Slip your arms into the sleeves and pull gown on (Fig. 5-14).

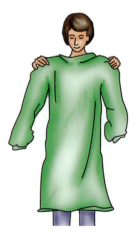

Fig. 5-14.

3. Tie the neck ties into a bow so they can be easily untied later.

4. Reach behind you. Pull the gown until it completely covers your clothing. Tie the back ties (Fig. 5-15).

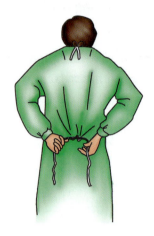

Fig. 5-15.

5. Use a gown only once and then remove and discard it. When removing a gown, roll the dirty side in and away from the body. If your gown ever becomes wet or soiled, remove it. Check clothing and put on a new gown. The Occupational Safety and Health Administration (OSHA) requires non-permeable gowns—gowns that liquids cannot penetrate—when working in a bloody situation.

6. Put on your gloves after putting on gown.

Masks and Goggles

Masks should also be worn when caring for residents with respiratory illnesses. Sometimes special masks are required for certain diseases, such as tuberculosis (TB). You will learn more about TB later in the chapter. Masks should fully cover your nose and mouth and prevent fluid penetration. Masks should fit snugly over the nose and mouth. Always change your mask between residents; do not wear the same mask from one resident to another.

Goggles provide protection for your eyes. Eyeglasses alone do not provide proper eye protection. Goggles should fit snugly over and around your eyes or eyeglasses.

Putting on mask and goggles

1. Wash your hands.

2. Pick up the mask by top strings or elastic strap. Be careful not to touch the mask where it touches your face.

3. Adjust the mask over your nose and mouth. Tie top strings first, then bottom strings. Masks must always be dry or they must be replaced. Never wear a mask hanging from only the bottom ties (Fig. 5-16).

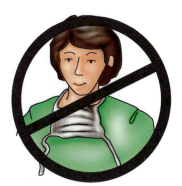

Fig. 5-16.

4. Put on the goggles.

5. Put on your gloves after putting on mask and goggles.

Face Shields

When additional skin protection is needed, a face shield can be used as a substitute for wearing a mask or goggles. Follow your facility's policies. The face shield should cover your forehead and go below the chin. It wraps around the sides of your face.

Your employer will give you PPE as needed. It is your responsibility to know where it is kept and how to use it (Fig. 5-17).

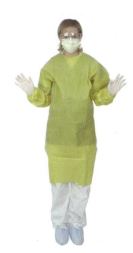

Fig. 5-17. *Using PPE is an important way to reduce the spread of infection.*

When applying PPE, remember this order:

1. Apply gown.

2. Apply mask.

3. Apply goggles or face shield.

4. Apply gloves last.

When removing PPE, remember this order:

1. Remove gloves.

2. Remove goggles or face shield.

3. Remove gown.

4. Remove mask.

Performing hand hygiene is always the final step after removing and disposing of PPE.

> **Tip**
>
> **Wearing PPE**
>
> OSHA states that it is the employer's responsibility to instruct the staff on how to properly wear (don) the PPE, how to wear the PPE effectively, and how to safely remove (doff) the PPE. This instruction needs to be given before the employee is in a situation where PPE is indicated, and as an annual review.

7. List guidelines for handling equipment and linen

Equipment, linen, and supplies are kept in special supply or utility rooms. There are separate rooms for supplies that are considered "clean" and for supplies that are considered "dirty" or contaminated. You will be told where these rooms are located and what types of equipment and supplies are found in each room. Perform hand hygiene before entering clean utility rooms and before leaving dirty utility rooms. This helps prevent the spread of pathogens.

Cleaning usually involves the use of water with or without detergents. General cleaning removes microorganisms but does not kill them. This type of cleaning is often adequate for equipment that does not touch residents or touches only skin that is intact (for example, crutches and blood pressure cuffs). **Sterilization** is a measure that destroys all microorganisms, including pathogens. It uses steam under pressure, liquid or gas chemicals, or dry heat to sterilize. Items that need to be sterilized are ones that go directly into the bloodstream or into other normally sterile areas of the body (for example, surgical instruments). **Disinfection** is a process that kills pathogens, but not all microorganisms; it reduces the organism count to a level that is generally not considered infectious. It is defined as a measure that falls between general cleaning and sterilization. Disinfection is carried out with pasteurization or chemical germicides. Examples of items that are usually disinfected are re-usable oxygen tanks, wall mounted blood pressure cuffs, and any re-usable resident care equipment.

Guidelines:
Handling Equipment, Linen, and Clothing

G   Handle all equipment in a way that prevents

- Skin/mucous membrane contact

- Contamination of your clothing

- Transfer of disease to other residents or areas

G   Do not use "re-usable" equipment again until it has been properly cleaned and reprocessed.

G   Dispose of all "single-use," or disposable, equipment properly. **Disposable** means it is discarded after one use. Disposable razors are an example of disposable equipment.

G   Clean and disinfect

- All environmental surfaces

- Beds, bedrails, all bedside equipment

- All frequently touched surfaces (such as doorknobs, call lights, handles on dressers and tables)

G   Handle, transport, and process soiled linens and clothing in a way that prevents

- Skin and mucous membrane exposure

- Contamination of clothing (hold linen and clothing away from uniform) (Fig. 5-18)

- Transfer of disease to other residents and areas (do not shake linen or clothes; fold or roll linen so that the dirtiest area is inside)

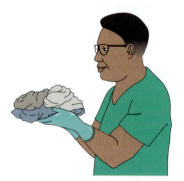

Fig. 5-18. Hold and carry dirty linen away from your uniform.

G   Bag soiled linen at point of origin.

G   Sort soiled linen away from resident care areas.

G   Place wet linen in leak-proof bags.

You will learn more about cleaning equipment and supplies in Chapter 12.

8. Explain how to handle spills

Spills, especially those involving blood, body fluids, or glass, can pose a serious risk of infection.

Long-term care facilities will have cleaning solutions for spills. Clean spills using proper equipment and procedure.

Guidelines:
Cleaning Spills Involving Blood, Body Fluids, or Glass

G Apply gloves before starting. In some cases, industrial-strength gloves are best.

G First, absorb the spill with whatever product is used by the facility. It may be an absorbing powder.

G Scoop up the absorbed spill, and dispose of in a designated container.

G Apply the proper disinfectant to the spill area and allow it stand wet for a minimum of 10 minutes.

G Clean up spills immediately with the proper cleaning solution.

G Do not pick up any pieces of broken glass, no matter how large, with your hands. Use a dustpan and broom or other tools.

G Waste containing broken glass, blood, or body fluids should be properly bagged. Waste containing blood or body fluids may need to be placed in a special biohazard container. Follow facility policy.

Tip
Cleaning Spills

Many facilities use special clean-up kits for spills. Follow directions when using these kits.

Sometimes staff members assume that the disinfectant should be placed directly on the spilled fluid before absorbing and removing the fluid. This is incorrect. The spilled fluid may neutralize the disinfectant upon contact. Absorb and remove the spill first.

9. Explain transmission-based precautions

The CDC set forth a second level of precautions beyond standard precautions. These precautions are used when caring for persons who are infected or suspected of being infected with a disease. These precautions are called **transmission-based**, or **isolation, precautions**. When ordered, these precautions are used in addition to standard precautions. These precautions will always be listed in the care plan and on your assignment sheet. It is for your safety and the safety of others that these precautions must be followed.

There are three categories of transmission-based precautions:

- Airborne precautions
- Droplet precautions
- Contact precautions

The category used depends on the disease and how it spreads to other people. They may also be used in combination for diseases that have multiple routes of transmission. Diseases that require isolation precautions in addition to standard precautions include the following:

- **Multidrug-resistant organisms (MDROs)** (microorganisms, mostly bacteria, that are resistant to one or more antimicrobial agents), such as methicillin-resistant *Staphylococcus aureus* (MRSA) and vancomycin-resistant *enterococcus* (VRE) *
- *Clostridium difficile* (C- diff or C. difficile) *
- Scabies (a skin disease that causes itching)
- Lice
- Influenza (during an outbreak)

* You will learn more about these infections later in the chapter.

Airborne Precautions

Airborne precautions are used for diseases that are transmitted through the air after being expelled (Fig. 5-19). The pathogens are so small that they can attach to moisture in the air and remain floating for some time. For certain care you may be required to wear a special mask, such as N-95 or HEPA masks, to avoid being infected. Airborne diseases include tuberculosis, measles, and chickenpox. More information on tuberculosis is found later in this chapter.

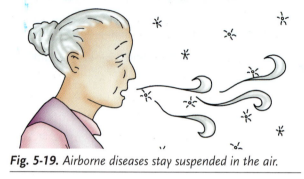

Fig. 5-19. Airborne diseases stay suspended in the air.

Droplet Precautions

Droplet precautions are used when the disease-causing microorganism does not stay suspended in the air and usually only travels short distances after being expelled. Droplets normally do not travel more than three feet. Droplets can be created by coughing, sneezing, talking, laughing, or suctioning (Fig. 5-20). Droplet precautions include wearing a face mask during care and restricting visits from uninfected people. Residents should wear masks, if they are able to do so, when being moved from room to room. Cover your nose and mouth with a tissue when you sneeze or cough, and ask residents, family, and others to do the same. Dispose of the tissue in the nearest waste container. If you sneeze on your hands, wash them promptly. An example of a droplet disease is the mumps.

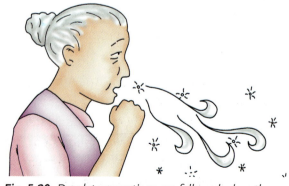

Fig. 5-20. Droplet precautions are followed when the disease-causing microorganism does not stay suspended in the air.

Respiratory Hygiene/Cough Etiquette in Healthcare Settings

The CDC has set forth special infection prevention measures for all respiratory infections in healthcare settings. They include the following:

1. Post visual alerts at the entrances of care facilities instructing that all patients and visitors inform staff of symptoms of respiratory infections and to practice respiratory hygiene/cough etiquette.

2. All individuals with signs and symptoms of a respiratory infection must:

* Cover their nose/mouth when coughing and sneezing.

* Use tissues for respiratory secretions and dispose of them in the nearest waste container.

* Perform hand hygiene after contact with respiratory secretions and contaminated objects.

Healthcare facilities must make these items available to staff, patients, and visitors:

* Tissues and no-touch receptacles for tissue disposal

* Conveniently located hand rub dispensers and handwashing supplies in areas where sinks are located

3. During times of increased respiratory infections, offer masks to anyone who is coughing and encourage coughing people to sit at least three feet away from others in waiting areas.

Contact Precautions

Contact precautions are used when there is a risk of transmitting or contracting a microorganism from touching an infected object or person (Fig. 5-21). Lice, scabies, and bacterial conjunctivitis (pink eye) are examples of situations that require contact precautions. Transmission can occur with skin-to-skin contact during transfers or bathing.

Contact precautions include wearing PPE and resident isolation. They require washing hands with antimicrobial soap and not touching infected surfaces with ungloved hands or uninfected surfaces with contaminated gloves.

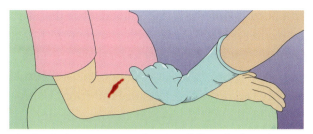

Fig. 5-21. *Contact precautions are followed when the person is at risk of transmitting or getting a microorganism from touching an infected object or person.*

Staff often refer to residents who need transmission-based precautions as being in "isolation." A sign should be on the door indicating "isolation" or "contact precautions" and alerting people to see the nurse before entering the room. Other guidelines to follow for isolation (contact) precautions include the following:

Guidelines:
Isolation

G   When they are indicated, transmission-based precautions are always used **in addition** to standard precautions.

G   Nurses will set up the isolation unit. Some facilities have a special room where isolation supplies are kept. Some facilities keep supplies within the room itself, while other facilities set up an isolation cart outside the room. Isolation supplies consist of gloves, masks, gowns, or aprons and, if indicated, goggles, face shields, respirator masks, or other forms of specialized personal protective equipment (PPE).

G   You will be told the proper PPE to wear for care of each resident in isolation. Make sure to put on the PPE properly and remove it safely. Remove PPE and place it in the appropriate container before exiting a resident's room. PPE cannot be worn outside the resident's room. Perform hand hygiene following removal of PPE and exiting the resident's room. In addition to handwashing areas

within the resident's room, there may be an alcohol-based hand rub dispenser mounted on the wall inside the room as you exit the door.

G   Do not share equipment between residents. Use disposable supplies that can be discarded after use whenever possible. Use dedicated (only for use by one resident) equipment when disposable is not an option. For example, a resident in isolation has her own (dedicated) blood pressure cuff and stethoscope. Disposable thermometers are used to take her temperature. When using disposable supplies, discard them in the resident's room before leaving. Be careful not to contaminate reusable equipment by setting it on furniture or counters in the resident's room. When the resident is discharged or no longer needs the additional precautions, properly dispose of dedicated equipment, if required. If the dedicated equipment is to be used for other residents, it should be cleaned and disinfected after use.

G   Some facilities will require that disposable dishes, glasses, cups, and eating utensils be used for residents in isolation. Wear the proper PPE, if indicated, when serving food and drink. Do not leave uneaten food uncovered in the resident's room. When the meal is completed, remove the meal tray and take it to the designated area, or put it back on the food cart. When the food carts are returned to the kitchen, all soiled trays will be handled with gloves by the dietary staff and the tray and dinnerware will be cleaned and sanitized.

G   Follow standard precautions when dealing with body waste removal. Wear gloves when touching or handling the resident's waste. Wear gowns and goggles when indicated. The waste must be disposed of in such a manner as to minimize splashing and spraying.

G   If required to take a specimen from a resident in isolation, wear the proper PPE. Collect the specimen following proper procedure, and place it in the appropriate container without the outside of the container coming into contact with the specimen. Properly remove your PPE and dispose of it in the room. Perform hand hygiene before leaving the room, and take the container holding the specimen to the nurse.

G   Residents need to feel that their circumstances and feelings are appreciated and understood by members of the care team without criticism or judgment. Listen to what your resident is telling you and allow time to talk with your resident about his concerns. Reassure residents that it is the disease, not the person, that is being isolated. Explain why these steps are being taken. Relay any requests outside your scope of practice to the nurse.

Residents' Rights

Isolation

Residents' basic needs remain the same while in isolation. Human basic needs do not change, even though physical conditions may change. Do not avoid a resident in isolation. Do not rush through care tasks or make the resident feel that he or she should be avoided. Being professional, caring and competent may help lessen a resident's worries or concerns and feelings of being isolated. If you have questions about the care you are giving, talk to the charge nurse.

10. Define "bloodborne pathogens" and describe two major bloodborne diseases

Bloodborne pathogens are microorganisms found in human blood that can cause infection and disease in humans. They may also be in body fluids, draining wounds, and mucous membranes. Bloodborne diseases can be transmitted by infected blood entering your bloodstream, or if infected semen or vaginal secretions contact your mucous membranes. You can become infected with a bloodborne disease by having sexual contact with someone with that disease. It is not necessary to have sexual intercourse to transmit disease. Other kinds of sexual activity can just as easily cause infection. Using a needle to inject drugs and sharing needles can also transmit bloodborne diseases. In addition, infected mothers may transmit bloodborne diseases to their babies in the womb or during birth.

In health care, contact with infected blood or certain other body fluids is the most common way to be infected with a bloodborne disease. This chapter explains work practices, such as standard precautions, hand hygiene, isolation, and using PPE to help prevent transmission of bloodborne diseases. Employers are required by law to help prevent exposure to bloodborne pathogens. You will learn more about that law in the next learning objective. Understand and follow standard precautions and other procedures to protect yourself from bloodborne diseases.

You can safely touch, hug, and spend time talking with residents who have a bloodborne disease (Fig. 5-22). They need the same thoughtful, personal attention you give to all your residents. Follow standard precautions but never isolate a resident emotionally because he or she has a bloodborne disease.

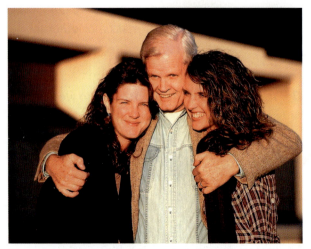

Fig. 5-22. *Hugs and touches cannot spread a bloodborne disease.*

The major bloodborne diseases in the United States are acquired immune deficiency syndrome (AIDS) and hepatitis. **HIV** stands for human immunodeficiency virus, and it is the virus that can cause AIDS. HIV weakens the immune system so that people cannot effectively fight infections. Some of these people will develop AIDS as a result of their HIV infection. People with AIDS lose all ability to fight infection. They can die from illnesses that a healthy body could handle. You will learn more about HIV and AIDS in Chapter 18.

Hepatitis is inflammation of the liver caused by infection. It begins with symptoms that resemble the flu (fever, fatigue, nausea, vomiting), but eventually jaundice appears. **Jaundice** is a condition in which the skin, whites of the eyes, and mucous membranes appear yellow. Liver function can be permanently damaged by hepatitis, which can lead to other chronic, life-long illnesses. Several different viruses can cause hepatitis: A, B, C, D, and E. The most common types of hepatitis are A, B, and C.

The virus causing hepatitis A is a result of fecal-oral contamination. For example, a person washes her hands improperly after having a bowel movement. She then prepares and eats food that has been contaminated by the fecal material left on her hands and/or under her nails.

Hepatitis B is contracted through blood or needles that are contaminated with the virus, or by sexual contact with an infected person. Hepatitis B (HBV) can cause short-term illness that leads to:

- Loss of appetite
- Diarrhea and vomiting
- Fatigue
- Jaundice (yellow skin or eyes)
- Pain in muscles, joints, and stomach

It can also cause long-term illness that leads to:

- Liver damage (cirrhosis)
- Liver cancer
- Death

Hepatitis C is also transmitted through blood and possibly sexual intercourse. Hepatitis B and C can lead to cirrhosis and liver cancer; they can even cause death. Many more people have hepatitis B (HBV) than HIV. The risk of acquiring hepatitis is greater than the risk of acquiring HIV. HBV poses a serious threat to healthcare workers.

Hepatitis D is caused by the hepatitis D virus (HDV) and is only found in people who carry the hepatitis B virus. It is uncommon in the United States. It is transmitted through contact with infectious blood. Hepatitis E caused by the hepatitis E virus (HEV) that usually results in an acute infection but does not lead to a chronic infection. HEV is rare in the United States, but is more common in many parts of the world. HEV is transmitted through ingestion of fecal matter, even in small amounts.

Your employer must offer you a free vaccine to protect you from hepatitis B. The HBV vaccine can prevent hepatitis B. Prevention is the best option for dealing with this disease. If you have not received the hepatitis B vaccine and you are exposed to a body fluid with the virus, your chances of acquiring infection are over 30%. Hepatitis B can remain capable of causing infection on an environmental surface for up to seven days in a dried state. Take the vaccine when it is offered. It is the best protection against HBV. There is no vaccine for hepatitis C, D, and E.

11. Explain OSHA's Bloodborne Pathogen Standard

The **Occupational Safety and Health Administration (OSHA)** is a federal government agency that makes rules to protect workers from hazards on the job. OSHA has set standards for special procedures that must be followed in healthcare facilities. One of these is the **Bloodborne Pathogens Standard**. This law requires that healthcare facilities protect employees from bloodborne health hazards. By law, employers must follow these rules to reduce or eliminate the risk of exposure to infectious diseases. The standard also guides employers and employees through the steps to follow if exposed to infectious material. Significant exposures include:

- Exposure by injection; a needle stick

- Mucous membrane contact

- Cut from an object containing a potentially infectious body fluid (includes human bites)

- Non-intact skin (OSHA includes acne as non-intact skin)

Guidelines employers must follow include:

- Employers must have a written **exposure control plan** designed to eliminate or reduce employee exposure to infectious material. This plan also identifies what to do if an employee is exposed to infectious material. This plan must be accessible to all employees, and they must receive training on the plan.

- Employers must give all employees, visitors, and residents proper personal protective equipment (PPE) to wear when needed at no cost. Employers must make sure the PPE is available in the appropriate sizes and is readily accessible.

- Employers must make biohazard containers available for disposal of sharps and other infectious waste. These containers must be puncture resistant, labeled or color-coded, and leakproof.

- Employers must provide a free hepatitis B vaccine to all employees after hire. This vaccine must be made available at no cost to the employee.

- Warning labels must be affixed to waste containers and refrigerators and freezers that contain blood or any other potentially infectious material (Fig. 5-23).

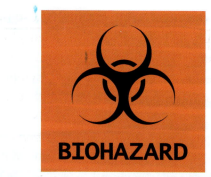

Fig. 5-23. *This label indicates that the material is potentially infectious.*

- Employers must keep a log of injuries from contaminated sharps. The information recorded must protect the confidentiality of the injured employee. Employers are also required to select safer needle devices and to involve employees in choosing these devices.

- Employers must provide training for employees to explain the standard and its contents.

If any potential exposures occur, you will need to fill out an incident report or a special exposure report form. Your employer will help you find out if you have been infected and will take steps to keep you from becoming sick. To protect your health and that of others, report any potential exposures right away. Steps will also be taken to help keep similar incidents from occurring again. Your facility may require tests and other measures to keep you healthy. For more information on OSHA, visit their website— osha.gov.

12. Define "tuberculosis" and list infection control guidelines

Tuberculosis, or TB, is an airborne disease carried on very small mucous droplets suspended in the air. When a person infected with TB talks, coughs, breathes, or sings, he may release mucous droplets carrying the disease. TB usually infects the lungs, causing coughing, trouble breathing, fever, weight loss, and fatigue. If left untreated, TB may cause death.

There are two types of TB: **latent TB**, also called TB infection, and **active TB**, also called TB disease. Someone with latent TB (TB infection) carries the disease but does not show symptoms and cannot infect others. A person with active TB (TB disease) shows symptoms of the disease and can spread TB to others. TB infection can progress to TB disease. The signs and symptoms of TB include the following:

- Fatigue
- Loss of appetite
- Weight loss
- Slight fever and chills
- Night sweats
- Prolonged coughing
- Coughing up blood
- Chest pain
- Shortness of breath
- Trouble breathing

Tuberculosis is more likely to be spread in small, confined, or poorly ventilated places. TB is more likely to develop in people whose immune systems are weakened by illness, malnutrition, alcoholism, or drug abuse. People with cancer or HIV/AIDS are more susceptible to developing active TB when exposed. This is due to their weakened immune systems.

Multidrug-resistant TB (MDR-TB) is a type of TB that can develop when a person with active TB does not take all the prescribed medication. **Resistant** means drugs no longer work to kill the specific bacteria. When the full course of medication is not taken, bacteria remains in the body and is less likely to be killed by the TB medication. If the TB bacilli develop a resistance to the drugs that treat TB, fighting the disease becomes more difficult. Surgery may be the only option for treatment. However, if the disease is widespread throughout both lungs, surgery may not be possible.

Guidelines:
Tuberculosis

G Follow standard precautions and airborne precautions.

G Wear a mask and gown during resident care. Special masks, such as N-95, high efficiency particulate air (HEPA), or other masks, may be needed (Fig. 5-24). These masks filter out very small particles, such as the germs that cause TB. You must be fit-tested for these special masks. You will also be trained on how to use the masks.

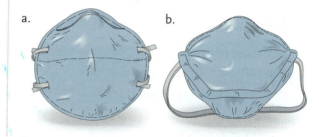

Fig. 5-24. a) N-95 respirator mask and b) PFR-95 respirator mask.

G Use special care when handling sputum or phlegm. **Phlegm** is thick mucus from the respiratory passage.

G Residents with TB will be placed in a special airborne infection isolation room (AIIR). Other names for the isolation room may be "Negative Air Pressure Room" or "Acid-Fast Bacillus (AFB) isolation room." In this type of room, the flow of air is carefully controlled. Airborne particles are not trapped in the room. The air is changed often through a special air system. The air is exhausted directly outside or forced through filters to remove particles. The room will be identified with a special sign identifying it as a special respiratory isolation room. When entering this room, do not open or close the door quickly. This pulls contaminated room air into the hallway. The door should remain closed.

G Follow isolation procedures for airborne diseases if directed.

G Help the resident remember to take all medication prescribed. Failure to take all medication is a major factor in the spread of TB.

13. Define the terms "MRSA," "VRE," and "C. Difficile"

Multidrug-resistant organisms (MDROs) are microorganisms, mostly bacteria, that are resistant to one or more antimicrobial agents that are commonly used for treatment. MDROs are increasing, and this is a serious problem. Two common types of MDROs are MRSA and VRE.

MRSA stands for methicillin-resistant *Staphylococcus aureus*. *Staphylococcus aureus* is a common type of bacteria that can cause illness. Methicillin is a powerful antibiotic drug. MRSA is an antibiotic-resistant infection often acquired by people in hospitals and other healthcare facilities who have weakened immune systems. However, MRSA infections also occur in otherwise healthy people who have not been recently hospitalized or had recent medical procedures. They are sometimes acquired in fitness centers when equipment has not been disinfected during use. These infections are known as community-associated MRSA infections (CA-MRSA) and are usually skin infections, such as pimples or boils.

MRSA can spread among people having close contact with infected people. MRSA is almost always spread by direct physical contact, and not through the air. This means if a person has MRSA on his skin, especially on the hands, and touches someone, he may spread MRSA. Spread also occurs through indirect contact by touching objects (for example, towels, sheets, wound dressings, clothes) contaminated by the infected skin of a person with MRSA.

You can help prevent MRSA by practicing good hygiene. Handwashing, using soap and warm water, is the single most important measure to control MRSA. Keep cuts and abrasions clean and covered with a proper dressing (e.g. bandage) until healed. Avoid contact with other people's wounds or material that is contaminated from wounds.

VRE stands for vancomycin-resistant *enterococcus*. *Enterococci* are bacteria that live in the digestive and genital tracts. They normally do not cause problems in healthy people. Vancomycin is a powerful antibiotic that is often the antibiotic of last resort. It is generally limited to use against bacteria that are resistant to other antibiotics. Vancomycin-resistant *enterococcus* is a genetically changed strain of *enterococcus* that originally developed in people who were exposed to the antibiotic vancomycin.

VRE is dangerous because it cannot be controlled with most of the antibiotics currently in use. It causes life-threatening infections in those with weakened immune systems—the very young, the very old, and the very ill. VRE is spread through direct and indirect contact. Once it establishes itself, it is very difficult to eliminate. Preventing VRE is much easier. You can help prevent its spread by washing your hands often. Wear PPE as directed. Disinfect items according to facility policy.

Clostridium difficile (C-diff, C. difficile) is a spore-forming bacteria which can be part of the normal intestinal flora. When the normal intestinal flora are altered, *C. difficile* can flourish in the intestinal tract. It produces a toxin that causes frequent, foul-smelling, watery stools. Other symptoms include diarrhea that contains blood and mucus and abdominal cramps. Enemas, nasogastric tube insertion, and GI tract surgery increase a person's risk of developing the disease. The overuse of antibiotics may also alter the normal intestinal flora and increase the risk of developing *C. difficile* diarrhea. *C. difficile* can also cause colitis, a more serious intestinal condition.

C. difficile is spread by spores in feces that are difficult to kill. These spores can be carried on the hands of people who have direct contact with infected residents or with environmental surfaces (floors, bedpans, toilets, etc.) contaminated with *C. difficile*. *C. difficile* spores can remain viable for months in the environment in a spore state. Most disinfectants cause *C. difficile* to go into a spore state without killing them. A bleach solution, if used before the spore formation, will eliminate the organism. However, once the organism has formed its spore state, the bleach solution is no longer effective. Frequently cleaning surfaces with a bleach solution will kill those *C. difficile* spores that change back to their vegetative form.

Proper handwashing and handling of contaminated wastes can help prevent the disease. Hand rubs have been shown to increase the risk of *C. difficile* transmission on the hands of healthcare workers. This is because many feel that a hand rub is all that is needed, rather than performing proper handwashing. Hand rubs effectively smear *C. difficile* all over the hands. The alcohol in hand rubs sends the *C. difficile* into an instant spore state, which makes the alcohol ineffective. Even though handwashing does not kill the *C. difficile*, it does get it off the hands and down the drain. Use a hand rub only after performing proper handwashing. Limiting the use of antibiotics also helps lower the risk of developing *C. difficile* diarrhea.

14. List employer and employee responsibilities for infection control

Several state and federal government agencies have guidelines and laws concerning infection prevention. OSHA requires employers to provide for the safety of their employees through rules and suggested guidelines. The CDC issues guidelines for healthcare workers to follow on the job. Some states have additional requirements. Facilities consider these rules very carefully when writing their policies and procedures. It is very important that you learn these and follow them. They exist to protect you. Some of the infection prevention requirements for you and your employer are listed below.

Employers' responsibilities for infection control include the following:

- Establish infection control procedures and an exposure control plan to protect workers.

- Provide continuing in-service education on infection control, including bloodborne and airborne pathogens.

- Have written procedures to follow should an exposure occur, including medical treatment and plans to prevent similar exposures.

- Provide PPE for employees to use and teach them when and how to properly use it.

- Provide free hepatitis B vaccinations for all employees.

Employees' responsibilities for infection control include the following:

- Follow standard precautions.

- Follow all of the facility's policies and procedures.

- Follow care plans and assignments.

- Use provided PPE as indicated or as appropriate.

- Take advantage of the free hepatitis B vaccination.

- Immediately report any exposure you have to infection.

- Participate in annual education programs covering the control of infection.

Chapter Review

1. Define the following terms: infection control, microorganism, healthcare-associated infections, medical asepsis, clean, and dirty.

2. How does infection occur?

3. What is the chain of infection?

4. What is direct contact? What is indirect contact?

5. Define "mucous membranes."

6. Why are elderly people at a higher risk for infection?

7. List four signs of a localized infection and four signs of a systemic infection.

8. Under standard precautions, what does the phrase "body fluids" include?

9. On whom should standard precautions be practiced?

10. Under standard precautions, when should gloves be worn?

11. What is the most important thing you can do to prevent the spread of disease?

12. What is hand hygiene? What is hand antisepsis?

13. List ten situations that require nursing assistants to wash their hands.

14. How many times can disposable gloves be worn?

15. In what order should PPE be applied? In what order should it be removed?

16. What is always the final step after removing PPE?

17. Define sterilization. Define disinfection.

18. How should soiled linen be carried?

19. Describe three guidelines for cleaning spills.

20. What are transmission-based precautions? List the three categories of transmission-based precautions.

21. What are bloodborne pathogens?

22. How are bloodborne diseases transmitted?

23. What does HIV do to the immune system?

24. What is hepatitis?

25. How is hepatitis B (HBV) contracted?

26. Describe what an exposure control plan is.

27. List four guidelines employers must follow under the Bloodborne Pathogen Standard.

28. In which people is tuberculosis more likely to develop?

29. In what kind of settings is TB most likely to spread?

30. What are multidrug-resistant organisms (MDROs)?

31. What is one of the best ways to prevent the spread of MRSA and VRE?

32. List the factors that increase a person's risk of developing *C. difficile* diarrhea.

33. List five employer responsibilities for infection control. List five employee responsibilities for infection control.

6
Safety and Body Mechanics

1. Identify the persons at greatest risk for accidents and describe accident prevention guidelines

All staff members, including you, are responsible for safety in a facility. Elderly people have more safety concerns due to dementia, confusion, illness, disability, and diminished senses. Walking aids, such as crutches, walkers, canes, or boots for foot or leg injuries, put persons at risk for falling. Residents who take medications that cause dizziness and light-headedness are likely to have accidents.

Our senses—sight, hearing, touch, smell, and taste—give us information about the world around us and help keep us safe. Normal changes of aging can cause sensory losses. The senses of vision, hearing, taste and smell decrease. Sensitivity to heat and cold decreases. In addition to normal aging changes, diseases can cause diminished senses. Diseases of the circulatory system, the integumentary system (the skin), and paralysis can reduce the skin's ability to feel. **Paralysis** is the loss of ability to move all or part of the body, and often includes loss of feeling in the affected area. Strokes and brain or spinal injuries affect sensation and awareness of surroundings. A loss of sensation can lead to burns or other accidents. Drowsiness, due to illness, lack of sleep, medications or even feeling depressed can also cause a lack of awareness. Being in pain or unconscious may reduce awareness. Individuals who are less aware may

not know the positions of their body parts. Their reflexes slow. It is more difficult to react in time to avoid accidents, such as falls. Visual or hearing problems can also cause falls. Residents with vision problems may not see hazards, such as an object or water on the floor. Those who cannot hear well may not understand directions.

It is very important to try to prevent accidents *before* they occur. Prevention is the key to safety. As you work, watch for safety hazards, and report unsafe conditions to your supervisor promptly.

There are many accidents and injuries that may occur in a facility, including falls, burns/scalds, not identifying a resident before performing care or serving food, choking, poisoning, and cuts. Below you will find guidelines for preventing common types of accidents.

Falls

The majority of accidents that occur in a facility are falls. Falls can be caused by an unsafe environment, loss of abilities, diseases, and medications. The consequences of falls can range from minor bruises to fractures and life-threatening injuries. A **fracture** is a broken bone. Older people are often more seriously injured by falls, as their bones are more fragile. Hip fractures are one of the most common type of fractures from falls. Hip fractures cause the greatest number of deaths and can lead to severe health problems. Be especially alert to the risk of falls.

Factors that raise the risk of falls include the following:

- Clutter
- Throw rugs
- Exposed electrical cords
- Slippery or wet floors
- Uneven floors or stairs
- Poor lighting
- Call lights that are out of reach or not promptly answered

Personal conditions that raise the risk of falls include medications, loss of vision, walking or balance problems, weakness, paralysis, and disorientation. **Disorientation** means confusion about person, place, or time.

Guidelines:
Preventing Falls

G Keep all walking areas are free of clutter, trash, throw rugs, and cords.

G Use rugs with a non-slip backing.

G Have residents wear non-slip, sturdy shoes. Make sure shoelaces are tied.

G Residents should avoid wearing clothing that is too long or drags on the floor.

G Keep frequently-used personal items close to residents, including call lights (Fig. 6-1).

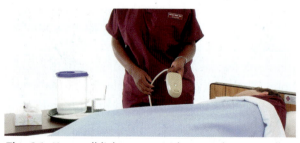

Fig. 6-1. Keep call lights near residents so they can call you when needed. Answer call lights promptly.

G Answer call lights right away.

G Immediately clean up spills on the floor.

G Report loose hand rails immediately.

G Mark uneven flooring or stairs with colored tape to indicate a hazard.

G Improve lighting where needed.

G Lock wheelchairs before helping residents into or out of them (Fig. 6-2).

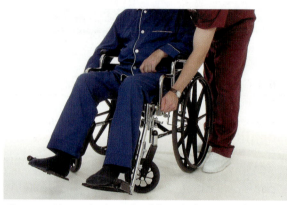

Fig. 6-2. Always lock a wheelchair before transferring a resident into or out of it.

G Lock bed wheels before helping a resident into and out of bed or when giving care (Fig. 6-3).

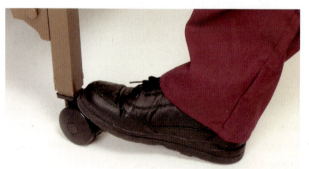

Fig. 6-3. Always lock the bed wheels before helping a resident into or out of bed, and before giving care.

G Before giving care, there are many times that you will need to raise beds to make your job easier and safer. After completing care, return beds to their lowest positions.

G Get help when moving a resident; do not assume you can do it alone. When in doubt, ask for help. Keep residents' walking aids, such as canes or walkers within their reach.

G Offer help with toileting regularly (Fig. 6-4). Respond to requests for help immediately. Think about how you would feel if you had to wait for help to go to the bathroom.

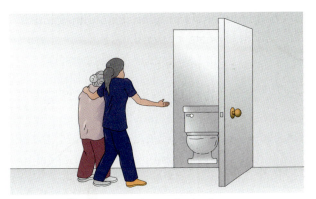

Fig. 6-4. Offer frequent trips to the bathroom.

G Leave furniture in the same place as you found it.

G Know which residents are at risk for falls and pay close attention so that you can give help often.

G If a resident starts to fall, be in a good position to help support her. Never try to catch a falling resident. Use your body to slide her to the floor. If you try to reverse a fall, you may hurt yourself and/or the resident.

Burns/Scalds

Burns can be caused by dry heat (e.g. hot iron, stove, other electrical appliances), wet heat (e.g. hot water or other liquids, steam), or chemicals (e.g. lye, acids). Small children, older adults, or people with loss of sensation due to paralysis are at the greatest risk of burns.

Scalds are burns caused by hot liquids. It takes five seconds or less for a serious burn to occur when the temperature of liquid is 140°F. Coffee, tea, and other hot drinks are usually served at 160°F to 180°F. These temperatures can cause almost instant burns that require surgery. Preventing burns is very important.

Guidelines:
Preventing Burns and Scalds

G Always check water temperature with a water thermometer or on your wrist before using.

G Report frayed electrical cords or unsafe-looking appliances immediately, and do not use them.

G Let residents know you are about to pour or set down a hot liquid.

G Pour hot drinks away from residents.

G Keep hot drinks and liquids away from edges of tables. Put a lid on them.

G Make sure residents are sitting down before serving hot drinks.

G If plate warmers or other equipment that produces heat are used, monitor them carefully.

Resident Identification

Residents must always be identified. Not identifying residents before giving care or serving food can cause serious problems, even death. Facilities have different methods of identification. Some have ID bracelets. Some have pictures to identify residents. Identify each resident before beginning any procedure or giving any care (Fig. 6-5). Always identify residents before placing meal trays or helping with feeding. Check the diet card against the resident's identification. Call the resident by name.

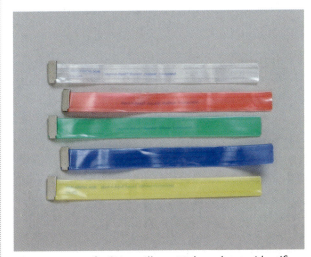

Fig. 6-5. Some facilities will use ID bracelets to identify residents; others will use other methods of identification. Identify all residents before giving care. (REPRINTED WITH PERMISSION OF BRIGGS CORPORATION, 800-247-2343, WWW.BRIGGSCORP.COM)

Choking

Choking can occur when eating, drinking, or swallowing medication. Babies and young children who put objects in their mouths are at great risk of choking. People who are weak, ill, or unconscious can choke on their own saliva. A person's tongue can also become swollen and obstruct the airway. To guard against choking, residents should eat sitting as upright as they can (Fig. 6-6). Residents with swallowing problems may have special diets with liquids thickened to the consistency of honey or syrup. Thickened liquids are easier to swallow. You will learn more about helping with feeding and thickened liquids in Chapter 15.

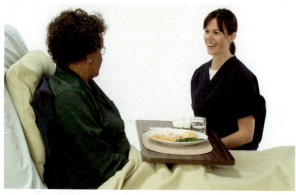

Fig. 6-6. *Residents must be sitting up straight when eating, whether in a bed or a chair.*

Poisoning

Facilities have many harmful substances that should not be swallowed. These include cleaners, paints, medicines, toiletries, and glues. These products should be stored or locked away from confused residents or those with limited vision. Do not leave cleaning products in residents' rooms. Residents with dementia may hide food and let it spoil in closets, drawers, or other places. Investigate any odors you notice. The number for the Poison Control Center should be posted by all telephones.

Cuts/Abrasions

Cuts or abrasions typically occur in the bathroom at a facility or in the kitchen or bathroom

when at home. An **abrasion** is an injury which rubs off the surface of the skin. Put any sharp objects, including scissors, nail clippers, or razors away after use. Take care when transferring residents into and out of beds, chairs, and wheelchairs. When moving a resident in a wheelchair, push the wheelchair forward. Do not pull it behind you. If using an elevator to get to another floor, turn the wheelchair around before entering the elevator, so the resident is facing forward.

Other general safety guidelines are:

- Do not run in halls, on stairs, or in the dining room.

- Keep paths clear and free of clutter.

- Wipe up spilled liquids right away.

- Discard trash properly.

- Follow instructions. Ask about anything you do not understand.

- Report injuries immediately.

Promoting safety is one of your responsibilities. Help make your workplace safer for everyone by reporting hazards immediately.

Residents' Rights

Safety

Residents have the right to a safe environment. Observe the environment carefully to eliminate safety hazards. If you see any safety hazards, such as a frayed electrical cord on a resident's radio, report them immediately. Residents have the right to have personal items and to have these items treated with respect. However, if a resident's possession is a potential safety hazard, report this to the nurse. The safety of all residents and staff members is most important.

2. List safety guidelines for oxygen use

Residents with breathing problems may receive oxygen that is more concentrated than what is in the air. Oxygen is prescribed by a doctor. Nursing assistants never stop, adjust, or administer oxygen. Oxygen may be piped into a resident's room through a central system. It may be in tanks or produced by an oxygen concentrator. An oxygen concentrator is a box-like device that changes air in the room into air with more oxygen. You will learn more about oxygen delivery in Chapter 14.

Oxygen is a very dangerous fire hazard because it makes other things burn. Oxygen itself does not burn; it merely supports combustion. **Combustion** means the process of burning. Working around oxygen requires special safety precautions.

Guidelines:
Working Safely Around Oxygen

G Remove all fire hazards from the room or area. Fire hazards include electric razors, hair dryers, other electrical appliances, cigarettes, matches, and flammable liquids (Fig. 6-7). **Flammable** means easily ignited and capable of burning quickly. Alcohol and gasoline are examples of flammable liquids. Notify the nurse if a fire hazard is present and the resident does not want it removed.

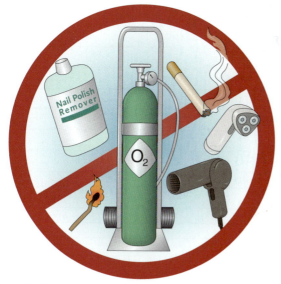

Fig. 6-7. Examples of fire hazards.

G Post "No Smoking" and "Oxygen in Use" signs. Never allow smoking where oxygen is used or stored.

G Do not burn candles, light matches, or use lighters around oxygen. Any type of open flame that is present around oxygen is a dangerous fire hazard.

G Learn how to turn oxygen off in case of fire if facility allows this. Never adjust the oxygen level.

G Report if the nasal cannula or face mask is causing skin irritation. Check behind ears for irritation from tubing (Fig. 6-8).

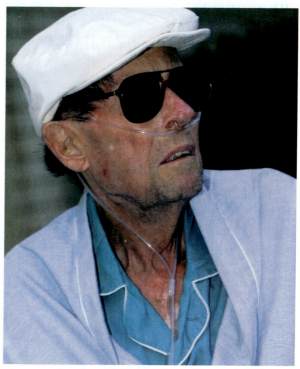

Fig. 6-8. A resident with a nasal cannula.

3. Explain the Material Safety Data Sheet (MSDS)

The Occupational Safety and Health Administration (OSHA) requires that all hazardous chemicals must have a Material Safety Data Sheet (MSDS) (Fig. 6-9). This sheet details the chemical ingredients, chemical dangers, emergency response actions to be taken, and safe handling procedures for the product (Fig. 6-10). Some facilities use a toll-free number to access MSDS information. MSDSs must be accessible in work areas for all employees.

Material Safety Data Sheet

May be used to comply with OSHA's Hazard Communication Standard, 29 CFR 1910 1200. Standard must be consulted for specific requirements.

U.S. Department of Labor

Occupational Safety and Health Administration (Non-Mandatory Form)
Form Approved
OMB No. 1218-0072

IDENTITY *(as Used on Label and List)*	Note: Blank spaces are not permitted. If any item is not applicable or no information is available, the space must be marked to indicate that.

Section I

Manufacturer's name	Emergency Telephone Number
Address *(Number, Street, City, State and ZIP Code)*	Telephone Number for Information
	Date Prepared
	Signature of Preparer *(optional)*

Section II—Hazardous Ingredients/Identity Information

Hazardous Components (Specific Chemical Identity, Common Name(s))	OSHA PEL	ACGIH TLV	Other Limits Recommended	% (optional)

Section III—Physical/Chemical Characteristics

Boiling Point		Specific Gravity (H_2O = 1)	
Vapor Pressure (mm Hg)		Melting Point	
Vapor Density (AIR = 1)		Evaporation Rate (Butyl Acetate = 1)	

Solubility in Water

Appearance and Odor

Section IV—Fire and Explosion Hazard Data

Flash Point (Method Used)		Flammable Limits	LEL	UEL

Extinguishing Media

Special Fire Fighting Procedures

Unusual Fire and Explosion Hazards

OSHA 174 Sept. 1985

Fig. 6-9. *A Material Safety Data Sheet.*

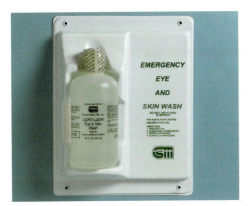

Fig. 6-10. *OSHA requires that emergency eyewashes be placed in all hazardous areas in case an eye injury occurs. Employees must know where the closest eyewash station is and how to get there with restricted vision.* (REPRINTED WITH PERMISSION OF BRIGGS CORPORATION, 800-247-2343, WWW.BRIGGSCORP.COM)

Important information about the MSDS includes the following:

- Your employer must have an MSDS for every chemical used.

- Your employer must provide easy access to the MSDS.

- You must know where your MSDSs are kept and how to read them. If you do not know how to read them, ask for help.

The list of hazardous chemicals that have to have an MSDS will be updated as new chemicals are purchased.

4. Define the term "restraint" and give reasons why restraints were used

A **restraint** is a physical or chemical way to restrict voluntary movement or behavior. Physical restraints are also called postural supports or protective devices. Examples of physical restraints are vests and jacket restraints, belt restraints, wrist/ankle restraints, and mitt restraints. Side rails on a bed and special chairs, such as geriatric chairs, are also considered physical restraints (Figs. 6-11 and 6-12). Chemical restraints are medications given to control a person's behavior.

In the past, restraints were commonly used to safeguard residents who wander, are prone to falls, are violent, or are at risk of hurting

themselves. Restraints were also used to keep residents from pulling out tubing that is needed for treatment. However, abuse by caregivers and injury to residents led to new restrictions and laws on the use of restraints. In many states, restraints are illegal, and in general, the use of any type of restraint has greatly decreased.

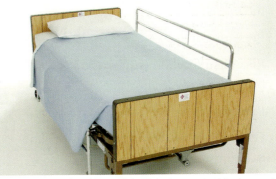

Fig. 6-11. *Side rails are considered restraints because they restrict movement.*

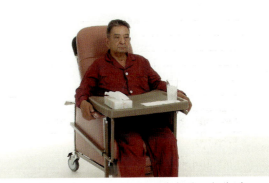

Fig. 6-12. *When the tray table is attached or locked, a geriatric chair, or geri-chair, is considered a restraint.*

Generally, restraints are only used as a last resort. If restraint use is legal, a doctor must prescribe it. Never use physical restraints unless a doctor has ordered it in the care plan and you have been trained in their use. It is against the law for staff to apply restraints for convenience or to discipline a resident. Check with the nurse for laws and policies on the use of restraints.

5. List physical and psychological problems associated with restraints

There are many negative effects of restraint use, including the following:

- Reduced blood circulation

- Stress on the heart

- Incontinence

- Constipation

- Weakened muscles and bones

- Loss of bone mass

- Muscle **atrophy** (weakening or wasting of the muscle)

- Pressure sores

- Risk of suffocation (**suffocation** is death from a lack of air or oxygen)

- Pneumonia

- Less activity, leading to poor appetite and malnutrition

- Sleep disorders

- Loss of dignity

- Loss of independence

- Increased agitation

- Increased depression and/or withdrawal

- Poor self-esteem

Some restraints have caused severe injury and even death. Never use a restraint unless your supervisor has told you to do so, and you have been instructed in the proper use of the restraint.

6. Define the terms "restraint-free" and "restraint alternatives" and list examples of restraint alternatives

Laws allow the use of restraints only when absolutely necessary for the safety of the person, others around that person, and the staff. State and federal agencies encourage facilities to take steps toward a restraint-free environment. **Restraint-free** care means that restraints are not used for any reason and are usually not kept in the facility. To reach this goal, many care facilities have developed creative ideas to use instead of using restraints. **Restraint alternatives** are any intervention used in place of a restraint or that reduces the need for a restraint. Many scientific studies have shown that the use of restraints is no longer needed. People tend to respond better to the use of creative ways to reduce tension, pulling at tubes, wandering, and boredom.

Examples of restraint alternatives include the following:

- Improve safety measures to prevent accidents and falls. Improve lighting.

- Make sure the call light is within the resident's reach, and answer call lights promptly.

- Ambulate the resident when he is restless. The doctor or nurse may add exercise into the care plan.

- Provide activities for those who wander at night.

- Encourage activities and independence. Escort the person to social activities. Increase visits and social interaction.

- Give frequent help with toileting. Help with cleaning immediately after an episode of incontinence.

- Offer food or drink. Offer reading materials.

- Distract or redirect interest. Give the resident a repetitive task.

- Decrease the noise level. Listen to soothing music. Offer back massages or use relaxation techniques.

- Reduce pain levels through medication. Monitor the resident closely and report complaints of pain to the nurse.

- Offer one-on-one time with a caregiver. Provide familiar caregivers, and increase the number of caregivers with family and volunteers.

- Use a team approach to meeting the person's needs. Offer training to teach gentle approaches to difficult people.

There are also several types of pads, belts, special chairs, and alarms that can be used instead of restraints (Fig. 6-13).

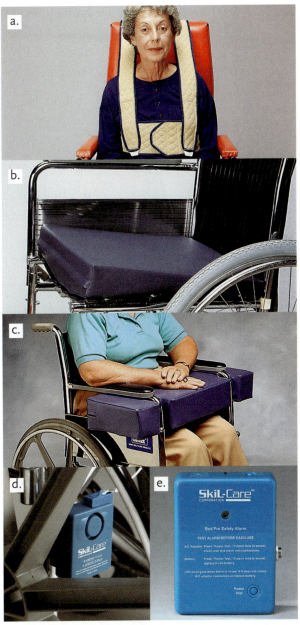

Fig. 6-13. a) A Posey Torso Support; b) A Posey Deluxe Wedge Cushion; c) A lap-top cushion; d) A chair alarm warns caregiver of chair exits; e) An under-mattress alarm warns if person gets out of bed (PHOTOS A, B, AND C COURTESY OF NORTH COAST MEDICAL, INC., WWW.NCMEDICAL.COM, 800-821-9319. PHOTOS D AND E REPRINTED WITH PERMISSION OF BRIGGS CORPORATION, 800-247-2343, WWW.BRIGGSCORP.COM)

7. Describe guidelines for what must be done if a restraint is ordered

Remember that a restraint can never be applied without a doctor's order. Do not use a restraint unless the charge nurse has told you to do so and you have been trained in its proper use. If you are asked to apply a restraint, follow these guidelines:

Guidelines:
Restraints

G Check to make sure there is a doctor's order for restraint use and that it is in the care plan before applying restraints.

G If you are asked to apply a restraint, follow the manufacturer's instructions.

G Restraints can only be tied to the movable part of a bed frame, not to the side rails or other areas on the bed.

G Check to make sure that the restraint is not too tight. Place an open hand flat between the resident and the restraint. This helps to ensure that the device fits properly and is comfortable.

G Make sure that the breasts or skin are not caught in the restraint.

G Place the call light where the resident can easily access it. Answer call lights immediately.

G Document restraint use according to facility policy.

A restrained resident must be monitored constantly; the resident must be checked at least every 15 minutes. At regular, ordered intervals, the following must be done:

G Release the restraint (or discontinue use).

G Offer help with toileting. Check for episodes of incontinence. Provide incontinence care.

G Offer fluids.

G Check the skin for signs of irritation. Report any red, purple, blue-tinged, gray, or pale skin or any discolored areas to the nurse immediately.

G Check for swelling of the body part and report swelling to the nurse immediately.

G Reposition the resident.

G Ambulate the resident if he is able.

If any problems occur with the restraint, especially resident injury, notify the nurse and complete an incident report as soon as possible.

8. Explain the principles of body mechanics

Back strain or injury is one of the greatest risks that nursing assistants face. In fact, the increasing injury rate is one reason why many long-term care facilities have decided to have "lift-free" or "zero-lift" policies. This means that these facilities have set strict guidelines on the use of lifts and transfers of residents in order to reduce injuries. Using proper body mechanics is an important step in preventing back strain and injury.

Body mechanics is the way the parts of the body work together whenever you move. Good body mechanics help save energy and prevent injury. Good body mechanics help you push, pull, and lift objects or people who cannot fully support or move their own bodies. Understanding some basic principles of body mechanics will help keep you and residents safe.

Alignment: Alignment is based on the word "line." When you stand up straight, a vertical line could be drawn through the center of your body and your center of gravity (Fig. 6-14). When the line is straight, the body is in alignment and you are exhibiting good posture. **Posture** is the way a person holds and positions his body. Whether standing, sitting, or lying down, try to have your body in alignment and to have good posture. This means that the two sides of the body are mirror images of each other, with body parts lined up naturally. Maintain correct body alignment when lifting or carrying an object by keeping it close to your body. Point your feet

and body in the direction you are moving. Avoid twisting at the waist.

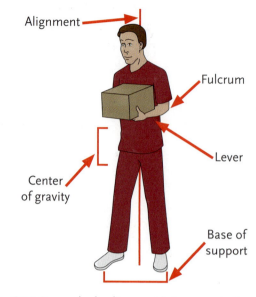

Fig. 6-14. *Proper body alignment is important when standing and sitting.*

Base of support: The base of support is the foundation that supports an object. The feet are the body's base of support. The wider your support, the more stable you are. Standing with your legs shoulder-width apart allows for a greater base of support. You will be more stable than someone standing with his feet together.

Fulcrum and lever: A **lever** moves an object by resting on a base of support, called a fulcrum. Think of a seesaw. The flat board you sit on is the lever. The triangular base the board rests on is the fulcrum. When two children sit on opposite sides of the seesaw, they easily move each other up and down. This is because the fulcrum and lever of the seesaw are doing the work.

If you think of your body as a set of fulcrums and levers, you can find smart ways to lift without working as hard. Think of your arm as a lever with the elbow as the fulcrum. When you lift something, rest it against your forearm. This will shorten the lever and make the item easier to lift than it would be if you were holding it in your hands.

Center of gravity: The center of gravity in your body is the point where the most weight is concentrated (Fig. 6-15). This point will depend on the position of the body. When you stand, your weight is centered in your pelvis. A low center of gravity gives a more stable base of support. Bending your knees when lifting an object lowers your pelvis and, therefore, lowers your center of gravity. This gives you more stability. It makes you less likely to fall or strain the working muscles.

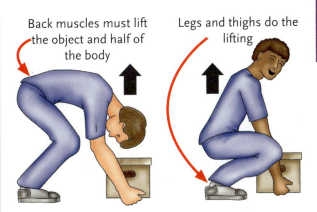

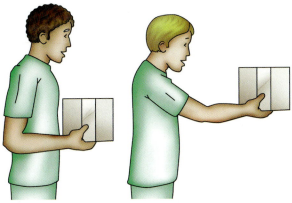

Fig. 6-15. *Holding things close to you moves weight toward your center of gravity. In this illustration, who is more likely to strain his back muscles?*

9. Apply principles of body mechanics to daily activities

By applying the principles of body mechanics to your daily activities, you can avoid injury and use less energy. Some examples of using good body mechanics include the following:

When lifting a heavy object from the floor, spread your feet shoulder-width apart. Bend your knees. Using the strong, large muscles in your thighs, upper arms, and shoulders, lift the object. Pull it close to your body, to a point level with your pelvis. By doing this, you keep the object close to your center of gravity and base of support. When you stand up, push with your strong hip and thigh muscles. Raise your body and the object together (Fig. 6-16).

Back muscles must lift the object and half of the body

Legs and thighs do the lifting

Fig. 6-16. *In this illustration, which person is lifting correctly?*

Do not twist when you are moving an object. Always face the object or person you are moving. Pivot your feet instead of twisting at the waist.

To help a resident sit up, stand up, or walk, protect yourself by assuming a good stance. Place your feet twelve inches, or shoulder-width, apart. Place one foot in front of the other, with your knees bent. Your upper body should stay upright and in alignment. Do this whenever you have to support a resident's weight. If the resident starts to fall, you will be in a good position to help support her. Never try to "catch" a falling resident. If the resident falls, assist her to the floor (Fig. 6-17). If you try to reverse a fall in progress, you will probably injure yourself and/or the resident.

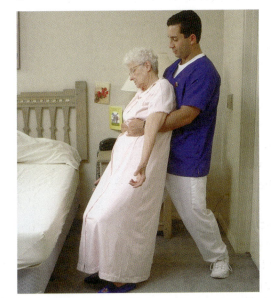

Fig. 6-17. *Maintaining a wide base of support and low center of gravity will enable you to help a falling resident.*

Bend your knees to lower yourself, rather than bending from the waist. When a task requires bending, use a good stance. This allows you to use the big muscles in your legs and hips rather than straining the smaller muscles in your back.

If you are making an adjustable bed, adjust the height to a safe working level, usually waist high. If you are making a regular bed, lean or kneel to support yourself at working level. Avoid bending at the waist.

Prevention of back strain and injury is very important. Throughout this text you will learn correct procedures for assisting with resident transfers, positioning, and ambulation. These procedures will include instructions for maintaining proper body mechanics. In addition, always keep the following tips in mind:

- Use both arms and hands to lift, pull, push, or carry objects.

- Hold objects close to you when you are lifting or carrying them.

- Push, slide, or pull objects rather than lifting them.

- Avoid bending and reaching as much as possible. Move or position furniture so that you do not have to bend or reach.

- Avoid twisting at the waist. Instead, turn your whole body. Your feet should point toward what you are lifting.

- Get help when possible for lifting or helping residents.

- When moving a resident, let him know what you will do so he can help if possible. Count to three. Lift or move on three so everyone moves together.

Report to the nurse any task you feel that you cannot safely do. Never try to lift an object or a resident that you feel you cannot handle.

10. Identify major causes of fire and list fire safety guidelines

In order for a fire to occur, it requires three elements: heat, fuel, and oxygen. A fire can be prevented or extinguished by removing any one of these elements.

Recognize and report any fire hazards you observe. There are many potential fire hazards in facilities and in the home, including the following:

- Careless smoking, smoking in bed, cigarettes left burning, or confused residents smoking

- Frayed or exposed electrical wires

- Damaged electrical equipment

- Oxygen use

- Flammable liquids stored near appliances

- Electrical sockets that are overloaded

In addition, in the home, these hazards may exist:

- Wood stoves and kerosene, gas, or electric heaters that appear old, damaged, or faulty

- Unvented heaters used in small, enclosed areas or sleeping areas

- Space heaters used near fabrics such as draperies, bedspreads, or towels, or used to dry clothing or towels

- Matches or lighters left within reach of children or incapacitated adults

- Careless cooking

All facilities have a fire safety plan, and all workers need to know this plan. Your facility's guidelines regarding fires and evacuations will be explained to you. Evacuation routes are posted in facilities. Read and review them often. Attend fire and disaster in-services when they are offered. They will help you learn what to do in an emergency. Get residents to safety first. A fast, calm and confident response by the staff saves lives.

Guidelines:
Reducing Fire Hazards and Responding to Fires

G Never leave smokers unattended. If residents smoke, make sure they are in the proper area for smoking. Be sure that cigarettes are extinguished. Empty ashtrays often. Before emptying ashtrays, make sure there are no hot ashes or hot matches in ashtray.

G Report frayed or damaged electrical cords immediately. Report electrical equipment in need of repair immediately.

G Fire alarms and exit doors should not be blocked. If they are, report this to the nurse.

G Every facility will have a fire extinguisher (Fig. 6-18). The PASS acronym will help you understand how to use it:

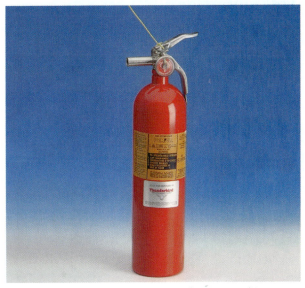

Fig. 6-18. Know where the extinguisher is stored in your facility and how to use it.

- Pull the pin.
- Aim at the base of fire when spraying.
- Squeeze the handle.

- Sweep back and forth at the base of the fire.

G In case of fire, the RACE acronym is a good rule to follow:

- Remove residents from danger.
- Activate 911.
- Contain fire if possible.
- Extinguish, or fire department will extinguish.

Follow these guidelines for helping residents exit the building safely:

G Know the facility's fire evacuation plan.

G Remain calm.

G Follow the directions of the fire department.

G Know which residents need one-on-one help or assistive devices. Immobile residents can be moved in several ways. If they have a wheelchair, help them into it. You can also use other wheeled transporters, such as carts, bath chairs, stretchers, or beds. A blanket can be used as a stretcher or even pulled across the floor with someone on it.

G Residents who can walk will also need assistance getting out of the building. Those who are hard of hearing or deaf may not hear the warnings and instructions. Staff will need to tell them directly what to do while guiding them to the nearest safe exit. Individuals with visual problems should be moved out of the way of the wheelchairs, carts, etc. and helped to the exit. Confused and disoriented residents will also need guidance.

G Remove anything blocking a window or door that could be used as a fire exit.

G Do not use elevators.

G If a door is closed, check for heat coming from it before opening it. If the door or doorknob feels hot to the touch, it is best to stay in the room if there is no safe exit. Plug the doorway (use wet towels or clothing) to prevent smoke from entering. Stay in the room until help arrives.

G Use the "stop, drop, and roll" fire safety technique to use to extinguish a fire on clothing or hair. Stop running or stay still. Drop to the ground, lying down if possible. Roll on the ground to try to extinguish the flames.

G Use a damp covering over the mouth and nose to reduce smoke inhalation.

G After leaving the building, move away from it.

Chapter Review

1. List five reasons that elderly people have more safety concerns than others do.

2. What type of accident occurs most frequently in long-term care facilities?

3. List eleven guidelines to prevent falls.

4. Describe five ways to guard against burns/scalds.

5. What should nursing assistants always do before giving care or serving meal trays?

6. In what position should residents eat to avoid choking?

7. What are three guidelines for working safely around oxygen?

8. What is the purpose of the MSDS?

9. When can a restraint be used?

10. Can restraints be used if staff do not have enough time to care for residents? Can restraints be used if the resident has made a staff member mad by arguing with the staff member or being in a bad mood?

11. List ten problems associated with restraint use.

12. Define the terms "restraint-free" and "restraint alternatives."

13. List six things that must be done at regular times if a resident is restrained.

14. What does the phrase "body mechanics" mean?

15. What is the name for the point in the body where most weight is concentrated?

16. When lifting a heavy object from the floor, how should the feet be placed? How should the knees be positioned?

17. When a task requires bending, which of the following demonstrates proper body mechanics: bending the knees or bending from the waist?

18. Is it better to push an object or to lift an object?

19. What three elements are needed for a fire to occur?

20. List nine fire hazards that may exist in a facility or at home.

21. List ten guidelines for reducing fire hazards and responding to fires.

7

Emergency Care and Disaster Preparation

1. Demonstrate how to recognize and respond to medical emergencies

Medical emergencies may be the result of accidents or sudden illnesses. This chapter discusses how to respond appropriately to medical emergencies. Heart attacks, strokes, diabetic emergencies, choking, automobile accidents, and gunshot wounds are all medical emergencies.

Falls, burns, and cuts can also be emergencies when they are severe. In an emergency situation, it is important to remain calm, act quickly, and communicate clearly. Knowing the following steps will help you respond calmly and quickly in an emergency:

Assess the situation. Try to determine what has happened. Make sure you are not in danger. Notice the time.

Assess the victim. Ask the injured or ill person what has happened. If the person is unable to respond, he may be unconscious. Being **conscious** means being mentally alert and having awareness of surroundings, sensations, and thoughts. To determine whether a person is conscious, tap the person and ask if he is all right. Speak loudly. Use the person's name if you know it. If there is no response, assume the person is unconscious and that you have an emergency situation. Call for help right away or send someone else to call.

If a person is conscious and able to speak, then he is breathing and has a pulse. Talk with the person about what happened. Obtain the person's permission to touch him or her. (Anyone who is unable to give consent for treatment, i.e. a child with no parent near or an unconscious or seriously injured person, may be treated with "implied consent," meaning that if the person was able or the parent was present, they would have given consent). Check the person for injury, checking for the following:

- Severe bleeding
- Changes in consciousness
- Irregular breathing
- Unusual color or feel to the skin
- Swollen places on the body
- Medical alert tags
- Anything the person says is painful

If any of these conditions exists, you may need professional medical help. Always get help/call the nurse before doing anything else.

If the injured or ill person is conscious, he may be frightened about his condition. Listen to the person. Tell him what actions are being taken to help him. Be calm and confident. Reassure him that you are taking care of him.

Once the emergency is over, you will need to document the emergency in your notes and complete an incident report. Try to remember as many details as possible. Remember, report the facts only. If you think a resident had a heart attack, write the signs and symptoms you observed and the actions you took. Knowing the kind of information you will have to document will help you remember the important facts during the emergency. For instance, it is especially important to remember the time at which a resident becomes unconscious.

Reporting Emergencies

If a resident needs emergency help, the nurse may ask you to call emergency services. Know the procedure for dialing an outside line. If you need to call emergency medical services, dial 911.

When calling emergency services, be prepared to give the following information:

- The phone number and address of the emergency, including exact directions or landmarks, and the location within the building, if necessary

- The person's condition, including any medical background you know

- Your name and position

- Details of any first aid being given

The dispatcher you speak with may need other information or may want to give you other instructions. Do not hang up the phone until the dispatcher hangs up or tells you to hang up. If you are in a home, unlock the front door so emergency personnel can get in when they arrive.

If you are a home health aide working in a home, remember this: when in doubt about calling for help, call! If you are alone, make the call yourself. If you are not alone, shout for help and have someone make the call for you and then return to you. After calling 911, notify your supervisor of what is happening and that you have called 911 or emergency services. She will be able to notify the family or friends who need to know this information.

2. Demonstrate knowledge of CPR and first aid procedures

First aid is emergency care given immediately to an injured person. **Cardiopulmonary resuscitation (CPR)** refers to medical procedures used when a person's heart or lungs have stopped working. CPR is used until medical help arrives.

Quick action is necessary. CPR must be started immediately after calling for help or sending someone to call for help. Brain damage may occur within four to six minutes after the heart stops beating and the lungs stop breathing. The person can die within ten minutes.

Only properly trained people should administer CPR. Your facility will probably arrange for you to be trained in CPR. If your facility does not do this, ask about American Heart Association or Red Cross CPR training or contact one of these agencies yourself. CPR is an important skill to learn. **If you are not trained, do not attempt to perform CPR.** Performing CPR incorrectly can further injure a person.

Beginning CPR

Know your facility's policies on whether you can initiate CPR if you have been trained. Some facilities do not allow nursing assistants to begin CPR without direction of the nurse. This is due, in part, to residents' advance directives. Some people have made the decision that they do not want CPR. Notify the nurse immediately if an emergency occurs.

This textbook is not a CPR course. The following is intended as a brief review for people who have had CPR training. It is based on the American Heart Association's training guidelines for healthcare providers (HCP).

1. After making sure that the scene is safe, check whether the person is responsive. Tap the person on the shoulder and shout, "Are you all right?"

2. If there is no response, call 911 immediately or send someone to call 911. Remain calm.

3. After calling 911, get an automated external defibrillator (AED) (if available and if trained in its use) and return to the person to provide CPR. More information on the AED is in step 10.

4. The person should be on his back on a hard surface (if he has no spinal injuries) before CPR is started.

5. Open the airway. Tilt the head back slightly by lifting the chin with one hand while pushing down on the forehead with the other hand (head tilt-chin lift method) (Fig. 7-1). This method is used if a neck injury is not suspected.

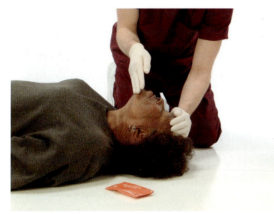

Fig. 7-1. *The head tilt-chin lift method.*

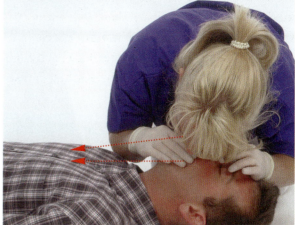

Fig. 7-2. *Give two rescue breaths while covering the person's mouth and pinching the nose to keep air from escaping.*

6. Look, listen, and feel for signs of life for no longer than 10 seconds:

- Look for the chest to rise and fall.

- Listen for sounds of breathing. Put your ear near the person's nose and mouth.

- Feel for the person's breath on your cheek.

7. If you do not detect adequate breathing within 10 seconds, you will have to breathe for the person. Give two rescue breaths. To give rescue breaths:

- Pinch the nose to keep air from escaping from the nostrils. Cover the person's mouth completely with your mouth.

- Blow into the person's mouth slowly, watching for the chest to rise (Fig. 7-2). Blow one breath for about one second, take a "regular" (not a deep) breath, and give a second rescue breath for about one second. Turn your head to the side to listen for air. If the chest does not rise when you give a rescue breath, reopen the airway using the head tilt-chin lift method. Try to give rescue breaths again. You can also use a barrier device, such as a special face mask, if available (Fig. 7-3).

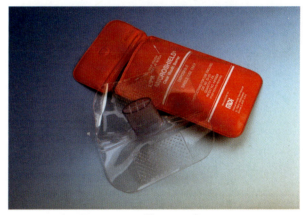

Fig. 7-3. *This is one type of face mask.*

8. After giving rescue breaths, look for signs of circulation. The person may start moving, breathing normally, or coughing. If they do not respond to the rescue breaths, give 30 chest compressions only if you have been trained to do so. Be sure the person is lying flat on a hard surface. To give chest compressions:

- Place the heel of one hand on the sternum in the center of the person's chest between the nipples. Place the heel of the other hand on top of the positioned hand. Interlace your fingers (Fig. 7-4).

- Position your body directly over your hands. Lock your elbows and shoulders. Look down at your hands.

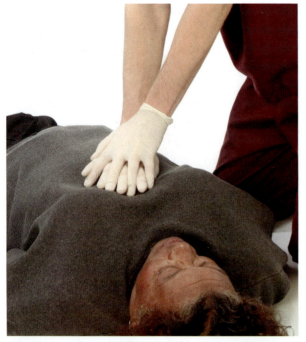

Fig. 7-4. *Interlace your fingers and keep your elbows locked.*

- Use the heels of your hands to give 30 chest compressions. Push in 2 inches with each compression. Push hard and fast. Allow the chest to recoil completely after each compression. Do not take your hands off the chest between compressions.

9. Continue giving CPR in cycles of 30 compressions to 2 breaths, with 5 cycles taking about two minutes. Do not stop CPR to recheck anything. Continue until the scene becomes unsafe, the person recovers, paramedics arrive with an AED and take over, help arrives to assist you, or you become too exhausted to continue. If you do see signs of life, stop compressions, maintain an open airway, and turn the person onto his side, in the recovery position.

10. The AED may be used together with CPR. AED stands for "automated external defibrillator." It is a computerized device that checks a person's heart rhythm. It is able to recognize a rhythm that requires a shock. The AED uses voice prompts, lights and text messages to relay instructions to the rescuer (Fig. 7-5). You must be trained in its use.

If you are not trained, do not try to use the AED.

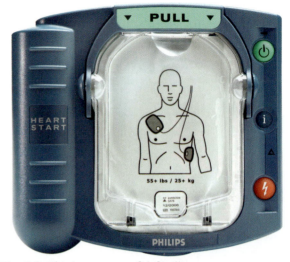

Fig. 7-5. *This is one type of defibrillator.* (REPRINTED WITH PERMISSION OF THE BRIGGS CORPORATION, 800-247-2343, WWW.BRIGGSCORP.COM)

When medical help arrives, follow their directions. Assist them as necessary. Report details of the incident.

Residents' Rights

CPR

Protect the privacy of residents who need CPR by pulling the privacy curtain around the bed and closing the door. Anyone who is not directly involved in giving care should leave the room. Remain calm and be professional. Remember that the resident may be able to hear what is being said. Some residents have do-not-resuscitate (DNR) orders in place, which means that no CPR may be given. This is a legal order; the resident's decision for a DNR order and other advance directives must be honored. Do not judge these very personal decisions.

Choking

When something is blocking the tube through which air enters the lungs, the person has an **obstructed airway**. When people are choking, they usually put their hands to their throats and cough (Fig. 7-6). As long as a person can speak, breathe, or cough, do nothing. Encourage him to cough as forcefully as possible to get the object out. Stay with the person at all times, until he stops choking or can no longer speak, cough, or breathe.

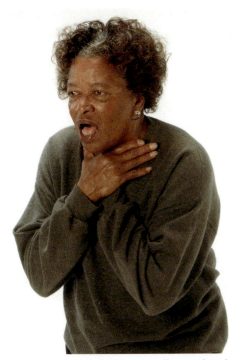

Fig. 7-6. *People who are choking usually put their hands to their throats and cough.*

If a person can no longer speak, cough, or breathe, have someone call 911. Use the call light or emergency cord to notify someone that you need help. Do not leave a choking victim to call for help.

Abdominal thrusts are a method of attempting to remove an object from the airway of someone who is choking. These thrusts work to remove the blockage upward, out of the throat. Make sure the person needs help before starting to give abdominal thrusts. Ask, "Can you cough? Can you speak? Can you breathe? Are you choking? I know what to do. Can I help you?" This is obtaining consent. If the person cannot speak or cough, or if his response is weak, start giving abdominal thrusts.

Performing abdominal thrusts for the conscious person

1. Obtain consent to treat the victim. Ask, "Can you cough? Can you speak? Can you breathe? Are you choking? I know what to do. Can I help you?"

2. Stand to one side of the person. Put one of your arms under his arm, and reach across the chest to the opposite shoulder. Have him lean forward on your arm.

3. With the other forearm and heel of your hand, give 5 sharp, separate blows to the person's back, between the shoulder blades (back blows).

4. If the object does not come out, stand behind the person and bring your arms under his arms. Wrap your arms around the person's waist.

5. Make a fist with one hand. Place the flat, thumb side of the fist against the person's abdomen, above the navel but below the breastbone.

6. Grasp the fist with your other hand. Pull both hands toward you and up, quickly and forcefully (Fig. 7-7).

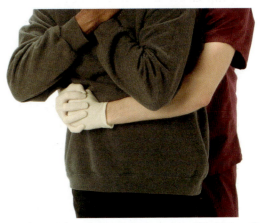

Fig. 7-7. *When giving abdominal thrusts, pull both hands toward you and up (inward and upward), quickly and forcefully.*

7. Repeat 5 times, then alternate 5 back blows and 5 abdominal thrusts until the object is pushed out or the person loses consciousness.

8. Report and document the incident properly.

Do not practice this procedure on a live person; this risks injury to the ribs or internal organs.

If the person becomes unconscious while choking, help him to the floor gently. Lie him on his back with his face up. Make sure help is on the way. He may have a completely blocked airway. He needs professional medical help immediately.

If you are a home health aide working in the home, you need to know how to clear an obstructed airway in an infant.

Clearing an obstructed airway in a conscious infant

1. Lie the infant face down on your forearm; if you are sitting, rest the arm holding the infant's torso on your lap or thigh. Support her jaw and head with your hand. Keep her head lower than the rest of her body.

2. Using the heel of your free hand, deliver up to 5 back blows. Back blows are performed by striking the infant between the shoulder blades (Fig. 7-8).

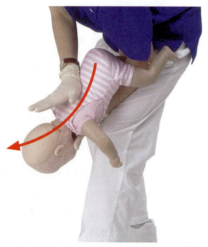

Fig. 7-8. *Keeping the infant's head below the rest of her body, deliver back blows.*

3. If the obstruction is not expelled with back blows, turn the infant onto her back while supporting the head. Deliver up to 5 chest thrusts by placing two or three fingers in the center of the breastbone (Fig. 7-9). This is the same position used for chest compression during CPR.

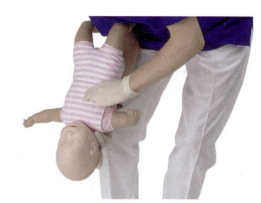

Fig. 7-9. *Turn the infant on her back to give chest thrusts if the obstruction is not expelled with back blows.*

4. Repeat alternating 5 back blows and 5 chest compressions until the object is pushed out or the infant loses consciousness.

5. Report and document the incident properly.

Call 911 immediately if the infant loses consciousness. Follow any instructions you are given.

Emergency Codes

Facilities often use codes to inform staff of emergencies while preventing panic and stress among residents and visitors. These codes are frequently coded by color. For example, "Code Red" usually means fire. "Code Blue" usually means cardiac arrest. However, the meanings of these codes vary from facility to facility. Know the codes for your facility. Do not panic when you hear codes announced. Respond calmly and professionally.

Shock

Shock occurs when organs and tissues in the body do not receive an adequate blood supply. Bleeding, heart attack, severe infection, and falling blood pressure can lead to shock. Shock can become worse when the person is frightened or in severe pain.

Shock is a dangerous, life-threatening situation. Signs of shock include pale or bluish skin, staring, increased pulse and respiration rates, low blood pressure, and extreme thirst. Always call for help if you suspect a person is experi-

Emergency Care and Disaster Preparation

encing shock. To prevent or treat shock, do the following:

Responding to shock

1. Have the person lie down on her back. If the person is bleeding from the mouth or vomiting, place her on her side (unless you suspect that the neck, back, or spinal cord is injured).

2. Control bleeding. This procedure is described later in the chapter.

3. Check pulse and respirations if possible (see Chapter 14).

4. Keep the person as calm and comfortable as possible.

5. Maintain normal body temperature. If the weather is cold, place a blanket around the person. If the weather is hot, provide shade.

6. Elevate the feet unless the person has a head or abdominal injury, breathing difficulties, or a fractured bone or back (Fig. 7-10). Elevate the head and shoulders if a head wound or breathing difficulties are present. Never elevate a body part if the person has a broken bone.

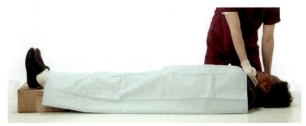

Fig. 7-10. If a person is in shock, elevate the feet unless he or she has head or abdominal injuries, breathing difficulties, or fractured bones or back.

7. Do not give the person anything to eat or drink.

8. Call for help immediately. Victims of shock should always receive medical care quickly.

9. Report and document the incident properly.

Myocardial Infarction or Heart Attack

Myocardial infarction (MI), or heart attack, occurs when the heart muscle itself does not receive enough oxygen because blood vessels are blocked. You will learn more about MI in Chapter 18. A myocardial infarction is an emergency that can result in serious heart damage or death. The following are signs and symptoms of MI:

- Sudden, severe pain in the chest, usually on the left side or in the center behind the sternum (breastbone)
- Pain or discomfort in other areas of the body, such as one or both arms, the back, neck, jaw, or stomach
- Indigestion or heartburn
- Nausea and vomiting
- **Dyspnea** or difficulty breathing
- Dizziness
- Skin color may be pale, gray, or bluish (cyanotic), indicating lack of oxygen
- Perspiration
- Cold and clammy skin
- Weak and irregular pulse rate
- Low blood pressure
- Anxiety and a sense of doom
- Denial of a heart problem

The pain of a heart attack is commonly described as a crushing, pressing, squeezing, stabbing, piercing pain, or, "like someone is sitting on my chest." The pain may go down the inside of the left arm. A person may also feel it in the neck and/or in the jaw. The pain usually does not go away.

As with men, women's most common symptom is chest pain or discomfort. But women are somewhat more likely than men to have shortness of breath, nausea/vomiting, and back, shoulder or jaw pain. Some women's symptoms seem more flu-like, and women are more likely to deny that they are having a heart attack.

You must take immediate action if a resident experiences any of these symptoms. Follow these steps:

Responding to a heart attack

1. Call for or have someone call the nurse. If working in the home, call 911 immediately.

2. Place the person in a comfortable position. Encourage him to rest, and reassure him that you will not leave him alone.

3. Loosen clothing around neck (Fig. 7-11).

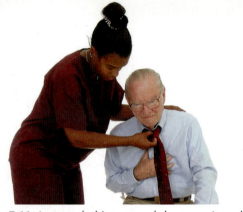

Fig. 7-11. Loosen clothing around the person's neck if you suspect he is having an MI.

4. Do not give the person liquids or food.

5. Monitor the person's breathing and pulse. If the person stops breathing or has no pulse, perform CPR only if you are trained and your facility permits you to do so.

6. Stay with the person until help arrives.

7. Report and document the incident properly.

Some states allow nursing assistants to offer heart medication, such as nitroglycerin, to a person having a heart attack. If you are allowed to do this, offer the medication only. Never place medication in someone's mouth.

Bleeding

Severe bleeding can cause death quickly and must be controlled. Call the nurse immediately, then follow these steps to control bleeding:

Controlling bleeding

1. Put on gloves. Take time to do this. If the resident is able, he can hold his bare hand over the wound until you can put on gloves.

2. Hold a thick sterile pad, a clean pad, or a clean cloth, handkerchief, or towel against the wound.

3. Press down hard directly on the bleeding wound until help arrives. Do not decrease pressure (Fig. 7-12). Put additional pads over the first pad if blood seeps through. Do not remove the first pad.

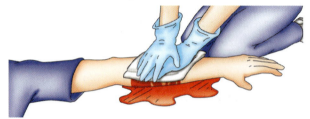

Fig. 7-12. Press down hard directly on the bleeding wound; do not decrease pressure.

4. If you can, raise the wound above the level of the heart to slow down the bleeding. If the wound is on an arm, leg, hand, or foot, and there are no broken bones, prop up the limb. Use towels, blankets, coats, or other absorbent material.

5. When bleeding is under control, secure the dressing to keep it in place. Check for symptoms of shock (pale skin, increased pulse and respiration rates, low blood pressure, and extreme thirst). Stay with the person until help arrives.

6. Remove gloves and wash hands thoroughly.

7. Report and document the incident properly.

Poisoning

As you learned in Chapter 6, facilities contain many harmful substances that should not be swallowed. Suspect poisoning when a resident suddenly collapses, vomits, and has heavy, labored breathing.

First aid kits in the home should contain syrup of ipecac, activated charcoal, and Epsom salts for the treatment of accidental poisoning (Fig. 7-13).

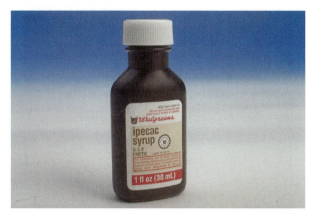

Fig. 7-13. *Ipecac syrup causes vomiting. It should only be used when directed by a doctor or by a poison control center.*

Always have the poison control center phone number available and know if syrup of ipecac is in the house.

If you suspect poisoning, take the following steps:

Responding to poisoning

1. Notify the nurse immediately.

2. Look for a container that will help you find out what the resident has taken or eaten. Using gloves, check the mouth for chemical burns and note the breath odor.

3. The nurse may have you call the local or state poison control center. Follow instructions from poison control.

4. Report and document the incident properly.

Burns

You first learned about preventing burns in Chapter 6. Care of a burn depends on its depth, size, and location. There are three types of burns: first degree, second degree, and third de-

gree burns (Fig. 7-14). First degree burns involve just the outer layer of skin. The skin becomes red, painful, and swollen, but no blisters occur. Second degree burns extend from the outer layer of skin to the next deeper layer of skin. The skin is red, painful, swollen, and blisters occur. Third degree burns involve all three layers of the skin. These burns may extend to the bone. If the nerves are destroyed, the person will not feel pain. The skin is shiny and appears hard. It may be white in color.

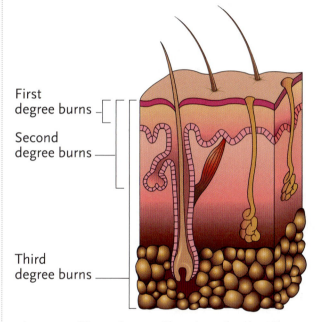

First degree burns
Second degree burns
Third degree burns

Fig. 7-14. *Different degrees of burns.*

Burns in the Home

When working in a home, you should call for emergency help in any of the following situations:

- An infant or child, or an elderly, ill, or weak person has been burned, unless burn is very minor.

- The burn occurs on the head, neck, hands, feet, face, or genitals, or burns cover more than one body part.

- The person who has been burned is having trouble breathing.

- The burn was caused by chemicals, electricity, or explosion.

Treating burns

To treat a minor burn:

1. Use cool, clean water (not ice) to decrease the skin temperature and prevent further injury (Fig. 7-15). Ice will cause further skin damage. Dampen a clean cloth and place it over the burn.

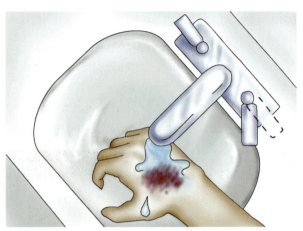

Fig. 7-15. *Use cool, clean water, not ice, on a minor burn.*

2. Once the pain has eased, you may cover the area with dry, sterile gauze.

3. Never use any kind of ointment, salve, or grease on a burn.

For more serious burns:

1. Remove the person from the source of the burn. If clothing has caught fire, smother it with a blanket or towel to put out flames. Protect yourself from the source of the burn.

2. Call for emergency help.

3. Check for breathing, pulse, and severe bleeding.

4. Do not apply water. It may cause infection.

5. Do not try to pull away any clothing from burned areas. Cover the burn with thick, dry, sterile gauze if available, or a clean cloth. Apply the gauze or cloth lightly. A dry, insulated cool pack may be used over the dress-

ing (Fig. 7-16). Again, never use any kind of ointment, salve, or grease on a burn.

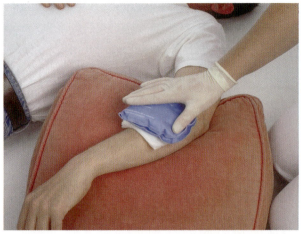

Fig. 7-16. *A dry cool pack may be used to treat a serious burn.*

6. Ask the person to lie down and elevate the affected part if this does not cause greater pain.

7. If the burn covers a larger area, wrap the person or the limb in a dry, clean sheet. Take care not to rub the skin.

8. Wait for emergency medical help.

9. Report and document the incident properly.

Chemical burns require special care. Call for help immediately. The chemical must be washed away thoroughly. A shower or a hose may be needed when the burns cover a large area.

Fainting

Fainting, also called syncope, occurs as a result of decreased blood flow to the brain, causing a loss of consciousness. Fainting may be the result of hunger, fear, pain, fatigue, standing for a long time, poor ventilation, or overheating. Signs and symptoms of fainting include dizziness, perspiration, pale skin, weak pulse, shallow respirations, and blackness in the visual field. If someone appears likely to faint, follow these steps:

Responding to fainting

1. Have the person lie down or sit down before fainting occurs.

2. If the person is in a sitting position, have her bend forward and place her head between her knees (Fig. 7-17). If the person is lying flat on her back, elevate the legs.

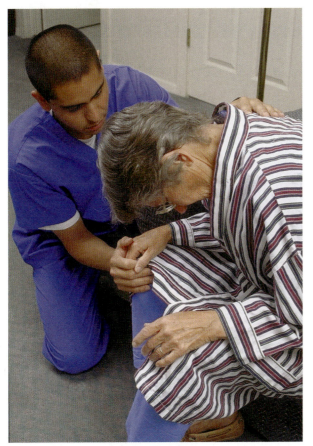

Fig. 7-17. Have the person bend forward and place her head between her knees if she is sitting.

3. Loosen any tight clothing.

4. Have the person stay in position for at least five minutes after symptoms disappear.

5. Help the person get up slowly. Continue to observe her for symptoms of fainting. Stay with the person until she feels better. If you need help but cannot leave the person, use the call light.

6. Report and document the incident properly.

If a person does faint, lower her to the floor or other flat surface. Position her on her back. Elevate her legs eight to twelve inches. Loosen any tight clothing. Check to make sure the person is breathing. She should recover quickly, but keep her lying down for several minutes. Report the incident to the nurse immediately. Fainting may be a sign of a more serious medical condition.

Nosebleed

A nosebleed can occur suddenly when the air is dry or when injury has occurred. The medical term for a nosebleed is epistaxis. If a resident has a nosebleed, notify the nurse and take the following steps:

Responding to a nosebleed

1. Elevate the head of the bed, or tell the person to remain in a sitting position, leaning forward slightly. Offer tissues or a clean cloth to catch the blood. Do not touch blood or bloody clothes, tissues, or cloths without gloves.

2. Put on gloves. Apply firm pressure over the bridge of the nose. Squeeze the bridge of the nose with your thumb and forefinger (Fig. 7-18). You can have the resident do this until you are able to put on gloves.

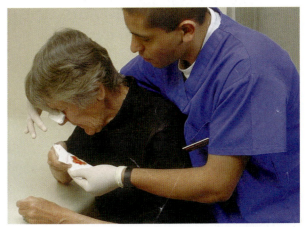

Fig. 7-18. With gloves on, squeeze the bridge of the nose with your thumb and forefinger.

3. Apply the pressure until the bleeding stops.

4. Use a cool cloth or ice wrapped in a cloth on the back of the neck, the forehead, or the upper lip to slow the flow of blood. Never apply ice directly to skin.

5. If the bleeding does not stop, tell the nurse immediately.

6. Report and document the incident properly.

Insulin Reaction and Diabetic Ketoacidosis

Insulin reaction and diabetic ketoacidosis are complications of diabetes that can be life-threatening. You will learn more about diabetes and related care in Chapter 18.

Insulin reaction (also called hypoglycemia) can result from either too much insulin or too little food. It occurs when insulin is given and the person skips a meal or does not eat all the food required. Even when a regular amount of food is eaten, physical activity may rapidly absorb the food. This causes too much insulin to be in the body. Vomiting and diarrhea may also lead to insulin shock in people with diabetes.

The first signs of insulin reaction include feeling weak or different, nervousness, dizziness, and perspiration. These signal that the resident needs food in a form that can be rapidly absorbed. A lump of sugar, a hard candy, or a glass of orange juice should be consumed right away. A diabetic should always have a quick source of sugar handy. Call the nurse if the resident has shown signs of insulin reaction. Signs and symptoms of insulin reaction include the following:

*   Hunger
*   Weakness
*   Rapid pulse
*   Headache
*   Low blood pressure
*   Perspiration
*   Cold, clammy skin
*   Confusion
*   Trembling
*   Nervousness
*   Blurred vision
*   Numbness of the lips and tongue
*   Unconsciousness

Diabetic ketoacidosis (DKA) (also called hyperglycemia or diabetic coma) is caused by having too little insulin. It can result from undiagnosed diabetes, going without insulin or not taking enough, eating too much food, not getting enough exercise, or physical or emotional stress. The signs of the onset of diabetic ketoacidosis include increased thirst or urination, abdominal pain, deep or labored breathing, and breath that smells sweet or fruity. Other signs and symptoms include the following:

*   Hunger
*   Weakness
*   Rapid, weak pulse
*   Headache
*   Low blood pressure
*   Dry skin
*   Flushed cheeks
*   Drowsiness
*   Slow, deep, and difficult breathing
*   Nausea and vomiting
*   Abdominal pain
*   Sweet, fruity breath odor
*   Air hunger, or resident gasping for air and being unable to catch his breath
*   Unconsciousness

Inform the nurse immediately if you think a resident is experiencing diabetic ketoacidosis.

Seizures

Seizures are involuntary, often violent, contractions of muscles. They can involve a small area or the entire body. Seizures are caused by an abnormality in the brain. They can occur in young children who have a high fever. Older children and adults who have a serious illness, fever, head injury, or a seizure disorder such as **epilepsy** may also have seizures.

The main goal of a caregiver during a seizure is to make sure the resident is safe. During a seizure, a person may shake severely and thrust arms and legs uncontrollably. He may clench his jaw, drool, and be unable to swallow. The following emergency measures should be taken if a resident has a seizure:

Responding to seizures

1. Lower the person to the floor. Lay him on his side.

2. Have someone call the nurse immediately or use the call light. Do not leave a person during a seizure unless you must do so to get medical help.

3. Move furniture away to prevent injury. If a pillow is nearby, place it under his or her head.

4. Do not try to restrain the person.

5. Do not force anything between the person's teeth. Do not place your hands in the person's mouth for any reason. You could be bitten.

6. Do not give liquids or food.

7. When the seizure is over, check breathing.

8. Report and document the incident properly, including how long the seizure lasted.

CVA or Stroke

You first learned about stroke, or cerebrovascular accident (CVA), in Chapter 4. A quick response to a suspected stroke is critical. Tests and treatment need to be given within a short time of the stroke's onset; early treatment may be able to reduce the severity of the stroke.

A **transient ischemic attack**, or TIA, is a warning sign of a CVA. TIA is also known as a "mini stroke." It is the result of a temporary lack of oxygen in the brain. Symptoms may last up to 24 hours and include difficulty speaking, weakness on one side of the body, temporary loss of vision, and numbness or tingling. These symptoms should not be ignored. Report them to the nurse immediately.

Signs that a CVA is occurring include the following:

- Facial numbness or weakness, especially on one side
- Arm numbness or weakness, especially on one side
- Slurred speech or difficulty speaking
- Use of inappropriate words
- Inability to understand spoken or written words
- Redness in the face
- Noisy breathing
- Dizziness
- Blurred vision
- Ringing in the ears
- Headache
- Nausea/vomiting
- Seizures
- Loss of bowel and bladder control
- Paralysis on one side of the body
- Elevated blood pressure
- Slow pulse rate
- Loss of consciousness

See Chapter 18 for more information on CVA and related care.

Falls

You learned about the risk of falls and ways to prevent falls in Chapter 6. Falls can be minor or severe. Report all falls to the nurse immediately. Complete an incident report. In the case of a severe fall, the nurse may ask you to call emergency medical services. Take the following steps to help a resident who is falling:

- Widen your stance. Bring the resident's body close to you to break the fall. Bend your knees. Support the resident as you lower her to the floor.

- Do not try to reverse or stop a fall. You or the resident can suffer worse injuries if you do.

- Call for help. Do not attempt to get the resident up or move the resident after the fall. Follow your facility's policies and procedures.

Vomiting

Vomiting, or **emesis**, is the act of ejecting stomach contents through the mouth. It can be a sign of a serious illness or injury. Because you may not know when a resident is going to vomit, you may not have time to explain what you will do and assemble supplies ahead of time. Talk to the resident soothingly as you help him clean up. Tell him what you are doing to help him. If a resident has vomited, notify the nurse and take the following steps:

Responding to vomiting

1. Put on gloves.

2. Place an emesis basin under the chin. Remove it when vomiting has stopped.

3. Remove soiled linens or clothes and set aside. Replace with fresh linens or clothes.

4. If resident's intake and output (I&O) is being monitored (Chapter 15), measure and note amount of vomitus.

5. Flush vomit down the toilet unless vomit is red, has blood in it, or looks like coffee

grounds. If these symptoms are observed, show this to the nurse before discarding the vomit. After disposing of vomit, wash and store basin.

6. Remove and discard gloves.

7. Wash your hands.

8. Put on fresh gloves.

9. Provide comfort to resident. Wipe face and mouth (Fig. 7-19). Position comfortably, and offer a drink of water. Provide oral care (see Chapter 13). It helps get rid of the taste of vomit in the mouth.

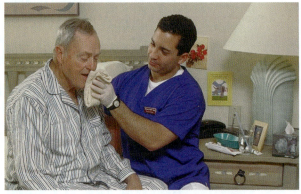

Fig. 7-19. Be calm and comforting when helping a client who has vomited.

10. Put soiled linen in proper containers.

11. Remove and discard gloves.

12. Wash your hands again.

13. Document time, amount, color, odor, and consistency of vomitus. Look for blood in vomitus, blood-tinged vomitus, or vomitus that looks like wet coffee grounds.

3. Describe disaster guidelines

Disasters can include fire, flood, earthquake, hurricane, tornado, or severe weather. Acts of terrorism may also be considered disasters. The disasters you may experience will depend on where you live. Nursing assistants need to be competent and professional when a disaster occurs. Facilities have disaster plans and you will be trained on these plans. Annual in-services and disaster drills are often held at facilities. Take advantage of these sessions when offered, and pay close attention to instructions.

During natural disasters, a nurse or the administrator will give directions. Listen carefully to all directions, and follow instructions. Facilities may rely on local or state management groups and the American Red Cross to assume overall responsibility for the ill and disabled.

The following guidelines apply in any disaster situation:

* Remain calm.
* Know the locations of all exits and stairways.
* Know where the fire alarms and extinguishers are located.
* Know the appropriate action to take in any situation.

In addition, you will be required to apply specific guidelines for the area in which you work. For example, an NA working where hurricanes are prevalent, such as Florida, needs to know the guidelines for hurricane preparedness as well as for storms and fires. The following general guidelines are separated by the type of disaster and can be applied to any particular geographical area. Keep the radio or television tuned to a local station to get the latest information.

Tornadoes

In the case of tornadoes, follow these guidelines:

* Seek shelter inside, ideally in a steel-framed or concrete building.
* Stay away from windows.
* Stand in the hallway or in a basement, or take cover under heavy furniture.
* Do not stay in a mobile home or trailer.
* Lie as flat as possible.

Lightning

If outdoors, follow these guidelines:

* Avoid the largest objects, such as trees, and avoid open spaces.
* Stay out of the water.
* Seek shelter in buildings.
* Stay away from metal fences, doors, or other objects.
* Avoid holding metal objects in your hands, such as golf clubs.
* Stay in automobiles.
* It is safe to perform CPR on lightning victims; they carry no electricity.

If indoors, stay inside and away from open doors and windows. Avoid the use of electrical equipment such as hair dryers and televisions, and do not use the phone.

Floods

In the case of floods, follow these guidelines:

* Fill the bathtub with fresh water.
* Board up windows.
* Evacuate if advised to do so.
* Check the fuel level in automobiles.
* Have a portable battery-operated radio, flashlight, and cooking equipment available.
* Do not drink water or eat food that has been contaminated with flood water.
* Do not handle electrical equipment.
* Do not turn off gas yourself, but ask the gas company to do so.

Blackouts

In the case of blackouts, follow these guidelines:

* Get a flashlight. Take prompt action to keep calm and provide light.

- Use a backup pack for electrical medical equipment such as an IV pump. Backup packs do not last more than 24 hours, so contact emergency personnel when instructed.

Hurricanes

In the case of hurricanes, follow these guidelines:

- Know what category the hurricane is and track the expected path.

- Know which residents or clients must go to shelters, hospitals, or other facilities, and which need assistance. Be aware of people with special needs. High-risk people include the elderly and those unable to evacuate on their own. High-risk areas include mobile homes or trailers.

- Call your employer for instructions.

- Fill the bathtub with fresh water.

- Board up windows.

- Evacuate if advised to do so.

- Check the fuel level in automobiles.

- Have a portable battery-operated radio, flash-light, and cooking equipment available.

In addition to the above, when working in the home, follow these guidelines for disasters:

- Listen to radio or television bulletins to keep informed. A battery-powered radio will help you to stay informed if power goes out.

- If a disaster is forecast (for example, a tornado or hurricane), be ready. Wear appropriate clothing and shoes. Have family members dressed and ready in case evacuation is necessary.

- Stay in contact with your supervisor or others if possible. Let someone know where you are, what conditions are, and where you will go if you must evacuate.

- Locate disaster supplies. Ideally, a disaster supply kit should meet your needs for at least three days. It should be assembled before disaster strikes and should include:

  - A three-day supply of water (one gallon per person per day) and food that will not spoil

  - One change of clothing and footwear per person, and one blanket or sleeping bag per person

  - A first aid kit that includes your family's prescription medications

  - Emergency tools, including a battery-powered radio, flashlight, and plenty of extra batteries

  - An extra set of car keys and a credit card, cash, or traveler's checks

  - Sanitation supplies

  - Special items for infant, elderly, or disabled family members

  - An extra pair of glasses

  - Important family documents in a waterproof container

Chapter Review

1. List two steps to follow when coming upon an emergency situation.

2. What information should a nursing assistant be prepared to give when calling emergency services?

3. Why should a nursing assistant not perform CPR if she is not trained to do so?

4. What is the correct number of chest compressions to rescue breaths when giving CPR?

5. How are abdominal thrusts used to help someone who is choking?

6. If the person becomes unconscious while choking, what should the nursing assistant do?

7. List the signs of shock.

8. List seven signs that a person is having a heart attack.

9. What can be done to a wound to slow the bleeding?

10. Why should ice not be applied to burns?

11. If a person feels like he is going to faint, in what position should he be placed?

12. Why should a nursing assistant put on gloves if a resident has a nosebleed?

13. What causes insulin reaction? What causes diabetic ketoacidosis?

14. Why should a nursing assistant not force anything into the mouth of a person who is having a seizure?

15. List symptoms of a transient ischemic attack (TIA).

16. List signs that a CVA/stroke is occurring.

17. What should a nursing assistant do if a resident starts to fall?

18. What are three things that a nursing assistant should observe for in a resident's vomit?

19. What are four guidelines that apply in any disaster situation?

8

Human Needs and Human Development

1. Identify basic human needs

People have different genes, physical appearances, cultural backgrounds, ages, and social or financial positions. But all human beings have the same basic physical needs:

- Food and water
- Protection and shelter
- Activity
- Sleep and rest
- Safety
- Comfort, especially freedom from pain

You will be helping residents meet these basic physical needs. Activities of daily living (ADLs), such as eating, toileting, bathing, and grooming, are the ways we meet our most basic physical needs. By assisting with ADLs or helping residents learn to perform them independently, you help residents meet their basic needs.

People also have **psychosocial** needs, which involve social interaction, emotions, intellect, and spirituality. Psychosocial needs are not as easy to define as physical needs. However, all human beings have the following psychosocial needs:

- Love and affection
- Acceptance by others
- Security

- Self-reliance and independence in daily living
- Contact with other people (Fig. 8-1)
- Success and self-esteem

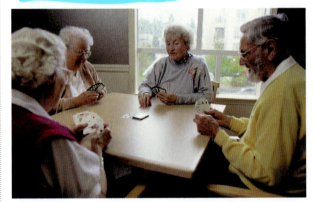

Fig. 8-1. *Interaction with other people is a basic psychosocial need. Encourage your residents to be with friends or relatives. Social contact is important.*

Health and well-being affect how well psychosocial needs are met. Stress and frustration occur when basic needs are not met. This can lead to fear, anxiety, anger, aggression, withdrawal, indifference, and depression. Stress can also cause physical problems that may eventually lead to illness.

Abraham Maslow, a researcher of human behavior, wrote about human physical and psychosocial needs. He arranged these needs into an order of importance. He thought that physical needs must be met before psychosocial needs can be met. His theory is called "Maslow's Hierarchy of Needs" (Fig. 8-2).

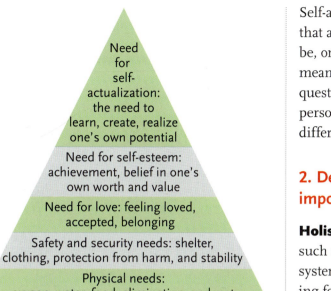

Fig. 8-2. Maslow's Hierarchy of Needs.

After meeting physical needs, safety and security needs must be met. Feeling safe means not feeling afraid and unstable. Residents need to feel safe in facilities. Many things can cause a person to feel unsafe. An illness or disability can be frightening and make a person feel fearful and insecure. Losing some independence and needing help from caregivers, such as NAs, may cause some uncertainty or discomfort. Residents need to feel safe with you and all other care team members; they need to know that they and their personal possessions will be protected.

After physical and safety needs are met, the need for love and belonging is important. This level involves feeling accepted, needed, and cared for. Regardless of their condition, residents need to know that their contributions are meaningful.

The need for self-esteem is the next level. This need involves respecting and valuing oneself, which comes from within, as well as from other people. Achievements that make a person feel valued are important. For residents, being able to do a task they were not able to do previously may satisfy this need. Hearing praise from NAs about this new achievement may also help meet this need.

Self-actualization is the highest level. It means that a person tries to be the best person he can be, or tries to reach his full potential. This may mean different things for each person. The quest to reach this need continues throughout a person's life and may change as a person enters different stages of life.

2. Define "holistic care" and explain its importance in health care

Holistic means considering a whole system, such as a whole person, rather than dividing the system up into parts. Holistic care means caring for the whole person—the mind as well as the body (Fig. 8-3). A simple example of holistic care is taking time to talk with your residents while helping them bathe. You are meeting the physical need with the bath and meeting the psychosocial need for interaction with others at the same time.

Another way of practicing holistic care is considering psychosocial factors in illness, as well as physical factors. For example, Mr. Hartman looks thin and tired. The cause might be depression rather than an infection. You do not need to determine the cause of his condition. However, by talking with him you might learn something that would help the rest of the care team. For example, you might learn that last year at this time his wife died, and he is still coping with that loss. You can and should share this information with the care team and document it.

3. Explain why independence and self-care are important

Any big change in lifestyle, such as moving into a long-term care facility, requires a huge emotional adjustment. Residents may be experiencing fear, loss, and uncertainty, along with a decline in health and independence. These feelings may cause them to behave differently than they have before. Be aware that dramatic

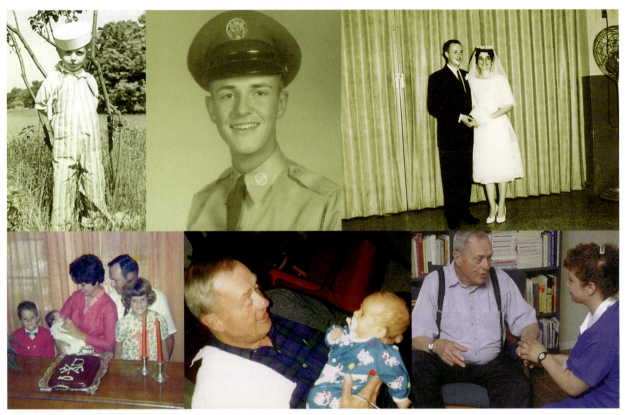

Fig. 8-3. *Remember that residents are people, not just lists of illnesses and disabilities. They have many needs, like you. Many have had rich and wonderful lives. Take time to know and care for your residents as whole people.*

changes in a resident's life may cause anger, hostility, or depression. It is important to remain supportive and encouraging. Be patient and empathic. Having empathy means being able to enter into the feelings of others.

To best understand feelings residents may be having, you must first understand how difficult it is to lose one's independence. Somebody else must now do what residents did for themselves all of their lives. Try to imagine what that would be like. Think about having to call someone to help every time you need to go to the bathroom. The loss of independence is also difficult for friends and family members. For example, a resident may have been the main provider for his or her family. A resident may have been the person who did all of the cooking for the family. Other losses residents may be experiencing include the following:

• Loss of spouse, family members, or friends due to death

• Loss of workplace and its relationships due to retirement

• Loss of ability to go to favorite places

• Loss of ability to attend services and meetings at their faith communities

• Loss of home and personal possessions (Fig. 8-4)

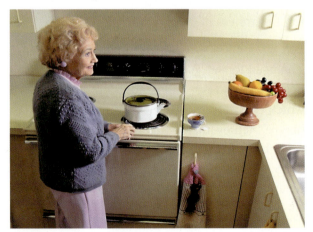

Fig. 8-4. *Understand and be sympathetic to the fact that many residents had to leave familiar places.*

- Loss of health and the ability to care for themselves

- Loss of ability to move freely

- Loss of pets

Independence often means not having to rely on others for money, daily routine care, or participation in social activities. Activities of daily living (ADLs) are the personal care tasks you do every day to care for yourself. People may take these activities for granted until they can no longer do them for themselves. ADLs include bathing or showering, dressing, caring for teeth and hair, toileting, eating and drinking, and moving from place to place.

A loss of independence can cause the following problems:

- Poor self-image

- Anger toward caregivers, others, and self

- Feelings of helplessness, sadness, and hopelessness

- Feelings of being useless

- Increased dependence

- Depression

To prevent these feelings, encourage residents to do as much as possible for themselves. Even if it seems easier for you to do things for residents, allow them to do tasks independently. Encourage self-care, regardless of how long it takes or how poorly they are able to do it. Be patient (Fig. 8-5).

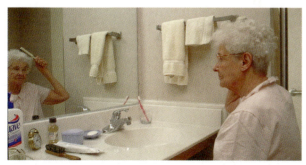

Fig. 8-5. *Even if personal care tasks take a long time, encourage residents to do what they can for themselves.*

Allowing residents to make choices is another way to promote independence. For example, residents can choose where to sit while they eat. They can choose what they eat and in what order. Respect a resident's right to make choices.

Residents' Rights

Dignity and Independence

Residents are adults; do not treat them like children. Encourage them to do self-care without rushing them. Remember that they have the right to refuse care and to make their own choices. Maintaining dignity and independence is your residents' legal right. It is also the proper and ethical way for you to work.

4. Explain ways to accommodate sexual needs

In addition to the needs discussed earlier, people also have sexual needs. These needs continue throughout their lives (Fig. 8-6). The ability to engage in sexual activity, such as intercourse and masturbation, continues unless a disease or injury occurs. **Masturbation** means to touch or rub sexual organs in order to give oneself or another person sexual pleasure.

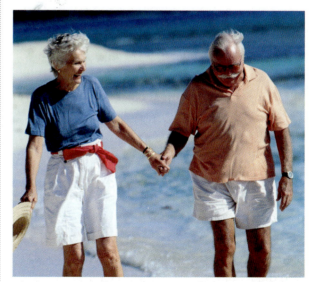

Fig. 8-6. *Human beings continue to have sexual needs throughout their lives.*

To meet and respect residents' sexual needs, you can do the following:

- Always knock or announce yourself before entering residents' rooms. Listen and wait for a response before entering.

- If you encounter a sexual situation, provide privacy and leave. However, if you see sexual abuse occurring, take the resident to a safe place, and notify the nurse immediately.

- Be open and nonjudgmental about residents' sexual attitudes. Do not judge residents' sexual orientation or any sexual behavior you see.

- Honor "Do Not Disturb" signs.

Residents have the right to choose how they express their sexuality. In all age groups, there is a variety of sexual behavior. This is true of your residents also. An attitude that any expression of sexuality by the elderly is "disgusting" or "cute" is inappropriate. It deprives residents of their right to dignity and respect.

Illness and disability can affect sexual desires, needs, and abilities. Residents may be sensitive about this. Sexual desire may not be lessened by a disability, although ability to meet sexual needs may be limited. Many people confined to wheelchairs can have sexual and intimate relationships, though adjustments may have to be made. Do not assume you know what impact a physical disability has had on sexuality.

Sexual needs may also be affected by residents' living environments. A lack of privacy and no available partner are often reasons for a lack of sexual expression in facilities. Be sensitive to privacy needs.

Sexual Identity

Terms defining sexual identity include the following:

Gay: 1. A person who has a desire for persons of the same sex. 2. A man whose sexual orientation is to men.

Heterosexual: A person who has a desire for persons of the opposite sex. This is also known as "straight."

Homosexual: A person who has a desire for persons of the same sex. The terms "gay" and "lesbian" are usually preferable.

Lesbian: A woman whose sexual orientation is to women.

Bisexual: A person who desires persons of both sexes.

Transsexual: 1. One who wishes to be accepted by society as a member of the opposite sex. 2. One who has undergone a sex change.

Residents' Rights

Sexual Abuse

Residents must be protected from unwanted sexual advances. If you see sexual abuse happening, remove the resident from the situation. Take him or her to a safe place. Report to the nurse immediately after making sure the resident is safe and secure.

5. Identify ways to help residents meet their spiritual needs

Residents have spiritual needs, and you can assist with these needs, too. **Spiritual** means of, or relating to, the spirit or soul. Helping residents meet their spiritual needs can help them cope with illness or disability. Remember that spirituality is a sensitive area. Do not offend residents by making judgments or imposing your beliefs.

Residents may have strong beliefs in God, or very little or no belief in God or a higher power. Residents may consider themselves spiritual, but may not believe in God or a higher power. The important thing for nursing assistants to remember is to respect all residents' beliefs, whatever they are. Do not make judgments about residents' spiritual beliefs or try to push your beliefs on residents. Following are some ways you can help residents meet their spiritual needs:

- Learn about residents' religions or beliefs (Fig. 8-7). Listen carefully to what residents say.

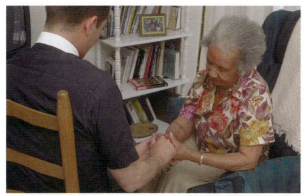

Fig. 8-7. *Be open to your residents' spiritual needs. Be welcoming when they receive visits from a spiritual leader.*

- Assist with practices such as dietary restrictions. Never make judgments about them. Also, respect your resident's decision to refrain from food-related rituals.

- If residents are religious, encourage participation in religious services.

- Respect all religious items.

- Report to the nurse (or social worker) if your resident expresses the desire to see clergy.

- Get to know the priest, rabbi, or minister who visits or calls your resident.

- Allow privacy for clergy visits.

- If asked, read religious materials aloud.

- If a resident asks you, help find spiritual resources available in the area. The yellow pages usually list churches, synagogues, and other houses of worship. You can also refer this request to the nurse or social worker.

You should never do any of the following:

- Try to change someone's religion

- Tell residents their belief or religion is wrong

- Express judgments about a religious group

- Insist residents join religious activities

- Interfere with religious practices

6. Identify ways to accommodate cultural and religious differences

You first learned about culture and cultural diversity in Chapter 4. Cultural diversity has to do with the wide variety of people living throughout the world. You will take care of residents with different backgrounds and traditions than your own. It is important to respect and value each person as an individual. Respond to differences and new experiences with acceptance, not prejudice. Sometimes it is easier to accept different practices or beliefs if you understand a little about them.

There are so many different cultures that they cannot all be listed here. One might talk about American culture being different from Japanese culture. But within American culture there are thousands of different groups with their own cultures: Japanese-Americans, African-Americans, and Native Americans, to name just a few. Even people from a particular region, state, or city can be said to have a different culture (Fig. 8-8). The culture of the South is not the same as the culture of New York City.

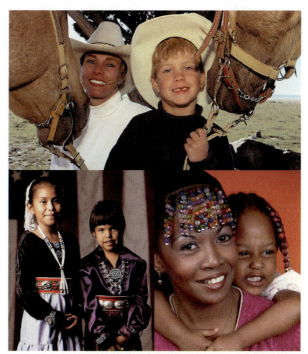

Fig. 8-8. *There are many different cultures in the United States.*

Cultural background affects how friendly people are to strangers. It can affect how close they want you to stand to them when talking. It can affect how they feel about you performing care for them or discussing their health with them. For example, a care team member asks a resident when he last had a bowel movement. One resident may freely answer this, while another may be embarrassed to have this discussion. A resident may be fine with you undressing him to help him bathe, while another may very uncomfortable with this. These reactions may also just be a part of a person's personality. Be sensitive to your residents' backgrounds. You may have to adjust your behavior around some residents. Regardless of their background, you must treat all residents with respect and professionalism. Expect them to treat you respectfully as well.

A resident's first language may be different from yours. If he or she speaks a different language, an interpreter may be necessary. Take time to learn a few common phrases in a resident's native language. Picture cards and flash cards can assist with communication.

Religious differences also influence the way people behave. Religion can be very important in people's lives, particularly when they are ill or dying. Some people belong to a religious group, but do not practice everything that religion teaches. Some people consider themselves spiritual but not religious. Others do not believe in any religion or god and do not consider themselves spiritual. You must respect the religious beliefs and practices of your residents, even if they are different from your own. Understanding a little bit about common religious groups in America may be useful. Common types of religions, listed alphabetically, follow:

Buddhism: Buddhism started in Asia but has many followers in other parts of the world. Buddhism is based on the teachings of Siddhartha Gautama, called "Buddha." Buddhists believe that life is filled with suffering that is caused by desire, and that suffering ends when desire ends. Buddhism emphasizes meditation. Proper conduct and wisdom release a person from desire, suffering, and a repeating sequence of births and deaths (reincarnation). Nirvana is the highest spiritual plane a person can reach. It is the state of peace and freedom from worry and pain. The Dalai Lama is considered to be the highest spiritual leader.

Christianity: Christians believe Jesus Christ was the son of God and that he died so their sins would be forgiven. Christians may be Catholic or Protestant. There are many subgroups or denominations (such as Baptists, Episcopalians, Evangelicals, Lutherans, Methodists, Mormons, and Presbyterians). Christians may go to church on Saturdays or Sundays. They may read the Bible, including the Old and New Testaments, take communion as a symbol of Christ's sacrifice, and be baptized. Some Christians may try to share their beliefs and convert others to their faith. Religious leaders may be called priests, ministers, pastors, or deacons.

Hinduism: Hinduism is the dominant faith of India; it is also practiced elsewhere. Hindus follow the teachings of ancient scriptures like the Vedas and Upanishads, as well as other major scriptures. Hindu beliefs vary widely; there may be a belief in only one God or in multiple gods. Worship can occur at a temple or at home. Hindus believe in **reincarnation**, which is a belief that some part of a living being survives death to be reborn in a new body. Hindus also believe in **karma**, which is the belief that all past and present deeds affect one's future and future lives. Hindus advocate respect for all life, and some Hindus are vegetarians. Vegetarians do not eat any meat. Hindus who do eat meat almost always refrain from eating beef.

Islam: Muslims, or followers of Mohammed, believe that Allah (God) wants people to follow the teachings of the prophet Mohammed as recorded in the Koran. Many Muslims pray five times a day facing Mecca, the holy city for their religion. Muslims worship at mosques and generally do not drink alcohol or eat pork. There are other dietary restrictions, too. There is a variety of Islamic religious leaders.

Judaism: Judaism is divided into Reform, Conservative, and Orthodox movements. Jews believe that God gave them laws through Moses and in the Bible, and that these laws should order their lives. Jewish services are held on Friday evenings and sometimes on Saturdays, in synagogues or temples. Some Jewish men wear a **yarmulke**, or small skullcap, as a sign of their faith. Some Jews follow special dietary restrictions. Jewish people may not do certain things, such as work or drive, on the Sabbath. This lasts from Friday sundown to Saturday sundown. Religious leaders are called **rabbis**.

Confucianism, which is practiced in China and Japan, is another major world religion. Native Americans follow many spiritual traditions.

As mentioned earlier, people have varying beliefs in religion, spirituality, and God. Some people may not believe in God or a higher power and identify themselves as "agnostic." **Agnostics** claim that they do not know or cannot know if God exists. They do not deny that God might exist, but they feel there is no true knowledge of God's existence. **Atheists** are people who claim that there is no God. This is different from what agnostics believe. Atheists actively deny the existence of God. For many atheists, this belief is as strongly held as any religious belief.

In addition to showing respect for different cultural and religious traditions, be aware of and respect specific practices that affect your work. Many religious beliefs include **dietary restrictions**. These are rules about what and when followers can eat. Some examples are listed below.

- Many Buddhists are vegetarians, though some include fish in their diet.

- Some Catholics do not eat meat on Fridays during Lent.

- Many Jewish people eat kosher foods, do not eat pork, and do not eat lobster, shrimp, and clams (shellfish). Kosher food is food prepared in accordance with Jewish dietary laws. Kosher and non-kosher foods cannot come into contact with the same plates. Jews may not eat meat products at the same meal with dairy products.

- Mormons may not drink alcohol, coffee or tea. They may not use tobacco in any form.

- Many Muslims do not eat pork or shellfish. Certain birds may need to be avoided, too. They may not drink alcohol. Muslims may have regular periods of fasting. **Fasting** means not eating food or eating very little food.

- Some people are vegetarians and do not eat any meat for religious, moral, or health reasons.

- Some people are vegans. **Vegans** do not eat any animals or animal products, such as eggs or dairy products. Vegans may also not use or wear any animal products, including wool and leather.

7. Describe the need for activity

Activity is an essential part of a person's life; it improves and maintains physical and mental health. Meaningful activities help promote independence, memory, self-esteem, and quality of life. In addition, physical activity can help manage illnesses, such as diabetes, high blood pressure, or high cholesterol. Regular physical activity can also help by:

- Lessening the risk of heart disease, colon cancer, diabetes, and obesity

- Relieving symptoms of depression

- Improving mood and concentration

- Improving body function

- Lowering the risk of falls

- Improving sleep quality

- Improving ability to cope with stress

- Increasing energy

- Increasing appetite and promoting better eating habits

Just as activity aids physical and mental health, inactivity and immobility can result in physical and mental problems, such as:

- Loss of self-esteem

- Depression

- Boredom

- Pneumonia

- Urinary tract infection

- Constipation

- Blood clots

- Dulling of the senses

Most facilities have an activity department. The activities are designed to help residents socialize and keep them physically and mentally active. Daily schedules are normally posted with activities for that particular day. Activities include exercise, arts and crafts, board games, newspapers, magazines, books, TV and radio, pet therapy, gardening, and group religious events. When activities are scheduled, help residents with grooming beforehand, as needed and requested. Assist with any personal care that the resident requires. Help residents with walking and wheelchairs, as necessary.

8. Discuss family roles and their significance in health care

Families are the most important unit within our social system (Fig. 8-9). Families play a huge role in many people's lives. Some examples of family types are listed below:

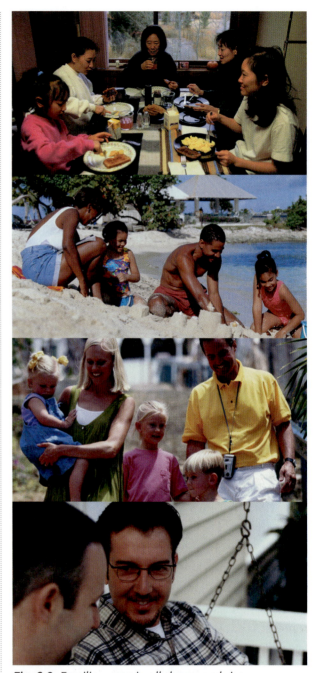

Fig. 8-9. *Families come in all shapes and sizes.*

- Single-parent families include one parent with a child or children.

- Nuclear families include two parents with a child or children.

- Blended families include widowed or divorced parents who have remarried. There may be children from previous marriages as well as from this marriage.

- Multigenerational families include parents, children, and grandparents.

- Extended families may include aunts, uncles, cousins, or even friends.

- Families may also be made up of unmarried couples of the same sex or opposite sexes, with or without children.

Today a family is defined more by supporting each other than by the particular people involved. Your residents' families may not look like the kind of family you are used to. Residents with no living relatives may have friends or neighbors who act as a family. Whatever kinds of families your residents have, recognize the important part they can play. Family members help in many ways:

- Helping residents make care decisions

- Communicating with the care team

- Giving support and encouragement

- Connecting the resident to the outside world

- Offering assurance to dying residents that family memories and traditions will be valued and carried on

Illness or disability requires residents and families to make adjustments. Making these adjustments may be difficult (Fig. 8-10). It depends on the family's emotional, spiritual, and financial resources. Some personal adjustments include the following:

- Accepting the illness or disability and its long-term consequences or results

- Finding money needed to pay the expenses of hospitalization, or long-term or home care

- Dealing with paperwork involved in insurance, Medicaid, or Medicare benefits

- Taking care of tasks the resident can no longer handle

- Understanding medical information and making difficult care decisions

- Caring for their children while caring for an elderly loved one (called the "sandwich generation"—being "sandwiched" between two generations)

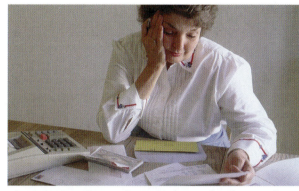

Fig. 8-10. Family members may have a hard time adjusting to the additional responsibilities when a loved one becomes ill or disabled.

Be sensitive to the big adjustments your residents and their families may be making. Help them by doing your job well. Be respectful and nice to friends and family members, and allow privacy for visits. After any visitor leaves, observe the effect the visit had on the resident. Report any noticeable effects to the nurse. Some residents have good relationships with their families; others do not. If you notice any abusive behavior from a visitor towards a resident, report it immediately to the charge nurse.

9. List ways to respond to emotional needs of residents and their families

Residents or family members may come to you with problems or needs. Changes in residents' health status can cause fear, uncertainty, stress, and anger. Your response will depend on many factors. These include how comfortable you feel with emotions in general, how well you know the person, and what the need or problem is. Try to empathize, or understand how the person feels. The following are good ways to respond to this situation:

Listen. Often just talking about a problem or concern can make it easier to handle. Sitting quietly and letting someone talk or cry may be the best help you can give (Fig. 8-11). Families often seek out nursing assistants because they are closest to the residents. This is an important responsibility. Show families that you have time for them, too.

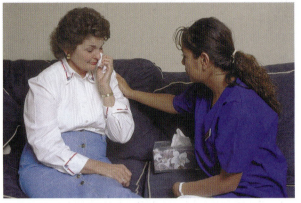

Fig. 8-11. *Sometimes listening to someone is the best way to provide emotional support.*

Offer support and encouragement. Saying things like, "You have really been under a lot of stress, haven't you?" or, "I can imagine that really is scary," can provide a lot of comfort. Avoid using clichés like, "It'll all work out." Things may not all work out. It is more comforting if you admit how hard the situation is. Do not simply dismiss feelings with a cliché.

Refer the problem to a nurse or social worker. When you feel that you cannot help the resident, get someone else on the care team to handle the situation. Say something like, "Mrs. Pfeiffer, I think my supervisor would be better at getting you the help you need."

10. Describe the stages of human growth and development and identify common disorders for each group

Throughout their lives, people change physically and psychologically. Physical changes occur in the body. Psychological changes occur in the mind and also in the person's behavior. These changes are called human growth and development.

Everyone will go through the same stages of development during their lives. However, no two people will follow the exact same pattern or rate of development. Each resident must be treated as an individual and a whole person who is growing and developing. He or she should not be treated as someone who is merely ill or disabled.

Infancy, Birth to 12 Months

Infants grow and develop very quickly. In one year a baby moves from total dependence to the relative independence of moving around, communicating basic needs, and feeding himself. Physical development in infancy moves from the head down. For example, infants gain control over the muscles of the neck before the muscles in their shoulders. Control over muscles in the trunk area, such as the shoulders, develops before control of arms and legs (Fig. 8-12). This head-to-toe sequence should be respected when caring for infants. For example, newborns must be supported at the shoulders, head, and neck. Babies who cannot sit or crawl should not be encouraged to stand or walk.

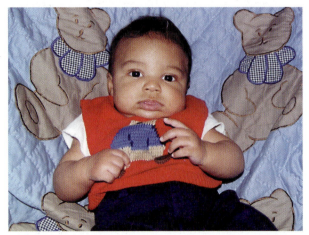

Fig. 8-12. *An infant's physical development moves from the head down.*

Common Disorders:
Infancy

C/D   Babies who are born before 37 weeks gestation (more than three weeks before the due date) are considered **premature**. These babies may weigh from one to six pounds, depending on how early they are born. Often, premature babies will remain in the hospital for some time after birth. At home, premature babies may need special care. This includes medication, heart monitoring, and frequent feedings to ensure weight gain.

C/D Babies born at full term but weighing less than five pounds are called low-birth-weight babies. Low-birth-weight babies can have many of the same problems premature babies have. They are cared for in much the same way as premature babies.

C/D The term "birth defects" is very general. It includes many different conditions that affect an infant from birth. Some birth defects are inherited from parents. Injury or disease during pregnancy causes others. Some of the conditions you may see when caring for infants in the home include cerebral palsy, Down syndrome, and cystic fibrosis.

C/D Viral or bacterial infections can cause fever, runny nose, coughing, rash, vomiting, diarrhea, or secondary infections of the sinuses or ears. Bacterial infections can be treated with antibiotics. Viral infections are treated with extra rest and fluids.

C/D **Sudden infant death syndrome (SIDS)** or crib death, is a condition in which babies stop breathing and die for no known reason while asleep. Doctors do not know how to prevent SIDS. However, studies have shown that putting the baby to sleep on its back can reduce the chances of SIDS. Because SIDS is more common among premature or low-birth-weight babies, these infants often wear apnea monitors to alert parents if breathing stops. Another factor that may contribute to SIDS is second-hand smoke. Parents and caregivers should never smoke around infants or children.

Childhood

The Toddler Period, Ages 1 to 3

During the toddler years, children gain independence. One part of this independence is new control over their bodies. Toddlers learn to speak, gain coordination of their limbs, and gain control over their bladders and bowels (Fig. 8-13). Toddlers assert their new independence by exploring. Poisons and other hazards, such as sharp objects, must be locked away. Psychologically, toddlers learn that they are individuals, separate from their parents. Children of this age may try to control their parents. They may try to get what they want by throwing tantrums, whining, or refusing to cooperate. This is a key time for parents to set rules and standards.

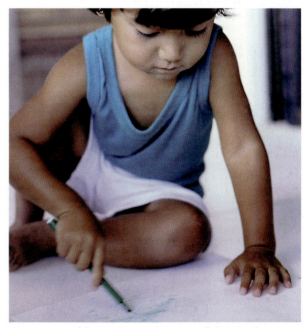

Fig. 8-13. *Toddlers gain coordination of their limbs.*

The Preschool Years, Ages 3 to 6

Children in their preschool years develop new skills. These will help them to become more independent and have social relationships (Fig. 8-14). They learn new words and develop language skills. They learn to play in groups. They become more physically coordinated and learn to care for themselves. Preschoolers also develop ways of relating to family members. They begin to learn right from wrong.

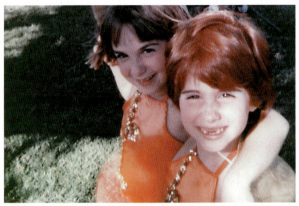

Fig. 8-14. *Children in their preschool years develop social relationships.*

School-Age Children, Ages 6 to 12

From ages 6 to about 12 years, children's development is centered on **cognitive** (related to thinking and learning) and social development. As children enter school, they also explore the world around them. They relate to other children through games, peer groups, and classroom activities. In these years, children learn to get along with each other. They also begin to behave in ways common to their sex. They begin to develop a conscience, morals, and self-esteem.

Common Disorders:
Childhood

C/D **Chickenpox** is a highly contagious viral illness that strikes nearly all children. It generally has no serious effects for healthy children. However, in adults or in anyone with a weakened immune system it can have more serious effects. Taking the varicella-zoster vaccine, commonly called the chickenpox vaccine, can prevent chickenpox.

C/D Children, as well as infants, may be susceptible to infections caused by viruses or bacteria. Bacterial infections can be treated with antibiotics. Viral infections are treated with extra rest, fluids, and over-the-counter medications for cough or congestion.

C/D **Leukemia** is a form of cancer. It refers to the inability of the body's white blood cells to fight disease. Children with leukemia may be susceptible to infections and other disorders. Chemotherapy can be used to fight this disease. See Chapter 18 for more information on cancer.

C/D Child abuse refers to physical, emotional, and sexual mistreatment of children, as well as neglect and maltreatment. Physical abuse includes hitting, kicking, burning, or intentionally causing injury to a child. Emotional abuse includes withholding affection, constantly criticizing, or ridiculing a child. Sexual abuse includes engaging in or allowing another person to engage in a sexual act with a child. Neglect and maltreatment include not providing adequate food, clothing, or support. They also include allowing children to use alcohol or drugs, leaving children alone, or exposing them to danger. See Chapters 3 and 27 for more information.

C/D Measles, mumps, rubella, diphtheria, smallpox, whooping cough, and polio are diseases that were once common during childhood. They can all be prevented now with vaccinations.

Adolescence

Puberty

During puberty, secondary sex characteristics, such as body hair, appear. Reproductive organs begin to function due to the secretion of the reproductive hormones. The start of puberty occurs between the ages of 10 and 16 for girls and 12 and 14 for boys.

Adolescence, Ages 12 to 18

Many teenagers have a hard time adapting to changes that occur in their bodies after puberty. Peer acceptance is important to them. Adolescents may be afraid that they are ugly or even abnormal. This concern for body image and acceptance, combined with changing hormones that influence moods, can cause rapid mood swings. Conflicting pressures develop as they remain dependent on their parents and yet need to express themselves socially and sexually. This causes conflict and stress. Social interaction between members of the opposite sex becomes very important (Fig. 8-15).

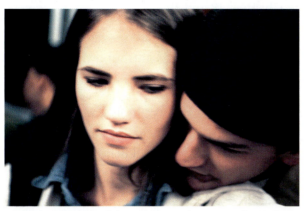

Fig. 8-15. *During adolescence, people express themselves socially and sexually.*

Common Disorders:
Adolescence

C/D As their bodies change, adolescents, especially girls, may develop eating disorders. **Anorexia** is a disease in which a person does not eat or exercises excessively to lose weight. A person with **bulimia** binges, eating huge amounts of foods or very fattening foods, and then purges, or eliminates the food by vomiting, using laxatives, or exercising excessively. Eating disorders can be serious and even life-threatening. These disorders must be treated with therapy and, in some cases, hospitalization.

C/D Teenagers can contract sexually transmitted diseases (STDs) and infections (STIs), such as chlamydia, herpes, and AIDS if they are sexually active. If teenagers are sexually active, only condoms offer some protection from sexually transmitted diseases and infections. See Chapter 18 for more information on STDs and STIs.

C/D Girls who are sexually active and do not use birth control, or do not use it properly, can become pregnant. Teenage pregnancy can have terrible consequences for adolescents, their families, and the babies born to teenage parents. Teenagers should understand that they can avoid pregnancy by using birth control or by not having sexual intercourse. Teenagers who choose to be sexually active should know what birth control methods are available and how to use them. Pregnancy puts a great deal of stress on teenage bodies. Adolescent girls are still children. Their bodies are still developing. In most cases they are not physically ready to bear a child. It is common for teenage mothers to give birth to premature or low-birth-weight babies.

C/D Because of the many physical and emotional changes they are experiencing, adolescents may become depressed and even attempt suicide. Parents, teachers, and friends should watch for the signs of depression. These include withdrawal, loss of appetite, weight gain or loss, sleep problems, moodiness, and apathy. Teenagers who are depressed should see a doctor, counselor, therapist, minister, or other trusted adult who can get them the help they need.

C/D Adolescents can sustain **trauma**, or severe injury, to the head or spinal cord in car accidents or sports injuries. These injuries can be temporarily or permanently disabling or even fatal.

Adulthood

Young Adulthood, Ages 18 to 40

By the age of 18, most young adults have stopped growing. Adopting a healthy lifestyle in these years can make life better now and prevent health problems in later adulthood. Psychological and social development continues, however. The tasks of these years include the following:

- Selecting an appropriate education

- Selecting an occupation or career
- Selecting a mate (Fig. 8-16)

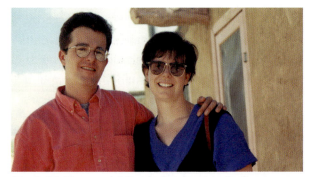

Fig. 8-16. Young adulthood often involves finding long-term mates.

- Learning to live with a mate or others
- Raising children
- Developing a satisfying sex life

Middle Adulthood: 40 to 65 Years

In general, people in middle adulthood are more comfortable and stable than they were in previous stages. Many of their major life decisions have already been made. In the early years of middle adulthood people sometimes experience a "mid-life crisis." This is a period of unrest centered on a subconscious desire for change and fulfillment of unmet goals.

Physical changes related to aging also occur in middle adulthood. Adults in this age group may notice that they have difficulty maintaining their weight or notice a decrease in strength and energy. Metabolism and other body functions slow down. Wrinkles and gray hair appear. Vision and hearing loss may begin. Women experience **menopause**, the end of menstruation. This occurs when the ovaries stop secreting hormones. Many diseases and illnesses can develop in these years. These disorders can become chronic and life-threatening.

Late Adulthood: 65 Years and Older

Persons in late adulthood must adjust to the effects of aging. These changes can include the loss of strength and health, the death of loved ones, retirement, and preparation for death. The developmental tasks of this age may seem to deal largely with loss. But solutions to these problems often involve new relationships, friendships, and interests. The disorders you are most likely to see (AIDS, arthritis, Alzheimer's disease, cancer, diabetes, and stroke) are discussed in Chapters 18 and 19.

11. Distinguish between what is true and what is not true about the aging process

Geriatrics is the study of health, wellness, and disease later in life. It includes the health care of older people and the well-being of their caregivers. **Gerontology** is the study of the aging process in people from mid-life through old age. Gerontologists look at the impact of the aging population on society.

Later adulthood covers an age range of as many as 25 to 35 years. People in this age category can have very different abilities, depending on their health. Some 70-year-old people enjoy active sports, while others are not active. Many 85-year-old people can still live alone. Others may live with family members or in long-term care facilities.

Ideas and stereotypes about older people are often false. They create prejudices against the elderly that are as unfair as prejudices against racial, ethnic, or religious groups. On television or in the movies older people are often shown as helpless, lonely, disabled, slow, forgetful, dependent, or inactive. However, research shows that most older people are active and engaged in work, volunteer activities, and learning and exercise programs. Aging is a normal process, not a disease. Most older people live independent lives and do not need assistance (Fig. 8-17). Prejudice toward, stereotyping of, and/or discrimination against older persons or the elderly is called **ageism**.

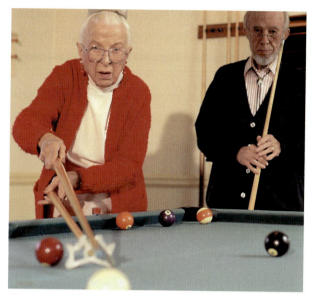

Fig. 8-17. Older adults often remain active and engaged.

You are likely to spend much of your time working with elderly residents. You must know what is true about aging and what is not true. While aging causes many changes, normal changes of aging do not mean an older person must become dependent, ill, or inactive. Knowing how to tell normal changes of aging from signs of illness or disability will allow you to better help residents. Normal changes of aging include the following:

- Skin is thinner, drier, more fragile, and less elastic.

- Muscles weaken and lose tone.

- Bones become more brittle.

- Sensitivity of nerve endings in the skin decreases.

- Responses and reflexes slow.

- Short-term memory loss occurs.

- Senses of vision, hearing, taste, and smell weaken.

- Heart works less efficiently.

- Oxygen in the blood decreases.

- Appetite decreases.

- Urinary elimination is more frequent.

- Digestion takes longer and is less efficient.

- Levels of hormones decrease.

- Immunity weakens.

- Lifestyle changes occur.

There are also changes that are NOT considered normal changes of aging and should be reported to the nurse. These include the following:

- Signs of depression

- Loss of ability to think logically

- Poor nutrition

- Shortness of breath

- Incontinence

Keep in mind that this is not a complete list. Your job includes reporting any change, normal or not. You will learn more about normal changes of aging in Chapter 9.

12. Explain developmental disabilities and list care guidelines

Developmental disabilities refer to disabilities that are present at birth or emerge during childhood. A developmental disability is a chronic condition. It restricts physical or mental ability. These disabilities prevent a child from developing at a "normal" rate. NAs help teach residents self-care and assist with ADLs.

Mental Retardation

According to the CDC, mental retardation is the most common developmental disorder. Approximately one percent of the population has mental retardation. It is neither a disease nor a psychiatric illness. People with mental retardation develop at a below-average rate. They have below-average mental functioning. They have difficulty in learning, communicating, moving, and may have problems adjusting socially. The ability to care for themselves may be affected. The potential for living independently and for financial independence may be limited. Despite their special needs, people who are mentally retarded have the same emotional and physical needs as others (Fig. 8-18). They experience the same emotions, such as anger, sadness, love, and joy, as others do. However, expression of their emotions may be limited, depending on their individual disabilities.

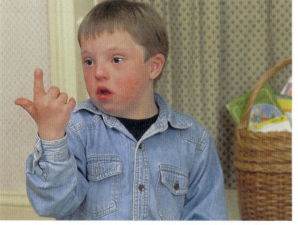

Fig. 8-18. People who are mentally retarded have the same emotional and physical needs as others do.

There are different degrees of mental retardation; the four degrees are mild, moderate, severe, and profound:

- Mild retardation usually causes a delay in walking and talking. With special support and education, the person can acquire academic skills up to the sixth grade level. With some assistance, he can become fairly independent and have some social skills and ability to work.

- Moderate mental retardation causes delays in speech and motor development. Simple communication skills may be acquired in childhood. With some support and supervision, the person can usually work and function successfully. He may be able to live alone, or may live in a facility or group home.

- Severe mental retardation causes noticeable delays in motor development, and the person has few communication skills. Very basic self-care skills, such as self-feeding, toileting, and dressing may be mastered. The person may live in a facility or group home.

- Profound mental retardation causes obvious delays in most areas of development. The person may not respond to his environment, and often there are physical problems as well. Walking may be mastered; communication skills are extremely basic. The person may need nursing care and require help in self-care. He will need a high level of support and supervision.

For residents who are mentally retarded, the main goal of care is to help them have as normal a life as possible. This means recognizing their individuality, basic human rights, and physical and emotional needs, as well as special needs.

Some residents and/or their families will prefer not to use the term "mental retardation" or "mentally retarded." Other terms that may be preferable are "intellectual disability" and "developmental disability." Respect the resident's wishes on which term or terms to use.

Guidelines:
Mental Retardation

G   Treat adult residents as adults, regardless of their behavior.

G   Praise and encourage often, especially positive behavior.

G   Help teach ADLs by dividing a task into smaller units.

G   Promote independence, but also assist residents with activities and motor functions that are difficult.

G   Encourage social interaction.

G   Repeat words to make sure they understand.

G   Be patient.

Down Syndrome

People who are born with Down syndrome have different degrees of mental retardation, along with physical symptoms. A person with Down syndrome typically has a small skull, a flattened nose, short fingers, and a wider space between the first two fingers and the first two toes. Some people with Down syndrome can become fairly independent.

Guidelines:
Down Syndrome

G Give the same type of care and instruction as for any other person with mental retardation.

G Praise and encourage often, especially positive behavior.

G Help teach ADLs by dividing a task into smaller units.

Cerebral Palsy

People with cerebral palsy have suffered brain damage while in the uterus or during birth. They may have both physical and mental disabilities. Damage to the brain stops the development of the child. It can cause disorganized or abnormal development. Muscle coordination and nerves are affected. People with cerebral palsy may lack control of the head, and have trouble using the arms and hands, and have poor balance or posture. They may be either stiff and spastic or limp and flaccid, and may have impaired speech. Gait and mobility may be affected. Intelligence may also be affected. With or without assistance, a person with cerebral palsy may be able to live independently.

Guidelines:
Cerebral Palsy

G Allow the resident to move slowly. People with cerebral palsy take longer to adjust their body position. They may repeat movements several times.

G Keep the resident's body in as normal an alignment as possible.

G Talk to the resident, even if he or she cannot speak. Be patient and listen.

G Use touch as a form of communication.

G Avoid activities that are tiring or frustrating.

G Be gentle when handling parts of the body that may be painful (Fig. 8-19).

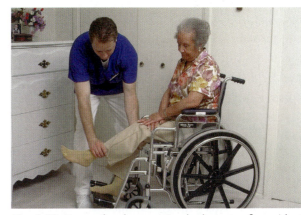

Fig. 8-19. *Be gentle when moving body parts of a resident who has cerebral palsy.*

G Promote independence and encourage socialization.

Spina Bifida

Spina bifida literally means "split spine." When part of the backbone is not well-developed at birth, the spinal cord may bulge out of the back. Spina bifida can cause a range of disabilities. Some babies born with spina bifida will be able to walk and will have no lasting disabilities. Others may be in a wheelchair. They may have little or no bladder or bowel control. In some cases, complications of spina bifida may cause brain damage.

Guidelines:
Spina Bifida

G If the resident is an adult, provide assistance with range of motion exercises and ADLs. If working in the home, help perform light housecleaning duties.

G If an infant or child has spina bifida, perform tasks that help the parents manage and stabilize the home.

G Be a positive role model for the resident and family in learning to deal with the resident's disabilities.

13. Identify community resources available to help the elderly

The larger community—the local government or social service agencies, church or synagogue—can provide resources to help the elderly. These resources can help them through difficult times and help solve problems. Some of these resources include the following:

- Local Area Agency on Aging
- Ombudsman program
- Alzheimer's Association
- Local Hospice organization
- Social workers
- Resident advocacy organizations
- Support groups
- Meal or transportation services (Fig. 8-20)

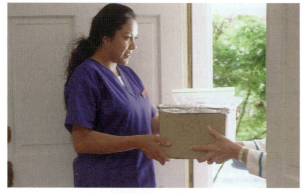

Fig. 8-20. "Meals on Wheels" and similar services provide nutritious meals to people unable to cook for themselves.

If residents ask you for help, refer them to the nurse or social worker. If no one asks but you think help is needed, speak to your supervisor.

Chapter Review

1. List six basic human needs.

2. What psychosocial needs do humans have?

3. According to Maslow, which needs must be met first, physical or emotional?

4. What does giving holistic care mean?

5. List six examples of losses that residents may experience.

6. What are six problems that a lack of independence can cause?

7. List four ways to accommodate residents' sexual needs.

8. How can nursing assistants help residents meet their spiritual needs?

9. What is never allowed regarding residents' spiritual or religious needs?

10. Pick three religions listed in Learning Objective 6 and briefly describe them. Feel free to add information that is not included in the Learning Objective.

11. If a resident is an atheist, but her NA believes in God, is it okay for the NA to ask the resident to pray with her?

12. List seven ways that regular physical activity can help a person.

13. List seven ways that inactivity and immobility can cause problems for a person.

14. List four ways that families can help residents.

15. Name three ways nursing assistants can meet emotional needs of residents and their families.

16. For each stage of human development—infancy, childhood, adolescence, adulthood—name two common disorders.

17. What is ageism?

18. What is true/factual about most older adults?

19. List ten normal changes of aging.

20. What are developmental disabilities?

21. What is the most common developmental disorder?

22. List four community resources that can help residents meet their needs.

9

The Healthy Human Body

1. Describe body systems and define key anatomical terms

Our bodies are organized into body systems. Each system has a condition under which it works best. **Homeostasis** is the name for the condition in which all of the body's systems are working at their best. To be in homeostasis, the body's **metabolism**, or physical and chemical processes, must be working at a steady level. When disease or injury occur, the body's metabolism is disturbed. Homeostasis is lost.

Changes in metabolic processes are called signs and symptoms. For instance, changes in body temperature could indicate that the body is fighting an infection. Noticing and reporting changes in your residents is a very important part of your job. The changes you notice could be signs of significant problems.

Each system in the body has its own unique structure and function. There are also normal age-related changes for each body system. Knowing normal changes of aging will help you be able to recognize any abnormal changes in your residents. This chapter also includes tips on how you can help residents with their normal changes of aging.

The body's systems can be broken down in different ways. In this book we divide the human body into ten systems:

1. Integumentary, or skin
2. Musculoskeletal
3. Nervous
4. Cardiovascular or circulatory
5. Respiratory
6. Urinary
7. Gastrointestinal
8. Endocrine
9. Reproductive
10. Immune and Lymphatic

Body systems are made up of **organs**. An organ has a specific function. Organs are made up of **tissues**. Tissues are made up of groups of cells that perform a similar task. For example, in the circulatory system, the heart is one of the organs. It is made up of tissues and cells. **Cells** are the building blocks of our bodies. Living cells divide, grow, and die, renewing the tissues and organs of our body systems.

Anatomical Terms of Location

Anatomical terms of location are descriptive terms to help identify positions or directions of the body. Here are some anatomical terms used to describe location in the human body:

- Anterior or ventral: the front of the body or body part
- Posterior or dorsal: the back of the body or body part
- Superior: toward the head
- Inferior: away from the head
- Medial: toward the midline of the body

- Lateral: to the side away from the midline of the body
- Proximal: closer to the torso
- Distal: farther away from the torso

This section discusses the structure and function, as well as age-related changes, of each body system. The bulk of information on diseases and disorders of each system and related care will be discussed in Chapter 18. Chapters 16, 17, and 19 also have information on diseases.

2. Describe the integumentary system

The largest organ and system in the body is the skin. The skin is a natural protective covering, or **integument**. Skin prevents injury to internal organs. It also protects the body against entry of bacteria. Skin also prevents the loss of too much water, which is essential to life. Skin is made up of tissues and glands (Fig. 9-1). **Glands** secrete hormones. **Hormones** are chemical substances created by the body that control numerous body functions.

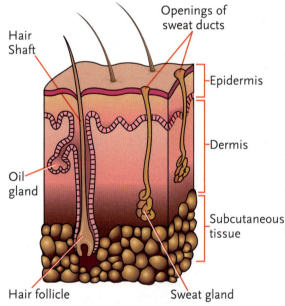

Fig. 9-1. *Cross-section showing details of the integumentary system.*

The skin is also a *sense organ* that feels heat, cold, pain, touch, and pressure. Body temperature is regulated in the skin. Blood vessels **dilate** or widen, when the outside temperature is too high. This brings more blood to the body surface to cool it off. The same blood vessels **constrict**, or narrow, when the outside temperature is too cold. By restricting the amount of blood reaching the skin, the blood vessels help the body retain heat.

The blood vessels, called capillaries, are located in the dermis, which is the inner layer of skin. The dermis also contains nerves, sweat glands, oil glands, and hair roots. Sweat glands help control body temperature by secreting sweat. Sweat is made up of mostly water, but it also contains salt and a small amount of waste products. Sweat comes to the body's surface through pores, or tiny openings in the skin. It cools the body as it evaporates. Oil glands in the dermis secrete oil. Oil comes to the skin surface through hair follicles, or roots. Oil keeps the skin and hair soft.

No blood vessels, and only a few nerve endings, are located in the epidermis, which is the outer layer of skin. Thinner than the dermis, the epidermis contains both dead and living cells. The dead cells begin deeper in the epidermis. They are pushed to the surface as other cells divide. They are eventually worn off. The epidermis also contains pigment cells that give the skin its color.

Hair grows from roots located in the dermis. It grows through hair follicles that extend through the epidermis to the outside of the body. Hair protects the body from heat and cold. Hair inside the nose and ears keeps out particles and bacteria trying to enter the body.

Normal changes of aging include the following:

- Skin is thinner, drier, and more fragile. It is more easily damaged.

- Skin is less elastic.

- Protective fatty tissue is lost, so person feels colder.

- Hair thins and may turn gray.

- Wrinkles and brown spots, or "liver spots" appear.

- Nails are harder and more brittle.

- Reduced circulation to the skin can cause dryness, itching, and irritation.

Observing and Reporting:
Integumentary System

During daily care, a resident's skin should be observed for changes that may indicate disease. Observe and report the following signs and symptoms:

O/R Pale, white or reddened, or purple areas, blisters or bruises on the skin

O/R Dry or flaking skin

O/R Rashes or any skin discoloration

O/R Cuts, boils, sores, wounds, abrasions

O/R Fluid or blood draining from the skin

O/R Changes in moistness/dryness

O/R Swelling

O/R Blisters

O/R Changes in wound or ulcer (size, depth, drainage, color, odor)

O/R Redness or broken skin between toes or around toenails

O/R Scalp or hair changes

O/R Skin that appears different from normal or that has changed

O/R In ebony complexions, also look for any change in the feel of the tissue, any change in the appearance of the skin, such as an "orange-peel" look, a purplish hue, and extremely dry, crust-like areas that might be covering a tissue break upon a closer look.

3. Describe the musculoskeletal system

Muscles, bones, ligaments, tendons, and cartilage give the body shape and structure. They work together to allow the body to move.

The skeleton, or framework, of the human body has 206 **bones** (Fig. 9-2). Besides allowing the body to move, bones also protect organs. For example, the skull protects the brain and the vertebrae protect the spinal cord. Bones are hard and rigid, but are made up of living cells. Blood vessels supply oxygen and nutrients to the bones, as well as other tissues of the body.

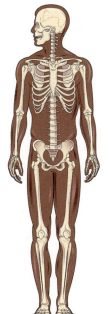

Fig. 9-2. *The skeleton is composed of 206 bones that help movement and protect organs.*

Two bones meet at a **joint** (Fig. 9-3). Some joints make movement possible in all directions, such as the ball and socket joint. This joint is a type of synovial joint. In this joint, the round end of one bone fits into the hollow end of the other bone, which allows it to move in all directions. The hip and shoulder joints are examples.

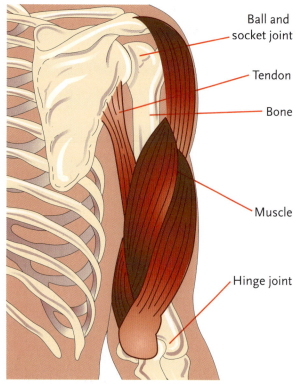

Ball and
socket joint

Tendon

Bone

Muscle

Hinge joint

Fig. 9-3. Muscles are connected to bone by tendons. Bones meet at different types of joints. The ball and socket joint and the hinge joint are shown here.

Other joints permit movement in one direction only. The hinge joint is another example of a synovial joint. Like the hinge of a door, a hinge joint permits movement in one direction only. The elbow and knee are hinge joints. They only bend in one direction.

Muscles provide movement of body parts to maintain posture and to produce heat. Muscles can be voluntary or involuntary. Voluntary muscles are also called skeletal muscles. They are attached to bones. They can be moved when a person wants them to move. Examples of voluntary muscles are the arm and leg muscles, which are consciously controlled. Involuntary muscles cannot be consciously controlled. They automatically regulate the movement of organs and blood vessels. Examples of involuntary muscles are the heart and the diaphragm. The diaphragm is the muscle that makes humans breathe.

Exercise is important for improving and maintaining physical and mental health. Inactivity and immobility can result in a loss of self-es-

teem, depression, pneumonia, and urinary tract infections. They can also lead to constipation, blood clots, dulling of the senses, and muscle atrophy or contractures. When atrophy occurs, the muscle wastes away, decreases in size, and becomes weak. When a **contracture** develops, the muscle shortens, becomes inflexible, and "freezes" in position. This can cause permanent disability of the limb.

Range of motion (ROM) exercises can help prevent these conditions. With ROM exercises, the joints are extended and flexed. Exercise increases circulation of blood, oxygen, and nutrients and improves muscle tone. See Chapter 21 for more information on ROM exercises.

Normal changes of aging include the following:

- Muscles weaken and lose tone.

- Body movement slows.

- Bones lose density. They become more brittle, making them more susceptible to breaks.

- Joints may stiffen and become painful.

- Height is gradually lost.

How You Can Help: NA's Role

Falls can cause life-threatening complications, including fractures. Prevent falls by keeping items out of residents' paths. Keep furniture in the same place. Keep walkers or canes where residents can easily reach them. Encourage regular movement and self-care. Encourage residents to perform as many ADLs as possible. To prevent or slow osteoporosis, the condition that is responsible for fragile bones, encourage residents to walk and do other light exercise. Exercise can strengthen bones as well as muscles. Help with range of motion (ROM) exercises as needed.

Observing and Reporting:
Musculoskeletal System

Observe and report the following signs and symptoms:

O/R Changes in ability to perform routine movements and activities

- **O/R** Any changes in residents' ability to perform ROM exercises
- **O/R** Pain during movement
- **O/R** Any new or increased swelling of joints
- **O/R** White, shiny, red, or warm areas over a joint
- **O/R** Bruising
- **O/R** Aches and pains reported to you

4. Describe the nervous system

The nervous system is the control and message center of the body. It controls and coordinates all body functions. The nervous system also senses and interprets information from outside the human body (Fig. 9-4).

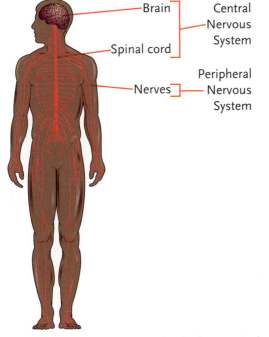

Fig. 9-4. *The nervous system includes the brain, spinal cord, and nerves throughout the body.*

The neuron, or nerve cell, is the basic unit of the nervous system. Neurons send messages or sensations from the receptors in different parts of the body, through the spinal cord, to the brain.

The nervous system has two main parts: the **central nervous system** (CNS) and the **peripheral nervous system** (PNS). The central nervous system is composed of the brain and spinal cord. The peripheral nervous system deals with the periphery, or outer part of the body, via the nerves that extend throughout the body.

The Central Nervous System

The brain is housed within the skull. The spinal cord is housed within the spinal column. The spinal column extends from the brain into the trunk of the body. Both the brain and the spinal cord are covered by a protective membrane made up of three layers. Between two of these layers is the cerebrospinal fluid. This fluid circulates around the brain and spinal cord. It provides a cushion against injuries.

The brain has three main sections: the cerebrum, the cerebellum, and the brainstem (Fig. 9-5). The largest section of the human brain is the cerebrum. The outside layer of the cerebrum is the cerebral cortex. The cerebral cortex is the part of the brain in which thinking, analysis, association of ideas, judgment, emotions, and memory occur. The cerebral cortex also:

- Directs speech and emotions
- Interprets messages from the eyes, ears, nose, tongue, and skin
- Controls voluntary muscle movement

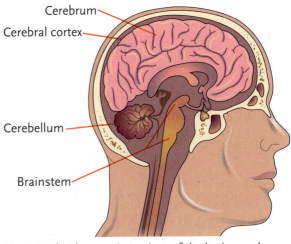

Fig. 9-5. *The three main sections of the brain: cerebrum, brainstem, and cerebellum.*

The cerebrum is divided into right and left hemispheres. The right hemisphere controls movement and function in the left side of the body. The left hemisphere controls movement and function in the right side of the body (Fig. 9-6). Any illness or injury to the right hemisphere affects functions on the left side of the body. Illness or injury to the left hemisphere disrupts function on the right side.

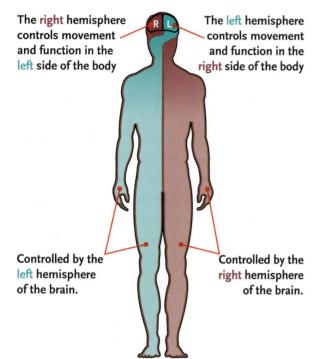

The **right** hemisphere controls movement and function in the **left** side of the body

The **left** hemisphere controls movement and function in the **right** side of the body

Controlled by the **left** hemisphere of the brain.

Controlled by the **right** hemisphere of the brain.

Fig. 9-6. The right hemisphere controls movement and function in the left side of the body. The left hemisphere controls movement and function in the right side of the body.

The cerebellum controls balance and regulates the body's voluntary muscles. It produces and coordinates smooth movements. Someone who has a problem in the cerebellum will be uncoordinated and have jerky movements and muscle weakness.

The cerebrum and cerebellum are connected to the spinal cord by the brainstem. The brainstem contains a kind of regulatory center. It controls heart rate, breathing, swallowing, coughing, vomiting, and closing or opening of blood vessels.

The spinal cord is connected to the brain. It is protected by the bones of the spinal column. Nerve pathways run through the spinal cord.

They conduct messages between the brain and the body. Cranial nerves attach to the brain and brain stem. Some of these nerves bring information from the sense organs to the brain. Some control muscles and others are connected to glands or organs, such as the lungs. There are 12 pairs of cranial nerves. Nerves that are attached to the spinal cord and connect the spinal cord with other parts of the body are called spinal nerves. The brain communicates with most of the body through the spinal nerves. There are 31 pairs of spinal nerves.

Normal changes of aging include the following:

- Responses and reflexes slow.

- Sensitivity of nerve endings in skin decreases.

- Person may show some memory loss, more often with short-term memory. Long-term memory, or memory for past events, usually remains sharp.

How You Can Help: NA's Role

Help with memory loss by suggesting residents make lists or write notes about things they want to remember. Placing a calendar nearby may help. If your residents enjoy reminiscing, take an interest in their past by asking to see photos or hear stories. Allow time for decision-making and avoid sudden changes in schedule. Allow plenty of time for movement; never rush the person. Encourage reading, thinking, and other mental activities.

Observing and Reporting:
Central Nervous System

Observe and report the following signs and symptoms:

O/R Fatigue or any pain with movement or exercise

O/R Shaking or trembling

O/R Inability to speak clearly

O/R Inability to move one side of body

- Disturbance or changes in vision or hearing
- Changes in eating patterns and/or fluid intake
- Difficulty swallowing
- Bowel and bladder changes
- Depression or mood changes
- Memory loss or confusion
- Violent behavior
- Any unusual or unexplained change in behavior
- Decreased ability to perform ADLs

The Nervous System: Sense Organs

The eyes, ears, nose, tongue, and skin are the body's major sense organs. They are considered part of the central nervous system because they receive impulses from the environment. They relay these impulses to the nerves.

The eye, which is about an inch in diameter, is located in a bony socket in the skull. The bony socket protects the eye, which is surrounded by muscles that control its movements (Fig. 9-7).

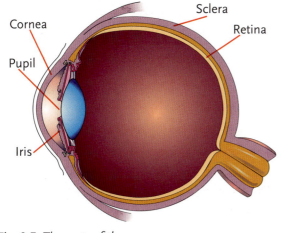

Fig. 9-7. *The parts of the eye.*

The outer part of the eye is called the sclera. The sclera appears white, except in front, where it is called the cornea. The cornea is actually clear, but it appears colored because it lies over the iris, or the colored part of the eye. The pupil, or black circle in the center of the iris, widens or narrows to adjust the amount of light that enters the eye. Inside the back of the eye is the retina. The retina contains cells that respond to light and send a message to the brain, where the picture is interpreted so you can "see."

The ear is a sense organ that provides balance and hearing. It is divided into three parts: the outer ear, the middle ear, and the inner ear (Fig. 9-8). The outer ear is the funnel-shaped outer part, sometimes called the auricle or pinna. It guides sound waves into the auditory canal. This canal is about one inch long and contains many glands that secrete earwax. Earwax and hair in the ear protect the ear from foreign objects. The eardrum, or tympanic membrane, separates the outer ear from the middle ear.

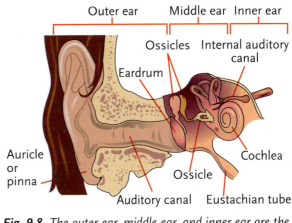

Fig. 9-8. *The outer ear, middle ear, and inner ear are the three main divisions of the ear.*

The middle ear consists of the eustachian tube and three ossicles, small bones that amplify sound. The ossicles transmit sound to the inner ear. The eustachian tube connects the middle ear to the throat. It functions to allow air into the middle ear to equalize pressure on the tympanic membrane. The inner ear contains fluid that carries sound waves from the middle ear to the auditory nerve. The auditory nerve then transmits the impulse to the brain. The inner ear also contains structures that help in maintaining balance.

Normal changes of aging include the following:

- Vision and hearing decreases. Sense of balance may be affected.

- Senses of taste, smell, and touch decrease.

- Sensitivity to heat and cold decreases.

How You Can Help: NA's Role

Encourage the use of eyeglasses and keep them clean. Bright colors and good lighting will also help. Encourage the use of hearing aids and keep them clean. Face the resident when speaking. Speak slowly and clearly in a low-pitched voice; do not shout. Repeat words when necessary. Loss of senses of taste and smell may lead to decreased appetite. Encourage good oral care. Foods with a variety of tastes and textures should be provided. Loss of smell may make resident unaware of increased body odor. Assist as needed with regular bathing. Due to decreased sense of touch, be careful with hot drinks and hot bath water. Residents may not be able to tell if something is too hot for them.

Observing and Reporting:
Eyes and Ears

Observe and report the following signs and symptoms:

O/R Changes in vision or hearing

O/R Signs of infection

O/R Dizziness

O/R Complaints of pain in eyes or ears

5. Describe the cardiovascular system

The cardiovascular, or circulatory, system is made up of the heart, blood vessels, and blood (Fig. 9-9). The heart pumps blood through the blood vessels to the cells. The blood carries food, oxygen, and other substances cells need to function properly. A healthy cardiovascular system is essential for life. Cells, tissues, and organs need good circulation to function well. If circulation is reduced, cells do not receive enough oxygen

and nutrients. Waste products of cell metabolism are not removed, and organs become diseased.

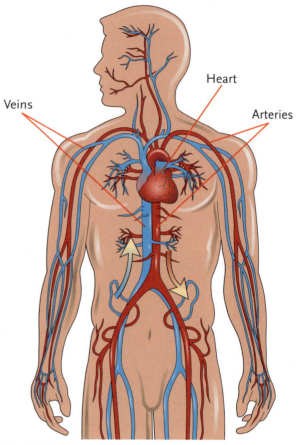

Fig. 9-9. *The heart, blood vessels, and blood are the main parts of the cardiovascular system.*

The cardiovascular system performs the following major functions:

- Supplies food, oxygen, and hormones to cells

- Produces and supplies antibodies and other infection-fighting blood cells

- Removes waste products from cells

- Controls body temperature

Blood contains blood cells and plasma. Plasma is the liquid portion of the blood. It carries many substances, including blood cells, nutrients, and waste products. Analyzing these parts of blood samples can help identify illness and infection:

- Red blood cells carry oxygen from the lungs to all parts of the body. Red blood cells are produced by bone marrow, a substance found inside hollow bones. Iron, found in bone marrow and red blood cells, is essential to blood. It gives it its red color. Red blood cells function for a short time, then die. They are filtered out of the blood by the liver and spleen. Iron in diets allows bodies to produce new red blood cells.

- White blood cells defend the body against foreign substances, such as bacteria and viruses. When the body becomes aware of these invaders, white blood cells rush to the site of infection. They multiply rapidly. The bone marrow, spleen, and thymus gland produce white blood cells.

- Platelets are also carried by the blood. They cause the blood to clot, preventing excess bleeding. Platelets are also produced by the bone marrow.

The heart is the pump of the circulatory system (Fig. 9-10). The heart is a muscle. It is located in the middle lower chest, on the left side. The heart muscle is made up of three layers: the pericardium, the myocardium and the endocardium.

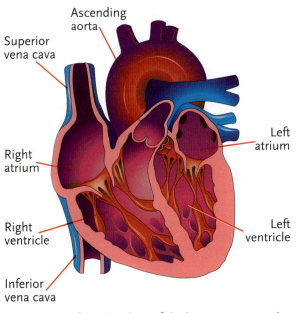

Fig. 9-10. *The four chambers of the heart connect to the body's largest blood vessels.*

The interior of the heart is divided into four chambers. The two upper chambers are called the left atrium and right atrium. They receive blood. The two lower chambers, or ventricles, pump blood. The right atrium receives blood from the veins. This blood, containing carbon dioxide, then flows into the right ventricle. It is pumped to the blood vessels in the lungs. Carbon dioxide is exchanged for oxygen. The heart's left atrium receives the oxygen-saturated blood. It then flows into the left ventricle. There it is pumped through the arteries to all parts of the body. Two valves, one located between the right atrium and right ventricle and the other between the left atrium and left ventricle, allow the blood to flow in only one direction (Fig. 9-11).

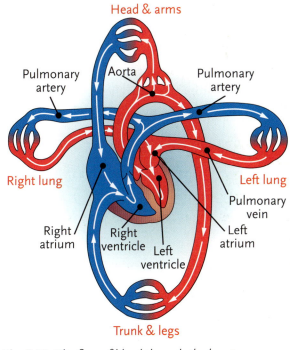

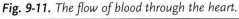

Fig. 9-11. *The flow of blood through the heart.*

The heart functions in two phases: the contracting phase or **systole**, when the ventricles pump blood through the blood vessels and the resting phase, or **diastole**, when the chambers fill with blood. When a person's blood pressure is taken, the numbers measure these two phases. See Chapter 14 for more information on how to take blood pressure.

Three types of blood vessels are found in the body: arteries, capillaries, and veins. Arteries carry oxygen-rich blood away from the heart.

The blood is pumped from the left ventricle, through the aorta, the largest artery. Blood is then pumped through other arteries that branch off from it. The coronary arteries carry blood to the heart itself.

Capillaries are tiny blood vessels that receive blood from the arteries. Nutrients, oxygen, and other substances in the blood pass from the capillaries to the cells. Waste products, including carbon dioxide, pass from the cells into the capillaries.

Veins carry the blood containing waste products from the capillaries back to the heart. Near the heart, the veins come together to form the two largest veins, the inferior vena cava and the superior vena cava. These empty into the right atrium. The inferior vena cava carries blood from the legs and trunk. The superior vena cava carries blood from the arms, head, and neck.

Normal changes of aging include the following:

- Heart pumps less efficiently.
- Blood flow decreases.
- Blood vessels narrow.

How You Can Help: NA's Role

Encourage movement and exercise. Walking, stretching, and even lifting light weights can help older people maintain strength and mobility. Range of motion exercises are important for residents who cannot get out of bed. Allow enough time to complete activities. Prevent residents from tiring. Layer clothing to keep residents warm. Use socks, slippers, or shoes to keep the feet warm.

Observing and Reporting:
Cardiovascular System

Observe and report the following signs and symptoms:

O/R Changes in pulse rate

O/R Weakness, fatigue

O/R Loss of ability to perform activities of daily living (ADLs)

O/R Swelling of hands and feet

O/R Pale or bluish hands, feet, or lips

O/R Chest pain

O/R Weight gain

O/R Shortness of breath, changes in breathing patterns, inability to catch breath

O/R Severe headache

O/R Inactivity (which can lead to cardiovascular problems)

6. Describe the respiratory system

Respiration, the body taking in oxygen and removing carbon dioxide, involves breathing in, **inspiration**, and breathing out, **expiration**. The lungs accomplish this process (Fig. 9-12). The functions of the respiratory system are to bring oxygen into the body and to eliminate carbon dioxide produced as the body uses oxygen.

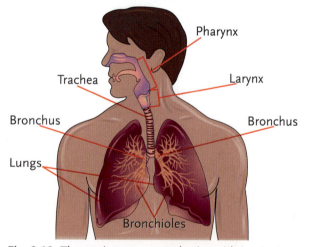

Fig. 9-12. *The respiratory process begins with inspiration through the nose or mouth. The air travels through the trachea and into the lungs via the bronchi, which then branch into bronchioles.*

As the lungs inhale, the air is pulled in through the nose and into the pharynx, a tubular passageway for both food and air. From the pharynx, air passes into the larynx, or voice box. The larynx is located at the beginning of the trachea, or windpipe. The trachea divides into two branches at its lower portion, the right bronchus and the left bronchus, or bronchi. Each bronchus leads into a lung and then subdivides into bronchioles. These smaller airways subdivide further. They end in alveoli: tiny, one-cell sacs that appear in grape-like clusters. Blood is supplied to the alveoli by capillaries. Oxygen and carbon dioxide are exchanged between the alveoli and capillaries.

Oxygen-saturated blood then circulates through the capillaries and venules (small veins) of the lung, into the pulmonary vein and left side of the heart. The carbon dioxide is exhaled through the alveoli into the bronchioles and bronchi of the lungs, the trachea, through the larynx, the pharynx, and out the nose and mouth.

Each lung is covered by the pleura, a membrane with two layers. One is attached to the chest wall. One is attached to the surface of the lung. The space between the layers is filled with a thin fluid that lubricates the layers, preventing them from rubbing together during breathing.

Normal changes of aging include the following:

- Lung strength decreases.
- Lung capacity decreases.
- Oxygen in the blood decreases.
- Voice weakens.

How You Can Help: NA's Role

Provide rest periods as needed. Encourage exercise and regular movement. Encourage and assist with deep breathing exercises, as ordered. Make sure people with acute or chronic upper respiratory conditions are not exposed to cigarette smoke or polluted air. People who have difficulty breathing will usually be more comfortable sitting up than lying down.

Observing and Reporting:
Respiratory System

Observe and report the following signs and symptoms:

- **o/R** Change in respiratory rate
- **o/R** Shallow breathing or breathing through pursed lips
- **o/R** Coughing or wheezing
- **o/R** Nasal congestion or discharge
- **o/R** Sore throat, difficulty swallowing, or swollen tonsils
- **o/R** The need to sit after mild exertion
- **o/R** Pale, bluish, or gray color of the lips and arms and legs
- **o/R** Pain in the chest area
- **o/R** Discolored **sputum**, or the fluid a person coughs up from the lungs (green, yellow, blood-tinged, or gray)

7. Describe the urinary system

The urinary system is composed of two kidneys, two ureters, one urinary bladder, and a single urethra. The urinary system has two important functions. Through urine, the urinary system eliminates waste products created by the cells. The urinary system also maintains the water balance in the body.

The kidneys are located in the upper part of the abdominal cavity on each side of the spine. These two bean-shaped organs are protected by the muscles of the back and the lower part of the rib cage. When blood flows through the kidneys, waste products and excess water are filtered out. Necessary water and substances are reabsorbed into the bloodstream. Waste and the remaining fluid form urine. The body must maintain a proper balance between water absorbed in the body and waste fluids that are released from the body. You will learn more about fluid intake and output in Chapter 15.

Each kidney has a ureter, which is attached to the bladder. Urine flows through the ureters to the bladder, a muscular sac in the lower part of the abdomen. Urine flows from the bladder through the urethra. It then passes out of the body through the meatus, the opening at the end of the urethra (Figs. 9-13 and 9-14). In the female, the meatus is located in the genital area just in front of the opening of the vagina. In the male, the meatus is located at the end of the penis.

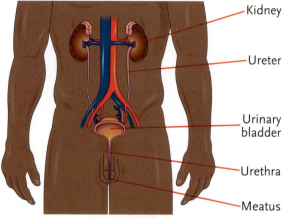

Fig. 9-13. *The urinary system consists of two kidneys and their ureters, the bladder, the urethra, and the meatus. This is an illustration of the male urinary system.*

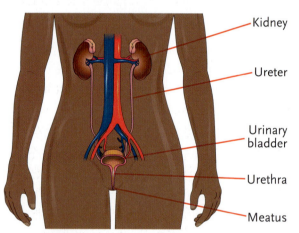

Fig. 9-14. *The female urethra is shorter than the male urethra. Because of this, the female bladder is more likely to become infected by bacteria traveling up the urethra.*

Normal changes of aging include the following:

*   The ability of kidneys to filter blood decreases.

*   Bladder muscle tone weakens.

*   Bladder holds less urine, which causes more frequent urination.

*   Bladder may not empty completely, causing more chance of infection.

How You Can Help: NA's Role

Encourage residents to drink plenty of fluids. Offer frequent trips to the bathroom. If residents are incontinent, do not show frustration or anger. **Urinary incontinence** is the inability to control the bladder, which leads to an involuntary loss of urine. Keep residents clean and dry.

Observing and Reporting:
Urinary System

Observe and report the following signs and symptoms:

O/R Weight loss or gain

O/R Swelling in the upper or lower extremities

O/R Pain or burning during urination

O/R Changes in urine, such as cloudiness, odor, or color

O/R Changes in frequency and amount of urination

O/R Swelling in the abdominal/bladder area

O/R Complaints that bladder feels full or painful

O/R Urinary incontinence/dribbling

O/R Pain in the kidney or back/flank region

O/R Inadequate fluid intake

8. Describe the gastrointestinal system

The gastrointestinal (GI) system, also called the digestive system, is made up of the gastrointestinal tract and the accessory digestive organs (Fig. 9-15). The gastrointestinal system has two functions: digestion and elimination. **Digestion** is the process of preparing food physically and chemically so that it can be absorbed into the cells. **Elimination** is the process of expelling solid wastes made up of the waste products of food that are not absorbed into the cells.

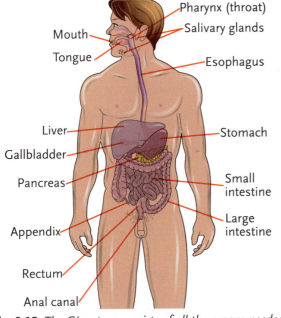

Fig. 9-15. *The GI system consists of all the organs needed to digest food and process waste.*

The gastrointestinal tract is a long passageway extending from the mouth to the anus, the opening of the rectum. Food passes from the mouth through the pharynx, esophagus, stomach, small intestine, large intestine, and out of the body as solid waste. The teeth, tongue, salivary glands, liver, gall bladder, and pancreas are the accessory organs to digestion. They help prepare the food so that it can be absorbed.

Food is first placed in the mouth. The teeth chew it by cutting it, then chopping and grinding it into smaller pieces that can be swallowed. Saliva moistens the food and begins chemical digestion. The tongue helps with chewing and swallowing by pushing the food around between the teeth and then into the pharynx.

The pharynx is a muscular structure located at the back of the mouth. It extends into the throat. It contracts with swallowing and pushes food into the esophagus. The muscles of the esophagus then move food into the stomach through involuntary contractions called peristalsis.

The stomach is a muscular pouch located in the upper left part of the abdominal cavity. It provides physical digestion by stirring and

churning the food to break it down into smaller particles. The glands in the stomach lining aid in digestion. They secrete gastric juices that chemically break down food. This process turns food into a semi-liquid substance called chyme. Peristalsis continues in the stomach, pushing the chyme into the small intestine.

The small intestine is about twenty feet long. Here enzymes secreted by the liver and the pancreas finish digesting the chyme. Bile, a green liquid produced by the liver, is stored in the gallbladder and released into the small intestine. Bile helps break down dietary fat. The liver converts fats and sugars into glucose, a sugar that can be carried to cells by the blood. The liver also stores glucose. The pancreas produces insulin, an enzyme that regulates the body's conversion of sugar into glucose.

The chyme is moved by peristalsis through the small intestine. There villi, tiny projections lining the small intestine, absorb the digested food into the capillaries.

Peristalsis moves the chyme that has not been digested through the large intestine. In the large intestine most of the water in the chyme is absorbed. What remains is feces, a semi-solid material of water, solid waste material, bacteria, and mucus. Feces passes by peristalsis through the rectum, the lower end of the colon. It moves out of the body through the anus, the rectal opening.

Normal changes of aging include the following:

- Decreased saliva production affects the ability to chew and swallow.

- Absorption of vitamins and minerals decreases.

- Process of digestion takes longer and is less efficient.

- Body waste moves more slowly through the intestines, causing more frequent constipation.

How You Can Help: NA's Role

Encourage fluids and nutritious, appealing meals. Allow time to eat. Make mealtime enjoyable. Provide good oral care. Make sure dentures fit properly and are cleaned regularly. Residents who have trouble chewing and swallowing are at risk of choking. Provide plenty of fluids with meals. Residents should eat a diet that contains fiber and drink plenty of fluids to help prevent constipation. Encourage daily bowel movements. Give residents the opportunity to have a bowel movement around the same time each day.

Observing and Reporting:
Gastrointestinal System

Observe and report the following signs and symptoms:

O/R Difficulty swallowing or chewing (including denture problems, tooth pain, or mouth sores)

O/R Fecal/**anal incontinence** (inability to control the bowels, leading to involuntary passage of stool)

O/R Weight gain/weight loss

O/R Anorexia (loss of appetite)

O/R Abdominal pain and cramping

O/R Diarrhea

O/R Nausea and vomiting (especially vomitus that looks like coffee grounds)

O/R Constipation

O/R Flatulence

O/R Hiccups, belching

O/R Abnormally-colored stool (bloody, black, or hard)

O/R Heartburn

O/R Poor nutritional intake

9. Describe the endocrine system

The endocrine system is made up of glands that secrete hormones. Hormones are chemi-cals that regulate essential body processes (Fig. 9-16). They are carried in the blood to the various organs, where they perform the following functions:

- Maintaining homeostasis
- Influencing growth and development
- Regulating levels of sugar in the blood
- Regulating levels of calcium in the bones
- Regulating the body's ability to reproduce
- Determining how fast cells burn food for energy

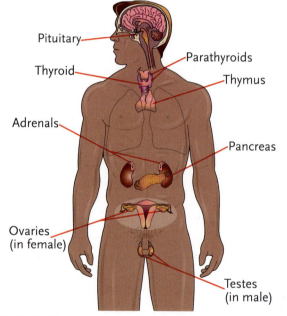

Fig. 9-16. *The endocrine system includes organs that produce hormones that regulate body processes.*

The pituitary gland is located behind the eyes at the base of the brain. It is called the "master" gland. It secretes key hormones that cause other glands to produce other hormones. Some hormones secreted by the pituitary gland are:

- Growth hormone, which regulates growth and development
- Antidiuretic hormone (ADH), which controls the balance of fluids in the body
- Oxytocin, which causes the uterus to contract during and after childbirth

The pituitary gland also produces hormones that regulate the thyroid gland and the adrenal glands. The thyroid gland is located in the neck in front of the larynx. It produces thyroid hormone, which regulates metabolism, the burning of food for heat and energy.

The parathyroid glands secrete a hormone that regulates the body's use of calcium. Nerves and muscles require calcium to function smoothly. A deficiency of this hormone can cause severe muscle contractions and spasms. It can be fatal if untreated.

The pancreas, a gland located in the upper mid-section of the abdomen, secretes insulin. Insulin is a hormone that regulates the amount of sugar (glucose) available to the cells for metabolism. The cells cannot absorb sugar without insulin.

Two adrenal glands are located at the tops of the kidneys. They produce hormones that are essential to life. These hormones are important because they help the body regulate carbohydrate metabolism. They also control the body's reaction to stress and regulate salt and water absorption in the kidneys. Adrenal glands also produce the hormone adrenaline. It regulates muscle power, heart rate, blood pressure, and energy levels during stressful situations or emergencies.

Gonads, or sex glands, produce hormones that regulate the body's ability to reproduce. The testes in the male secrete testosterone. The ovaries in the female secrete estrogen and progesterone.

Normal changes of aging include the following:

- Levels of hormones, such as estrogen and progesterone, decrease.
- Insulin production lessens.
- Body is less able to handle stress.

How You Can Help: NA's Role

Encourage proper nutrition. Try to eliminate or reduce stressors. Stressors are anything that causes stress. Offer encouragement and listen to residents.

Observing and Reporting:
Endocrine System

Observe and report the following signs and symptoms:

- O/R Headache*
- O/R Weakness*
- O/R Blurred vision*
- O/R Dizziness*
- O/R Hunger*
- O/R Irritability*
- O/R Sweating/excessive perspiration*
- O/R Change in "normal" behavior*
- O/R Confusion*
- O/R Weight gain/weight loss
- O/R Loss of appetite/increased appetite
- O/R Increased thirst
- O/R Frequent urination
- O/R Dry skin
- O/R Sluggishness or fatigue
- O/R Hyperactivity

* indicates signs and symptoms that should be reported immediately

10. Describe the reproductive system

The reproductive system is made up of the reproductive organs, which are different in men and women. The reproductive system allows human beings to **reproduce**, or create new human life. Reproduction begins when a male's and female's sex cells (sperm and ovum) join. These sex cells are formed in the male and female sex glands. These sex glands are called the **gonads**.

The Male Reproductive System

In the male, the sex glands or gonads are the testes or testicles. The two oval glands are located outside the body in the scrotum. The scrotum is a sac made of skin and muscle and it is suspended between the thighs. The testes produce the male sex cells, called sperm, and testosterone (Fig. 9-17). Testosterone is the male hormone needed for the reproductive organs to function properly. Testosterone also promotes development of male secondary sex characteristics, which include:

- Facial hair

- Pubic and underarm hair

- Hair on the chest, legs, and arms

- Deepening of the voice

- Development of muscle mass

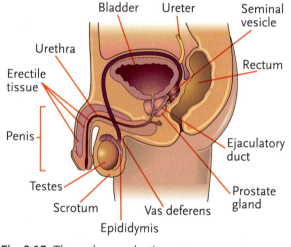

Fig. 9-17. *The male reproductive system.*

Sperm travel from the testes through a coiled tube, the epididymis, and another tube called the vas deferens. Sperm then pass into the seminal vesicle where semen is produced. Semen carries sperm out of the body.

The ducts coming from each seminal vesicle unite to form the ejaculatory ducts. They pass through the prostate gland, where more fluid is added to the semen. In the prostate, the ejaculatory ducts join the urethra, the tube through which both urine and semen pass. The urethra continues through the penis, the sex organ located outside the body, in front of the scrotum. The penis is composed of erectile tissue that

becomes filled with blood during sexual excitement. As the penis fills with blood, it becomes enlarged and erect. It then can enter the vagina, the female reproductive tract, where it releases semen containing sperm.

The Female Reproductive System

In the human female, the gonads are two oval glands called the ovaries. There are two ovaries, one on each side of the uterus (Fig. 9-18). The ovaries make the female sex cells or eggs (ova). They release the female hormones, estrogen and progesterone. Each month from puberty to menopause, an egg is released from an ovary. This cycle is maintained by estrogen and progesterone. These hormones control development of female secondary sex characteristics, which include:

- Increased breast size

- Wider and rounder hips

- Axillary and pubic hair

- A slightly deeper voice

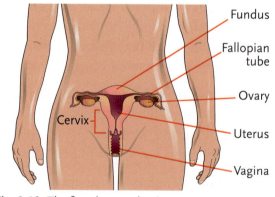

Fig. 9-18. *The female reproductive system.*

Once an egg is released from an ovary, it travels through the fallopian tube to the uterus. The uterus is a hollow, pear-shaped, muscular organ that is located within the pelvis. It lies behind the bladder and in front of the rectum. If sexual intercourse takes place while the egg is in the fallopian tube, the egg may be fertilized by sperm in the fallopian tube. The fertilized egg then travels down into the uterus. It implants in the endometrium, the lining of the uterus. Stimulated by hormones, the endometrium builds up during the menstrual cycle. It has many blood vessels supplying it for the growth and feeding of an embryo. If the egg is not fertilized, the hormones decrease. The blood supply to the endometrium decreases. The endometrium then breaks up in a process called menstruation.

The main section of the uterus is the fundus. This is where a baby develops after the fertilized egg is implanted. The narrow neck of the uterus extending into the vagina is the cervix. The cervix has an opening through which menstrual fluid can pass and semen can enter the vagina. The vagina is the muscular canal that opens to the outside of the body. The external vaginal opening is partially closed by the hymen membrane. The vagina is kept moist by secretions from glands in the vaginal walls. The vagina receives the penis during sexual intercourse. It also serves as the birth canal. The baby passes through the cervix, which is made thin by pressure from the baby's head during contractions. Once the cervix opens, the baby can then move out through the vagina.

Normal changes of aging include the following:

Female

- Menstruation ends. Menopause is when a female stops having menstrual periods.
- Decrease in estrogen may lead to a loss of calcium. This can cause brittle bones and, potentially, osteoporosis.
- Vaginal walls become drier and thinner.

Male

- Sperm production decreases.
- Prostate gland enlarges.

How You Can Help: NA's Role

Sexual needs and desires continue as people age. Provide privacy when necessary for sexual activity. Respect your residents' sexual needs. Never make

fun of or judge any sexual behavior. Do report any behavior that makes you uncomfortable or seems inappropriate. Inappropriate behavior is not a normal sign of aging, and could be a sign of illness.

Observing and Reporting:
Reproductive System

Observe and report the following signs and symptoms:

- O/R Discomfort or difficulty with urination
- O/R Discharge from the penis or vagina
- O/R Swelling of the genitals
- O/R Changes in menstruation
- O/R Blood in urine or stool
- O/R Breast changes, including size, shape, lumps, or discharge from the nipple
- O/R Sores on the genitals
- O/R Resident reports of impotence, or inability of male to have sexual intercourse
- O/R Resident reports of painful intercourse

Residents' Rights

Sexual Expression and Privacy

Residents have the right to sexual freedom and expression. Residents have the right to privacy and to meet their sexual needs.

11. Describe the immune and lymphatic systems

The immune system protects the body from disease-causing bacteria, viruses, and organisms in two ways. **Nonspecific immunity** protects the body from disease in general. **Specific immunity** protects against a particular disease that is invading the body at a given time.

Nonspecific Immunity

To protect itself against disease in general, the body has several defenses:

- Anatomic barriers include the skin and the mucous membranes. They provide a physical barrier to keep foreign materials—bacteria, viruses, or organisms—from invading the body. Saliva, tears, and mucous secretions also help protect the body by washing away substances.

- Physiologic barriers include body temperature and acidity of certain organs. Most organisms that cause disease cannot survive high temperatures or high acidity. When the body senses foreign organisms, it can raise its temperature (by running a fever) to kill off the invaders. The acidity of organs like the stomach keeps harmful bacteria from growing there.

- Inflammatory response refers to the body's ability to fight infection by inflammation or swelling of an infected area. When inflammation occurs, it indicates that the body has sent extra disease-fighting cells and extra blood to the infected area to fight the infection.

Specific Immunity

To protect itself against specific diseases, the body makes different types of cells that will fight a range of different invaders. Once it has successfully eliminated an invader, the immune system records the invasion in the form of antibodies. Antibodies are carried within cells. They prevent a disease from threatening the body a second time.

Acquired immunity is a kind of specific immunity. The body acquires it either by fighting an infection or by vaccination. For example, you can acquire immunity to a disease like the measles in two ways:

1. You get the measles. Your body forms antibodies to the disease to make sure you will not get it again; or

2. You get a vaccine for the measles. This causes your body to produce the same antibodies to protect you from the disease.

The lymphatic system removes excess fluids and waste products from the body's tissues. It also helps the immune system fight infection. It is closely related to both the immune and the circulatory systems (Fig. 9-19). The lymphatic system consists of lymph vessels and lymph capillaries in which a fluid called lymph circulates. **Lymph** is a clear yellowish fluid that carries disease-fighting cells called lymphocytes.

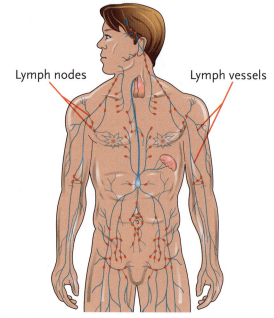

Lymph nodes   Lymph vessels

Fig. 9-19. *Lymph nodes are located throughout the body.*

When the body is fighting an infection, swelling may occur in the lymph nodes. These are oval-shaped bodies that can be as small as a pinhead or as large as an almond. Located in the neck, groin, and armpits, the lymph nodes filter out germs and waste products carried from the tissues by the lymph fluid. After lymph fluid has been purified in the lymph nodes, it flows into the bloodstream.

Unlike the circulatory system, in which the heart functions as a pump to move the blood, the lymph system has no pump. Lymph fluid is circulated by muscle activity, massage, and breathing. A sore muscle may feel better if you rub it. The rubbing action helps the lymph fluid circulate, carrying waste products away from the tired muscle.

Normal changes of aging include the following:

- Immune system weakens, increasing the risk of all types of infections

- Decreased response to vaccines

How You Can Help: NA's Role

Follow rules for preventing infection. Wash hands often. Keep the resident's environment clean to prevent infection. Encourage and help with good personal hygiene. Encourage proper nutrition and fluid intake to help residents stay healthy. A slight temperature increase may indicate that a person is fighting an infection. Take accurate vital sign measurements.

Observing and Reporting:
Immune and Lymphatic Systems

Observe and report these signs and symptoms:

- O/R Recurring infections (such as fevers and diarrhea)

- O/R Swelling of the lymph nodes

- O/R Increased fatigue

Chapter Review

1. What is homeostasis?

2. What are three functions of the skin, or integument?

3. List ten signs and symptoms to observe and report about the integumentary system.

4. How many bones make up the skeleton of the human body?

5. What type of exercises can help prevent contractures and muscle atrophy?

6. List five signs and symptoms to observe and report about the musculoskeletal system.

7. What are two functions of the nervous system?

8. List ten signs and symptoms to observe and report about the central nervous system.

9. List three signs and symptoms to observe and report about the eyes and ears.

10. What are four functions of the cardiovascular system?

11. List seven signs and symptoms to observe and report about the cardiovascular system.

12. What does "respiration" mean? What are the two parts involved in respiration?

13. List seven signs and symptoms to observe and report about the respiratory system.

14. What are two functions of the urinary system?

15. List seven signs and symptoms to observe and report about the urinary system.

16. What does digestion mean? What does elimination mean?

17. List nine signs and symptoms to observe and report about the gastrointestinal system.

18. List eight signs and symptoms to observe and report immediately about the endocrine system.

19. What is the function of the reproductive system?

20. List seven signs and symptoms to observe and report about the reproductive system.

21. What is nonspecific immunity? What is specific immunity?

22. What is the function of the lymphatic system?

23. List three signs and symptoms to observe and report about the immune and lymphatic systems.

10
Positioning, Lifting, and Moving

1. Review the principles of body mechanics

This chapter deals with moving and positioning residents. It is important to always use good body mechanics when assisting with moving or positioning. This helps prevent injury and protects both you and your residents. You first learned about body mechanics in Chapter 6. The following guidelines will help you review what you have learned to remember to use good body mechanics:

Guidelines:
Proper Body Mechanics

G   Assess the load. Before lifting, assess the weight of the load. Determine if you can safely move the object without help. Know the lift policies at your facility. Never attempt to lift someone you are not sure you can lift.

G   Think ahead, plan, and communicate the move. Check for any objects in your path. Look for any potential risks, such as a wet floor. Make sure the path is clear. Watch for hazards, such as high-traffic areas, combative residents, or loose toilet seats or hand rails. Decide exactly what you and the resident are going to do together. Agree on the verbal cues you will use before attempting to transfer.

G   Check your base of support. Be sure you have firm footing. Use a wide but balanced stance to increase support. Keep this stance when walking. Make sure you and your resident are wearing non-skid shoes.

G   Face what you are lifting. Your feet should always face the direction you are moving. Do not twist; twisting at the waist increases the likelihood of injury. Twisting should always be avoided. Turn and face the area you are moving the object to, then set the object down.

G   Keep your back straight, your head up, and your shoulders back. This will keep the back in the proper position. Take a deep breath to help you regain correct posture.

G   Begin in a squatting position. Bend at the hips and knees. Use the strength of your leg muscles to stand and lift the object. You will need to push your buttocks out to do this. Before you stand with the object you are lifting, remember that your legs, not your back, will enable you to lift. You should be able to feel your leg muscles working. Lifting with the large leg muscles decreases stress on your back.

G   Tighten your stomach muscles when beginning the lift. This will help to take weight off the spine and maintain alignment.

G   Keep the object close to your body. This decreases stress to your back. Lift objects to your waist. Carrying them any higher can affect your balance.

G   Push or pull when possible rather than lifting. When you lift an object, you must overcome gravity to balance the load. Try to push or pull the object instead. Then you only need to overcome the friction between the surface and the object. Use your body weight to move the object, not your lifting muscles. Push rather than pull whenever possible. Stay close to the object.

2. Explain beginning and ending steps in care procedures

Within most care procedures, there are beginning and ending steps that need to be repeated. Understanding why each step is important will help you remember to perform it every time care is provided.

Beginning Steps

Wash your hands. Handwashing provides for infection control. Nothing fights infection like consistent, proper handwashing.

Identify yourself by name. Identify the resident by name. Residents have the right to know the identity of their caregivers. Addressing residents by name shows respect (Fig. 10-1). It also establishes correct identification. This prevents care from being performed on the wrong person.

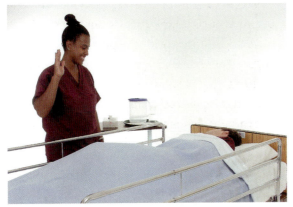

Fig. 10-1. Addressing resident by name shows respect and establishes correct identification. This must be done each time before care is performed.

Explain procedure to the resident. Speak clearly, slowly, and directly. Maintain face-to-face contact whenever possible. Residents have a legal right to know exactly what care you will provide. Doing this also promotes understanding, cooperation, and independence. Encouraging residents' independence is important. Residents are more able to do things for themselves if they know what needs to happen.

Provide for the resident's privacy with curtain, screen, or door. Doing this maintains residents' rights to privacy and dignity. Providing for privacy is not simply a courtesy; it is a legal right.

If the bed is adjustable, adjust bed to a safe level, usually waist high. If the bed is movable, lock bed wheels. This prevents injury to you and to residents. Locking bed wheels is an important safety measure. It ensures that the bed will not move as you are performing care.

Ending Steps

Make resident comfortable. Make sure sheets are free from wrinkles and the bed free from crumbs. Sheets that are damp, wrinkled, or bunched up are uncomfortable. They may prevent the resident from resting or sleeping well. Sheets that do not lie flat under the resident's body increase the risk of pressure sores because they cut off circulation. Other comfort measures include replacing bedding and pillows.

Return bed to lowest position. Remove privacy measures. Lowering the bed provides for residents' safety. Remove any extra privacy measures added during the procedure. This includes anything you may have draped over and around residents, as well as privacy screens.

Before leaving, place call light within resident's reach. A call light allows residents to communicate with staff as necessary. Remember that the decision not to respond to a call light is considered neglect. Unless residents are on fluid restrictions, provide fresh water before leaving the room. Keeping beverages close by encourages residents to drink more often. Make sure that the pitcher and cup are light enough for residents to lift.

Wash your hands. Again, handwashing is the most important thing you can to do to prevent the spread of infection. Always wash your hands after removing gloves and other PPE.

Report any changes in resident to the nurse. Reporting promptly and accurately provides the nurse with information to assess resident. Care plans are made based on your reports.

Document procedure using facility guidelines. What you write is a legal record of what you did. If you do not document it, legally it did not happen.

3. Explain positioning and describe how to safely position residents

Residents who spend a lot of time in bed often need help getting into comfortable positions. They also need to change positions periodically to avoid muscle stiffness and skin breakdown or pressure sores. Too much pressure on one area for too long can cause a decrease in circulation, which can lead to the formation of pressure sores, a serious condition. You will learn much more about pressure sores and prevention guidelines in Chapter 13.

Positioning means helping residents into positions that will be comfortable and healthy for them. Bed-bound residents should be repositioned at least every two hours. Document the position and time every time there is a change. Which positions a resident uses will depend on the diagnosis, the condition, and the resident's preference. The care plan will give specific instructions. Always keep principles of body mechanics and alignment in mind when positioning residents. Also, check skin for whiteness or redness, especially around bony areas, each time you reposition a resident.

The following are tips for positioning residents in the five basic body positions:

1. In the **supine** position, the resident lies flat on his back. To maintain correct body position, support the head and shoulders with a pillow

(Fig. 10-2). You may also use pillows, rolled towels, or washcloths to support his arms (especially a weak or immobilized arm) or hands. The heels should be "floating." This means you must place a firm pillow under the calves so the heels do not touch the bed. Pillows or a footboard can be used to keep the feet flexed.

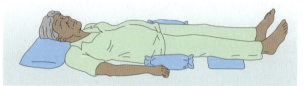

Fig. 10-2. *A person in the supine position is lying flat on his or her back.*

2. A resident in the **lateral** position is lying on either side. There are many variations in this position. Pillows can be used to support the arm and leg on the upper side, the back, and the head (Fig. 10-3). Ideally, the knee on the upper side of the body should be flexed. The leg is brought in front of the body and supported on a pillow. There should be a pillow under the bottom foot so that the toes are not touching the bed. If the top leg cannot be brought forward, it rests on the bottom leg. Pillows should be used between the two legs. This relieves pressure and helps to avoid skin breakdown.

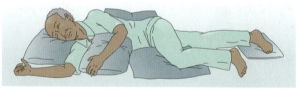

Fig. 10-3. *A person in the lateral position is lying on his or her side.*

3. A resident in the **prone** position is lying on the stomach, or front side of the body (Fig. 10-4). This is not comfortable for many people, especially elderly people. Never leave a resident in a prone position for very long. In this position, the arms are either at the sides or raised above the head. The head is turned to one side. A small pillow may be used under the head and under the legs. This keeps the feet from touching the bed.

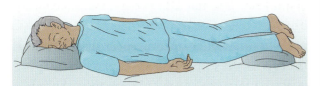

Fig. 10-4. *A person lying in the prone position is lying on his or her stomach.*

4. A resident in the **Fowler's** position is in a semi-sitting position (45 to 60 degrees). The head and shoulders are elevated. The resident's knees may be flexed and elevated using a pillow or rolled blanket as a support (Fig. 10-5). The feet may be flexed and supported using a footboard or other support. The spine should be straight. In a true Fowler's position, the upper body is raised halfway between sitting straight up and lying flat. In a high Fowler's position, the head is raised 80 to 90 degrees. In a semi-Fowler's position, head is elevated 30 to 45 degrees.

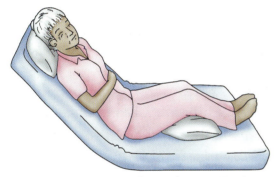

Fig. 10-5. *A person lying in the Fowler's position is partially reclined.*

5. The **Sims'** position is a left side-lying position. The lower arm is behind the back and the upper knee is flexed and raised toward the chest, using a pillow as support. There should be a pillow under the bottom foot so that the toes are not touching the bed (Fig. 10-6).

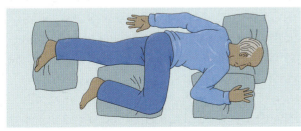

Fig. 10-6. *A person in the Sims' position is lying on his or her left side with one leg drawn up.*

Helping a resident sit up using the arm lock

1. Wash your hands.

2. Identify yourself by name. Identify the resident by name.

3. Explain procedure to the resident. Speak clearly, slowly, and directly. Maintain face-to-face contact whenever possible.

4. Provide for the resident's privacy with curtain, screen, or door.

5. If the bed is adjustable, adjust bed to a safe level, usually waist high. Lock bed wheels (Fig. 10-7).

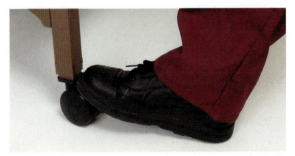

Fig. 10-7. *Always lock bed wheels if bed is movable before positioning or transferring a resident.*

6. Stand facing the head of the bed, with your legs about 12 inches apart and your knees bent. The foot that is further from the bed should be slightly ahead of the other foot (Fig. 10-8).

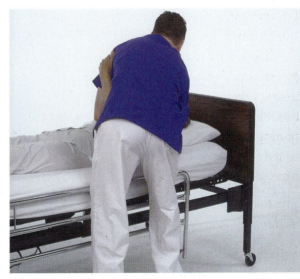

Fig. 10-8.

7. Place your arm under the resident's armpit and grasp the resident's shoulder. Have the resident grasp your shoulder in the same manner. This hold is called the **arm lock** or **lock arm** (Fig. 10-9).

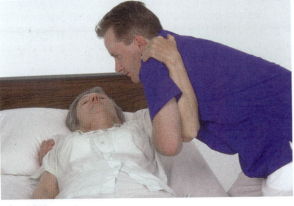

Fig. 10-9.

8. Reach under the resident's head and place your other hand on the resident's far shoulder. Have the resident bend her knees. Bend your knees.

9. At the count of three, rock yourself backward and pull the resident to a sitting position. Use pillows or a bed rest to support the resident in the sitting position.

10. Check the resident for dizziness or weakness.

11. Make resident comfortable. Make sure sheets are free from wrinkles and the bed free from crumbs.

12. Return bed to lowest position. Remove privacy measures.

13. Place call light within resident's reach.

14. Wash your hands.

15. Report any changes in resident to the nurse.

16. Document procedure using facility guidelines.

Helping a resident move up in bed helps prevent skin irritation that can lead to pressure sores. You can use a helper if one is available. Get help if you think it is not safe to move the resident by yourself. If a resident is unable to help you, use a draw sheet or turning sheet (Fig. 10-10). A **draw sheet** is an extra sheet placed on top of the bottom sheet. It allows you to reposition the resident without causing shearing. **Shearing** is rubbing or friction that results from the skin moving one way and the bone underneath it remaining fixed or moving in the opposite direction.

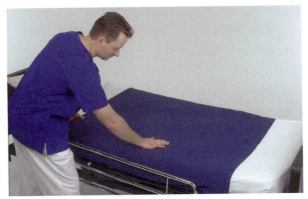

Fig. 10-10. A draw sheet is a special sheet (or a regular bed sheet folded in half) that is used to help move residents in bed without causing shearing on the skin.

Moving a resident up in bed

For residents who can help you move them up in bed, follow these steps:

1. Wash your hands.

2. Identify yourself by name. Identify the resident by name.

3. Explain procedure to the resident. Speak clearly, slowly, and directly. Maintain face-to-face contact whenever possible.

4. Provide for the resident's privacy with curtain, screen, or door.

5. If the bed is adjustable, adjust bed to a safe level, usually waist high. Lock bed wheels.

6. Lower the head of bed to make it flat. Remove the pillow from under the head and place it standing upright against the head of the bed.

7. If the bed has side rails, raise the rail on the far side of the bed.

8. Stand by bed with your feet apart, facing the resident.

9. Place one arm under resident's shoulder blades. Place the other arm under resident's thighs. Use good body mechanics.

10. Ask resident to bend her knees, brace feet on the mattress, and push her feet and hands on the count of three (Fig. 10-11).

11. On the count of three, shift your body weight, and help move resident while she pushes with her feet. Always allow her to do all she can for herself.

12. Make resident comfortable and replace pillow under resident's head. Make sure sheets are free from wrinkles and the bed free from crumbs.

13. Return bed to lowest position. Remove privacy measures.

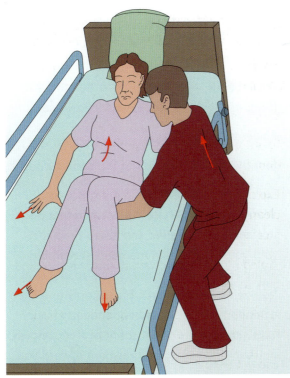

Fig. 10-11. *Keep your back straight and your knees bent.*

14. Place call light within resident's reach.

15. Wash your hands.

16. Report any changes in resident to the nurse.

17. Document procedure using facility guidelines.

When the resident cannot assist and there is no one else around to help you move her up in bed, follow these steps:

1. Follow steps 1 through 6 above.

2. Stand behind the head of the bed with your feet shoulder-width apart and one foot slightly in front of the other.

3. Roll and grasp the top edge of the draw sheet.

4. With your knees bent and your back straight, rock your weight from the front foot to the back foot in one smooth motion (Fig. 10-12).

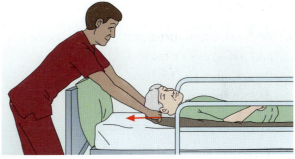

Fig. 10-12.

5. Make resident comfortable and replace pillow under resident's head. Unroll the draw sheet and leave it in place for the next repositioning.

6. Return bed to lowest position. Remove privacy measures.

7. Place call light within resident's reach.

8. Wash your hands.

9. Report any changes in resident to the nurse.

10. Document procedure using facility guidelines.

When you have help from another person, you can modify the procedure as follows:

1. Follow steps 1 through 6 above.

2. Stand on the opposite side of the bed from your helper. Each of you should be turned slightly toward the head of the bed. For each of you, the foot that is closest to the head of the bed should be pointed in that direction. Stand with your feet shoulder-width apart and bend your knees slightly.

3. Roll the draw sheet up to the resident's side, and have your helper do the same on his side of the bed. Grasp the sheet with your palms up, and have your helper do the same.

4. Shift your weight to your back foot (the foot closer to the foot of the bed) and have your helper do the same (Fig. 10-13). On the count of three, you and your helper both shift your weight to your forward feet as you slide the draw sheet toward the head of the bed (Fig. 10-14).

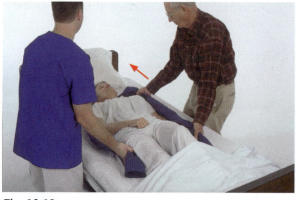

Fig. 10-13.

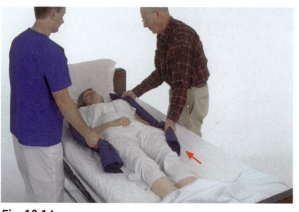

Fig. 10-14.

5. Make resident comfortable and replace pillow under the head. Unroll the draw sheet and leave it in place for the next repositioning.

6. Return bed to lowest position. Remove privacy measures.

7. Place call light within resident's reach.

8. Wash your hands.

9. Report any changes in resident to the nurse.

10. Document procedure using facility guidelines.

Moving a resident to the side of the bed

Equipment: draw sheet

1. Wash your hands.

2. Identify yourself by name. Identify the resident by name.

3. Explain procedure to the resident. Speak clearly, slowly, and directly. Maintain face-to-face contact whenever possible.

4. Provide for the resident's privacy with curtain, screen, or door.

5. If the bed is adjustable, adjust bed to a safe level, usually waist high. Lock bed wheels.

6. Lower the head of bed.

7. Stand on the same side of the bed to where you are moving the resident.

8. **With a draw sheet**: Roll the draw sheet up to the resident's side, and grasp the sheet with your palms up. One hand should be at the resident's shoulders, the other about level with the resident's hips. Apply one knee against the side of the bed, and lean back with your body. On the count of three, slowly pull the draw sheet and resident toward you.

   Without a draw sheet: Gently slide your hands under the head and shoulders and move toward you (Fig. 10-15). Gently slide your hands under the midsection and move toward you. Gently slide your hands under the hips and legs and move them toward you (Fig. 10-16).

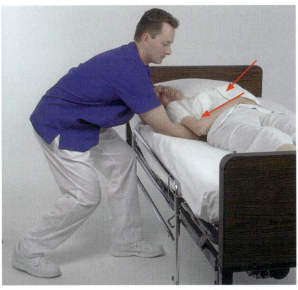

Fig. 10-15.

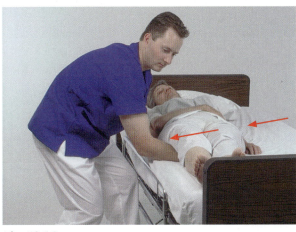

Fig. 10-16.

9. Make resident comfortable. Make sure sheets are free from wrinkles and the bed free from crumbs.

10. Return bed to lowest position. Remove privacy measures.

11. Place call light within resident's reach.

12. Wash your hands.

13. Report any changes in resident to the nurse.

14. Document procedure using facility guidelines.

Residents may be turned on their sides in preparation for sitting up or to change position and take pressure off their backs. This helps prevent skin irritation and pressure sores.

Turning a resident

1. Wash your hands.

2. Identify yourself by name. Identify the resident by name.

3. Explain procedure to the resident. Speak clearly, slowly, and directly. Maintain face-to-face contact whenever possible.

4. Provide for the resident's privacy with curtain, screen, or door.

5. If the bed is adjustable, adjust bed to a safe level, usually waist high. Lock bed wheels.

6. Lower the head of bed.

7. Stand on side of bed opposite to where resident will be turned. If the bed has side rails, raise the far side rail. Lower side rail nearest you if it is up.

8. Move resident to side of bed nearest you using previous procedure.

9. *Turning resident away from you:*

a. Cross resident's arm over his or her chest. Move arm on side resident is being turned to out of the way. Cross the leg nearest you over the far leg (Fig. 10-17).

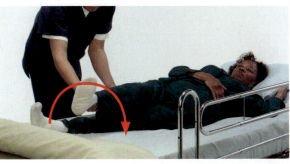

Fig. 10-17.

b. Stand with feet about 12 inches apart. Bend your knees.

c. Place one hand on the resident's shoulder. Place the other hand on the resident's nearest hip.

d. Gently push the resident toward the other side of the bed. Shift your weight from your back leg to your front leg (Fig. 10-18).

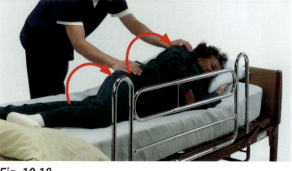

Fig. 10-18.

Turning resident toward you:

a. Cross resident's arm over his or her chest. Move arm on side resident is being turned to out of the way. Cross the leg furthest from you over the near leg.

b. Stand with feet about 12 inches apart. Bend your knees.

c. Place one hand on the resident's far shoulder. Place the other hand on the far hip.

d. Gently roll the resident toward you (Fig. 10-19). Your body will block resident and prevent her from rolling out of bed.

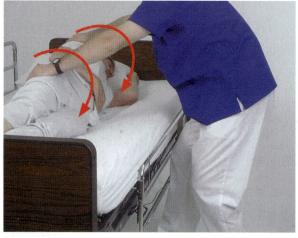

Fig. 10-19.

10. Position the resident properly and comfortably, in good alignment. Proper positioning includes the following:

- head supported by pillow

- shoulder adjusted so resident is not lying on arm

- top arm supported by pillow

- back supported by supportive device

- top knee flexed

- supportive device between legs with top knee flexed; knee and ankle supported

11. Make resident comfortable. Make sure sheets are free from wrinkles and the bed free from crumbs.

12. Return bed to lowest position. Remove privacy measures.

13. Place call light within resident's reach.

14. Wash your hands.

15. Report any changes in resident to the nurse.

16. Document procedure using facility guidelines.

Some residents' spinal columns must be kept in alignment. To turn these residents in bed, you will use a procedure called logrolling. **Logrolling** means moving a resident as a unit, without disturbing the alignment of the body. The head, back, and legs must be kept in a straight line. This is necessary in cases of neck or back problems, spinal cord injuries, or after back or hip surgeries. It is safer for two people to perform this procedure together. A draw sheet assists with moving.

Logrolling a resident with one assistant

Equipment: draw sheet, co-worker

1. Wash your hands.

2. Identify yourself by name. Identify the resident by name.

3. Explain procedure to the resident. Speak clearly, slowly, and directly. Maintain face-to-face contact whenever possible.

4. Provide for the resident's privacy with curtain, screen, or door.

5. If the bed is adjustable, adjust bed to a safe level, usually waist high. Lock bed wheels.

6. Lower the head of bed to make it flat.

7. If the bed has side rails and they are raised, lower the side rail on side closest to you.

8. Both workers stand on the same side of the bed. One person stands at the resident's head and shoulders. The other stands near the resident's midsection.

9. Place the resident's arms across his or her chest. Place a pillow between the knees.

10. Stand with your feet about 12 inches apart. Bend your knees.

11. Grasp the draw sheet on the far side (Fig. 10-20).

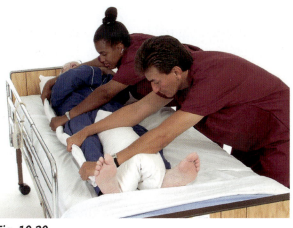

Fig. 10-20.

12. On the count of three, gently roll the resident toward you. Turn the resident as a unit (Fig. 10-21).

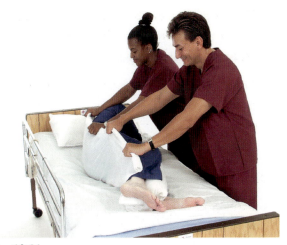

Fig. 10-21.

13. Make resident comfortable. Make sure sheets are free from wrinkles and the bed free from crumbs.

14. Return bed to lowest position. Return side rails to ordered position. Remove privacy measures.

15. Place call light within resident's reach.

16. Wash your hands.

17. Report any changes in resident to the nurse.

18. Document procedure using facility guidelines.

Before a resident who has been lying down moves to a standing position, she should dangle. To **dangle** means to sit up with the feet over the side of the bed for a moment to regain balance. It gives the resident time to adjust to being in an upright position after lying down. For some residents who are unable to walk, dangling the legs for a few minutes may be ordered.

Assisting a resident to sit up on side of bed: dangling

1. Wash your hands.

2. Identify yourself by name. Identify the resident by name.

3. Explain procedure to the resident. Speak clearly, slowly, and directly. Maintain face-to-face contact whenever possible.

4. Provide for the resident's privacy with curtain, screen, or door.

5. Adjust bed height to lowest position. Lock bed wheels.

6. Fanfold (fold into pleats) the top covers to the foot of the bed. Ask the resident to turn onto her side, facing you. Assist as needed (a procedure earlier in this chapter describes how to help a resident turn over).

7. Tell the resident to reach across her chest with her top arm and place her hand on the edge of the bed near her opposite shoulder. Ask her to push down on that hand to raise her shoulders up while swinging her legs over the side of the bed (Fig. 10-22).

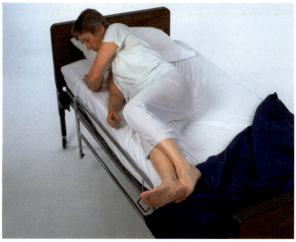

Fig. 10-22.

8. Always allow the resident to do all she can for herself. However, if the resident needs assistance, raise the head of the bed to a sitting position.

9. Stand with your legs about 12 inches apart, with one foot six to eight inches in front of the other. Bend your knees.

10. Place one arm under resident's shoulder blades. Place the other arm under resident's thighs (Fig. 10-23).

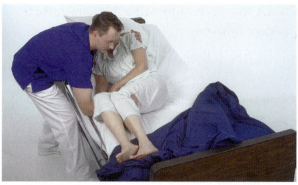

Fig. 10-23.

11. On the count of three, slowly turn resident into sitting position with legs dangling over side of bed. The weight of the resident's legs hanging down from the bed helps the resident sit up (Fig. 10-24).

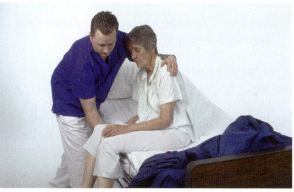

Fig. 10-24.

12. Ask resident to hold onto the edge of mattress with both hands. Assist resident to put on non-skid shoes or slippers.

13. Have resident dangle as long as ordered. The care plan may direct you to allow the resident to dangle for several minutes and then return her to lying down, or it may direct you to allow the resident to dangle in preparation for walking or a transfer. Follow the instructions in the care plan. Do not leave the resident alone. If the resident is dizzy for more than a minute, have her lie down again and report to the nurse.

14. Take vital signs as ordered (you will learn how to take vital signs in Chapter 14).

15. Remove slippers or shoes.

16. Gently assist resident back into bed. Place one arm around resident's shoulders. Place the other under resident's knees. Slowly swing resident's legs onto bed.

17. Make resident comfortable. Make sure sheets are free from wrinkles and the bed free from crumbs.

18. Leave bed in lowest position. Remove privacy measures.

19. Place call light within resident's reach.

20. Wash your hands.

21. Report any changes in resident to the nurse.

22. Document procedure using facility guidelines.

Residents' Rights

Moving, Lifting and Transferring

When moving, lifting, and transferring residents, make sure they are not unnecessarily exposed. Keep them properly covered, dressed, or draped to protect their privacy and to promote dignity. Pull the privacy curtain around the bed when moving residents in bed.

4. Describe how to safely transfer residents

Transferring a resident means that you are moving him from one place to another. Transfers can move a resident from a wheelchair to a bed or stretcher, from a bed to a chair, from a wheelchair to a shower or toilet, and so on.

Safety is one of the most important things to consider during transfers. In 2002, OSHA announced new ergonomic guidelines for transfers. **Ergonomics** is the science of designing equipment and work tasks to suit the worker's abilities. OSHA now says that manual lifting of residents should be reduced in all cases and eliminated when possible. Manual lifting, transferring, and repositioning of residents may increase risks of pain and injury.

To that end, many facilities today have adopted "zero-lift" or "lift-free" policies. These policies set strict guidelines for lifting and transferring of residents. Lift-free polices vary; facilities decide how they want to address reducing lifting and transferring of residents. Some allow no lifting at all and require that mechanical equipment be used on every resident who needs to be transferred.

The more restrictions placed on lifting, the less chance there is of injury. The amount and type of equipment available also factor into reducing workplace injuries. This learning objective teaches procedures for manual lifting and transferring of residents. It is important for nursing assistants to carefully follow facility policies on lifting and to use equipment properly. If you are unsure how to use equipment, ask for help. Always get help when you need it.

A **transfer belt** is a safety device used to transfer residents who are weak, unsteady, or uncoordinated. It is called a **gait belt** when used to help residents walk. The belt is made of canvas or other heavy material. It sometimes has handles and fits around the resident's waist outside the clothing. The transfer belt is a safety device that gives you something firm to hold on to. Transfer belts cannot be used if a resident has fragile bones or recent fractures.

Residents' Rights

Communicate!

Any time you help residents transfer, talk to them about what you would like to do. Promote their independence by letting them do what they can. The two of you must work together, especially during transfers.

Applying a transfer belt

1. Wash your hands.

2. Identify yourself by name. Identify the resident by name.

3. Explain procedure to the resident. Speak clearly, slowly, and directly. Maintain face-to-face contact whenever possible.

4. Provide for the resident's privacy with curtain, screen, or door.

5. Assist the resident to a sitting position.

6. Place the belt over the resident's clothing and around the waist. Do not put it over bare skin.

7. Tighten the buckle until it is snug. Leave enough room to insert two fingers comfortably into the belt.

8. Check to make sure that a female's breasts are not caught under the belt.

9. For comfort, place the buckle off-center in the front or back.

A **slide** or **transfer board** may be used to help transfer residents who are unable to bear weight on their legs. Slide boards can be used for almost any transfer that involves moving from one sitting position to another. For example, slide boards can be helpful for transfers from bed to chair or wheelchair to car (Fig. 10-25.)

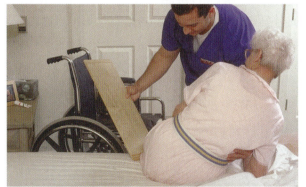

Fig. 10-25. *A sliding board can help with bed-to-chair transfers.*

Guidelines:
Wheelchairs

G   Learn how each wheelchair works. Residents may use manual (require human power to move them) or electric wheelchairs. Know how to apply and release the brake and how to operate the armrests and footrests. Always lock a wheelchair before helping a resident into or out of it (Fig. 10-26). After a transfer, unlock the wheelchair.

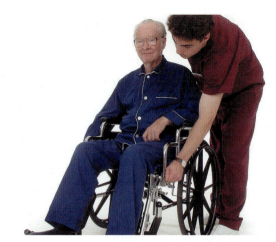

Fig. 10-26. *You must always lock the wheelchair before a resident gets into or out of it.*

G   To unfold a standard wheelchair, tilt the chair slightly to raise the wheels on the opposite side. Press down on one or both seat rails until the chair opens and the seat is flat. To fold a standard wheelchair, lift up under the center edge of the seat.

G   To remove an armrest, release the arm lock by the armrest, and lift the arm from the center. To replace the armrest, simply reverse the procedure.

G   To move a footrest out of the way, press or pull the release lever and swing the footrest out towards the side of the wheelchair. To remove the footrest, lift it off when it is towards the side of the wheelchair (Fig. 10-27). To replace a footrest, simply put it back in the side position, then swing it back to the front position, where it should lock into place.

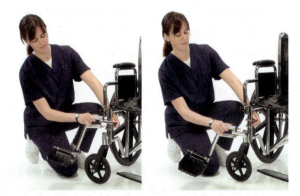

Fig. 10-27. *To remove a footrest, swing the footrest toward the side of the wheelchair and lift it off.*

G To transfer to or from a wheelchair, the resident must use the side or areas of the body that can bear weight to support and lift the side or areas that cannot bear weight. Residents who can bear no weight with their legs may use leg braces or an overhead trapeze to support themselves during transfers.

G Before any transfer, make sure the resident is wearing non-skid footwear which is securely fastened. This promotes residents' safety and reduces the risk of falls.

G During wheelchair transfers make sure the resident is safe and comfortable. Ask the resident how you can assist. Some may only want you to bring the chair to the bedside. Others may want you to be more involved. Always be sure the chair is as close as possible to the resident and is locked in place. Use a transfer belt if you are going to assist with the transfer. Be sure the transfer is done slowly, allowing time for the resident to rest. Check the resident's alignment in the chair when the transfer is complete.

G When a resident is in a wheelchair, he or she should be repositioned every two hours or as needed. The reasons for doing this are:

- It promotes comfort.
- It reduces pressure.
- It increases circulation.
- It exercises the joints.
- It promotes muscle tone.

G The resident's body should be kept in good alignment while in the wheelchair. Special cushions, pillows, and soft blankets can be used for support. The hips should be positioned well back in the chair. If the resident needs to be moved back in the wheelchair, go to the back of the chair. Gently reach forward and down under the resident's arms. Ask the resident to place his feet on the ground and push up. Gently pull the resident up in the chair while the resident pushes.

Falls

Remember the following tips if a resident starts to fall during a transfer:

- Widen your stance. Bring the resident's body close to you to break the fall. Bend your knees and support the resident as you lower her to the floor. You may need to drop to the floor with the resident to avoid injury to you or the resident.
- Do not try to reverse or stop a fall. You or the resident can be injured if you try to stop a fall rather than break the fall.
- Call for help. Do not try to get the resident up after the fall.

Some residents have one-sided weakness due to paralysis or stroke. When transferring these residents, move their stronger side first. The weaker (also called "involved" or "affected") side follows.

Transferring a resident from bed to wheelchair

Equipment: wheelchair, transfer belt, non-skid footwear

1. Wash your hands.
2. Identify yourself by name. Identify the resident by name.
3. Explain procedure to the resident. Speak clearly, slowly, and directly. Maintain face-to-face contact whenever possible.
4. Provide for the resident's privacy with curtain, screen, or door. Check the area to be certain it is uncluttered and safe.
5. Remove wheelchair footrests close to the bed.
6. Place wheelchair near the head of the bed with arm of the wheelchair almost touching the bed. The wheelchair should be placed on resident's stronger, or unaffected, side.
7. Lock wheelchair wheels.
8. Raise the head of the bed. Adjust bed level so that the height of the bed is equal to or slightly higher than the chair. Lock bed wheels.
9. Assist resident to sitting position with feet flat on the floor.

10. Put non-skid footwear on resident and fasten.

11. **With transfer (gait) belt:**

a. Stand in front of resident.

b. Stand with feet about 12 inches apart. Bend your knees.

c. Place belt around resident's waist. Grasp belt securely on both sides.

Without transfer belt:

a. Stand in front of resident.

b. Stand with feet about 12 inches apart. Bend your knees.

c. Place your arms around resident's torso under the arms. Ask resident to use the bed to push up (or your shoulders, if possible).

12. Provide instructions to allow resident to help with transfer. Instructions may include:

"When you start to stand, push with your hands against the bed."

"Once standing, if you're able, you can take small steps in the direction of the chair."

"Once standing, reach for the chair with your stronger hand."

13. With your legs, brace resident's lower legs to prevent slipping (Fig. 10-28).

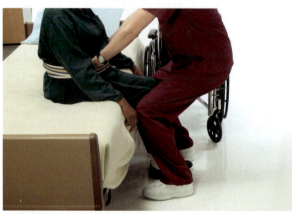

Fig. 10-28. *Use your legs to brace the resident's lower legs to prevent slipping.*

14. Count to three to alert resident. On three, slowly help resident to stand.

15. Tell the resident to take small steps in the direction of the chair while turning her back toward the chair. If more assistance is needed, help the resident to pivot to front of wheelchair with back of resident's legs against wheelchair (Fig. 10-29). Always allow the resident to do all she can for herself.

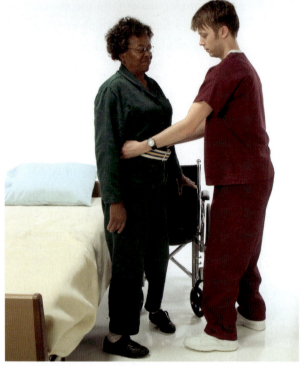

Fig. 10-29. *Pivoting is safer than twisting.*

16. Ask the resident to put hands on wheelchair arm rests if able. When the chair is touching the back of the resident's legs, help the resident lower herself into the chair.

17. Reposition resident with hips touching back of wheelchair. Remove transfer belt, if used.

18. Attach footrests and place the resident's feet on the footrests. Check that the resident is in good alignment. Make resident comfortable. Place a lap robe or folded blanket over the resident's lap as appropriate.

19. Remove privacy measures.

20. Place call light within resident's reach.

21. Wash your hands.

22. Report any changes in resident to the nurse.

Positioning, Lifting, and Moving

23. Document procedure using facility guidelines.

Stretchers

A stretcher, also called a gurney, is a medical device used to move injured or ill persons from one place to another. Stretchers may be used for serious injuries and illnesses and/or when a person cannot or should not walk but needs to be transported somewhere. Stretchers transfer residents within facilities or to other facilities.

Guidelines:
Safe Use of a Stretchers

G Lock the stretcher wheels before transferring a resident onto or off of a stretcher.

G Secure resident with the safety belt while in the stretcher.

G Raise the safety rails.

G Cover the resident with a sheet. Hands, feet, fingers, etc. should remain inside the sheet during transport.

G Keep the wheels locked at all times except when moving the stretcher.

G Get help if you cannot move the stretcher alone.

G Move slowly and carefully.

G Push the stretcher from the head end.

G Go through doorways by opening the door, entering first, and pulling the stretcher through.

G Avoid hitting walls or doorways.

G Be cautious going down sloping areas.

G Stay with the resident at all times.

A draw sheet is used to transfer a resident to a stretcher. The next procedure shows how to transfer a resident to a stretcher from a bed using four workers. At least three workers are necessary to safely transfer a resident to a stretcher.

1. Wash your hands.

2. Identify yourself by name. Identify the resident by name.

3. Explain procedure to the resident. Speak clearly, slowly, and directly. Maintain face-to-face contact whenever possible.

4. Provide for the resident's privacy with curtain, screen, or door.

5. Lower the head of bed so that it is flat. Lock bed wheels.

6. If the bed has side rails, lower the side rail on side to which you will move resident.

7. Move the resident to the side of the bed. Have your co-workers help you do this. Refer to the procedure "Moving a resident to the side of the bed" in this chapter.

8. Lower the side rail on the other side of the bed. Keep a hand on the resident at all times.

9. Place stretcher solidly against the bed, and lock stretcher wheels. Bed height should be equal to the height of the stretcher. Remove stretcher safety belts.

10. Two workers should be on one side of resident. Two workers should be standing behind the stretcher.

11. Each worker should roll up the sides of the draw sheet and prepare to move the resident (Fig. 10-30). Protect the resident's arms and legs during the transfer.

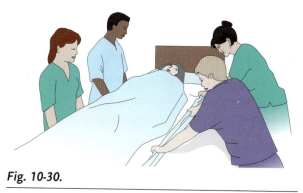

Fig. 10-30.

12. On the count of three, the workers lift and move the resident to the stretcher. All should move at once. Make sure the resident is centered on the stretcher (Fig. 10-31).

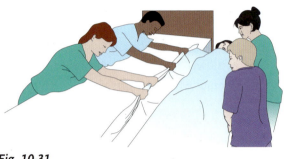

Fig. 10-31.

13. Place a pillow under the resident's head, and cover the resident.

14. Place the safety straps across the resident. Raise side rails on stretcher.

15. Unlock stretcher's wheels. Move resident to proper place, staying with him until another staff member takes over.

16. Wash your hands.

17. Report any changes in resident to the nurse.

18. Document procedure using facility guidelines.

To return the resident to bed, reverse the above procedure.

Mechanical Lifts

Facilities may have mechanical, or hydraulic, lifts available to transfer residents. This equipment avoids wear and tear on your body. Lifts help prevent injury to you and the resident.

If you are trained to do so, you may assist residents with many types of transfers using a mechanical lift. Never use equipment you have not been trained to use. You or your resident could get hurt if you use lifting equipment improperly.

There are many different types of mechanical lifts (Fig. 10-32). You must be trained on the specific lift you will be using. Using these devices

helps prevent common workplace injuries and may be mandatory at your facility if it has a lift-free policy. Ask questions if there is anything that you do not understand about the provided lift equipment.

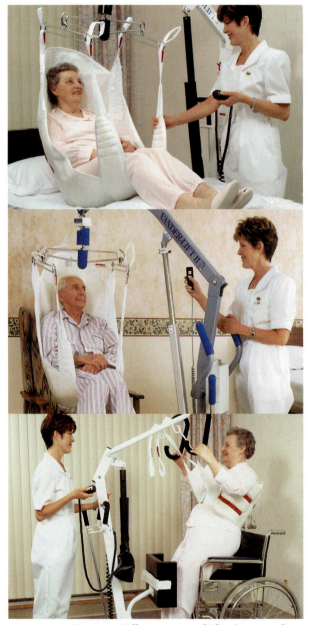

Fig. 10-32. There are different types of lifts that transfer completely dependent residents and residents who can bear some weight. (PHOTOS COURTESY OF VANCARE INC., 800-694-4525)

Guidelines:
Mechanical or Hydraulic Lifts

Be very careful when moving a resident by mechanical lift. Use these safety precautions when assisting a resident with the use of a hydraulic lift:

G   Keep the chair or wheelchair to which the resident is to be moved close to the bed so that the resident is only moved a short distance in the lift.

G   Check that the valves are working on the lift before using it.

G   Check the sling and straps for any fraying or tears. Do not use the lift if there are tears or holes.

G   Open the legs of the stand to the widest position before helping the resident into the lift.

G   Once the resident is in the sling and the straps are connected, pump up the lift only to the point where the resident's body clears the bed or chair.

Transferring a resident using a mechanical lift

This is a basic procedure for transferring using a mechanical lift. Ask someone to help you before starting.

Equipment: wheelchair or chair, co-worker, mechanical or hydraulic lift

1. Wash your hands.

2. Identify yourself by name. Identify the resident by name.

3. Explain procedure to the resident. Speak clearly, slowly, and directly. Maintain face-to-face contact whenever possible.

4. Provide for the resident's privacy with curtain, screen, or door.

5. Lock bed wheels.

6. Position wheelchair next to bed. Lock brakes.

7. Help the resident turn to one side of the bed. Position the sling under the resident, with the edge next to the resident's back, fanfolding if necessary. Make the bottom of the sling even with the resident's knees. Help the resident

roll back to the middle of the bed. Spread out the fanfolded edge of the sling.

8. Roll the mechanical lift to bedside. Make sure the base is opened to its widest point. Push the base of the lift under the bed.

9. Position the overhead bar directly over the resident (Fig. 10-33).

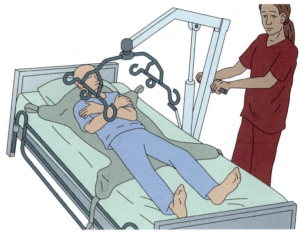

Fig. 10-33.

10. With the resident lying on his back, attach one set of straps to each side of the sling. Attach one set of straps to the overhead bar. If available, have a co-worker support the resident at the head, shoulders, and knees while being lifted. The resident's arms should be folded across his chest (Fig. 10-34). If the device has "S" hooks, they should face away from resident (Fig. 10-35). Make sure all straps are connected properly.

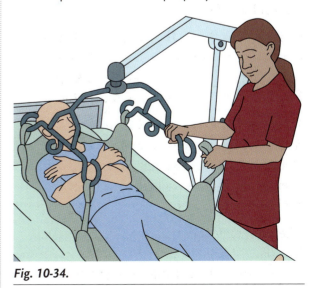

Fig. 10-34.

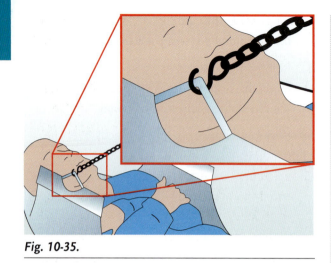

Fig. 10-35.

11. Following manufacturer's instructions, raise the resident two inches above the bed. Pause a moment for the resident to gain balance.

12. If available, a lifting partner can help support and guide the resident's body while you roll the lift so that the resident is positioned over the chair or wheelchair (10-36).

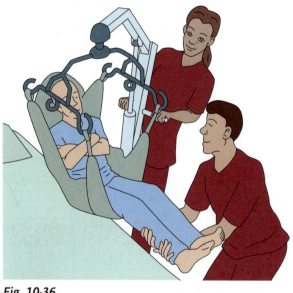

Fig. 10-36.

13. Slowly lower the resident into the chair or wheelchair. Push down gently on the resident's knees to help the resident into a sitting, rather than reclining, position.

14. Undo the straps from the overhead bar. Leave the sling in place for transfer back to bed.

15. Be sure the resident is seated comfortably and correctly in the chair or wheelchair. Remove privacy measures.

16. Place call light within resident's reach.

17. Wash your hands.

18. Report any changes in resident to the nurse.

19. Document procedure using facility guidelines.

Toilet Transfers

The bladder empties more efficiently when a person is able to use the toilet. In order to use the toilet, residents must be able to bear some weight on their legs. Falls may occur if a resident has to wait to go to the bathroom. Offer trips to the toilet often and respond to call lights quickly. You will learn more about assisting with toileting in Chapter 16.

Transferring a resident onto and off of a toilet

Equipment: disposable gloves, toilet tissue, wheelchair, transfer belt

1. Wash your hands.

2. Identify yourself by name. Identify the resident by name.

3. Explain procedure to the resident. Speak clearly, slowly, and directly. Maintain face-to-face contact whenever possible. Make sure resident is wearing non-skid shoes.

4. Provide for the resident's privacy with curtain, screen, or door.

5. Position wheelchair at a right angle to the toilet to face the hand bar/wall rail.

6. Remove wheelchair footrests. Lock wheels.

7. Apply a transfer belt around the resident's waist. Grasp the belt. Put one of your hands toward the resident's back and one toward the resident's front.

8. Ask resident to push against the armrests of the wheelchair and stand, reaching for and grasping the hand bar (Fig. 10-37).

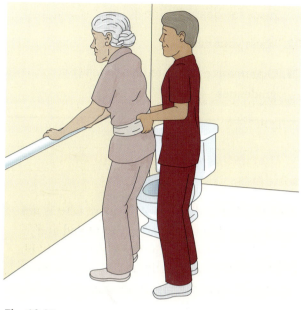

Fig. 10-37.

9. Ask resident to pivot her foot and back up so that she can feel the front of the toilet with the back of her legs (Fig. 10-38).

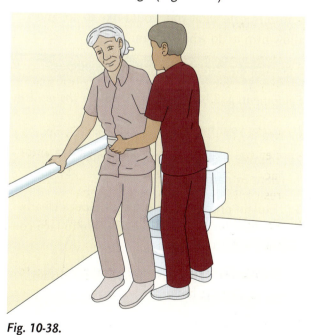

Fig. 10-38.

10. Help resident to pull down underwear and pants. You may need to keep one hand on the transfer belt while helping to remove clothing.

11. Help resident to slowly sit down onto the toilet. Allow privacy unless resident cannot be left alone.

12. When the resident is finished, apply gloves. Assist with perineal care as necessary (see Chapter 13). Ask her to stand and reach for the hand bar.

13. Use toilet tissue or damp cloth to clean the resident. Make sure he or she is clean and dry before pulling up clothing. Remove and dispose of gloves. Wash your hands.

14. Pull up resident's clothing. Help resident to the sink to wash hands.

15. Help resident back into wheelchair.

16. Wash your hands again.

17. Help resident to leave the bathroom. Make sure resident is comfortable. Remove privacy measures.

18. Place call light within resident's reach.

19. Report any changes in resident to the nurse.

20. Document procedure using facility guidelines.

Car Transfers

When a resident is leaving a facility, you may need to help him or her into a car. The front seat is wider and is usually easier to get into.

Transferring a resident into a car

Equipment: car, wheelchair

1. Wash your hands.

2. Identify yourself by name. Identify the resident by name.

3. Explain procedure to the resident. Speak clearly, slowly, and directly. Maintain face-to-face contact whenever possible.

4. Place wheelchair close to the car at a 45-degree angle. Open the door on the resident's stronger side.

5. Lock wheelchair.

6. Ask the resident to push against the arm rests of the wheelchair and stand (Fig. 10-39).

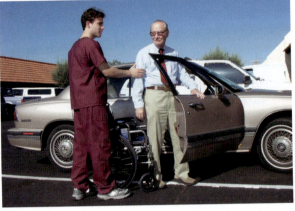

Fig. 10-39.

7. Ask the resident to stand, grasp the car, and pivot his foot so the side of the car seat touches the back of the legs.

8. The resident should then sit in the seat and lift one leg, and then the other, into the vehicle (Fig. 10-40).

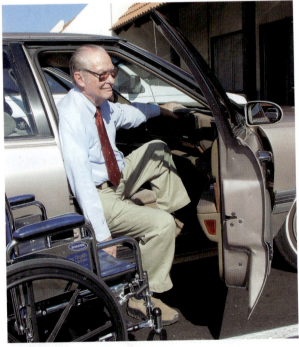

Fig. 10-40.

9. Carefully position the resident comfortably in the car. Help secure seat belt.

10. See that door can be safely shut and shut the door.

11. Return the wheelchair to the appropriate place for cleaning.

12. Wash your hands.

13. Document procedure using facility guidelines.

5. Discuss how to safely ambulate residents

Ambulation is walking. A resident who is **ambulatory** is one who can get out of bed and walk. Many older residents are ambulatory, but need assistance to walk safely. Several tools, including transfer or gait belts, canes, walkers, and crutches, assist with ambulation.

Check the care plan before helping a resident ambulate. Discuss the resident's abilities and disabilities with the nurse, and know the resident's limitations. Any time you help a resident, communicate what you would like to do, and allow him to do what he can.

Assisting a resident to ambulate

Equipment: gait belt, non-skid shoes for the resident

1. Wash your hands.

2. Identify yourself by name. Identify the resident by name.

3. Explain procedure to resident. Speak clearly, slowly, and directly. Maintain face-to-face contact whenever possible.

4. Provide for resident's privacy with curtain, screen, or door.

5. Before ambulating, properly fasten non-skid footwear on the resident.

6. Adjust bed to low position so that the feet are flat on the floor. Lock bed wheels.

7. Stand in front of and face the resident.

8. Brace the resident's lower extremities. Bend your knees. Place one foot between the resident's knees. If the resident has a weak knee, brace it against your knee.

9. **With gait (transfer) belt**: Place belt around resident's waist. Bending your knees and leaning forward, grasp the belt. Hold her close to your center of gravity. Tell the resident to lean forward, push down on the bed with her hands, and stand, on the count of three. When you start to count, begin to rock. At three, rock your weight onto your back foot and assist the resident to a standing position.

   Without transfer belt: Place arms around resident's torso under armpits, while assisting resident to stand.

10. **With transfer belt**: Walk slightly behind and to one side of resident for the full distance, while holding onto the transfer belt (10-41).

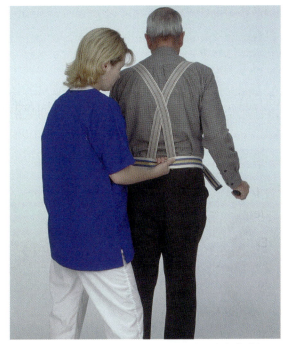

Fig. 10-41. Walk behind and to one side while holding onto the gait belt when assisting with ambulation.

   Without transfer belt: Walk slightly behind and to one side of resident for the full distance. Support the resident's back with your arm.

If the resident has a weaker side, stand on that side. Use the hand that is not holding the belt or the arm not on the back to offer support on the weak side.

11. Observe the resident's strength while you walk together. Provide a chair if the resident becomes dizzy or tired.

12. After ambulation, remove gait belt if used. Help resident to the bed or chair and make resident comfortable.

13. Return bed to lowest position. Remove privacy measures.

14. Place call light within resident's reach.

15. Wash your hands.

16. Report any changes in resident to nurse.

17. Document procedure using facility guidelines.

When helping a visually-impaired resident walk, let the person walk beside and slightly behind you, as he rests a hand on your elbow. Walk at a normal pace. Let the person know when you are about to turn a corner, or when a step is approaching. Tell him whether you will be stepping up or down.

Residents who have difficulty walking may use adaptive or assistive devices, such as canes, walkers, or crutches to help themselves (Fig. 10-42). Understanding the purpose of each device will help you know how to use it properly.

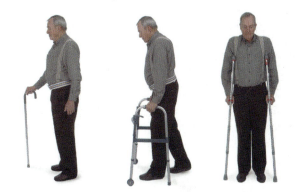

Fig. 10-42. Residents who have difficulty walking may use canes, walkers, or crutches to help themselves.

The purpose of a cane is to help with balance. Residents using canes should be able to bear weight on both legs. If one leg is weaker, the cane should be held in the hand on the strong side.

Types of canes include the C cane, the functional grip cane, and the quad cane. The **C cane** is a straight cane with a curved handle at the top. It has a rubber-tipped bottom to prevent slipping. A C cane is used to improve balance. A **functional grip cane** is similar to the C cane, except that it has a straight grip handle, rather than a curved handle. The grip handle helps improve grip control and provides a little more support than the C cane. A **quad cane**, with four rubber-tipped feet and a rectangular base, is designed to bear more weight than the other canes.

A **walker** is used when the resident can bear some weight on the legs. The walker provides stability for residents who are unsteady or lack balance. The metal frame of the walker may have rubber-tipped feet and/or wheels. Crutches are used for residents who can bear no weight or limited weight on one leg. Some people use one crutch, and some use two.

Whichever device is being used, your role is to ensure safety. Stay near the person, on the weak side. Make sure the equipment is in proper condition. It must be sturdy, and it must have rubber tips or wheels on the bottom.

When a resident uses a walker or cane, follow these guidelines. They will help keep the resident safe.

Guidelines:
Cane or Walker Use

G Be sure the walker or cane is in good condition. It must have rubber tips on bottom. The tips should not be cracked. Walkers may have wheels. If so, roll the walker to make sure the wheels are moving properly.

G Be sure the resident is wearing securely fastened non-skid shoes.

G When using a cane, the resident should place it on his stronger side.

G When using a walker, have the resident place both hands on the walker. The walker should not be over-extended; it should be placed no more than 12 inches in front of the resident.

G Stay near the resident on the weaker side.

G Do not hang purses or clothing on the walker.

G If the height of the cane or walker does not appear to be correct (too short, too tall, etc.), inform the nurse.

Assisting with ambulation for a resident using a cane, walker, or crutches

Equipment: transfer belt, non-skid shoes for resident, cane, walker, or crutches

1. Wash your hands.

2. Identify yourself by name. Identify resident by name.

3. Explain procedure to resident. Speak clearly, slowly, and directly. Maintain face-to-face contact whenever possible.

4. Provide for resident's privacy with curtain, screen, or door.

5. Before ambulating, properly fasten non-skid footwear on resident.

6. Adjust bed to low position so that the feet are flat on the floor. Lock bed wheels.

7. Stand in front of and face the resident.

8. Brace the resident's lower extremities. Bend your knees. Place one foot between the resident's knees. If the resident has a weak knee, brace it against your knee.

9. Place gait belt around resident's waist. Grasp the belt while helping the resident to stand as previously described.

10. Help as needed with ambulation.

a. **Cane**. Resident places cane about 12 inches in front of his stronger leg. He brings weaker leg even with cane. He then brings stronger leg forward slightly ahead of cane. Repeat (Fig. 10-43).

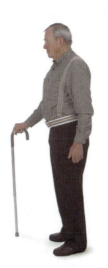

Fig. 10-43. The cane moves in front of the stronger leg first.

b. **Walker**. Resident picks up or rolls the walker and places it about 12 inches in front of him. All four feet or wheels of the walker should be on the ground before resident steps forward to the walker. The walker should not be moved again until the resident has moved both feet forward and is steady (Fig. 10-44). The resident should never put his feet ahead of the walker.

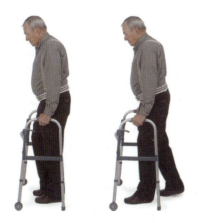

Fig. 10-44. The walker can be moved after the resident is steady and both feet are forward.

c. **Crutches**. Resident should be fitted for crutches and taught to use them correctly by a physical therapist or nurse. The resident may use the crutches several different ways, depending on what his weakness is. No matter how they are used, weight should be on the hands and arms. Weight should not be on the underarm area (Fig. 10-45).

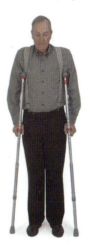

Fig. 10-45. When using crutches, weight should be on the hands and arms, not on the underarms.

11. Whether the resident is using a cane, walker, or crutches, walk slightly behind and to one side of resident. Stay on the weaker side if resident has one. Hold the gait belt if one is used.

12. Watch for obstacles in the resident's path. Ask the resident to look ahead, not down at his feet.

13. Encourage the resident to rest if he is tired. When a resident is tired, it increases the chance of a fall. Let the resident set the pace. Discuss how far he plans to go based on the care plan.

14. After ambulation, remove gait belt. Help resident to a position of comfort and safety.

15. Leave bed in lowest position. Remove privacy measures.

16. Place call light within resident's reach.

17. Wash your hands.

18. Report any changes in resident to nurse.

19. Document procedure using facility guidelines.

Chapter Review

1. List nine guidelines for using proper body mechanics.

2. Why is handwashing an important step at the beginning and at the end of care procedures?

3. Why are beds usually adjusted to a low position at the end of care procedures?

4. What is positioning?

5. How often should bedbound residents be repositioned?

6. In which position is a resident lying on his/her side?

7. In which position is a resident lying on his/her stomach?

8. In which position is a resident lying flat on his/her back?

9. In which position is a resident lying on his/her left side with the lower arm behind the back and the upper knee bent and raised toward the chest?

10. In which position is a resident in a semi-sitting position (45 to 60 degrees) with the head and shoulders up?

11. What is a draw sheet?

12. What is shearing?

13. When is logrolling necessary?

14. How does dangling benefit a resident?

15. How should a transfer belt be applied to a person?

16. Before helping a resident into or out of a wheelchair, what should a nursing assistant do?

17. Describe what a nursing assistant should do if a resident starts to fall.

18. If a resident has a weaker side, which side moves first in a transfer—the weaker or stronger side?

19. When may stretchers be used for residents?

20. List five safety guidelines for using a mechanical lift.

21. What is one benefit of using the toilet rather than a bedpan or urinal?

22. Define "ambulation."

23. What is the purpose of canes?

24. Which type of adaptive device for walking can be used when a resident can bear no weight on one leg—cane, walker, or crutches?

25. Which side should a nursing assistant stay by when a resident is using adaptive equipment—the weaker or stronger side?

11
Admitting, Transferring, and Discharging

1. Describe how residents may feel when entering a facility

Chapter 8 described some of the many feelings residents may be having as they make the transition into a care facility. Losses, such as the loss of a familiar environment, or the loss of independence, can cause a person to feel scared, angry, sad, lonely, worried, helpless, or depressed. A new resident may yell at caregivers, or may cry often. He or she may refuse to join in activities and want to be left alone. A new resident may want to talk to staff members as much as possible until he becomes more comfortable. These are just a few of the ways that new residents may show their emotions.

Moving always requires an adjustment, but as a person ages, it can be even harder (Fig. 11-1). This is especially true if illness, disability, and mobility problems are present. Imagine that at age 45 you began to live alone as your children left the house. Then you lived alone, happily, for 25 years before having a stroke. You were no longer able to live alone safely, and your children did not live nearby to help you with your daily care. And living with your children was not an option. You might have to move into a care facility. You might feel worried and scared because you have never known any other home but the one you lived in for so many years. You might feel angry or depressed about moving into a new place filled with people you do not know. If

independence is restricted, and health declines, people may be faced with difficult decisions about care. Moving into a facility is not an easy choice to make.

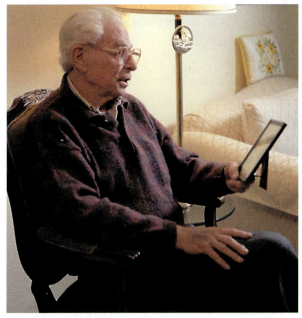

Fig. 11-1. *A new resident must leave familiar places and things. He may have just lost someone very close to him. He may be experiencing other losses as well. Be supportive and welcoming.*

Nursing assistants play an important role in helping residents make a successful transition to a long-term care facility. Giving emotional support is a big part of this. Listening and being kind, compassionate, and helpful may make new residents feel better about their new homes. More guidelines on assisting new residents are found in the next learning objective.

2. Explain the nursing assistant's role in the admission process

When a new resident is admitted, he or she is first directed to the admitting office. Paperwork is signed. The admission staff member makes copies of insurance information, Medicare cards, and other types of information. Both parties sign an agreement or contract, agreeing to the services provided and the costs for them. Emergency contact information and names of doctors are obtained. Staff is required to explain information on advance directives and to find out if the resident has advance directives in place or wants to create them. A copy of the resident's rights is given to the new resident and his or her family. The rights are explained in a language the resident can understand. A facility handbook of policies and procedures may be given. The procedure on how to file grievances and complaints is explained. Pictures of new residents may be taken, which are used to identify them and may be posted outside of their rooms.

Admission is often the first time you meet a new resident. This is a time of first impressions. Make sure a resident has a good impression of you and your facility. Because change is difficult, staff must communicate with new residents. Explain what to expect during the process, and answer any questions that are within your scope of practice. If residents have questions you cannot answer, find the nurse. Ask questions to find out a resident's personal preferences and routines.

Your facility will have a procedure for admitting residents to their new home. These guidelines will help make the experience pleasant and successful.

Guidelines:
Admission

G   Prepare the room before the resident arrives. This helps him or her to feel expected and welcome. Make sure the bed is made and the

room is tidy. Restock supplies that are low. Make sure there is an admission kit available, if used. Admission kits often contain personal care items, such as bath basin, emesis basin, water pitcher, drinking glass, toothpaste, soap, comb, lotion, and tissues (Fig. 11-2). They may also contain a urine specimen cup, label, and transport bag.

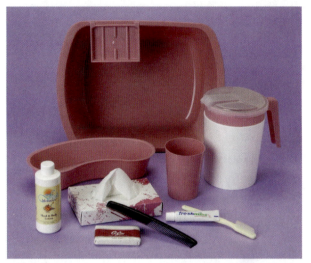

Fig. 11-2. *An admission kit is usually placed in a resident's room before he or she is admitted. It may contain personal care items that the resident will need.* (REPRINTED WITH PERMISSION OF BRIGGS CORPORATION, 800-247-2343, WWW.BRIGGSCORP.COM)

G   When a new resident arrives at the facility, note the time and her condition. Is she using a wheelchair, on a stretcher, or walking? Who is with her? Observe the new resident for level of consciousness and if she seems confused. She will probably be feeling anxiety; look for signs of nervousness. Note any tubes she has, such as IVs or catheters.

G   Introduce yourself and state your position. Smile and be friendly. Always call the person by her formal name until she tells you what she wants to be called.

G   Never rush the process or the new resident. He should not feel like he is an inconvenience. Make sure that the new resident feels welcome and wanted.

G   Explain day-to-day life in the facility. Offer to take the resident on a tour (Fig. 11-3).

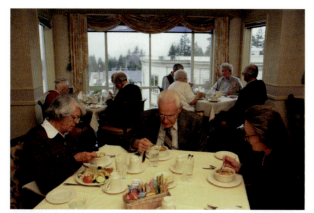

Fig. 11-3. Make sure you include the location of the dining room when taking a new resident on a tour. Go over posted dining schedules.

G Introduce the resident to other residents and staff members you see (Fig. 11-4). Introduce the roommate if there is one.

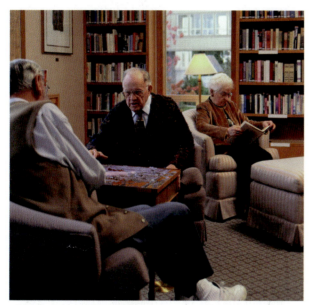

Fig. 11-4. Introduce new residents to all other residents you see.

G Handle personal items with care and respect. A resident has a legal right to have his personal items treated carefully. These are the items he has chosen to bring with him. Some items may be stored in bags marked specifically for personal belongings (Fig. 11-5). Ask the new resident if she brought any valuables with her. If so, offer to have them safely stored according to your facility's policy. If she refuses, follow the procedure to write an inventory, and get the necessary signatures.

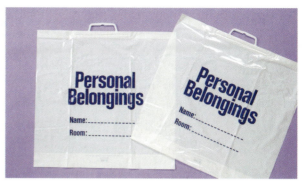

Fig. 11-5. Some personal items may be stored in special bags. Follow facility policy. (REPRINTED WITH PERMISSION OF BRIGGS CORPORATION, 800-247-2343, WWW.BRIGGSCORP.COM)

G When setting up the room, ask her what she likes. Place personal items where the resident wants them (Fig. 11-6).

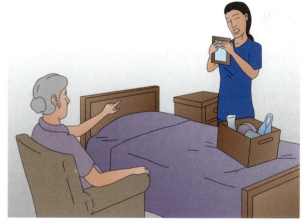

Fig. 11-6. Handle personal items carefully, and set up the room as she prefers.

G Admission is a stressful time. Be sure to observe the resident as she could have a problem that is missed with the emphasis on transporting, paperwork, etc. It is important to observe the new resident's condition in order to recognize any changes that may take place later. Report to the nurse if you notice any of the following:

• Tubes that need to be reconnected

• Resident seems confused, combative, and/or unaware of surroundings

• Resident is having difficulty breathing or any other signs of distress

• Resident has missed a meal during admission process

G Follow facility policy on any other tasks that are required during the admission process.

G New residents may have good days followed by not-so-good days. Let residents adapt to their new homes at their own pace. Everyone is different. Getting used to a new home may take quite some time.

Residents' Rights

Rights during Admission

Upon admission, residents must be told of their rights. They must be provided with a written copy of these rights. This includes rights about their funds and the right to file a complaint with the state survey agency.

Admitting a resident

Equipment: may include admission paperwork (checklist and inventory form), gloves and vital signs equipment

Often an admission kit will contain a urine specimen cup and transport bag, and personal care items, such as bath basin, water pitcher, drinking glass, toothpaste and soap.

1. Wash your hands.

2. Identify yourself by name. Identify the resident by name.

3. Explain procedure to the resident. Speak clearly, slowly, and directly. Maintain face-to-face contact whenever possible.

4. Provide for the resident's privacy with curtain, screen, or door. If the family is present, ask them to step outside until the admission process is over.

5. If part of facility procedure, do these things:

- Take the resident's height and weight (see procedures below).

- Take the resident's baseline vital signs (see Chapter 14). **Baseline** signs are initial values that can then be compared to future measurements.

- Obtain a urine specimen if required (see Chapter 16).

- Complete the paperwork. Take an inventory of all the personal items.

- Help the resident put personal items away.

- Provide fresh water (Fig. 11-7).

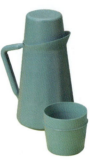

Fig. 11-7. *Providing fresh water is something you should do every time you leave a resident's room, unless he is on a fluid restriction. Doing this helps prevent dehydration. Make sure the pitcher and glass are light enough for the resident to lift.* (REPRINTED WITH PERMISSION OF BRIGGS CORPORATION, 800-247-2343, WWW.BRIGGSCORP.COM)

6. Show the resident the room and bathroom. Explain how to work the bed (and television if there is one). Show the resident how to work the call light and explain its use.

7. Introduce the resident to his roommate, if there is one. Introduce other residents and staff.

8. Make sure resident is comfortable. Remove privacy measures. Bring the family back inside if they were outside.

9. Place call light within resident's reach.

10. Wash your hands.

11. Document procedure using facility guidelines.

In addition to measuring weight and height at admission, you will check them often as part of your care. Height is checked less frequently than weight. Weight changes can be signs of illness, so you must report any weight loss or gain, no matter how small.

Admitting, Transferring, and Discharging

Measuring and recording weight of an ambulatory resident

Equipment: standing scale or bathroom scale, pen and paper

1. Wash your hands.

2. Identify yourself by name. Identify the resident by name.

3. Explain procedure to the resident. Speak clearly, slowly, and directly. Maintain face-to-face contact whenever possible.

4. Provide for resident's privacy with curtain, screen, or door.

5. If using a bathroom scale, set the scale on a hard surface in a place the resident can get to easily.

6. Start with scale balanced at zero before weighing resident.

7. Help resident to step onto the center of the scale, as needed. Be sure she is not holding, touching, or leaning against anything. This interferes with weight measurement. Do not force someone to let you go. If you are unable to obtain a weight, notify the nurse.

8. Determine the resident's weight. **Using a standing scale**: this is done by balancing the scale. Make the balance bar level by moving the small and large weight indicators until the bar balances (Fig. 11-8). Add these two numbers together. **Using a bathroom scale**: read the weight when the dial has stopped moving.

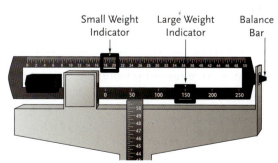

Fig. 11-8. Move the small and large weight indicators until the bar balances.

9. Help resident to safely step off scale before recording weight.

10. Record weight.

11. Remove privacy measures.

12. Place call light within resident's reach.

13. Wash your hands.

14. Report any changes in resident's weight (when weighing resident after admission) to the nurse.

15. Document procedure using facility guidelines.

Some residents will not be able to get out of a wheelchair easily and may be weighed on a wheelchair scale. With this scale, wheelchairs are rolled onto the scale (Fig. 11-9). On some wheelchair scales, you will need to subtract the weight of the wheelchair from a resident's weight. In this case, weigh the empty wheelchair first. Then subtract the wheelchair's weight from the total. Some wheelchairs are marked with their weight.

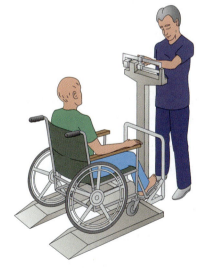

Fig. 11-9. A type of wheelchair scale.

Some residents will not be able to get out of bed. Weighing these residents requires a special scale (Fig. 11-10). Before using a bed scale, know how to use it properly and safely. Follow your facility's procedure and any manufacturer's instructions.

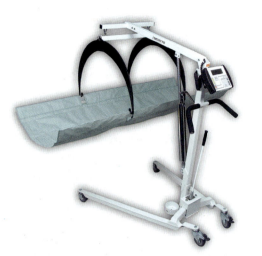

Fig. 11-10. *A type of bed scale.* (PHOTO COURTESY OF DETECTO, WWW.DETECTO.COM, 800-641-2008)

Measuring and recording height of a resident

Some residents will be unable to get out of bed. If so, height can be measured using a tape measure (Fig. 11-11).

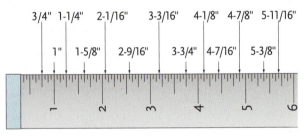

Fig. 11-11. *A tape measure.*

Equipment: tape measure, pencil, pen and paper

1. Wash your hands.

2. Identify yourself by name. Identify the resident by name.

3. Explain procedure to the resident. Speak clearly, slowly, and directly. Maintain face-to-face contact whenever possible.

4. Provide for resident's privacy with curtain, screen, or door.

5. Position the resident lying straight in bed, flat on his back with arms and legs at his sides. Be sure the bed sheet is smooth underneath the resident.

6. Make a pencil mark on the sheet at the top of the head.

7. Make another mark at the resident's heel (Fig. 11-12).

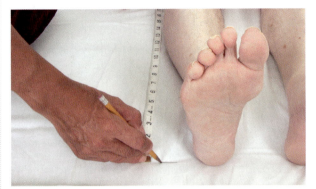

Fig. 11-12. *Make marks on the sheet at the resident's head and feet.*

8. With the tape measure, measure the distance between the marks.

9. Record height.

10. Remove privacy measures. Store equipment.

11. Place call light within resident's reach.

12. Wash your hands.

13. Document procedure using facility guidelines.

For residents who can get out of bed, you will measure height using a standing scale.

Equipment: standing scale, pen and paper

1. Wash your hands.

2. Identify yourself by name. Identify the resident by name.

3. Explain procedure to the resident. Speak clearly, slowly, and directly. Maintain face-to-face contact whenever possible.

4. Provide for resident's privacy with curtain, screen, or door.

5. Help resident to step onto scale, facing away from the scale.

6. Ask resident to stand straight, if possible. Help as needed.

7. Pull up measuring rod from back of the scale and gently lower the rod until it rests flat on the resident's head (Fig. 11-13).

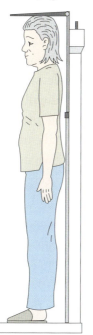

Fig. 11-13. *To determine height on a standing scale, gently lower the measuring rod until it rests flat on the resident's head.*

8. Determine the resident's height.

9. Assist the resident in stepping off scale before recording height. Make sure that the measuring rod does not hit the resident in the head.

10. Record height.

11. Remove privacy measures.

12. Place call light within resident's reach.

13. Wash your hands.

14. Document procedure using facility guidelines.

The rod measures height in inches and fractions of inches. Record the total number of inches. If you have to change inches into feet, remember that there are 12 inches in a foot.

3. Explain the nursing assistant's role during an in-house transfer of a resident

Residents may be transferred to a different area of the facility. In cases of acute illness, they may be transferred to a hospital. Change is difficult, and this is especially true when a person has an illness or her condition gets worse. Make the transfer as smooth as possible for the resident. Try to lessen the stress. Inform the resident of the transfer as soon as possible so that she can then begin to adjust to the idea. Explain how, where, when, and why the transfer will occur.

For example, "Mrs. Jones, you will be moving to a private room. You will be transferred to your new room in a wheelchair. This will happen on Wednesday around 10 a.m. The staff will take good care of you and your things. We will make sure you are comfortable. Do you have any questions?"

Assist residents with packing their personal items. Residents often worry about losing their belongings. Involve them with the packing process if appropriate. For example, let them see the empty closet, drawers, etc.

The resident may be transferred in a bed, in a stretcher, or in a wheelchair. Find out the method from the nurse so that you can plan the move ahead of time. After the resident is in her new room or area, make sure to introduce her to all staff members you see. You want her to feel welcome, settled, and comfortable.

Residents' Rights

Changing Rooms or Roommates
Residents have the right to receive notice of any room or roommate change.

Transferring a resident

Equipment: may include a wheelchair, cart for belongings, the medical record, all of the resident's personal care items and packed personal items

1. Wash your hands.

2. Identify yourself by name. Identify the resident by name.

3. Explain procedure to the resident. Speak clearly, slowly, and directly. Maintain face-to-face contact whenever possible.

4. Provide for resident's privacy with curtain, screen, or door.

5. Collect the items to be moved onto the cart. Take them to the new location. If the resident is going into the hospital, the facility may want them placed in temporary storage.

6. Help the resident into the wheelchair (stretcher may be used for some residents). Take him or her to proper area.

7. Introduce new residents and staff.

8. Help the resident to put personal items away.

9. Make sure that the resident is comfortable. Remove privacy measures.

10. Place call light within resident's reach.

11. Wash your hands.

12. Report any changes in resident to the nurse.

13. Document procedure using facility guidelines.

In addition to the above, when residents are being transferred out of the facility, make sure their clothing is clean and appropriate for the weather. In addition, observe and report the following to the nurse:

- How did the resident leave the facility?

- Who was with her?

- Did she leave by stretcher or wheelchair?

- Did she seem to understand where she was going?

- What belongings did she take with her?

- What were her vital signs before the transfer?

If the resident will be returning soon, change the bed linens, tidy the room, and restock supplies.

4. Explain the nursing assistant's role in the discharge of a resident

The day of discharge is usually a happy day for a resident who is going home. When a resident is discharged, he is released from the facility's care by the doctor. You will collect the resident's belongings and pack them carefully. Ask the resident which personal care items to bring, and pack those, too. Know what the resident's condition is at the time of discharge; find out if she will be using a wheelchair or stretcher.

When residents are discharged they may experience doubts or fear about not being cared for at the facility anymore. They may be concerned that their health will suffer. Be positive; assure her that she is ready for this important change. Remind her that her doctor believes she is ready. However, if she has specific questions about care, inform the nurse.

Before the resident is discharged, the nurse may cover important information with the resident and her family and friends. Some of the following areas may be discussed:

- Future doctor or physical, speech, and occupational therapy appointments (Fig. 11-14)

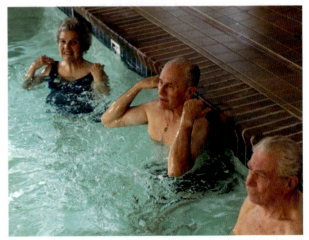

Fig. 11-14. After a resident is discharged, she may continue to receive physical therapy.

- Home care, skilled nursing care
- Medications
- Ambulation instructions from the doctor
- Medical equipment needed
- Medical transportation
- Any restrictions on activities
- Special exercises to keep the resident functioning at the highest level
- Special nutrition or dietary requirements
- Community resources

Discharging a resident

Equipment: may include a wheelchair, cart for belongings, the discharge paperwork, including the inventory list done on admission, all of the resident's personal care items

1. Wash your hands.

2. Identify yourself by name. Identify the resident by name.

3. Explain procedure to the resident. Speak clearly, slowly, and directly. Maintain face-to-face contact whenever possible.

4. Provide for resident's privacy with curtain, screen, or door.

5. Compare the checklist to the items there. If all items are there, ask the resident to sign.

6. Put the items to be taken onto the cart and take them to pick-up area.

7. Help the resident dress and then into the wheelchair or stretcher, if used.

8. Help the resident to say his goodbyes to the staff and residents.

9. Take resident to the pick-up area. Help her into vehicle. You are responsible for the resident until she is safely in the car and the door is closed.

10. Wash your hands.

11. Document procedure using facility guidelines. Include the following:

- Time of discharge
- Method of transport
- Who was with the resident
- The vital signs at discharge
- What items the resident took with her (inventory checklist)

Residents' Rights

Privacy during Discharges

It is important to always be aware of residents' privacy. Close the door before talking about medical matters or other private things. Pull the privacy curtain before the resident changes clothes or is bathed before transfer or discharge.

5. Describe the nursing assistant's role in physical exams

When arriving at a facility, a resident may have a physical exam to help determine the resident's needs and the care plan. Doctors or nurses will perform the exam. Nursing assistants may help by bringing the resident to the proper area, gathering equipment, and providing emotional support. People can be scared about having physical exams. They may fear what the examiner will do or what he or she will find. Exams can cause discomfort and embarrassment. Assist residents during this process. Be comforting and answer questions they have that are within your scope of practice.

Your responsibilities will include gathering equipment for the nurse or doctor. Examples of equipment that may be needed include the following:

- Sphygmomanometer (used to measure blood pressure; you will learn about this in Chapter 14)
- Stethoscope
- Alcohol wipes (Fig. 11-15)

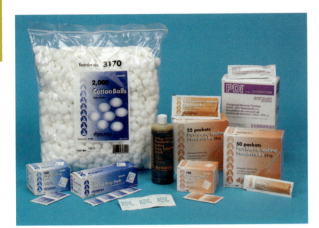

Fig. 11-15. *Alcohol wipes can be used for infections and for minor wound care, among other uses. You may be required to gather other supplies as well.* (REPRINTED WITH PERMISSION OF BRIGGS CORPORATION, 800-247-2343, WWW.BRIGGSCORP.COM)

- Flashlight
- Thermometer
- Tongue depressor
- Eye chart
- Tuning fork (tests hearing with vibrations)
- Reflex, or percussion, hammer (taps body parts to test reflexes) (Fig. 11-16)

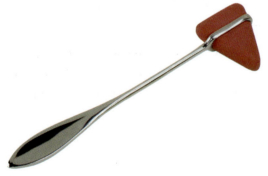

Fig. 11-16. *A reflex, or percussion, hammer is used to test reflexes.* (REPRINTED WITH PERMISSION OF BRIGGS CORPORATION, 800-247-2343, WWW.BRIGGSCORP.COM)

- Otoscope (lighted instrument that examines the outer ear and eardrum)
- Ophthalmoscope (lighted instrument that examines the eye)
- Specimen containers
- Lubricant
- Special card to test for blood in stool

- Vaginal speculum for females (opens the vagina so that it and the cervix can be examined)
- Gloves
- Drapes

You may be asked to position and drape residents in the correct position for the exam. Some positions are embarrassing and uncomfortable. You can help by explaining why the position is needed and how long the resident can expect to stay in the position.

The **dorsal recumbent** position is used to examine the breasts, chest, and abdomen. It is also used to examine the perineal area (Fig. 11-17). A resident in the dorsal recumbent position is flat on her back with her knees flexed and feet flat on the bed. The drape is put over the resident, covering her body. Her head remains uncovered.

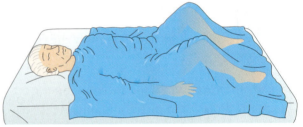

Fig. 11-17. *The dorsal recumbent position.*

A **lithotomy** position is used to examine the vagina (Fig. 11-18). The resident lies on her back. Her hips are brought to the edge of the exam table. Her legs are flexed, and her feet are in padded stirrups. The drape is put over the resident, covering her body. Her head remains uncovered. The drape is also brought down to cover the perineal area and tops of the thighs.

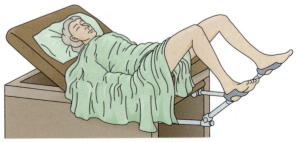

Fig. 11-18. *The lithotomy position.*

The **knee-chest** position is used to examine the rectum, or sometimes, the vagina (Fig. 11-19). A resident in the knee-chest position is lying on her abdomen. The knees are pulled towards the abdomen and legs are separated. Arms are pulled up and flexed. The head is turned to one side. In the knee-chest position, the resident will be wearing a gown and possibly socks. The drape should be applied in a diamond shape to cover the back, buttocks and thighs.

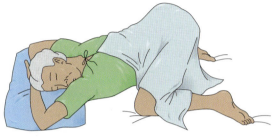

Fig. 11-19. *The knee-chest position.*

Before exams, offer residents drapes and other privacy measures, such as closing the privacy screen or curtain and closing the door to the room. Promote the resident's right to privacy. Tell the resident that he or she will not be exposed more than necessary during the exam.

Guidelines:
Physical Exams

G   Wash your hands before and after the exam.

G   Ask the resident to urinate before the exam. Collect any urine needed for a specimen at this time.

G   Provide privacy throughout the exam. Use drapes and privacy screens for privacy. Expose only the body part being examined.

G   Listen to and calm the resident throughout the exam.

G   Follow the directions of the examiner.

G   Help the resident into the proper positions as needed.

G   Protect the resident from falling.

G   Provide enough light for the examiner.

G   Put instruments in the proper place for the examiner. Hand instruments to the examiner as needed.

G   Take and label specimens as needed.

G   Follow standard precautions.

G   For vision screenings, you may be asked to check that needed equipment is in place. Follow directions. Assist the screener to set up any equipment, such as the eye chart. If you transport residents to the site for screening, make sure to take their current eyeglasses or contact lenses with them. The screener will instruct you where to seat the residents or to have them stand. Operate the light switch as instructed. Make sure that the residents have their eyeglasses and other belongings when returned to their rooms.

G   After the exam, the NA's responsibilities include:

- Help the resident clean up and get dressed. Help the resident safely back to his or her room.

- Dispose of any trash and disposable equipment in the exam area.

- Bring all reusable equipment to the appropriate cleaning room. Clean and store reusable equipment according to facility policy.

- Label and bring any specimens to the desk to take to the lab.

Residents' Rights

Exams

Residents have the right to know why exams are being done and who is doing them. Residents have the right to choose examiners and to have family members present during the exam.

Chapter Review

1. How can nursing assistants help residents feel better about moving to a long-term care facility?

2. List eight guidelines for helping residents during the admission process.

3. Why is it important to report any weight loss or gain that a resident has, no matter how small?

4. How many inches are in a foot?

5. How can nursing assistants make transfers as smooth as possible for residents?

6. List eight types of information that the nurse may cover with the resident and her family and friends during the discharge process.

7. What are two ways that nursing assistants can provide emotional support to residents who are having a physical exam?

8. In which position is a resident lying on her abdomen with her knees pulled towards the abdomen, her arms pulled up and flexed, and her head turned to one side?

9. Which position is generally used to examine the vagina, with the woman's feet in padded stirrups?

10. In which position is a resident lying flat on her back with her knees flexed and feet flat on the bed?

12

The Resident's Unit

1. Explain why a comfortable environment is important for the resident's well-being

Illness and disability cause great stress. It helps residents feel better physically and psychologically if their environments are clean and comfortable. A comfortable and clean environment aids in relaxation and helps to reduce stress. A soothing environment may also help relieve pain and promote healing. Many things affect residents' comfort within their rooms. The more you pay attention and try to improve their environments, the more positive impact it may have on residents' health and well-being.

Many things can affect comfort level, such as noise, odors, temperature, lighting, diet, medications, illness, fear, and anxiety. Below are some guidelines for avoiding problems and promoting comfort.

Guidelines:
Promoting Comfort

G Common noises in facilities can upset and/or irritate residents. You can help keep the noise level low by:

- Not banging equipment or meal trays
- Keeping your voice low
- Promptly answering ringing telephones and call lights
- Closing doors when residents ask you to

- Turning off televisions when they are not in use

G Odors may be caused by urine, feces, vomit, certain diseases, and wound drainage. Body and breath odors may be offensive, too. You can help control odors by:

- Promptly cleaning up after episodes of incontinence
- Changing incontinent briefs as soon as they are soiled and disposing of them properly
- Emptying and cleaning bedpans, urinals, commodes, and emesis basins promptly
- Changing soiled bed linens and clothing as soon as possible
- Giving regular oral care and personal care to help avoid body and breath odors

G As people age and lose protective fatty tissue, they may feel cold often. Illness can cause a person to feel cold, too. You can help residents stay comfortable by:

- Layering clothing and bed covers for warmth
- Keeping residents away from drafty areas, such as by doors and windows
- Offering blankets to persons in wheelchairs
- Keeping residents covered while giving personal care

G Good lighting is important to promote safety and prevent falls. It also helps make a room pleasant. Residents may prefer darker rooms when they are ill, have a headache, or are sleeping. Keep lighting controls within the resident's reach.

G Foods ordered in special diets for residents may cause them discomfort. Heavy meals can also cause discomfort. Report resident complaints about food to the nurse. You will learn more about nutrition and special diets in Chapter 15.

G Foods and drinks that contain caffeine can prevent sleep or sleeping well. Caffeine may need to be decreased to promote better rest (Fig. 12-1).

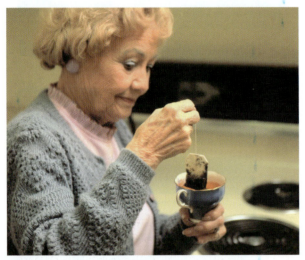

Fig. 12-1. *Caffeinated drinks, such as coffee or some teas, can prevent sleep and cause fatigue and irritability. They may need to be limited if they cause problems.*

G If residents seem sad, anxious, or fearful, help them by talking with them and listening to their concerns. Provide emotional support. If you think residents require more assistance than you can give, discuss this with the nurse.

2. Describe a standard resident unit

A resident's unit is the room or area where the resident lives. It contains the resident's furniture and personal possessions. The unit is the resident's home and must be treated with respect.

Always knock and wait to receive permission before entering.

You will need to keep a resident's unit neat and clean. After providing care for the resident, you will tidy the area. Clean and put equipment away. Providing a clean, safe, and orderly environment is an essential part of your job.

Equipment that you will generally find in each resident's unit includes the following:

- **Electric or manual bed**: Electric beds, also called hospital beds, are operated by controls that hang on or near the side of the bed (Fig. 12-2). One pair of buttons operates the head section and the other pair operates the foot section. By using the arrows, you can move these sections up or down (Fig. 12-3). The middle pair of buttons operate the bed height. Most electric beds have a way to insert a crank so that they can be adjusted if there is a power failure. Manual beds have cranks to move them. The left crank usually raises and lowers the head of the bed. The right crank raises and lowers the foot of the bed. If the bed has a center crank, it will adjust the bed height. Normally, beds are kept in their lowest horizontal position. Lowering the bed provides for residents' safety and helps reduce the risk of falls.

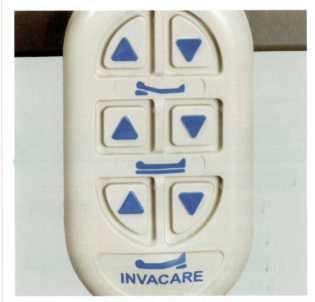

Fig. 12-2. *Controls for an electric bed.* (PHOTO COURTESY OF INVACARE CONTINUING CARE GROUP, 1-800-347-5440, WWW.INVACARE-CCG.COM)

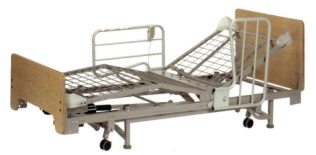

Fig. 12-3. The head, foot and height of an electric bed are generally easily adjusted. (PHOTO COURTESY OF INVACARE CONTINUING CARE GROUP, 1-800-347-5440, WWW.INVACARE-CCG.COM.)

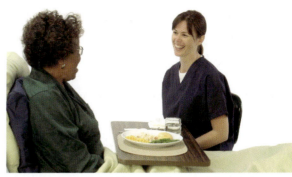

Fig. 12-5. Overbed tables are often used for residents' meals; they must be kept clean. Do not place bedpans, urinals, or soiled linens on overbed tables.

- **Bedside stand**: Small items are usually stored in bedside stands. The water pitcher and cup are often placed on top of the bedside stand. A telephone and/or a radio, and other items, such as photos, may also be placed there. These items may be stored inside the bedside stand:

  - Urinal/bedpan and covers
  - Wash basin
  - Emesis basin (Fig. 12-4)
  - Soap dish and soap
  - Bath blanket
  - Toilet paper
  - Personal hygiene items

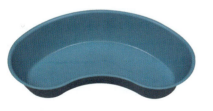

Fig. 12-4. An emesis basin is a kidney-shaped basin often used when giving mouth care. (REPRINTED WITH PERMISSION OF BRIGGS CORPORATION, 800-247-2343, WWW.BRIGGSCORP.COM)

- **Overbed table**: The overbed table may be used for meals or personal care. It is a clean area and it must be kept clean and free of clutter (Fig. 12-5). Bedpans, urinals, soiled linen, and other contaminated items should not be placed on overbed tables.

- **Call light**: The intercom system is the most common call system used. When the resident presses the button, a light will be seen and/or a bell will be heard at the nurses' station. The call light allows the resident to communicate with staff whenever necessary. It is important to always place the call light within the resident's reach and to answer all call lights immediately.

- **Privacy screen or curtain**: All residents in a facility have the right to personal privacy. This means that they must always be protected from public view when receiving care. Each bed in the facility usually has a privacy curtain that extends all the way around the bed. Screens and curtains keep others from seeing a resident undressed or while having care procedures done. Keep this curtain closed when you are giving care to protect the resident's privacy. Although curtains and screens block vision, they do not block sound. Take care not to violate the resident's right to confidentiality through careless conversation. Close the door when possible to provide more complete privacy.

Tip

Bed Positions

You first learned about body positions in Chapter 10. You may be asked to position electric beds in specific positions. To position the bed in the Fowler's position, raise the head of the bed 45 to 60 degrees. To position the bed in the semi-Fowler's position, raise the head of the bed 30 to 45 degrees.

3. Discuss how to care for and clean unit equipment

You will be taught the correct way to use many pieces of equipment. It is important to know how to use and care for all equipment properly. This prevents infection and injury. If you do not know how to use a particular piece of equipment, ask for assistance. Do not try to use equipment that you do not know how to use.

Some equipment you will use will be disposable or "single-use." This means it is discarded after one use. Disposable razors and latex gloves are examples of this type of equipment. Disposable equipment is used to prevent the spread of microorganisms. Discard disposable equipment in proper containers.

Some equipment will need to be cleaned after each use. Bedpans, urinals, and wash basins are examples of this. Wear gloves while rinsing and cleaning this equipment so that you do not come into contact with infectious wastes. Rinse them with water before cleaning them. After cleaning reusable equipment, you may need to disinfect or sterilize it. Follow facility policy.

Guidelines:
Resident's Unit

G Clean the overbed table after use. Place it within the resident's reach before leaving.

G Keep equipment clean and in good condition. If any equipment appears broken or damaged, report it to the nurse and/or file the proper paperwork to get it repaired. Do not use broken or damaged equipment.

G Keep the call light within the resident's reach at all times. Check to see that the resident can reach the call light every time you are going to leave the room.

G Remove meal trays right after meals. Check to make sure that there are no crumbs in the bed. Straighten bed linens as needed. Change linens if they become wet, soiled, or wrinkled.

G Report signs of insects or pests immediately to the nurse.

G Check to see if any personal supplies need to be restocked. Make sure the resident has fresh drinking water and a clean cup within reach and is able to lift the pitcher and the cup. Make sure that tissues, paper towels, toilet paper, soap and other supplies that are used daily are stocked before you leave.

G If trash needs to be emptied or the bathroom needs to be cleaned, notify the housekeeping department. Trash should be emptied at least daily.

G Do not move resident's belongings or discard any personal items. Respect the resident's things. Ask residents where they want items stored. Offer to help residents arrange their space in a way that is pleasing to them. If residents control the heat and air conditioning in their rooms, do not change it for your comfort.

G Clean equipment and return it to proper storage. Tidy the area. Providing a clean, safe, and orderly environment is part of your job.

4. Explain the importance of sleep and factors affecting sleep

Sleep is a natural period of rest for the mind and body. As a person sleeps, the mind and body's energy is restored. During sleep, vital functions are performed, such as repairing and renewing cells, processing information, and organizing memory. Sleep is essential to a person's health and well-being.

The circadian rhythm is an important factor in determining sleep patterns of humans. The **circadian rhythm** is the 24-hour day-night cycle. It also affects body temperature and hormone production, among other things.

When a person is sleep-deprived or suffers from **insomnia** (lack of ability to fall asleep or stay asleep), or other sleep disorders, problems result. These include decreased mental function, reduced reaction time, and irritability. Sleep deprivation also decreases immune system function.

The elderly may take longer to go to sleep and can have more irregular sleep patterns. Some will take short naps during the day. Many elderly persons, especially those who are living away from their homes, have sleep problems. Many things can affect sleep, such as fear, stress, noise, diet, medications, and illness. Sharing a room with another person can disturb sleeping.

Observing and Reporting:
Sleep Issues

When a resident complains that he or she is not sleeping well, observe and report the following:

O/R Sleeping too much in daytime

O/R Eating or drinking items that contain too much caffeine late in the day

O/R Wearing night clothes during the day

O/R Eating heavy meals late at night

O/R Refusing to take medication ordered for sleep

O/R Taking new medications

O/R TV, radio, or light on late at night

O/R Pain

5. Describe bedmaking guidelines and perform proper bedmaking

When residents spend much or all of their time in bed, careful bedmaking is essential to their comfort, cleanliness, and health (Fig. 12-6). Linens should always be changed after personal care procedures such as bed baths, or any time bedding or sheets are damp, soiled, or in need of straightening. The following are three reasons why it is important that bed linens be changed frequently:

1. Sheets that are damp, wrinkled, or bunched up under a resident are uncomfortable. They may keep the resident from sleeping well.

2. Microorganisms thrive in moist, warm places. Bedding that is damp or unclean may cause infection and disease.

3. Residents who spend long hours in bed are at risk for pressure sores. Sheets that do not lie flat increase this risk by cutting off circulation.

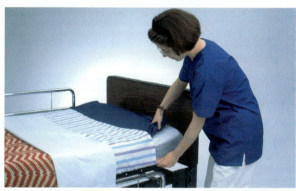

Fig. 12-6. *Multiple layers of bedding, including a draw sheet, are used for residents who spend a lot of time in bed.*

Guidelines:
Bedmaking

G Keep linens wrinkle-free and tidy. Change linen whenever wet, damp, wrinkled, or dirty.

G Wash your hands before handling clean linen.

G Hold soiled linens away from your body and place it in the proper container immediately. If dirty linen touches your uniform, your uniform becomes contaminated (Fig. 12-7).

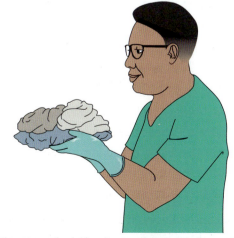

Fig. 12-7. *Carry dirty linen away from your uniform.*

G   Do not shake linen or clothes.

G   Put on gloves before removing bed linens from beds.

G   Look for personal items, such as dentures, hearing aids, jewelry, and glasses, before removing linens.

G   When removing linen, fold or roll linen so that the dirtiest area is inside. Rolling puts the dirtiest surface of the linen inward. This lessens contamination.

G   Bag soiled linen at the point of origin. Do not take it to other residents' rooms.

G   Sort soiled linen away from resident care areas.

G   Place wet linen in leak-proof bags.

G   Disposable bed protectors or pads are used for residents who are incontinent. Change the bed protectors as soon as they are soiled or wet, and dispose of them in the proper container. Put a clean bed protector on the bed when you change linens. (Fig. 12-8).

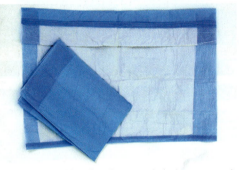

Fig. 12-8. *Disposable absorbent pads help protect sheets from sweat, urine, feces, or other fluids.*

If a resident cannot get out of bed, you must change the linens with the resident in bed. An **occupied bed** is a bed made while the resident is in the bed. When making the bed, use a wide stance. Bend your knees to avoid injury. Avoid bending from the waist, especially when tucking sheets or blankets under the mattress. Raise the height of the bed to make it easier and safer.

Mattresses can be heavy. It is easier to make an empty bed than one with a resident in it. An **unoccupied bed** is a bed made while no resident is in the bed. If the resident can be moved, your job will be easier.

Making an occupied bed

Equipment: clean linen—mattress pad, fitted or flat bottom sheet, waterproof bed protector if needed, cotton draw sheet, flat top sheet, blanket(s), bath blanket, pillowcase(s), gloves

1. Wash your hands.

2. Identify yourself by name. Identify the resident by name.

3. Explain procedure to the resident. Speak clearly, slowly, and directly. Maintain face-to-face contact whenever possible.

4. Provide for the resident's privacy with curtain, screen, or door.

5. Place clean linen on clean surface within reach (e.g., bedside stand, overbed table, or chair).

6. Adjust bed to a safe working level, usually waist high. Lower head of bed. Lock bed wheels.

7. Put on gloves.

8. Loosen top linen from the end of the bed on the working side. Unfold bath blanket over the top sheet to cover the resident, and remove the top sheet.

9. You will make the bed one side at a time. If the bed has side rails, raise the side rail on far side of bed. After raising side rail, go to the other side. Help resident to turn onto her side, moving away from you toward the raised side rail (Fig. 12-9).

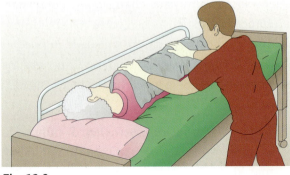

Fig. 12-9.

10. Loosen bottom soiled linen, mattress pad and protector if present on the working side.

11. Roll bottom soiled linen toward resident. Tuck it snugly against the resident's back.

12. Place and tuck in clean bottom linen. Finish with bottom sheet free of wrinkles. If you are using a flat bottom sheet, leave enough overlap on each end to tuck under the mattress. If the sheet is only long enough to tuck in at one end, tuck it in securely at the top of the bed. Make hospital corners to keep bottom sheet wrinkle-free (Fig. 12-10).

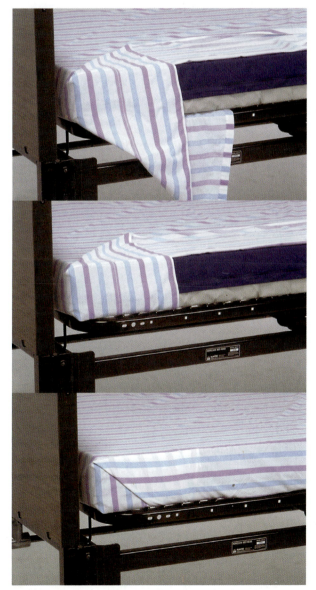

Fig. 12-10. *Hospital corners help keep the flat sheet smooth under the resident. They help prevent a resident's feet from being restricted by or tangled in linen when getting in and out of bed.*

13. Smooth the bottom sheet out toward the resident. Be sure there are no wrinkles in the mattress pad. Roll the extra material toward the resident. Tuck it under the resident's body (Fig. 12-11).

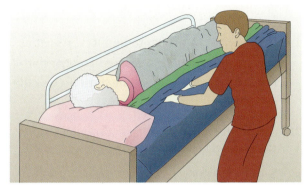

Fig. 12-11.

14. If using a waterproof pad, unfold it and center it on the bed. Tuck the side near you under the mattress. Smooth it out toward the resident. Tuck as you did with the sheet.

15. If using a draw sheet, place it on the bed. Tuck in on your side, smooth, and tuck as you did with the other bedding.

16. Raise side rail nearest you. Go to the other side of the bed and lower the side rail. Help resident to turn onto clean bottom sheet (Fig. 12-12). Protect the resident from any soiled matter on the old linens.

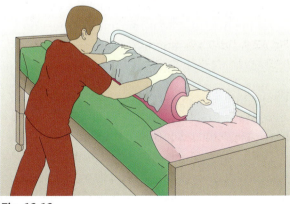

Fig. 12-12.

17. Loosen the soiled linen. Check for any personal items. Roll linen from head to foot of the bed. Avoid contact with your skin or clothes. Place it in a hamper or bag. Never

shake it. Soiled bed linens are full of microorganisms that should not be spread to other parts of the room.

18. Pull and tuck in clean bottom linen just like the other side. Finish with bottom sheet free of wrinkles.

19. Ask resident to turn onto her back. Assist as needed. Keep resident covered and comfortable, with a pillow under the head. Raise side rail.

20. Unfold the top sheet. Place it over the resident. Ask the resident to hold the top sheet. Slip the blanket or old sheet out from underneath (Fig. 12-13). Put it in the hamper or bag.

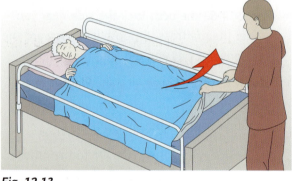

Fig. 12-13.

21. Place a blanket over the top sheet, matching the top edges. Tuck the bottom edges of top sheet and blanket under the bottom of the mattress. Make hospital corners on each side. Loosen the top linens over the resident's feet. This prevents pressure on the feet. At the top of the bed, fold the top sheet over the blanket about six inches.

22. Remove the pillow. Do not hold it near your face. Remove the soiled pillowcase by turning it inside out. Place it in the hamper or bag. Remove your gloves.

23. With one hand, grasp the clean pillowcase at the closed end. Turn it inside out over your arm. Next, using the same hand that has the pillowcase over it, grasp one narrow edge

of the pillow. Pull the pillowcase over it with your free hand (Fig. 12-14). Do the same for any other pillows. Place them under resident's head with open end away from door.

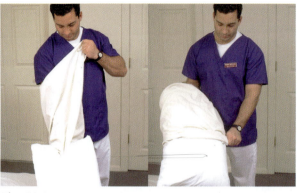

Fig. 12-14.

24. Make resident comfortable.

25. Return bed to lowest position. Remove privacy measures.

26. Place call light within resident's reach.

27. Take laundry bag or hamper to proper area.

28. Wash your hands.

29. Report any changes in resident to the nurse.

30. Document procedure using facility guidelines.

Making an unoccupied bed

Equipment: clean linen—mattress pad, fitted or flat bottom sheet, waterproof bed protector if needed, blanket(s), cotton draw sheet, flat top sheet, pillowcase(s), gloves

1. Wash your hands.

2. Place clean linen on clean surface within reach (e.g., bedside stand, overbed table, or chair).

3. Adjust bed to a safe working level, usually waist high. Put bed in flattest position. Lock bed wheels.

4. Put on gloves.

5. Loosen soiled linen. Roll soiled linen (soiled side inside) from head to foot of bed. Avoid contact with your skin or clothes. Place it in a hamper or bag.

6. Remove and discard gloves. Wash your hands.

7. Remake the bed. Spread mattress pad and bottom sheet, tucking under mattress. Make hospital corners to keep the bottom sheet wrinkle-free. Put on mattress protector and draw sheet. Smooth and tuck under sides of bed.

8. Place top sheet and blanket over bed. Center these, tuck under end of bed and make hospital corners. Fold down the top sheet over the blanket about six inches. Fold both top sheet and blanket down so resident can easily get into bed. If resident will not be returning to bed immediately, leave bedding up.

9. Remove pillows and pillowcases. Put on clean pillowcases. Replace pillows.

10. Return bed to lowest position.

11. Take laundry bag or hamper to proper area.

12. Wash your hands.

13. Document procedure using facility guidelines.

A **closed bed** is a bed completely made with the bedspread and blankets in place. It is made for residents who will be out of bed most of the day. It is also made when a resident is discharged. A closed bed is converted to an **open bed** by fanfolding the linen down to the foot of the bed. An open bed is a bed that is ready to receive a resident who has been out of bed all day or who is being admitted to the facility.

A **surgical bed** is made to accept residents who are returning to bed on stretchers, or gurneys. These residents may be coming from a hospital or returning from a test or procedure. A surgical bed is opened to receive residents by loosening the linens on one side and folding them to the other side. This leaves one side open. See Chapter 10 for information on transferring residents into bed from a stretcher.

Making a surgical bed

Equipment: clean linen (see procedure: Making an unoccupied bed), gloves

1. Wash your hands.

2. Place clean linen on clean surface within reach (e.g., bedside stand, overbed table, or chair).

3. Adjust bed to a safe working level, usually waist high. Lock bed wheels.

4. Put on gloves.

5. Remove all soiled linen, rolling it (soiled side inside) from head to foot of bed. Avoid contact with your skin or clothes. Place it in a hamper or bag.

6. Remove and discard gloves. Wash your hands.

7. Make an unoccupied, closed bed. See procedure: Making an unoccupied bed.

8. Loosen linens on the side of bed that is away from the door (where the stretcher will be).

9. Fanfold linens lengthwise to the side away from door (Fig. 12-15). Fanfolded means folded several times into pleats.

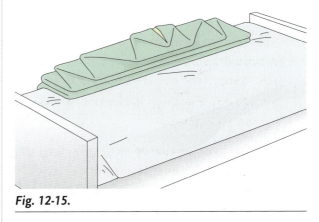

Fig. 12-15.

10. Put on clean pillowcases (as described above). Replace pillows.

11. Leave bed in its locked position with both side rails down.

12. Make sure the pathway to the bed is clear.

13. Take laundry bag or hamper to proper area.

14. Wash your hands.

15. Document procedure using facility guidelines.

Chapter Review

1. What are three ways that nursing assistants can keep the noise level low in facilities?

2. What are three ways that nursing assistants can help control odors in facilities?

3. How do electric bed controls usually work?

4. Why are beds usually kept in their lowest positions?

5. What is the overbed table used for? Can bedpans and soiled linen be placed on an overbed table?

6. Where should call lights always be placed?

7. How do screens and curtains help protect residents' privacy?

8. What can the use of disposable equipment help prevent?

9. List two functions that sleep performs for the body.

10. What problems can result from not getting enough sleep?

11. What are three reasons why bed linens should be changed often?

12. Define the following terms: occupied bed, unoccupied bed, closed bed, open bed, and surgical bed.

13. Which way should pillows face while under residents' heads?

13
Personal Care Skills

1. Explain personal care of residents

Personal care is different from taking vital signs or tidying a resident's unit, which are other tasks that NAs may perform for residents. The term "personal" refers to tasks that are concerned with the person's body, appearance, and hygiene, and suggests privacy may be important. **Hygiene** is the term used to describe practices to keep our bodies clean and healthy. Bathing and brushing teeth are two examples. **Grooming** refers to practices like caring for fingernails and hair. Hygiene and grooming activities, as well as dressing, eating, transferring, and toileting are called activities of daily living (ADLs).

Some people who are recovering from an illness or an accident may not have the energy to care for themselves. Other reasons someone may need personal care include the following:

- A person has a long-term, chronic condition
- A person is frail because of advanced age
- A person is permanently disabled
- A person is dying

These residents may need assistance with their personal care, or they may need you to provide it for them entirely. You may provide any or all of the personal care, including bathing, perineal care (care of genitals and anal area), toileting, mouth care, shampooing and combing the hair, nail care, shaving, dressing, eating, walking, and transferring. You will assist residents with these tasks every day. These activities are often called "a.m. care" or "p.m. care," which refers to the time of day when they are done.

Assisting with a.m. care includes the following:

- Offering a bedpan or urinal or helping the resident to the bathroom
- Helping the resident to wash face and hands
- Assisting with mouth care before or after breakfast, as the resident prefers

Assisting with p.m. care includes the following:

- Offering a bedpan or urinal or helping the resident to the bathroom
- Helping the resident to wash face and hands
- Giving a snack
- Assisting with mouth care
- Giving a back rub

Some residents may never be able to care for themselves, and you will assist them as needed. However, some residents will regain strength and be able to perform their own personal care. An important part of your job is to help residents be as independent as possible. This means encouraging residents to care for themselves. Promoting independence is part of your care.

We all have routines for personal care and activities of daily living. We also have preferences for how they are done. These routines remain important even when we are elderly, sick, or disabled. Be aware of your residents' individual preferences concerning their personal care. Residents may prefer certain soaps or skin care products. They may choose to bathe in the morning or at night. It is important to ask residents about their routines and preferences.

Many people have been doing personal care tasks for themselves their entire lives. They may feel embarrassed or uncomfortable about having anyone do or help them do these tasks. Some residents may not like to be touched by someone else. It is important to understand how stressful it may be for some people to have help with personal care. Be sensitive to this. Be professional when helping with these tasks.

Before you begin any task, explain to the resident exactly what you will be doing. Explaining care to a resident is not only his legal right, but it may also help lessen anxiety. Ask if he or she would like to use the bathroom or bedpan first. Provide the resident with privacy. Let him or her make as many decisions as possible about when, where, and how a procedure will be done (Fig. 13-1). This promotes dignity and independence. Encourage residents to do as much as they are able to do while giving care. Other ways to promote respect, dignity, and privacy include:

- Knocking before entering the resident's room

- Not interrupting residents while they are in the bathroom

- Leaving the room when residents receive or make phone calls

- Respecting residents' private time and personal things

- Not interrupting residents while they are dressing

- Encouraging residents to do things for themselves and being patient

- Keeping residents covered whenever possible when you help with dressing

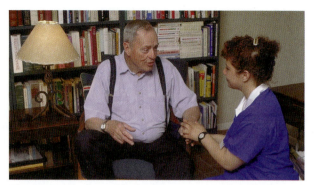

Fig. 13-1. *Let the resident make as many decisions as possible about the personal care you will perform.*

Personal care gives you the opportunity to observe your resident's skin, mental state, mobility, flexibility, comfort level, and ability to perform ADLs. While assisting with personal care, look for any problems or changes that have occurred. Communication is especially important during personal care. Some residents will talk about symptoms they are experiencing during personal care. They may tell you that they have been itching or their skin feels dry. They may complain of numbness and tingling in a certain part of the body. Keep a small note pad in a pocket to jot down exactly how the resident describes these symptoms. Make notes right after the procedure. Report these comments to the nurse and document them properly.

Observe the resident's mental and emotional state at this time. Is the resident depressed or confused? Can the resident concentrate on the activity or hold a conversation? Is the resident short of breath? Does the resident tremble or shake? Focus on changes from the resident's normal state. Is there a change in behavior, level of activity, skin color, movement, or anything else? You are in the best position to observe, report, and document any small change in your resident. No matter what care task is assigned to you, performing it is only half the job.

During the procedure, if the resident appears tired, stop and take a short rest. Never rush a resident. After care, always ask if the resident would like anything else. Leave the resident's area clean and tidy. Make sure the call light is within reach. Check to see that the room has good lighting and is a comfortable temperature. Make sure that there are not electrical cords or other objects in the walkways. Leave the bed in its lowest position unless instructed otherwise.

Observing and Reporting:
Personal Care

O/R Skin color, temperature, redness (more information listed in next learning objective)

O/R Mobility

O/R Flexibility

O/R Comfort level, or pain or discomfort

O/R Strength and the ability to perform ADLs

O/R Mental and emotional state

O/R Resident complaints

2. Identify guidelines for providing good skin care and preventing pressure sores

Immobility reduces the amount of blood that circulates to the skin. Residents who have restricted mobility have a higher risk of skin deterioration at pressure points. **Pressure points** are areas of the body that bear much of its weight. Pressure points are mainly located at bony prominences. **Bony prominences** are areas of the body where the bone lies close to the skin. These areas include elbows, shoulder blades, tailbone, hip bones, ankles, heels, and the back of the neck and head. The skin here is at a much higher risk for skin breakdown.

Other areas at risk are the ears, the area under the breasts, and the scrotum (Fig. 13-2). The pressure on these areas reduces circulation, decreasing the amount of oxygen the cells receive. Warmth and moisture also contribute to skin breakdown. Once the surface of the skin is weakened, pathogens can invade and cause infection. When infection occurs, the healing process is slower.

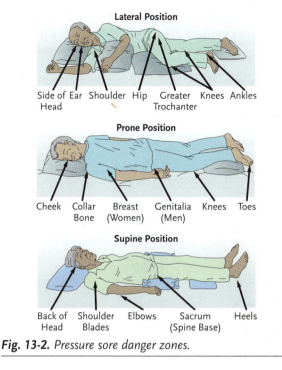

Fig. 13-2. *Pressure sore danger zones.*

When skin begins to break down, it becomes pale, white, or a reddened color. Darker skin may look purple. The resident may also feel tingling or burning in the area. This discoloration does not go away, even when the resident's position is changed. If pressure is allowed to continue, the area will further break down. The resulting wound is called a **pressure sore**, bed sore, or decubitus ulcer. Once a pressure sore forms, it can get bigger, deeper, and infected. Pressure sores are painful and difficult to heal. They can lead to life-threatening infections. Prevention is the key to skin health.

There are four accepted stages of pressure sores (Fig. 13-3):

- Stage 1: Skin is intact but there is redness that is not relieved within 15 to 30 minutes after removing pressure.

- Stage 2: There is partial skin loss involving the outer and/or inner layer of skin. The ulcer is superficial. It looks like a blister or a shallow crater.

- Stage 3: There is full skin loss involving damage or death of tissue that may extend down to but not through the tissue that covers muscle. The ulcer looks like a deep crater.

- Stage 4: There is full skin loss with major destruction, tissue death, damage to muscle, bone, or supporting structures.

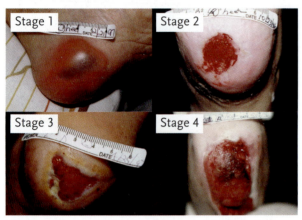

Fig. 13-3. *Pressure sores are categorized by four stages.*
(PHOTOS COURTESY OF DR. TAMARA D. FISHMAN AND THE WOUND CARE INSTITUTE, INC.)

Observing and Reporting:
Resident's Skin

Report any of these to the nurse:

- **O/R** Pale, white, reddened, or purple areas, blisters or bruises on the skin
- **O/R** Complaints of tingling, warmth, or burning of the skin
- **O/R** Dry or flaking skin
- **O/R** Itching or scratching
- **O/R** Rash or any skin discoloration
- **O/R** Swelling
- **O/R** Fluid or blood draining from skin
- **O/R** Broken skin
- **O/R** Wounds or ulcers on the skin
- **O/R** Changes in wound or ulcer (size, depth, drainage, color, odor)
- **O/R** Redness or broken skin between toes or around toenails

In darker complexions, also look for:

- **O/R** Any change in the feel of the tissue

- **O/R** Any change in the appearance of the skin, such as the "orange-peel" look or a purplish hue
- **O/R** Extremely dry, crust-like areas that might be covering a tissue break upon closer look

Breaks in the skin can cause serious, even life-threatening, complications. It is much better to prevent skin problems and keep the skin healthy than it is to treat skin problems. The following are guidelines for basic skin care:

Guidelines:
Basic Skin Care

- **G** Report any changes in a resident's skin.
- **G** Provide regular, daily care for skin to keep it clean and dry. When complete baths are not taken every day, check the resident's skin.
- **G** Reposition immobile residents often (at least every two hours).
- **G** Give frequent and thorough skin care as often as needed for incontinent residents. Change clothing and linens often as well. Check on them every two hours or as needed.
- **G** Do not scratch or irritate the skin in any way. Keep rough, scratchy fabrics away from the resident's skin. Report to the nurse if a resident wears shoes that cause blisters or sores.
- **G** Massage the skin often. Use light, circular strokes to increase circulation. Use little or no pressure on bony areas. Do not massage a white, red, or purple area or put any pressure on it. Massage the healthy skin and tissue around the area.
- **G** Be careful during transfers. Avoid pulling or tearing fragile skin.
- **G** Residents who are overweight may have poor circulation and extra folds of skin. The skin under the folds may be difficult to clean and to keep dry. Pay careful attention to these areas and give regular skin care. Report signs of skin irritation.

G Residents should eat well-balanced meals. Proper nutrition is important for keeping skin healthy. Nutrition affects the color and texture of the skin. Very thin residents may be malnourished, which puts them at risk for skin injuries. Be gentle when moving and positioning them. You will learn more about nutrition in Chapter 15.

G Keep plastic or rubber materials from coming into contact with the resident's skin. These materials prevent air from circulating, which causes the skin to sweat.

G The care plan may include instructions on giving special skin care for dry, closed wounds or other conditions. The skin may have to be washed with a special soap, or a brush may have to be used on the skin. Follow the care plan and nurse's instructions.

For residents who are not mobile or cannot change positions easily, remember:

G Keep the bottom sheet tight and free from wrinkles. Keep the bed free from crumbs. Keep clothing or gowns free of wrinkles, too.

G Do not pull the resident across sheets during transfers or repositioning. This causes shearing, which can lead to skin breakdown.

G Place a sheepskin, chamois skin, or bed pad under the back and buttocks to absorb moisture or perspiration that may build up and to protect the skin from irritating bed linens (Fig. 13-4).

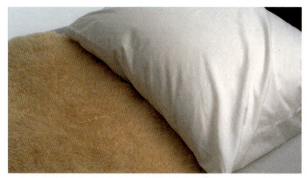

Fig. 13-4. *A sheepskin or chamois skin may be placed under the resident to absorb moisture.* (REPRINTED WITH PERMISSION OF BRIGGS CORPORATION, 800-247-2343, WWW.BRIGGSCORP.COM)

G Relieve pressure under bony prominences. Place foam rubber or sheepskin pads under them. Heel and elbow protectors made of foam and sheepskin are available (Fig. 13-5).

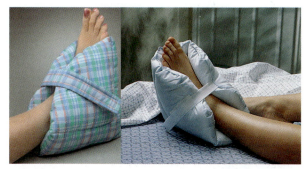

Fig. 13-5. *Padded heel protectors help keep feet properly aligned and prevent pressure sores.* (REPRINTED WITH PERMISSION OF BRIGGS CORPORATION, 800-247-2343, WWW.BRIGGSCORP.COM)

G A bed or chair can be made softer with flotation pads.

G Use a bed cradle to keep top sheets from rubbing the resident's skin.

G Residents seated in chairs or wheelchairs need to be repositioned often, too. Reposition residents every 15 minutes if they are in a wheelchair or chair and cannot change positions easily.

Applying Nonprescription Ointments, Lotions or Powders

You may be assigned to apply ointments, lotions or powders to a resident's skin (Fig. 13-6). Not all nursing assistants are allowed to do this. Make sure you understand the rules in your facility. If instructed to apply an ointment, lotion, or powder by the nurse, follow these rules. Ask questions if anything is unclear.

- Read the directions.

- Know exactly where it is to be applied

- Know if it should be rubbed in or left on the top of the skin.

- Wash your hands before and after application

- Wear gloves.

- Avoid getting any on clothing as it may stain.

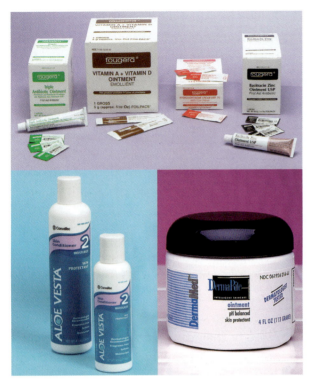

Fig. 13-6. There are many types of ointments, creams, and lotions that are used to treat, soften, and protect the skin. (REPRINTED WITH PERMISSION OF BRIGGS CORPORATION, 800-247-2343, WWW.BRIGGSCORP.COM)

Many positioning devices are available to help make residents more comfortable and safe.

Guidelines
Positioning Devices:

G   Backrests provide support and can be regular pillows or special wedge-shaped foam pillows.

G   Bed cradles are used to keep the bed covers from pushing down on a resident's feet.

G   Use draw sheets, or turning sheets, under residents who cannot help with turning, lifting, or moving up in bed. Draw sheets help prevent skin damage from shearing. A regular bed sheet folded in half can be used as a draw sheet.

G   Footboards are padded boards placed against the resident's feet to keep them properly aligned and to prevent foot drop (Fig. 13-7). **Foot drop** is a weakness of muscles in the

feet and ankles that causes difficulty with the ability to flex the ankles and walk normally. Rolled blankets or pillows can also be used as footboards.

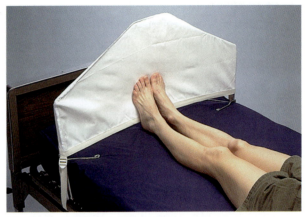

Fig. 13-7. Footboards help prevent pressure sores. (REPRINTED WITH PERMISSION OF BRIGGS CORPORATION, 800-247-2343, WWW.BRIGGSCORP.COM)

G   Handrolls keep the fingers from curling tightly. A rolled washcloth, gauze bandage, or a rubber ball placed inside the palm may be used to keep the hand in a natural position (Fig. 13-8).

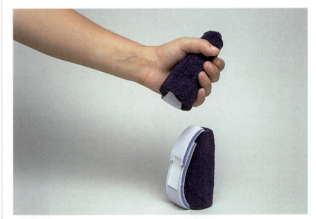

Fig. 13-8. Handrolls help keep fingers from curling too tightly. (REPRINTED WITH PERMISSION OF BRIGGS CORPORATION, 800-247-2343, WWW.BRIGGSCORP.COM)

G   Splints are a type of orthotic device (Fig. 13-9). An **orthotic device** is a device, such as a splint or brace, that helps support and align a limb and improve its functioning. Orthotics also help prevent or correct deformities. Splints and the skin area around them should be cleaned at least once daily and as needed.

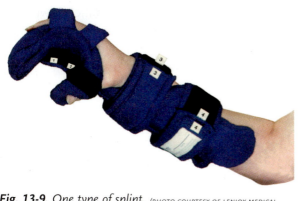

Fig. 13-9. One type of splint. (PHOTO COURTESY OF LENJOY MEDICAL ENGINEERING "COMFY SPLINTS TM" 800-582-5332, WWW.COMFYSPLINTS.COM)

G Trochanter rolls keep a resident's hips from turning outward (Fig. 13-10). A rolled towel works well, too.

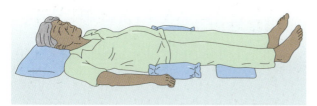

Fig. 13-10. Trochanter rolls help keep the hips in their proper position.

G Knee pillows can help keep spine, hips, and knees in the proper position and ease pain in the back, leg, hip and knee areas (Fig. 13-11).

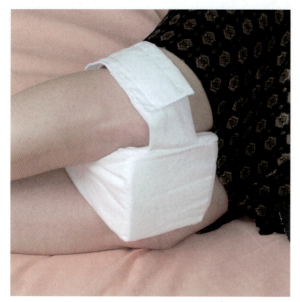

Fig. 13-11. Knee pillows help keep the knees, hip, and spine in the proper alignment. (REPRINTED WITH PERMISSION OF BRIGGS CORPORATION, 800-247-2343, WWW.BRIGGSCORP.COM)

3. Explain guidelines for assisting with bathing

Bathing promotes good health and well-being. It removes perspiration, dirt, oil, and dead skin cells that collect on the skin. It helps to prevent skin irritation and body odor. Bathing can also be relaxing. The bed bath is an excellent time for moving arms and legs and increasing circulation. Bathing gives you an opportunity to observe residents' skin carefully.

Residents may be given a complete bath in bed, or they may take a shower or have a tub bath. They may have a **partial bath**, which is a bath given on days when a complete bed bath, tub bath, or shower is not done. It includes washing the face, hands, **axillae** (underarms), and perineum. The **perineum** is the genital and anal area.

Most people have specific preferences for bathing. Some like to take long hot baths, while others prefer a quick shower. Usually they have been bathing the same way most of their lives. Doctors have factors to consider about whether or not to honor residents' personal preferences regarding bathing. They include the resident's capabilities and his or her safety, as well as the safety of the caregiver. The doctor, along with the resident, will decide which type of bath is appropriate.

A doctor may order a special bath using an additive. An **additive** is a substance added to another substance, changing its effect. Examples of some common bath additives and their purpose include the following:

*   Bran helps to relieve itching.

*   Oatmeal baths are used for inflamed skin. Oatmeal helps in relieving itching and irritation and is soothing.

*   Sodium bicarbonate (baking soda) is used to treat psoriasis (non-contagious skin disorder that causes red scaly patches on the skin) and helps relieve itching.

- Epsom salts baths or soaks reduce pain and swelling and relax muscles.

- Pine products help refresh, calm and cool.

- Tar coal baths are used to treat eczema and other skin conditions.

- Sulfur baths may be used for skin rashes, eczema, and to help relieve inflammation related to arthritis.

Guidelines:
Bathing

G The face, hands, underarms, and perineum should be washed every day. A complete bath or shower can be taken every other day or even less often.

G Older skin produces less perspiration and oil. Elderly people with dry and fragile skin should bathe only once or twice a week. This prevents further dryness. Be gentle with the skin when bathing residents.

G Use only products approved by the facility or that the resident prefers.

G Before bathing a resident, make sure the room is warm enough.

G Be familiar with available safety and assistive devices.

G Before bathing, make sure the water temperature is safe and comfortable. Test the water temperature to make sure it is not too hot, then have the resident test the water temperature. His or her sense of touch may be different than yours. The resident is best able to choose a comfortable water temperature.

G Gather supplies before giving a bath so the resident is not left alone.

G Make sure all soap is removed from the skin before completing the bath.

G Keep a record of the bathing schedule for each resident. Follow the care plan.

Giving a complete bed bath

Equipment: bath blanket, bath basin, soap, bath thermometer, 2-4 washcloths, 2-4 bath towels, clean gown or clothes, gloves, orangewood stick or emery board, lotion, deodorant

1. Wash your hands.

2. Identify yourself by name. Identify the resident by name.

3. Explain procedure to the resident. Speak clearly, slowly, and directly. Maintain face-to-face contact whenever possible.

4. Provide for the resident's privacy with curtain, screen, or door. Be sure the room is a comfortable temperature and there are no drafts.

5. Adjust bed to a safe level, usually waist high. Lock bed wheels.

6. Place a bath blanket or towel over resident (Fig. 13-12). Ask him to hold onto it as you remove or fold back top bedding. Remove gown, while keeping resident covered with bath blanket (or top sheet).

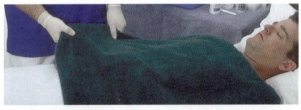

Fig. 13-12. *Cover the resident with a cotton blanket before removing top bedding.*

7. Fill the basin with warm water. Test water temperature with thermometer or your wrist and ensure it is safe. Water temperature should be 105° to 110° F. It cools quickly. Have resident check water temperature. Adjust if necessary. Change the water when it becomes too cool, soapy, or dirty.

8. Put on gloves.

9. Ask and assist resident to participate in washing.

10. Uncover only one part of the body at a time. Place a towel under the body part being washed.

11. Wash, rinse, and dry one part of the body at a time. Start at the head. Work down, and complete the front first. Fold the washcloth over your hand like a mitt and hold it in place with the thumb (Fig. 13-13).

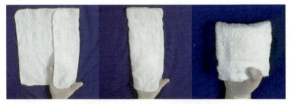

Fig. 13-13. Fold the washcloth to make a mitt.

Eyes and Face: Wash face with wet washcloth (no soap). Begin with the eye farther away from you. Wash inner aspect to outer aspect (Fig. 13-14). Use a different area of the washcloth for each eye. Wash the face from the middle outward. Use firm but gentle strokes. Wash the neck and ears and behind the ears. Rinse and pat dry.

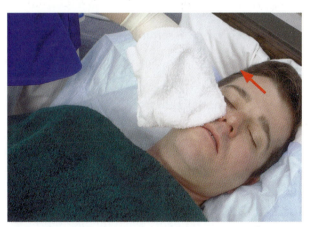

Fig. 13-14. Wash the eye from the inner part to the outer part.

Arms: Remove the resident's top clothing. Cover him with the bath blanket or towel. With a soapy washcloth, wash the upper arm and underarm. Use long strokes from the shoulder down to the wrist (Fig. 13-15). Rinse and pat dry.

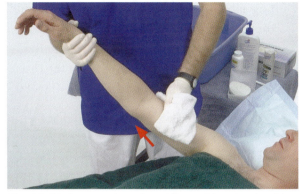

Fig. 13-15. Support the wrist while washing the shoulder, arm, underarm, and elbow.

Wash the hand in a basin: Clean under the nails with an orangewood stick or nail brush if available (Fig. 13-16). Rinse and pat dry. Give nail care (see procedure later in this chapter) if it has been assigned. Do not give nail care to a diabetic resident. Repeat for the other arm. Put lotion on the resident's elbows and hands if ordered.

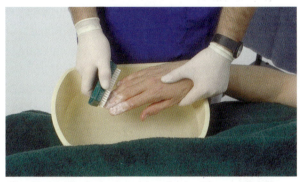

Fig. 13-16. Wash the hand in a basin. Thoroughly clean under the nails with a nail brush.

Chest: Place the towel again across the resident's chest. Pull the blanket down to the waist. Lift the towel only enough to wash the chest. Rinse it, and pat dry. For a female resident, wash, rinse, and dry breasts and under breasts. Check the skin in this area for signs of irritation and chafing.

Abdomen: Fold the blanket down so that it still covers the pubic area. Wash the abdomen, rinse, and pat dry. If the resident has an ostomy, or opening in the abdomen for getting rid of body wastes, give skin care around the opening (Chapter 17 includes more information about ostomies). Cover with the towel. Pull the cotton blanket up to the resident's chin. Remove the towel.

Legs and Feet: Expose one leg and place a towel under it. Wash the thigh. Use long downward strokes. Rinse and pat dry. Do the same from the knee to the ankle (Fig. 13-17).

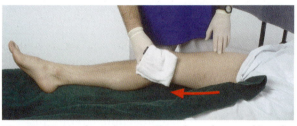

Fig. 13-17. *Use long downward strokes when washing the legs.*

Place another towel under the foot. Move the basin to the towel. Place the foot into the basin. Wash the foot and between the toes (Fig. 13-18). Rinse foot and pat dry. Make sure area between toes is dry. Give nail care (see procedure later in this chapter) if it has been assigned. Do not give nail care to a diabetic resident. Never clip a resident's toenails. Apply lotion to the foot if ordered, especially at the heels. Do not apply lotion between the toes. Repeat steps for the other leg and foot.

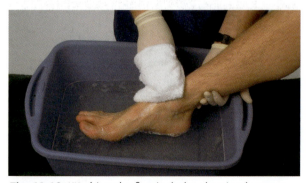

Fig. 13-18. *Washing the feet includes cleaning between the toes.*

Back: Help resident move to the center of the bed. Ask resident to turn onto his side so his back is facing you. If the bed has rails,

raise the rail on the far side for safety. Fold the blanket away from the back. Place a towel lengthwise next to the back. Wash the back, neck, and buttocks with long, downward strokes. Rinse and pat dry (Fig. 13-19). Apply lotion if ordered.

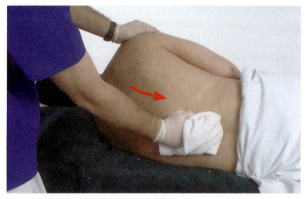

Fig. 13-19. *Wash the back with long downward strokes.*

12. Place the towel under the buttocks and upper thighs. Help the resident turn onto his back. Ask if he is able to wash the perineal area. If the resident is able to do this, place a basin of clean, warm water and a washcloth and towel within reach. Leave the room if the resident desires. If the resident has a urinary catheter in place, remind him not to pull it.

13. If the resident is unable to provide perineal care, you must do so. Put on gloves first (if you have not already done so). Provide privacy at all times.

14. **Perineal area and buttocks**: Change the bath water. Wash, rinse, and dry perineal area, working from front to back.

    For a female resident: Wash the perineum with soap and water. Work from front to back, using single strokes (Fig. 13-20). Do not wash from the back to the front. This may cause infection. Use a clean area of washcloth or a clean washcloth for each stroke. First wipe the center of the perineum, then each side. Then spread the labia majora, the outside folds of perineal skin that protect the urinary meatus and the vaginal opening. Wipe from front to back on each side. Rinse the area in the same way. Dry entire perineal area moving from front to back. Use a blotting motion with towel. Ask resident to turn on her side. Wash, rinse, and dry buttocks and anal area. Cleanse the anal area without contaminating the perineal area.

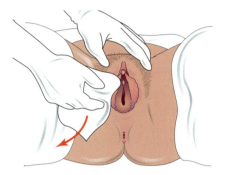

Fig. 13-20. *Always work from front to back when performing perineal care. This helps prevent infection.*

For a male resident: If the resident is uncircumcised, pull back the foreskin first. Gently push skin towards the base of penis. Hold the penis by the shaft. Wash in a circular motion from the tip down to the base. Use a clean area of washcloth or clean washcloth for each stroke (Fig. 13-21). Rinse the penis. If resident is uncircumcised, gently return foreskin to normal position. Then wash the scrotum and groin. The **groin** is the area from the pubis (area around the penis and scrotum) to the upper thighs. Rinse and pat dry. Ask the resident to turn on his side. Wash, rinse, and dry buttocks and anal area. Cleanse the anal area without contaminating the perineal area.

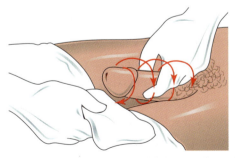

Fig. 13-21. *Wash the penis in a circular motion from the tip down to the base.*

15. Cover the resident with the blanket.

16. Empty, rinse, and dry bath basin. Place basin in designated dirty supply area or return to storage, depending on facility policy.

17. Place soiled clothing and linens in proper containers.

18. Remove and dispose of gloves properly. Wash your hands.

19. Put clean gown on resident. Provide resident with deodorant. Brush or comb the resident's hair (see procedure later in this chapter).

20. Make resident comfortable. Make sure sheets are free from wrinkles and the bed free from crumbs.

21. Return bed to lowest position. Remove privacy measures.

22. Place call light within resident's reach.

23. Wash your hands.

24. Report any changes in resident to the nurse.

25. Document procedure using facility guidelines.

A back rub can help relax residents. It can make them more comfortable and increase circulation. Back rubs are often given after baths. After giving a back rub, make sure to note any changes in a resident's skin.

Giving a back rub

Equipment: cotton blanket or towel, lotion

1. Wash your hands.

2. Identify yourself by name. Identify the resident by name.

3. Explain procedure to the resident. Speak clearly, slowly, and directly. Maintain face-to-face contact whenever possible.

4. Provide for resident's privacy with curtain, screen, or door.

5. Adjust bed to a safe working level, usually waist high. Lower the head of the bed. Lock bed wheels.

6. Position resident in the prone position (lying on his stomach). If this is uncomfortable, have him lie on his side. Cover with a cotton blanket, then fold back bed covers. Expose the back to the top of the buttocks. Back rubs can also be given with the resident sitting up.

7. Warm lotion by putting bottle in warm water for five minutes. Run your hands under warm water. Pour lotion on your hands and rub them together. Always put lotion on your hands rather than on resident's skin.

8. Place your hands on each side of upper part of the buttocks. Make long, smooth upward strokes with both hands. Move along each side of the spine, up to the shoulders (Figs. 13-22 and 13-23). Circle your hands outward. Then move back along outer edges of the back. At buttocks, make another circle. Move your hands back up to the shoulders. Without taking your hands from resident's skin, repeat this motion for three to five minutes.

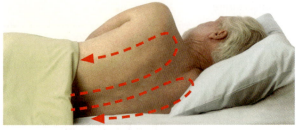

Fig. 13-22. A resident on his side.

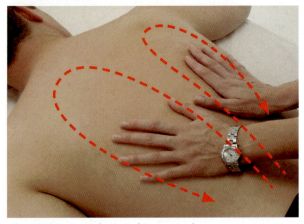

Fig. 13-23. A resident on his stomach.

9. Knead with the first two fingers and thumb of each hand. Place them at base of the spine.

Move upward together along each side of the spine. Apply gentle downward pressure with fingers and thumbs. Follow same direction as with the long smooth strokes, circling at shoulders and buttocks.

10. Gently massage bony areas (spine, shoulder blades, hip bones). Use circular motions of fingertips. If any of these areas are red, massage around them, rather than on them. The redness indicates that the skin is already irritated and fragile. Include this information in your report to the nurse.

11. Let the resident know when you are almost through. Finish with some long smooth strokes, like the ones you used at the beginning of the massage.

12. Dry the back if extra lotion remains on it.

13. Remove blanket and towel.

14. Help the resident get dressed. Make resident comfortable. Make sure sheets are free from wrinkles and the bed free from crumbs.

15. Store supplies. Place soiled clothing and linens in proper containers.

16. Return bed to lowest position. Remove privacy measures.

17. Place call light within resident's reach.

18. Wash your hands.

19. Report any changes in resident to the nurse.

20. Document procedure using facility guidelines.

Hair care is an important part of cleanliness. Shampooing the hair removes dirt, bacteria, oils, and other materials from the hair. Residents who can get out of bed may have their hair shampooed in the sink, tub, or shower. For residents who cannot get out of bed, special troughs exist for shampooing hair in bed. Troughs fit under the resident's head and neck and have a spout or hose that drains the water into a basin at the side of the bed (Fig. 13-24). There are also special types of shampoo that do not require the use of water (Fig. 13-25). Follow the care plan on what type of shampoo to use.

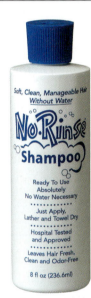

Fig. 13-24. *An inflatable bed shampoo trough can be used to shampoo hair while the person is in bed.* (REPRINTED WITH PERMISSION OF BRIGGS CORPORATION, 800-247-2343, WWW.BRIGGSCORP.COM)

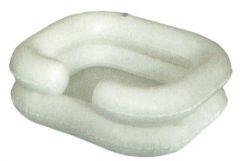

Fig. 13-25. *One type of shampoo that does not require water.* (REPRINTED WITH PERMISSION OF BRIGGS CORPORATION, 800-247-2343, WWW.BRIGGSCORP.COM)

Shampooing hair

Equipment: shampoo, hair conditioner (if requested), 2 bath towels, washcloth, bath thermometer, pitcher or handheld shower or sink attachment, waterproof pad (if washing hair in bed), bath blanket (if washing hair in bed), trough and catch basin (for washing hair in bed), protective plastic sheet or drape (if washing hair in sink) comb and brush, hair dryer

1. Wash your hands.

2. Identify yourself by name. Identify the resident by name.

3. Explain procedure to the resident. Speak clearly, slowly, and directly. Maintain face-to-face contact whenever possible.

4. Provide for the resident's privacy with curtain, screen, or door. Be sure the room is a comfortable temperature and there are no drafts.

5. Test water temperature with thermometer or your wrist. Ensure it is safe. Water temperature should be 105° F. Have resident check water temperature. Adjust if necessary.

6. Position the resident and wet the resident's hair.

a. **For washing hair in the sink**, seat the resident in a chair covered with a protective plastic drape or sheet. Use a pillow under the plastic to support the head and neck. Have the resident lean her head back toward the sink. Give the resident a folded washcloth to hold over her forehead or eyes. Wet hair using a plastic cup or a hand-held sink attachment (Fig. 13-26).

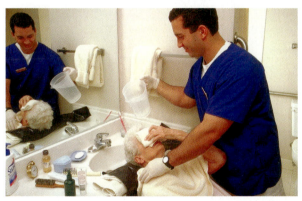

Fig. 13-26. *Make sure the resident's head and neck are supported and her eyes covered when washing hair in the sink.*

b. **For washing hair in bed**, arrange the supplies within reach on a nearby table. Remove all pillows, and place the resident in a flat position. Adjust bed to a safe level, usually waist high. Lock bed wheels. Place a waterproof pad beneath the resident's head and shoulders. Cover the resident with the blanket, and fold back the top sheet and regular blankets.

Place the trough under the resident's head and connect trough to the catch basin. Place one towel across the resident's shoulders. Protect resident's eyes with a dry washcloth. Using the pitcher or attachment, pour enough water on the resident's hair to make it thoroughly wet.

7. Apply a small amount of shampoo to your hands and rub them together. Using both hands, massage the shampoo to a lather in the resident's hair. With your fingertips, massage the scalp in a circular motion, from front to back (Fig. 13-27). Do not scratch the scalp.

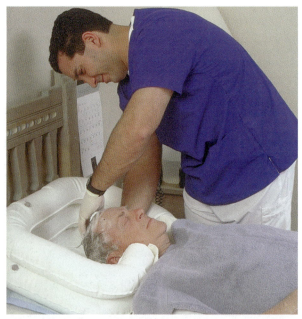

Fig. 13-27. Use your fingertips to work shampoo into a lather. Be gentle so that you do not scratch the scalp.

8. Rinse the hair in the same way you wet it. Rinse until water runs clear. Repeat the shampoo, rinse again, and use conditioner if the resident wants it. Be sure to rinse the hair thoroughly to prevent the scalp from getting dry and itchy.

9. Wrap the resident's hair in a towel. If shampooing at the sink, return the resident to an upright position. If shampooing in bed, remove the trough. Using the washcloth or a face towel, wipe water from the head and neck.

10. Remove the hair towel and gently rub scalp and hair with the towel. Comb or brush hair (see procedure later in the chapter).

11. Dry hair with a hair dryer on the low setting. Style hair as the resident prefers.

12. Make resident comfortable. Make sure sheets are free from wrinkles and the bed free from crumbs.

13. Return bed to lowest position. Remove privacy measures.

14. Place call light within resident's reach.

15. Empty, rinse, and wipe bath basin/pitcher. Take to proper area.

16. Clean comb/brush. Return hair dryer and comb/brush to proper storage.

17. Place soiled linen in proper container.

18. Wash your hands.

19. Report any changes in resident to nurse.

20. Document procedure using facility guidelines.

Many people prefer showers or tub baths to bed baths (Fig. 13-28). Check with the nurse first to make sure a shower or tub bath is allowed.

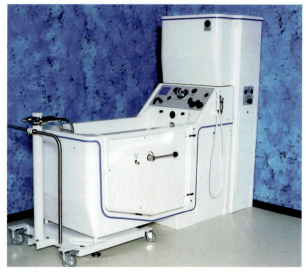

Fig. 13-28. A common style of tub in nursing homes.
(PHOTO COURTESY OF LEE PENNER OF PENNER TUBS)

Guidelines:
Safety for Showers and Tub Baths

G Clean tub or shower before and after use.

G Make sure bathroom or shower room floor is dry.

G Be familiar with available safety and assistive devices. Check that hand rails, grab bars, and lifts are in working order.

G Have resident use safety bars to get into or out of the tub or shower.

G Place all needed items within reach.

G Do not leave the resident alone.

G Bath oils and lotions are used to moisturize dry skin. Powders are drying and may be applied to moist or oily skin. Both lotions and powders reduce friction. They help protect the skin from injury when it is in contact with bed sheets or in skin folds. However, do not use bath oils, lotions, or powders in showers or tubs. They make surfaces slippery and dangerous.

G Test water temperature with thermometer or your wrist before resident gets into shower. Water temperature should be no more than 105° F. Make sure temperature is comfortable for resident.

Residents' Rights

Privacy when Bathing

Privacy is very important when transporting residents to the shower or tub room and during the shower or tub bath. Keep residents covered and make sure their bodies are not unnecessarily exposed.

Giving a shower or tub bath

Equipment: bath blanket, soap, shampoo, bath thermometer, 2-4 washcloths, 2-4 bath towels, clean gown and robe or clothes, non-skid footwear, gloves, lotion, deodorant

1. Wash your hands.

2. Place equipment in shower or tub room. Clean shower or tub area and shower chair.

3. Wash your hands.

4. Go to resident's room. Identify yourself by name. Identify the resident by name.

5. Explain procedure to the resident. Speak clearly, slowly, and directly. Maintain face-to-face contact whenever possible.

6. Provide for resident's privacy with curtain, screen, or door.

7. Help resident to put on nonskid footwear. Transport resident to shower or tub room.

For a shower:

8. If using a shower chair, place it into position. Lock wheels (Fig. 13-29). Safely transfer resident into shower chair.

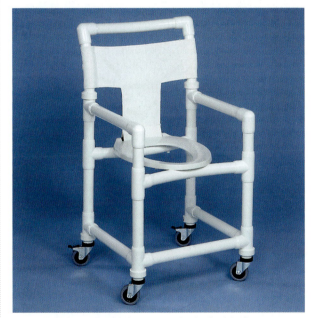

Fig. 13-29. A shower chair must be locked before transferring a resident into it. (PHOTO COURTESY OF INNOVATIVE PRODUCTS UNLIMITED)

9. Turn on water. Test water temperature with thermometer. Water temperature should be no more than 105° F. Have resident check water temperature.

For a tub bath:

8. Safely transfer resident onto chair or tub lift.

9. Fill the tub halfway with warm water. Test water temperature with thermometer. Water temperature should be no more than 105°F. Have resident check water temperature.

Remaining steps for either procedure:

10. Put on gloves.

11. Help resident remove clothing and shoes.

12. Help the resident into shower or tub. Put shower chair into shower and lock wheels.

13. Stay with resident during procedure.

14. Let resident wash as much as possible. Help to wash his or her face.

15. Help resident shampoo and rinse hair.

16. Help to wash and rinse the entire body. Move from head to toe.

17. Turn off water or drain the tub. Cover resident with bath blanket while tub drains.

18. Unlock shower chair wheels, if used. Roll resident out of shower, or help resident out of tub and onto a chair.

19. Give resident towel(s) and help to pat dry. Pat dry under the breasts, between skin folds, in the perineal area, and between toes.

20. Apply lotion and deodorant as needed.

21. Place soiled clothing and linens in proper containers.

22. Remove gloves and dispose of them.

23. Wash your hands.

24. Help resident dress and comb hair before leaving shower room. Put on non-skid footwear. Return resident to room.

25. Make sure resident is comfortable.

26. Place call light within resident's reach.

27. Report any changes in resident to nurse.

28. Document procedure using facility guidelines.

Tip

Shower Chairs

A **shower chair** is a sturdy chair designed to be placed in a bathtub or shower. It is water- and slip-resistant. The chair or bench enables a person who is unable to get into a tub or is too weak to stand in a shower to bathe in the tub or shower, rather than in bed. The types used in the home may look different than ones in care facilities (Fig. 13-30).

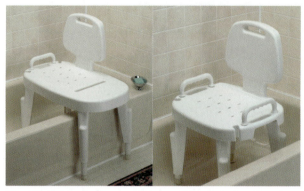

Fig. 13-30. *In the home, showers chairs can be placed directly into the tub.* (REPRINTED WITH PERMISSION OF BRIGGS CORPORATION, 800-247-2343, WWW.BRIGGSCORP.COM)

Some residents will have whirlpool baths. In a whirlpool bath, the action of the water cleanses and helps stimulate circulation and wound healing. To take a whirlpool bath, a resident is covered, placed in a chairlift, and lowered into the whirlpool. If you assist with this type of bath, do not leave the resident alone. The resident may feel faint or dizzy after the bath. Help as needed, and do not rush him or her. The tub and chair must be cleaned after use.

4. Explain guidelines for assisting with grooming

Grooming affects the way people feel about themselves and how they look to others. A well-groomed person is more likely to feel better physically and emotionally (Fig. 13-31). When helping with grooming, always let residents do all they can for themselves. Let them make as many choices as possible. Follow the care plan's instructions for what care to give. Remember that some residents may be embarrassed or depressed because they need help with grooming tasks they have done for themselves most their lives. Be sensitive to this. Be professional and respectful while assisting your residents with grooming. Your attitude can go a long way toward helping residents maintain self-respect and feel good about themselves.

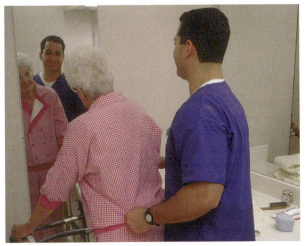

Fig. 13-31. A well-groomed appearance helps a person feel good about herself.

Fingernails can harbor bacteria. It is important to keep hands and nails clean to help prevent infection. Nail care should be given when assigned and when nails are dirty or have jagged edges. Never cut a resident's toenails. Poor circulation can lead to infection if skin is accidentally cut while caring for nails. In a diabetic resident, such an infection can lead to a severe wound or even amputation. See Chapter 18 for more information on diabetes. If you are told to give nail care, know exactly what care you are to provide. Never use the same nail equipment on more than one resident.

Providing fingernail care

Equipment: orangewood stick, emery board, lotion, basin, soap, washcloth, 2 towels, bath thermometer, gloves

1. Wash your hands.

2. Identify yourself by name. Identify the resident by name.

3. Explain procedure to the resident. Speak clearly, slowly, and directly. Maintain face-to-face contact whenever possible.

4. Provide for resident's privacy with curtain, screen, or door.

5. If resident is in bed, adjust bed to a safe level, usually waist high. Lock bed wheels.

6. Fill the basin halfway with warm water. Test water temperature with thermometer or your wrist to ensure it is safe. Water temperature should be 105° F. Have resident check water temperature. Adjust if necessary.

7. Place basin at a comfortable level for the resident. Soak the resident's nails in the water. Soak all 10 fingertips for at least five minutes.

8. Remove hands. Wash hands with soapy washcloth. Rinse. Pat hands dry with towel, including between fingers. Remove the hand basin.

9. Put on gloves.

10. Place the resident's hands on the towel. Use the pointed end of the orangewood stick or a nail brush to remove dirt from under the nails (Fig. 13-32).

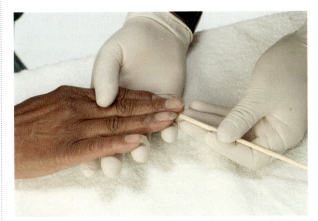

Fig. 13-32. Be gentle when removing dirt from under the nails with an orangewood stick.

11. Wipe orangewood stick on towel after cleaning under each nail. Wash resident's hands again. Dry them thoroughly.

12. Shape nails with file or emery board. File in a curve. Finish with nails smooth and free of rough edges.

13. Apply lotion from fingertips to wrist.

14. Empty, rinse, and dry basin. Place basin in designated dirty supply area or return to storage, depending on facility policy.

15. Place soiled clothing and linens in proper containers.

16. Remove and dispose of gloves properly. Wash your hands.

17. Make resident comfortable. Make sure sheets are free from wrinkles and the bed free from crumbs.

18. Return bed to lowest position. Remove privacy measures.

19. Place call light within resident's reach.

20. Wash your hands.

21. Report any changes in resident to the nurse.

22. Document procedure using facility guidelines.

Careful foot care is extremely important; it should be a part of daily care of residents. Keeping the feet clean and dry helps prevent complications, especially for diabetic residents. When providing foot care, observe the feet for any of the following:

Observing and Reporting:
Foot Care

Report any of these to the nurse:

- ^O/R Dry, flaking skin
- ^O/R Non-intact or broken skin
- ^O/R Discoloration of the feet, such as reddened, gray, white, or black areas
- ^O/R Blisters
- ^O/R Bruises
- ^O/R Blood or drainage
- ^O/R Long, ragged toenails
- ^O/R Ingrown toenails
- ^O/R Differences in temperature of the feet

Providing foot care

Equipment: basin, bath mat, soap, lotion, washcloth, 2 towels, bath thermometer, clean socks, gloves

Support the foot and ankle throughout procedure.

1. Wash your hands.

2. Identify yourself by name. Identify the resident by name.

3. Explain procedure to the resident. Speak clearly, slowly, and directly. Maintain face-to-face contact whenever possible.

4. Provide for resident's privacy with curtain, screen, or door.

5. If resident is in bed, adjust bed to a safe level, usually waist high. Lock bed wheels.

6. Fill the basin halfway with warm water. Test water temperature with thermometer or your wrist to ensure it is safe. Water temperature should be 105° F. Have resident check water temperature. Adjust if necessary.

7. Place basin on a bath mat or bath towel on the floor (if the resident is sitting in a chair) or on a towel at the foot of the bed (if the resident is in bed).

8. Remove resident's socks. Completely submerge resident's feet in water. Soak the feet for five to ten minutes. Add warm water to the basin as necessary.

9. Put on gloves.

10. Remove one foot from water. Wash entire foot, including between the toes and around nail beds, with soapy washcloth (Fig. 13-33).

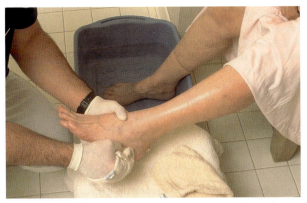

Fig. 13-33. Soak the resident's feet before washing the entire foot, including the nail beds.

11. Rinse entire foot, including between the toes.

12. Dry entire foot, including between the toes.

13. Repeat steps 10 through 12 for the other foot.

14. Put lotion in one hand and warm lotion by rubbing hands together.

15. Massage lotion into entire foot (top and bottom), except between the toes. Remove excess, if any, with a towel.

16. Empty, rinse, and dry basin. Place basin in designated dirty supply area or return to storage, depending on facility policy.

17. Place soiled clothing and linens in proper containers.

18. Remove and dispose of gloves properly. Wash your hands.

19. Make resident comfortable. Make sure sheets are free from wrinkles and the bed free from crumbs.

20. Return bed to lowest position. Remove privacy measures.

21. Place call light within resident's reach.

22. Wash your hands.

23. Report any changes in resident to the nurse.

24. Document procedure using facility guidelines.

Before assisting with shaving, make sure the resident wants you to shave him or help him shave. Respect personal preferences for shaving. Always wear gloves when shaving a resident. If you nick or cut a resident during shaving, there is chance you could come into contact with blood. Wearing gloves when shaving residents is a part of following standard precautions; it helps prevent infection.

If a resident has a beard or mustache, it will need daily care. Washing and combing a beard or mustache every day is usually enough. Ask the resident how he would like it done. Do not trim or shave a beard or mustache without his permission.

Check with the nurse to know which type of razor the resident uses:

- A **safety razor** has a sharp blade, but with a special safety casing to help prevent cuts. This type of razor requires shaving cream or soap.

- A **disposable razor** requires shaving cream or soap. It is discarded in a biohazard container after use.

- An **electric razor** is the safest and easiest type of razor to use. It does not require soap or shaving cream. Do not use an electric razor near any water, when oxygen is in use, or if resident has a pacemaker. Electricity near water may cause electrocution. Electricity near oxygen may cause an explosion. Electricity near some pacemakers may cause an irregular heartbeat.

Shaving a resident

Equipment: razor, basin filled halfway with warm water (if using a safety or disposable razor), 2 towels, washcloth, bath thermometer, mirror, shaving cream or soap (if using a safety or disposable razor), after-shave lotion, gloves, razor

1. Wash your hands.

2. Identify yourself by name. Identify the resident by name.

3. Explain procedure to the resident. Speak clearly, slowly, and directly. Maintain face-to-face contact whenever possible.

4. Provide for resident's privacy with curtain, screen, or door.

5. If resident is in bed, adjust bed to safe level, usually waist high. Raise the head of the bed so that the resident is sitting up. Lock bed wheels.

6. Place towel across the resident's chest, under his chin.

7. Put on gloves.

8. ***Shaving using a safety or disposable razor:***

8. If using a safety or disposable razor, use a blade that is sharp. A dull blade is hard on the skin. Soften the beard with a warm, wet washcloth on the face for a few minutes before shaving. Lather the face with shaving cream or soap and warm water. Warm water and lather make shaving more comfortable.

9. Hold skin taut. Shave in the direction of hair growth. Shave beard in downward strokes on face and upward strokes on neck (Fig. 13-34). Rinse the blade often in the basin to keep it clean and wet.

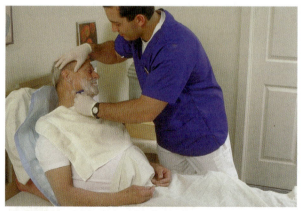

Fig. 13-34. *Holding the skin taut, shave in downward strokes on face and upward strokes on neck.*

10. When you have finished, wash, rinse, and dry the resident's face with a warm, wet washcloth or let him use the washcloth himself. Offer a mirror to the resident.

Shaving using an electric razor:

8. If using an electric razor, use a small brush to clean it. Do not use an electric razor near any water source, when oxygen is in use, or if resident has a pacemaker.

9. Turn on the razor and hold skin taut. Shave with smooth, even movements (Fig. 13-35). Shave beard with back and forth motion in direction of beard growth with foil shaver. Shave beard in circular motion with three-head shaver. Shave the chin and under the chin.

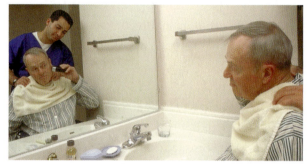

Fig. 13-35. *Shave, or have the resident shave, with smooth, even movements.*

10. When you have finished, offer a mirror to the resident.

Final steps:

11. If the resident wants after-shave lotion, moisten your palms with the lotion and pat it onto the resident's face.

12. Remove the towel. Place the towel and washcloth in proper container.

13. Clean the equipment and store it. For safety razor: rinse the razor. For disposable razor: dispose of it in a biohazard container if available. For electric razor: clean head of razor. Remove whiskers from razor. Recap shaving head and return razor to case.

14. Remove and dispose of gloves properly. Wash your hands.

15. Make resident comfortable. Make sure sheets are free from wrinkles and the bed free from crumbs.

16. Return bed to lowest position. Remove privacy measures.

17. Place call light within resident's reach.

18. Report any changes in resident to the nurse.

19. Document procedure using facility guidelines.

Nursing assistants help keep residents' hair clean and styled. Use hair ornaments only as requested. Do not comb or brush residents' hair into a childish style. When assisting with combing, brushing, or styling hair, handle it gently.

Pediculosis is an infestation of lice. Lice are tiny bugs that bite into the skin and suck blood to live and grow. Three types of lice are head lice, body lice, and crab or pubic lice. Head lice are usually found on the scalp. Lice are hard to see. Symptoms include itching, bite marks on the scalp, skin sores, and matted, bad-smelling hair and scalp. If you notice any of these symptoms, tell the nurse immediately. Lice can spread very quickly. Special lice cream, shampoo, or lotion may be used to treat the lice. People who have lice spread it to others. To help prevent the spread of lice, do not share residents' combs, brushes, clothes, wigs, or hats.

Dandruff is an excessive shedding of dead skin cells from the scalp. It is the result of the normal growing process of the skin cells of the scalp. The most common symptom is flaking of small, round, white patches from the head. Itching can also occur. Dandruff is a natural process. It cannot be stopped; it can only be controlled. Residents who have dandruff may use a special medicated dandruff shampoo to help control it.

Combing or brushing hair

Equipment: comb, brush, towel, mirror, hair care items requested by resident.

Use hair care products that the resident prefers for his or her type of hair.

1. Wash your hands.

2. Identify yourself by name. Identify the resident by name.

3. Explain procedure to the resident. Speak clearly, slowly, and directly. Maintain face-to-face contact whenever possible.

4. Provide for resident's privacy with curtain, screen, or door.

5. If the bed is adjustable, adjust bed to a safe level, usually waist high. Lock bed wheels.

6. Raise head of bed so the resident is sitting up. Place a towel under the head or around the shoulders.

7. Remove any hair pins, hair ties, and clips.

8. Remove tangles first by dividing hair into small sections. Hold lock of hair just above the tangle so you do not pull at the scalp. Gently comb or brush through the tangle. If resident agrees, you can use a small amount of detangler or leave-in conditioner on the tangle.

9. After tangles are removed, brush two-inch sections of hair at a time. Brush from roots to ends (Fig. 13-36). Residents who have dry, brittle hair may require a special treatment with oil or hair lotion. Residents whose hair is tightly curled may use a comb with large teeth, or a pick.

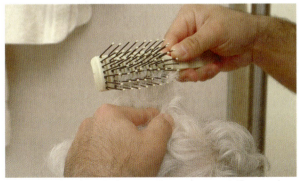

Fig. 13-36. *Gently brush hair from roots to ends.*

10. Each resident may prefer a different hairstyle. Style hair in the way the resident prefers (Fig. 13-37). Avoid childish hairstyles. Offer mirror to the resident.

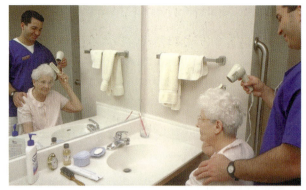

Fig. 13-37. Assist the resident in styling her hair as she prefers it.

11. Make resident comfortable. Make sure sheets are free from wrinkles and the bed free from crumbs.

12. Return bed to lowest position. Remove privacy measures.

13. Place call light within resident's reach.

14. Return supplies to proper storage. Clean hair from brush/comb.

15. Dispose of soiled linen in the proper container.

16. Wash your hands.

17. Report any changes in resident to nurse.

18. Document procedure using facility guidelines.

5. List guidelines for assisting with dressing

When helping a resident with dressing, know what limitations he or she has. If he has a weakened side from a stroke or injury, that side is called the **affected side**. It will be weaker. Never refer to the weaker side as the "bad side," or talk about the "bad" leg or arm. Use the terms weaker or **involved** to refer to the affected side. The weaker arm is usually placed through a sleeve first (Fig. 13-38). When a leg is weak, it is easier if the resident sits down to pull the pants over both legs.

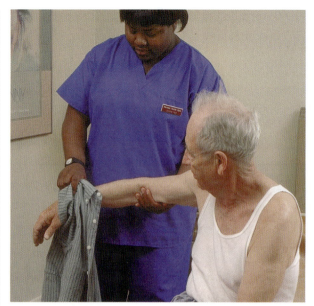

Fig. 13-38. When dressing, start with the involved (weaker) side first.

Guidelines:
Dressing and Undressing

G As with all care, the resident's wishes should be asked and followed. Remember: resident-directed care is the resident's legal right and your responsibility.

G Let the resident to choose clothing for the day. However, check to see if it is clean, appropriate for the weather, and in good condition.

G Encourage the resident to dress in regular clothes rather than nightclothes. Wearing regular daytime clothing encourages more activity and out-of-bed time. Elastic-waist pants or skirts are easy to pull on over legs and hips. Be sure the waistband of underpants, slip, pantyhose, pants, or skirt fits comfortably at the waist. Clothing that is a size larger than the resident would normally wear is easier to put on.

G The resident should do as much to dress or undress himself as possible. It may take longer, but it helps maintain independence and regain self-care skills. Ask where your help is needed.

G Provide privacy. If the resident has just had a bath, cover him with the bath blanket. Put on undergarments first. Never expose more than you need to.

G When putting on socks or stockings, roll or fold them down. They can then be slipped over the toes and foot, then unrolled up into place. Make sure toes, heels, and seams of socks or stockings are in the right place.

G For a female resident, make sure bra cups fit over the breasts. Front-fastening bras are easier for residents to work by themselves. Bras that fasten in back can be put around the waist and fastened first. Then rotate around and move bra up. Put arms through the straps last. This can be reversed for undressing.

G For residents who have weakness or paralysis on one side, place the weaker, or affected, arm or leg through the garment first. Then help with the strong arm or leg. When undressing, do the opposite—start with the stronger, or unaffected side.

G Several types of adaptive aids for dressing are available. These help residents maintain independence in dressing themselves (Fig. 13-39). An occupational therapist may teach residents to perform ADLs using adaptive equipment.

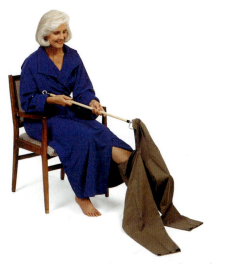

Fig. 13-39. Special dressing aids promote independence by helping residents dress themselves. (PHOTO COURTESY OF NORTH COAST MEDICAL, INC., WWW.NCMEDICAL.COM, 800-821-9319)

Dressing a resident with an affected (weak) right arm

Equipment: clean clothes of resident's choice, non-skid footwear

When putting on all items, move resident's body gently and naturally. Avoid force and over-extension of limbs and joints.

1. Wash your hands.

2. Identify yourself by name. Identify the resident by name.

3. Explain procedure to the resident. Speak clearly, slowly, and directly. Maintain face-to-face contact whenever possible.

4. Provide for resident's privacy with curtain, screen, or door.

5. Ask resident what she would like to wear. Dress her in outfit of choice (Fig 13-40).

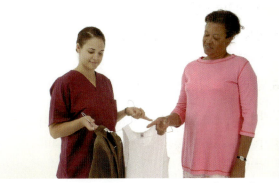

Fig. 13-40. Residents have a legal right to choose the clothing they want to wear for the day.

6. Remove resident's gown without completely exposing the resident. Remove from the stronger (unaffected) side first when undressing. Then remove gown from the weaker (affected) side.

7. Help resident to put the right (affected/weaker) arm through the right sleeve of the shirt, sweater, or slip before placing garment on left (unaffected) arm.

8. Help resident put on skirt, pants, or dress.

9. Place bed at the lowest position. Lock bed wheels.

10. Have resident sit down and help to apply non-skid footwear. Tie laces.

11. Finish with resident dressed appropriately. Make sure clothing is right-side-out and zippers/buttons are fastened.

12. Place gown in soiled linen container.

13. Keep bed in lowest position. Remove privacy measures.

14. Place call light within resident's reach.

15. Wash your hands.

16. Report any changes in resident to the nurse.

17. Document procedure using facility guidelines.

6. Identify guidelines for good oral care

Oral care, or care of the mouth, teeth, and gums, is performed at least twice each day. Oral care should be done after breakfast and after the last meal or snack of the day. It may also be done before a resident eats. Oral care includes brushing teeth, tongue, and gums; flossing teeth; and caring for dentures (Fig. 13-41). When giving oral care, wear gloves. Follow standard precautions.

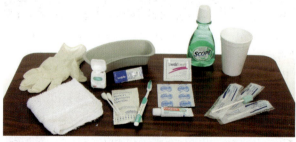

Fig. 13-41. *Some supplies needed for oral care.*

Proper, regular oral care can help prevent disease and bad breath (**halitosis**). Oral care also helps by preventing poor appetite and malnutrition. Cleaning the mouth removes particles and leftover food, and makes eating more pleasant. Residents who are unconscious, are on oxygen, or have tubes in their nose or mouths need fre-

quent oral care. Also, if they are not taking any fluids by mouth or are taking medications which dry their mouths, they will need oral care more often. When you perform oral care, observe the resident's mouth carefully.

Observing and Reporting:
Oral Care

Report any of these to the nurse:

- %R Irritation
- %R Infection
- %R Raised areas
- %R Coated or swollen tongue
- %R Ulcers, such as canker sores or small, painful, white sores
- %R Flaky, white spots
- %R Dry, cracked, bleeding, or chapped lips
- %R Loose, chipped, broken, or decayed teeth
- %R Swollen, irritated, bleeding, or whitish gums
- %R Breath that smells bad or fruity
- %R Resident reports of mouth pain

Providing oral care

Equipment: toothbrush, toothpaste, emesis basin, gloves, towel, glass of water

1. Wash your hands.

2. Identify yourself by name. Identify the resident by name.

3. Explain procedure to the resident. Speak clearly, slowly, and directly. Maintain face-to-face contact whenever possible.

4. Provide for resident's privacy with curtain, screen, or door.

5. Adjust bed to a safe level, usually waist high. Lock bed wheels. Make sure resident is in an upright sitting position.

6. Put on gloves.

7. Place towel across the resident's chest.

8. Wet toothbrush and put on small amount of toothpaste.

9. Clean entire mouth (including tongue and all surfaces of teeth). Use gentle strokes. First brush upper teeth, then lower teeth, using short strokes. Brush back and forth.

10. Give the resident water to rinse the mouth and place the emesis basin under the resident's chin. Have resident spit water into emesis basin (Fig. 13-42). Wipe resident's mouth and remove towel.

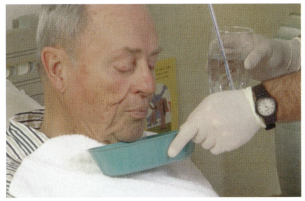

Fig. 13-42. Rinsing and spitting removes food particles and toothpaste.

11. Dispose of soiled linen in the proper container.

12. Clean and return supplies to proper storage.

13. Remove gloves and dispose of gloves properly. Wash your hands.

14. Make resident comfortable.

15. Return bed to lowest position. Remove privacy measures.

16. Place call light within resident's reach.

17. Wash your hands.

18. Report any problems with teeth, mouth, tongue, and lips to nurse. This includes odor, cracking, sores, bleeding, and any discoloration.

19. Document procedure using facility guidelines.

Oral care does not just involve taking care of the teeth. Residents who do not have teeth will need oral care performed too. **Edentulous** means having no teeth. You will clean the mouth, tongue, and gums using mouthwash or other solution on gauze or swabs. The gauze can be wrapped on a tongue blade and moistened with mouthwash or solution if swabs are not available.

Although residents who are unconscious cannot eat, breathing through the mouth causes saliva to dry in the mouth. Good mouth care needs to be performed more frequently to keep the mouth clean and moist. Swabs with a mixture of lemon juice and glycerine or other solutions are sometimes used to soothe the gums. Some solutions further dry the gums if used too often. Follow the care plan regarding the use of swabs.

With unconscious residents, it is important to use as little liquid as possible when giving mouth care. Because the person's swallowing reflex is weak, he or she is at risk for aspiration. **Aspiration** is the inhalation of food, fluid, or foreign material into the lungs. Aspiration can cause pneumonia or death.

Providing oral care for the unconscious resident

Equipment: sponge swabs, padded tongue blade (Fig. 13-43), towel, emesis basin, gloves, lip moisturizer, cleaning solution (check the care plan)

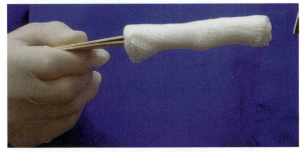

Fig. 13-43. To make a padded tongue blade, place two wooden tongue blades together and wrap the upper portion with gauze. Tape the gauze in place.

1. Wash your hands.

2. Identify yourself by name. Identify the resident by name. Even residents who are unconscious may be able to hear you. Always speak to them as you would to any resident.

3. Explain procedure to the resident. Speak clearly, slowly, and directly. Maintain face-to-face contact whenever possible.

4. Provide for resident's privacy with curtain, screen, or door.

5. Adjust bed to a safe level, usually waist high. Lock bed wheels.

6. Put on gloves.

7. Turn resident's head to the side. Place a towel under his cheek and chin. Place an emesis basin next to the cheek and chin for excess fluid.

8. Hold mouth open with padded tongue blade.

9. Dip swab in cleaning solution. Wipe teeth, gums, tongue, and inside surfaces of mouth. Change swab often. Repeat until the mouth is clean (Fig. 13-44).

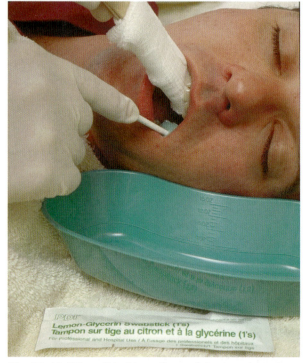

Fig. 13-44. *Wipe all inside surfaces of the mouth to clean the mouth, stimulate the gums, and remove mucus.*

10. Rinse with clean swab dipped in water.

11. Remove the towel and basin. Pat lips or face dry if needed. Apply lip moisturizer.

12. Dispose of soiled linen in the proper container.

13. Clean and return supplies to proper storage.

14. Remove and dispose of gloves properly. Wash your hands.

15. Make sure sheets are free from wrinkles and the bed free from crumbs.

16. Return bed to lowest position. Remove privacy measures.

17. Place call light within resident's reach.

18. Wash your hands.

19. Report any problems with teeth, mouth, tongue, and lips to nurse. This includes odor, cracking, sores, bleeding, and any discoloration.

20. Document procedure using facility guidelines.

Dental floss is a special kind of string used to clean between teeth. Flossing the teeth removes plaque and tartar buildup around the gum line and between the teeth. Teeth may be flossed right after or before they are brushed, as the resident prefers. Flossing should not be done for certain residents. Follow the care plan's instructions.

Flossing teeth

Equipment: floss, cup with water, emesis basin, gloves, towel

1. Wash your hands.

2. Identify yourself by name. Identify the resident by name.

3. Explain procedure to the resident. Speak clearly, slowly, and directly. Maintain face-to-face contact whenever possible.

4. Provide for resident's privacy with curtain, screen, or door.

5. Adjust the bed to a safe level, usually waist high. Lock bed wheels. Make sure the resident is in an upright sitting position.

6. Put on gloves.

7. Wrap the ends of floss securely around each index finger (Fig. 13-45).

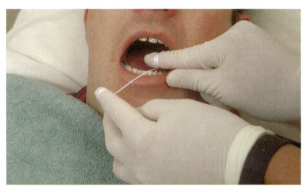

Fig. 13-45. Before beginning, wrap floss securely around each index finger.

8. Starting with the back teeth, place floss between teeth. Move it down the surface of the tooth. Use a gentle sawing motion (Fig. 13-46).

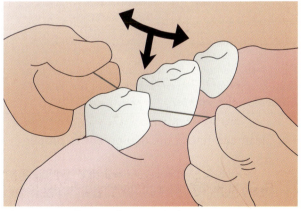

Fig. 13-46. Being gentle protects the gums.

Continue to the gum line. At the gum line, curve the floss into a letter C. Slip it gently into the space between the gum and tooth. Then go back up, scraping that side of the tooth (Fig. 13-47). Repeat this on the side of the other tooth.

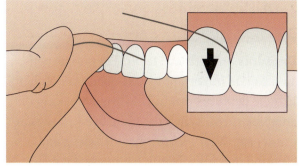

Fig. 13-47. Floss gently in the space between the gum and tooth. This removes food and prevents tooth decay.

9. After every two teeth, unwind floss from your fingers. Move it so you are using a clean area. Floss all teeth.

10. Occasionally offer water so that the resident can rinse the mouth. Ask the resident to spit it into the basin.

11. Offer resident a face towel when done flossing all teeth.

12. Discard floss. Empty basin into the toilet. Clean and store basin and supplies.

13. Dispose of soiled linen in the proper container.

14. Remove and dispose of gloves properly. Wash your hands.

15. Make resident comfortable. Make sure sheets are free from wrinkles and the bed free from crumbs.

16. Return bed to lowest position. Remove privacy measures.

17. Place call light within resident's reach.

18. Wash your hands.

19. Report any problems with teeth, mouth, tongue, and lips to nurse. This includes odor, cracking, sores, bleeding, and any discoloration.

20. Document procedure using facility guidelines.

7. Define "dentures" and explain how to care for dentures

Dentures are artificial teeth. They are expensive, so it is important to take good care of them. Handle dentures carefully to avoid breaking or chipping them. When dentures break, a person cannot eat. Wear gloves when handling and cleaning dentures. Notify the nurse if a resident's dentures do not fit properly, are chipped, or are missing.

Ask the resident how you can assist with denture care. Each person has his own preference about when and how it should be done. When storing dentures, place them in a denture cup labeled with the resident's name and room number. Make sure you match the dentures to the correct resident. Store them in solution or cool water. Hot water may damage dentures.

Residents' Rights

Oral Care

Oral care is very personal. Always pull the privacy curtain and close the door before beginning. Many people who have dentures do not want to be seen without their teeth in place. When you remove the teeth, clean and return them immediately.

Cleaning and storing dentures

Equipment: denture brush or toothbrush, denture cleanser or tablet, labeled denture cup, 2 towels, gloves

1. Wash your hands.

2. Put on gloves.

3. Line the sink or a basin with towels and fill with water. The towel and water will prevent the dentures from breaking if they slip from your hands and fall into the sink.

4. Rinse dentures in cool running water before brushing them. Do not use hot water.

5. Apply toothpaste or cleanser to toothbrush.

6. Brush dentures on all surfaces (Fig. 13-48).

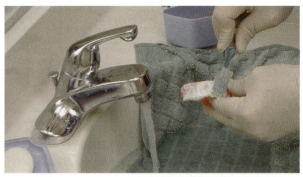

Fig. 13-48. Brush dentures on all surfaces to properly clean them.

7. Rinse all surfaces of dentures under cool running water. Do not use hot water.

8. Rinse denture cup before placing clean dentures in it.

9. Place dentures in clean denture cup with solution or cool water. Make sure cup is labeled with resident's name and room number (Fig. 13-49). Put denture cup where it is normally stored.

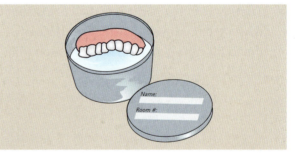

Fig. 13-49. Dentures should be stored in solution in a denture cup that is properly labeled with the resident's name and room number.

10. Clean and return the equipment to proper storage.

11. Drain sink. Dispose of towels in proper container.

12. Remove and dispose of gloves properly. Wash your hands.

13. Report any changes in appearance of dentures to the nurse.

14. Document procedure using facility guidelines.

Removing and reinserting dentures

If you are allowed to do so, and if a resident cannot remove his or her dentures, you must do it. Ask resident to sit upright, and apply gloves. Remove the lower denture first. The lower denture is easier to remove because it floats on the gum line of the lower jaw. Grasp the lower denture with a gauze square (for a good grip) and remove it. Place it in a denture cup filled with solution or cool water.

The upper denture is sealed by suction. Firmly grasp the upper denture with a gauze square. Give a slight downward pull to break the suction. Turn it at an angle to take it out of the mouth.

When inserting dentures, ask resident to sit as upright as possible. Apply gloves. Apply denture cream or adhesive to the dentures if needed. When the resident's mouth is open, place upper denture into the mouth by turning it at an angle. Straighten it and press it onto the upper gum line firmly and evenly (Fig. 13-50). Insert the lower denture onto the gum line of the lower jaw. Press firmly.

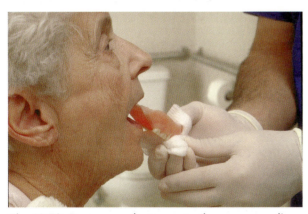

Fig. 13-50. Press upper denture onto the upper gum line firmly and evenly.

Chapter Review

1. List four examples of activities of daily living (ADLs).

2. List five reasons that a resident may need help with personal care.

3. Give four examples of how to promote dignity and independence while giving personal care.

4. What are five things about a resident that a nursing assistant should observe during personal care?

5. Why is preventing pressure sores extremely important?

6. When skin begins to break down, what does it look like?

7. List ten signs to observe and report about a resident's skin.

8. At a minimum, how often should residents be repositioned?

9. List four examples of positioning devices and explain how they can help.

10. Why is it unnecessary for many elderly people to have a complete bath or shower every day?

11. How often should the perineum be washed?

12. Why should residents, as well as NAs, test the water temperature before bathing?

13. Why should the nursing assistant wipe from front to back when giving perineal care?

14. List two benefits of back rubs.

15. Why should bath oils, lotions, or powders NOT be used in showers or tubs?

16. In what ways can good grooming affect a person?

17. Explain why NAs must be especially careful while giving nail care to diabetic residents.

18. Why should gloves be worn while shaving residents?

19. List the reasons why electric razors should not be used near water, when oxygen is in use, or if a resident has a pacemaker.

20. What are the symptoms of head lice?

21. If a resident has an affected side due to a stroke or an injury, how should an NA refer to that side?

22. When dressing a resident with a weaker side, which arm is usually placed through the sleeve first—the weaker or stronger arm?

23. What is the minimum number of times per day that oral care is done?

24. List nine signs and symptoms that should be observed and reported during oral care.

25. How can NAs help prevent aspiration during oral care of unconscious residents?

26. Explain why hot water should not be used when handling or cleaning dentures.

14
Basic Nursing Skills

1. Explain the importance of monitoring vital signs

Nursing assistants monitor, document, and report residents' **vital signs**. Vital signs are important. They show how well the vital organs of the body, such as the heart and lungs, are working. They consist of the following:

- Taking the body temperature

- Counting the pulse

- Counting the rate of respirations

- Taking the blood pressure

- Observing and reporting the level of pain

Watching for changes in vital signs is very important. Changes can indicate a resident's condition is worsening. You will not make diagnoses based on vital signs, but you will record accurate measurements and report changes and observations to the nurse. You should always notify the nurse if:

- The resident has a fever (temperature is above average for the resident or outside the normal range)

- The resident has a respiratory or pulse rate that is too rapid or too slow

- The resident's blood pressure changes

- The resident's pain is worse or is not relieved by pain management

Normal Ranges for Adult Vital Signs		
Temperature	**Fahrenheit**	**Celsius**
Oral	97.6°–99.6°	36.5°–37.5°
Rectal	98.6°–100.6°	37.0°–38.1°
Axillary	96.6°–98.6°	36.0°–37.0°
Pulse: 60–100 beats per minute		
Respirations: 12–20 respirations per minute		
Blood Pressure		
Normal:	Systolic 100–139	Diastolic 60–89
High:	140/90 or above	
Low:	Below 100/60	

Residents' Rights

Vital Signs

Protect residents' privacy while taking vital signs by not exposing them. If you need to take blood pressure or move clothing out of the way, pull the privacy curtain around the bed and close the door. Do not discuss residents' vital signs measurements while in earshot of other people. Report the information to the nurse.

2. List guidelines for taking body temperature

Body temperature is normally very close to 98.6°F (Fahrenheit) or 37°C (Celsius). Body temperature reflects a balance between the heat created by our bodies and the heat lost to the environment. Many factors affect temperature; age, illness, stress, environment, exercise, and the circadian rhythm can all cause changes in body temperature. The circadian rhythm is the 24-hour day-night cycle. Average temperature readings change throughout the day. People tend to have lower temperatures in the morning. Increases in body temperature may indicate an infection or disease.

There are four sites for taking body temperature:

1. The mouth (oral)

2. The rectum (rectal)

3. The armpit (axillary)

4. The ear (tympanic)

The different sites require different thermometers. Temperatures are most often taken orally. Do not take an oral temperature on a person who:

• Is unconscious

• Has recently had facial or oral surgery

• Is younger than 5 years old

• Is confused

• Is heavily sedated

• Is coughing

• Is being administered oxygen

• Has facial paralysis

• Has a nasogastric tube (a feeding tube that is inserted through the nose and goes into the stomach)

There are several types of thermometers, such as the following:

• Mercury-free glass

• Mercury glass (glass bulb)

• Battery-powered, digital, or electronic

• Disposable

• Tympanic

• Temporal artery

Using mercury glass or glass bulb thermometers to take oral or rectal temperatures used to be common. However, because mercury is a dangerous, toxic substance, thousands of healthcare facilities now discourage the use of products containing mercury. In fact, many states have passed laws to ban the sale of mercury thermometers. Today, mercury-free glass thermometers are more common (Fig. 14-1). They can be used to take an oral or rectal temperature, and they are considered much safer.

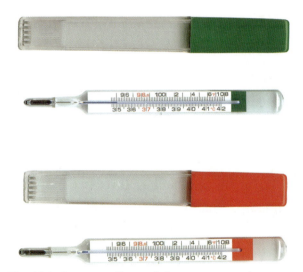

Fig. 14-1. *A mercury-free oral thermometer and a mercury-free rectal thermometer. Thermometers are usually color-coded to show which is for oral and which is for rectal use. Oral thermometers are usually green or blue; rectal thermometers are usually red.* (PHOTOS PROVIDED BY RG MEDICAL DIAGNOSTICS OF SOUTHFIELD, MI.)

Although some mercury-free thermometers are slightly larger than glass bulb thermometers, they operate identically. Numbers on the thermometer let you read the temperature after it registers. Most thermometers show the temperature in degrees Fahrenheit (F). Each long line represents one degree and each short line represents two-tenths of a degree. Some thermometers show the temperature in degrees Celsius (C), with the long lines representing one degree and the short lines representing one-tenth of a degree. The small arrow points to the normal temperature: 98.6°F and 37°C (Fig. 14-2).

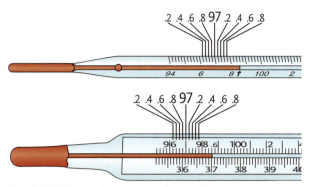

Fig. 14-2. *You read a mercury-free and a mercury glass thermometer the same way.*

Home Care Focus

Mercury glass thermometers may still be used in the home, so you may benefit from knowing a little bit about them. Mercury glass thermometers have a stem and a bulb. The stem has a column for the mercury to go up and down; the bulb stores the mercury. The bulb is available in either a long, slim shape or a blunt shape.

It is very important that you never use a thermometer that has the long, slim bulb to take a rectal or axillary temperature. This is because the slender bulb could break in the rectum or armpit and cause injuries. Only use the thermometers with long, slim bulbs to take oral temperatures.

The thermometers with the blunt bulbs should be used to take rectal and axillary temperatures. You can also use the blunt bulb for oral temperatures. However, if you typically use a thermometer with a blunt bulb to take a rectal temperature, never use the same thermometer to take an oral temperature.

If you must use a mercury glass thermometer, be careful. If you break a glass thermometer, never touch the mercury or broken glass. Know your agency's policies and procedures regarding safe disposal of mercury.

When cleaning a mercury glass thermometer, wipe it with alcohol wipes from clean to dirty (stem to bulb). Never use hot water on a mercury thermometer because hot water can heat the mercury and break the thermometer.

Battery-powered, digital, or electronic thermometers are other types of thermometers (Figs. 14-3 and 14-4). These thermometers display results digitally. They register the temperature more quickly than mercury-free or glass bulb thermometers. Digital thermometers usually take two to sixty seconds to register the temperature.

The thermometer will beep or flash when the temperature has registered. Digital thermometers may be used to take oral, rectal, or axillary temperatures. Follow the manufacturer's guide for proper use of these thermometers.

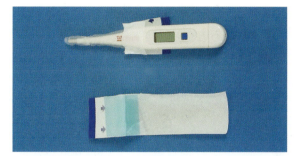

Fig. 14-3. *A digital thermometer with a disposable sheath underneath it.*

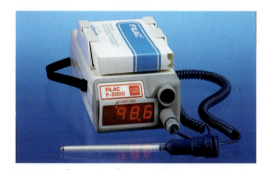

Fig. 14-4. *An electronic thermometer.*

The tympanic thermometer, or ear thermometer, also registers a temperature quickly (Fig. 14-5). These thermometers may not be as common. They also require more practice to be able to take accurate temperatures.

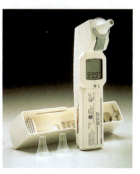

Fig. 14-5. *A tympanic thermometer.*

Disposable thermometers register temperatures in 60 seconds. Usually a colored dot shows the temperature. Disposable thermometers are often individually wrapped. They are only used once and then discarded in the proper container.

Disposable, or single-use, equipment helps prevent infection.

Temporal artery thermometers determine temperature readings by measuring the heat from the skin over the temporal artery. This is done by a gentle stroke or scan across the forehead (Fig. 14-6). Temporal artery thermometers are non-invasive, which means that they are not inserted into the body.

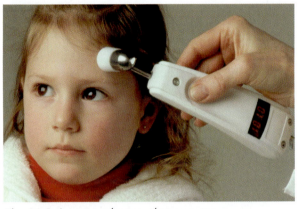

Fig. 14-6. *A temporal artery thermometer.* (PHOTO COURTESY OF EXERGEN CORPORATION, 800-422-3006, WWW.EXERGEN.COM)

Remember that there is a range of normal temperatures. Some people's temperatures normally run low. Others in good health will run slightly higher temperatures. Normal temperature readings also vary by the method used to take the temperature. A rectal temperature is considered to be the most accurate, but taking a rectal temperature on an uncooperative person, such as a resident with dementia or a small child, can be dangerous. An axillary temperature is considered the least accurate.

Taking and recording an oral temperature

Do not take an oral temperature on a resident who has smoked, eaten or drunk fluids, chewed gum, or exercised in the last 10-20 minutes.

Equipment: clean mercury-free, glass, digital, or electronic thermometer, gloves, disposable plastic sheath/cover for thermometer, tissues, pen and paper

1. Wash your hands.

2. Identify yourself by name. Identify the resident by name.

3. Explain procedure to the resident. Speak clearly, slowly, and directly. Maintain face-to-face contact whenever possible.

4. Provide for resident's privacy with curtain, screen, or door.

5. Put on gloves.

6. *Mercury-free thermometer*: Hold the thermometer by the stem. Before inserting the thermometer in the resident's mouth, shake thermometer down to below the lowest number (at least below 96°F or 35°C). To shake the thermometer down, hold it at the side opposite the bulb with the thumb and two fingers. With a snapping motion of the wrist, shake the thermometer (Fig. 14-7). Stand away from furniture and walls while doing so.

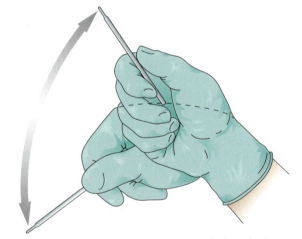

Fig. 14-7. *Shake thermometer down to below the lowest number before inserting in a resident's mouth.*

Digital thermometer: Put on the disposable sheath. Turn on thermometer and wait until "ready" sign appears.

Electronic thermometer: Remove the probe from base unit. Put on probe cover.

7. *Mercury-free thermometer*: Put on disposable sheath, if available. Insert bulb end of the thermometer into resident's mouth, under tongue and to one side (Fig. 14-8).

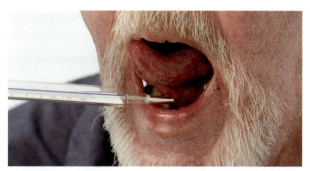

Fig. 14-8. *Insert thermometer under the resident's tongue and to one side.*

Digital thermometer: Insert the end of digital thermometer into resident's mouth, under tongue and to one side.

Electronic thermometer: Insert the end of electronic thermometer into resident's mouth, under tongue and to one side.

8. **Mercury-free thermometer**: Tell the resident to hold the thermometer in mouth with lips closed. Assist as necessary. Resident should breathe through his nose. Ask the resident not to bite down or to talk. Leave the thermometer in place for at least three minutes.

Digital thermometer: Leave in place until thermometer blinks or beeps.

Electronic thermometer: Leave in place until you hear a tone or see a flashing or steady light.

9. **Mercury-free thermometer**: Remove the thermometer. Wipe with a tissue from stem to bulb or remove sheath. Dispose of the tissue or sheath. Hold the thermometer at eye level. Rotate until line appears, rolling the thermometer between your thumb and forefinger. Read the temperature. Remember the temperature reading.

Digital thermometer: Remove the thermometer. Read temperature on display screen. Remember the temperature reading.

Electronic thermometer: Read the temperature on the display screen. Remember the temperature reading. Remove the probe.

10. **Mercury-free thermometer**: Rinse the thermometer in lukewarm water and dry. Return it to a plastic case or container.

Digital thermometer: Using a tissue, remove and dispose of sheath. Replace the thermometer in case.

Electronic thermometer: Press the eject button to discard the cover (Fig. 14-9). Return the probe to the holder.

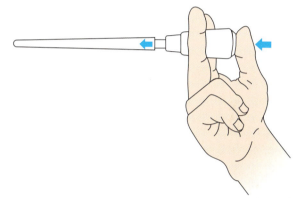

Fig. 14-9. *Eject the probe cover and dispose of it properly after use.*

11. Remove gloves and discard.

12. Wash your hands.

13. Immediately record the temperature, date, time and method used (oral).

14. Place call light within resident's reach.

15. Report any changes in resident to the nurse.

You may need to take a rectal temperature. Rectal temperatures can be necessary for unconscious residents, residents who have seizures, residents with poorly-fitted dentures or missing teeth, infants and young children, and anyone having trouble breathing through the nose. Always explain what you will do before starting this procedure. You need the resident's cooperation to take a rectal temperature. Ask the resident to hold still. Reassure him or her that the task will only take a few minutes. Keep your hand on the thermometer the entire time you are taking the temperature.

Taking and recording a rectal temperature

Equipment: clean rectal mercury-free, glass, or digital thermometer, lubricant, gloves, tissue, disposable sheath/cover, pen and paper

1. Wash your hands.

2. Identify yourself by name. Identify the resident by name.

3. Explain procedure to the resident. Speak clearly, slowly, and directly. Maintain face-to-face contact whenever possible.

4. Provide for resident's privacy with curtain, screen, or door.

5. If the bed is adjustable, adjust to a safe level, usually waist high. If the bed is movable, lock bed wheels.

6. Help the resident to the left-lying (Sims') position (Fig. 14-10).

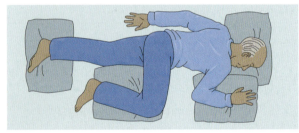

Fig. 14-10. *The resident must be in the left-lying (Sims') position.*

7. Fold back the linens to expose only the rectal area.

8. Put on gloves.

9. **Mercury-free thermometer**: Hold thermometer by stem. Shake the thermometer down to below the lowest number.

    Digital thermometer: Put on the disposable sheath. Turn on thermometer and wait until "ready" sign appears.

10. Apply a small amount of lubricant to tip of bulb or probe cover (or apply pre-lubricated cover).

11. Separate the buttocks. Gently insert thermometer into rectum 1 inch (1/2 inch for a child). Stop if you meet resistance. Do not force the thermometer in (Fig. 14-11).

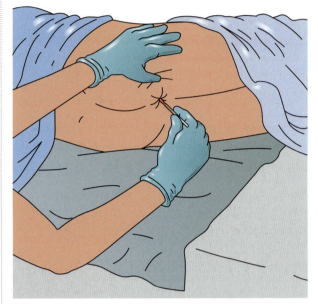

Fig. 14-11. *Gently insert a rectal thermometer one inch into the rectum. Do not force it into the rectum.*

12. Replace the sheet over buttocks while holding on to the thermometer. Hold on to the thermometer at all times.

13. **Mercury-free thermometer**: Hold thermometer in place for at least three minutes.

    Digital thermometer: Hold thermometer in place until thermometer blinks or beeps.

14. Gently remove the thermometer. Wipe with tissue from stem to bulb or remove sheath.

    Dispose of tissue or sheath.

15. Read the thermometer at eye level as you would for an oral temperature. Remember the temperature reading.

16. **Mercury-free thermometer**: Rinse the thermometer in lukewarm water and dry. Return it to plastic case or container.

    Digital thermometer: Discard probe cover. Replace the thermometer in case.

17. Remove gloves and discard.

18. Wash your hands.

19. Assist the resident to a position of safety and comfort.

20. Immediately record the temperature, date, time and method used (rectal).

21. Place call light within resident's reach.

22. Report any changes in resident to the nurse.

Tympanic thermometers can take fast and accurate temperature readings. As always, explain what you will do before beginning the procedure. Tell the resident that you will be placing a thermometer in the ear canal. Reassure the resident that this is painless. The short tip of the thermometer will only go into the ear one-quarter to one-half inch. Thermometer models vary. Follow the manufacturer's instructions.

Taking and recording a tympanic temperature

Equipment: tympanic thermometer, gloves, disposable probe sheath/cover, pen and paper

1. Wash your hands.

2. Identify yourself by name. Identify the resident by name.

3. Explain procedure to the resident. Speak clearly, slowly, and directly. Maintain face-to-face contact whenever possible.

4. Provide for resident's privacy with curtain, screen, or door.

5. Put on gloves.

6. Put a disposable sheath over earpiece of the thermometer.

7. Position the resident's head so that the ear is in front of you. Straighten the ear canal by pulling up and back on the outside edge of the ear (Fig. 14-12). Insert the covered probe into the ear canal. Press the button.

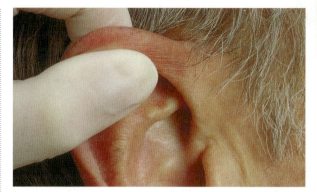

Fig. 14-12. *Straighten the ear canal by pulling up and back on the outside edge of the ear.*

8. Hold thermometer in place either for one second or until thermometer blinks or beeps (depends on model).

9. Read temperature. Remember the temperature reading.

10. Dispose of sheath. Return the thermometer to storage or to the battery charger if thermometer is rechargeable.

11. Remove gloves and discard.

12. Wash your hands.

13. Immediately record the temperature, date, time and method used (tympanic).

14. Place call light within resident's reach.

15. Report any changes in resident to the nurse.

Axillary temperatures are much less reliable than temperatures taken at other sites. The axillary site is usually used as a last resort.

Taking and recording an axillary temperature

Equipment: clean mercury-free, glass, digital, or electronic thermometer, gloves, tissues, disposable sheath/cover, pen and paper

1. Wash your hands.

2. Identify yourself by name. Identify the resident by name.

3. Explain procedure to the resident. Speak clearly, slowly, and directly. Maintain face-to-face contact whenever possible.

4. Provide for resident's privacy with curtain, screen, or door.

5. Put on gloves.

6. Remove resident's arm from sleeve of gown or top to allow skin contact with the end of the thermometer. Wipe axillary area with tissues before placing the thermometer.

7. *Mercury-free thermometer*: Hold the thermometer by the stem. Shake the thermometer down to below the lowest number.

   Digital thermometer: Put on the disposable sheath. Turn on thermometer and wait until "ready" sign appears.

   Electronic thermometer: Remove the probe from base unit. Put on probe cover.

8. Position thermometer (bulb end for mercury-free) in center of the armpit. Fold resident's arm over her chest.

9. *Mercury-free thermometer*: Hold the thermometer in place, with the arm close against the side, for eight to 10 minutes (Fig. 14-13).

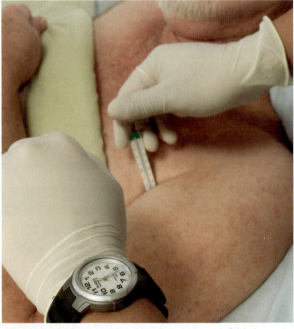

Fig. 14-13. *After inserting the thermometer, fold the resident's arm over his chest and hold it in place for eight to 10 minutes.*

Digital thermometer: Leave in place until thermometer blinks or beeps.

Electronic thermometer: Leave in place until you hear a tone or see a flashing or steady light.

10. *Mercury-free thermometer*: Remove the thermometer. Wipe with a tissue from stem to bulb or remove sheath. Dispose of the tissue or sheath. Read the thermometer at eye level as you would for an oral temperature. Remember the temperature reading.

    Digital thermometer: Remove the thermometer. Read temperature on display screen. Remember the temperature reading.

    Electronic thermometer: Read the temperature on the display screen. Remember the temperature reading. Remove the probe.

11. *Mercury-free thermometer*: Rinse the thermometer in lukewarm water and dry. Return it to plastic case or container.

    Digital thermometer: Using a tissue, remove and dispose of sheath. Replace the thermometer in case.

    Electronic thermometer: Press the eject button to discard the cover. Return the probe to the holder.

12. Remove gloves and discard.

13. Wash your hands.

14. Put resident's arm back into sleeve of gown.

15. Immediately record the temperature, date, time and method used (axillary).

16. Place call light within resident's reach.

17. Report any changes in resident to the nurse.

3. List guidelines for taking pulse and respirations

The pulse is the number of heartbeats per minute. The beat that you feel at certain pulse points in the body represents the wave of blood moving as a result of the heart pumping. The most common site for monitoring the pulse is on the inside of the wrist, where the radial artery runs just beneath the skin. This is called the **radial pulse**. The procedure for taking this pulse is located later in this chapter. The **brachial pulse** is the pulse inside the elbow, about 1 - 1 1/2 inches above the elbow. The radial and brachial pulses are involved in taking blood pressure. Blood pressure is explained later in this chapter. Other common pulse sites are shown in Fig. 14-14.

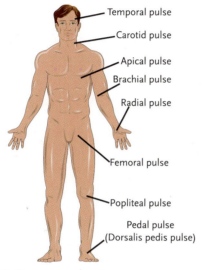

Temporal pulse
Carotid pulse
Apical pulse
Brachial pulse
Radial pulse
Femoral pulse
Popliteal pulse
Pedal pulse (Dorsalis pedis pulse)

Fig. 14-14. Common pulse sites.

For adults, the normal pulse rate is 60–100 beats per minute. Small children have more rapid pulses, in the range of 100–120 beats per minute. A newborn baby's pulse may be as high as 120–140 beats per minute. Many things can affect the pulse rate, including exercise, fear, anger, anxiety, heat, medications, and pain. An unusually high or low rate does not necessarily indicate disease. However, sometimes the pulse rate can be a signal that serious illness exists. For example, a rapid pulse may result from fever, infection, or heart failure. A slow or weak pulse may indicate dehydration, infection, or shock.

The **apical pulse** is heard by listening directly over the heart with a stethoscope. This is often the easiest method for measuring the pulse in infants and small children because their pulse points are harder to find. A **stethoscope** is an instrument designed to listen to sounds within the body, such as the heart beating or air moving through the lungs (Fig. 14-15). For adults, the apical pulse may be taken when the person

has heart disease or takes drugs that affect the heart. It may also be taken on residents who have a weak radial pulse or an irregular pulse.

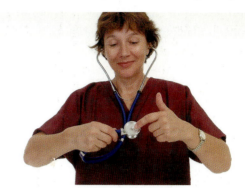

Fig. 14-15. For adults, use the larger round side of the stethoscope to hear a pulse and to take blood pressure. The smaller side is used for children or infants.

Taking and recording apical pulse

Equipment: stethoscope, watch with second hand, alcohol wipes, pen and paper

1. Wash hands.

2. Identify yourself by name. Identify the resident by name.

3. Explain procedure to the resident. Speak clearly, slowly, and directly. Maintain face-to-face contact whenever possible.

4. Provide for resident's privacy with curtain, screen, or door.

5. Fit the earpieces of the stethoscope snugly in your ears. Place the flat metal diaphragm on the left side of the chest, just below the nipple (Fig. 14-16). Listen for the heartbeat.

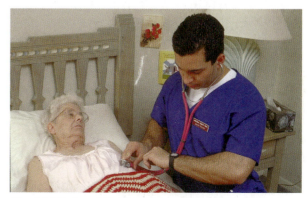

Fig. 14-16. Count the heartbeats for one full minute to measure the apical pulse.

6. Use the second hand of your watch. Count beats for one full minute. Each "lubdub" that you hear is counted as one beat. A normal heartbeat is rhythmical. Leave the stethoscope in place to count respirations (see procedure later in chapter).

7. Record pulse rate, date, time, and method used (apical). Note any irregularities in the rhythm.

8. Clean earpieces and diaphragm of stethoscope with alcohol wipes. Store stethoscope.

9. Wash your hands.

10. Place call light within resident's reach.

11. Report any changes in resident to the nurse.

Respiration is the process of breathing air into the lungs, or **inspiration**, and exhaling air out of the lungs, or **expiration**. Each respiration consists of an inspiration and an expiration. The chest rises during inspiration and falls during expiration.

The normal respiration rate for adults ranges from 12 to 20 breaths per minute. Infants and children have a faster respiratory rate. Infants normally breathe at a rate of 30 to 40 respirations per minute. People may breathe more quickly if they know they are being observed. Because of this, count respirations immediately after taking the pulse. Keep your fingers on a resident's wrist or on the stethoscope over the heart. Do not make it obvious that you are watching the resident's breathing.

Taking and recording radial pulse and counting and recording respirations

Equipment: watch with a second hand, pen and paper

1. Wash your hands.

2. Identify yourself by name. Identify the resident by name.

3. Explain procedure to the resident. Speak clearly, slowly, and directly. Maintain face-to-face contact whenever possible.

4. Provide for resident's privacy with curtain, screen, or door.

5. Place fingertips on the thumb side of resident's wrist. Locate pulse (Fig. 14-17).

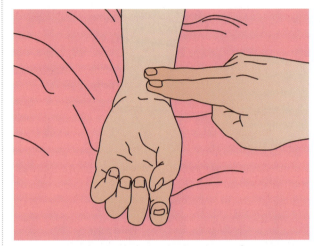

Fig. 14-17. *Take the radial pulse by placing fingertips on the thumb side of the wrist.*

6. Count the beats for one full minute.

7. Keep your fingertips on the resident's wrist. Count respirations for one full minute (Fig. 14-18). Observe for the pattern and character of the resident's breathing. Normal breathing is smooth and quiet. If you see signs of troubled breathing, shallow breathing, or noisy breathing, such as wheezing, report it.

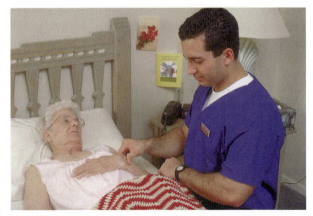

Fig. 14-18. *Count the respiratory rate directly after taking the radial pulse. Do not make it obvious that you are watching her breathing.*

8. Record pulse rate, date, time, and method used (radial). Record the respiratory rate and the pattern or character of breathing.

9. Place call light within resident's reach.

10. Wash your hands.

11. Report to the nurse if the pulse is less than 60 beats per minute, over 100 beats per minute, if the rhythm is irregular, or if breathing is irregular.

4. Explain guidelines for taking blood pressure

Blood pressure is an important measure of a person's health. Blood pressure is measured in millimeters of mercury (mmHg). The measurement shows how well the heart is working. There are two parts of blood pressure, the systolic measurement and the diastolic measurement.

In the **systolic** phase, the heart is at work. It contracts and pushes the blood from the left ventricle of the heart. The reading shows the pressure on the walls of arteries as blood is pumped through the body. The normal range for systolic blood pressure is 100–119 mmHg.

The second measurement reflects the **diastolic** phase—when the heart relaxes. The diastolic measurement is always lower than the systolic measurement. It shows the pressure in the arteries when the heart is at rest. The normal range for adults is 60–79 mmHg.

People with high blood pressure, or **hypertension**, have elevated systolic and/or diastolic blood pressures. A blood pressure level of 140/90 mmHg or higher is considered high.

However, if blood pressure is between 120/80 mmHg and 139/89 mmHg, it is called **prehypertension**. This means that the person does not have high blood pressure now but is likely to have it in the future. Report to the nurse if a resident's blood pressure is 140/90 or above.

Many factors can increase blood pressure. These include aging, exercise, physical or emotional stress, pain, medications, and the volume of blood in circulation. Loss of blood will lead to abnormally low blood pressure, or **hypotension**. Hypotension can be life-threatening if not corrected.

Blood pressure is taken using a stethoscope and a blood pressure cuff, or **sphygmomanometer** (Fig. 14-19). Inside the cuff is an inflatable balloon. It expands when air is pumped into the cuff. Two pieces of tubing are connected to the cuff. One leads to a rubber bulb that pumps air into the cuff. A pressure control button lets you control the release of air from the cuff after it is inflated. The other piece of tubing is connected to a pressure gauge with numbers. The gauge is either a mercury column or a round dial.

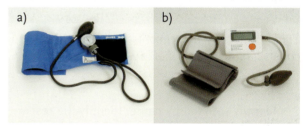

Fig. 14-19. a) A sphygmomanometer and b) an electronic sphygmomanometer.

There may be an electronic sphygmomanometer available. The systolic and diastolic pressure readings and pulse are displayed digitally. Some units automatically inflate and deflate. You do not need a stethoscope with an electronic sphygmomanometer. Ask for instructions on the proper use of the equipment.

When taking blood pressure, the first clear sound you will hear is the systolic pressure (top number). When the sound changes to a soft muffled thump or disappears, this is the diastolic pressure (bottom number). Blood pressure is recorded as a fraction. The systolic reading is on top, and the diastolic reading is on the bottom (for example: 120/80).

Never measure blood pressure on an arm that has an IV, a dialysis shunt, or any medical equipment. Avoid a side that has a cast, recent trauma, paralysis from a stroke, burn(s), or breast surgery (mastectomy).

This textbook includes two methods for taking blood pressure: the one-step method and the two-step method. If using the two-step method, you will get an estimate of the systolic blood pressure before you start. After getting an estimated systolic reading, you will deflate the cuff and begin again. If using the one-step method, you will not get an estimated systolic reading before obtaining the blood pressure reading. Your state may require that you know one or both of these methods. Some states do not allow NAs to measure blood pressure. Know your scope of practice and follow your facility's policies.

Taking and recording blood pressure (one-step method)

Equipment: sphygmomanometer (blood pressure cuff), stethoscope, alcohol wipes, pen and paper

1. Wash your hands.

2. Identify yourself by name. Identify the resident by name.

3. Explain procedure to the resident. Speak clearly, slowly, and directly. Maintain face-to-face contact whenever possible.

4. Provide for resident's privacy with curtain, screen, or door.

5. Ask the resident to roll up his or her sleeve. Do not measure blood pressure over clothing.

6. Position resident's arm with palm up. The arm should be level with the heart.

7. With the valve open, squeeze the cuff. Make sure it is completely deflated.

8. Place blood pressure cuff snugly on resident's upper arm. The center of the cuff is placed over the brachial artery (1-1½ inches above the elbow toward inside of elbow) (Fig. 14-20).

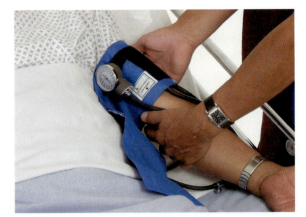

Fig. 14-20. *Place the center of the cuff over the brachial artery.*

9. Before using stethoscope, wipe diaphragm and earpieces with alcohol wipes.

10. Locate brachial pulse with fingertips.

11. Place diaphragm of stethoscope over brachial artery.

12. Place earpieces of stethoscope in ears.

13. Close the valve (clockwise) until it stops. Do not tighten it (Fig. 14-21).

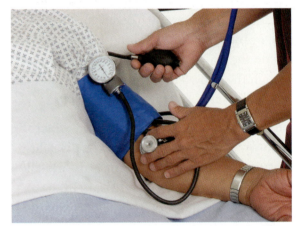

Fig. 14-21. *Close the valve, but do not tighten it; tight valves are difficult to release.*

14. Inflate cuff to 30 mmHg above the point at which the pulse is last heard or felt.

15. Open the valve slightly with thumb and index finger. Deflate cuff slowly.

16. Watch gauge. Listen for sound of pulse.

17. Remember the reading at which the first clear pulse sound is heard. This is the systolic pressure.

18. Continue listening for a change or muffling of pulse sound. The point of change or the point the sound disappears is the diastolic pressure. Remember this reading.

19. Open the valve to deflate cuff completely. Remove cuff.

20. Record both the systolic and diastolic pressures. Write the numbers like a fraction, with the systolic reading on top and the diastolic reading on the bottom (for example: 120/80). Note which arm was used. Write "RA" for right arm and "LA" for left arm.

21. Wipe diaphragm and earpieces of stethoscope with alcohol. Store equipment.

22. Place call light within resident's reach.

23. Wash your hands.

24. Report any changes in resident to the nurse.

Taking and recording blood pressure (two-step method)

Equipment: sphygmomanometer (blood pressure cuff), stethoscope, alcohol wipes, pen and paper

1. Wash your hands.

2. Identify yourself by name. Identify the resident by name.

3. Explain procedure to the resident. Speak clearly, slowly, and directly. Maintain face-to-face contact whenever possible.

4. Provide for resident's privacy with curtain, screen, or door.

5. Ask the resident to roll up his or her sleeve. Do not measure blood pressure over clothing.

6. Position resident's arm with palm up. The arm should be level with the heart.

7. With the valve open, squeeze the cuff. Make sure it is completely deflated.

8. Place blood pressure cuff snugly on resident's upper arm. The center of the cuff is placed over the brachial artery (1-1½ inches above the elbow toward inside of elbow).

9. Locate the radial (wrist) pulse with your fingertips.

10. Close the valve (clockwise) until it stops. Inflate cuff while watching gauge.

11. Stop inflating when you can no longer feel the pulse. Note the reading. The number is an estimate of the systolic pressure. This estimate helps you not to inflate the cuff too high later in this procedure. Inflating the cuff too high is painful and may damage small blood vessels.

12. Open the valve to deflate cuff completely. Remove cuff.

13. Write down the estimated systolic reading.

14. Before using stethoscope, wipe diaphragm and earpieces of stethoscope with alcohol wipes.

15. Locate brachial pulse with fingertips.

16. Place the earpieces of the stethoscope in your ears.

17. Place the diaphragm of the stethoscope over the brachial artery.

18. Close the valve (clockwise) until it stops. Do not tighten it.

19. Inflate the cuff to 30 mmHg above your estimated systolic pressure.

20. Open the valve slightly with thumb and index finger. Deflate cuff slowly. Releasing the valve slowly allows you to hear beats accurately.

21. Watch the gauge. Listen for sound of pulse.

22. Remember the reading at which the first clear pulse sound is heard. This is the systolic pressure.

23. Continue listening for a change or muffling of pulse sound. The point of change or the point the sound disappears is the diastolic pressure. Remember this reading.

24. Open the valve to deflate cuff completely. Remove cuff.

25. Record both the systolic and diastolic pressures. Write the numbers like a fraction, with the systolic reading on top and the diastolic reading on the bottom (for example: 120/80). Note which arm was used. Write "RA" for right arm and "LA" for left arm.

26. Wipe diaphragm and earpieces of stethoscope with alcohol. Store equipment.

27. Place call light within resident's reach.

28. Wash your hands.

29. Report any changes in resident to the nurse.

Tip

Orthostatic Blood Pressures
You may be asked by the nurse to take an orthostatic blood pressure measurement. To do this, the resident must first lie down. Take the blood pressure reading with the resident lying down. Record the systolic and diastolic pressures. Next, have the resident stand up. Wait two minutes, and take the blood pressure measurement again. Record both pressures again. Orthostatic blood pressures must be checked in this order: lying down first, then standing up.

5. Describe guidelines for pain management

Pain is often referred to as vital sign because it is so important to monitor. Pain is uncomfortable. It is also a personal experience, which means it is different for each person. Because you spend the most time with residents, you play an important role in pain monitoring and prevention. Care plans are made based on your reports. It is important to observe and report carefully on a resident's pain.

Pain is not a normal part of aging. When residents complain of pain, treat their complaints seriously (Fig. 14-22). Listen to what residents are saying about the way they feel. Take action to help them. If a resident says he or she is in

pain, ask the following questions to get the most accurate information. Immediately report the information to the nurse. Sustained pain may lead to withdrawal, depression, and isolation.

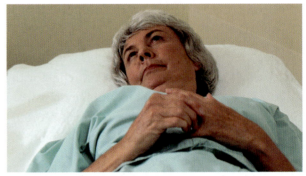

Fig. 14-22. *Believe residents when they say they are in pain and take quick action to help them. Being in pain is unpleasant. Be empathetic.*

- Where is the pain?

- When did the pain start?

- Is the pain mild, moderate, or severe? To help find out, ask the resident to rate the pain on a scale of 1 to 10, with 10 being the most severe.

- Ask the resident to describe the pain. Make notes if you need to. Use the resident's words when reporting to the nurse.

- Ask the resident what he or she was doing before the pain started.

- Ask the resident how long the pain lasts and how often it occurs.

- Ask the resident what makes the pain better and what makes the pain feel worse.

Residents may have concerns about managing their pain. These concerns may make them hesitant to report their pain. Some barriers to managing pain include the following:

- Fear of addiction to pain medication

- Feeling that pain is a normal part of aging

- Worrying about constipation and fatigue from pain medication

- Feeling that caregivers are too busy to deal with their pain

- Feeling that too much pain medication will cause death

Be patient and caring when helping residents who are in pain. If they are worried about the effects of pain medication or if they have questions about it, tell the nurse.

Understand that some people do not feel comfortable saying that they are in pain. A person's culture affects how he or she responds to pain. Some cultures believe that it is best not to react to pain. Other cultures believe in expressing pain freely. Watch for body language or other messages that residents may be in pain. Signs and symptoms of pain are important to observe and report.

Observing and Reporting:
Pain

Report any of these to the nurse:

- ^O/R Increased pulse, respirations, and/or blood pressure
- ^O/R Sweating
- ^O/R Nausea
- ^O/R Vomiting
- ^O/R Tightening the jaw
- ^O/R Squeezing eyes shut
- ^O/R Holding a body part tightly
- ^O/R Frowning
- ^O/R Grinding teeth
- ^O/R Increased restlessness
- ^O/R Agitation or tension
- ^O/R Change in behavior
- ^O/R Crying
- ^O/R Sighing
- ^O/R Groaning
- ^O/R Breathing heavily
- ^O/R Difficulty moving or walking

Use the following measures to help reduce pain:

- Report complaints of pain immediately.

- Gently position the body in good alignment. Use pillows for support. Assist in frequent changes of position if the resident desires it.

- Give back rubs.

- See if the resident would like to take a warm bath or shower.

- Assist the resident to the bathroom or commode or offer the bedpan or urinal.

- Encourage slow, deep breathing.

- Provide a calm and quiet environment. Use soft music to distract the resident.

- Be patient, gentle, kind, and responsive to residents who are in pain.

6. Explain the benefits of warm and cold applications

Applying heat or cold to injured areas can have several good effects. Heat relieves pain and muscular tension. It reduces swelling, elevates the temperature in the tissues, and increases blood flow. Increased blood flow brings more oxygen and nutrients to the tissues for healing. Cold applications can help stop bleeding. They help prevent swelling, reduce pain, and bring down high fevers.

Warm and cold applications may be dry or moist. Moisture strengthens the effect of heat and cold. This means that moist applications are more likely to cause injury. Paralysis, numbness, disorientation, confusion, dementia, and other conditions may cause a person not to be able to feel, notice, or understand damage that is occurring from a warm or cold application. For example, a resident recovering from a stroke who has paralysis on one side may not be able to feel if a warm pack is burning his skin. A resident with Alzheimer's disease may not understand that he is being burned and/or be able to communicate pain clearly. Be very careful when using these applications. Know how long the application should be performed. Use the correct temperature as given in the care plan. Check on the application often, especially for residents who have conditions that may make them unaware of possible injury.

Types of moist applications are:

- Compresses (warm or cold)
- Soaks (warm or cold)
- Tub baths (warm)
- Sponge baths (warm or cold)
- Sitz baths (warm)
- Ice packs (cold)

Types of dry applications are:

- Aquamatic K-pad ® (warm or cold)
- Electric heating pad (warm)
- Disposable warm pack (warm)
- Ice bag (cold)
- Disposable cold pack (cold)

Some states allow nursing assistants to prepare and apply warm and cold applications. Never perform a procedure you are not trained or allowed to do. Only perform procedures that are assigned to you.

Observing and Reporting:
Warm and Cold Applications

Report the following to the nurse:

O/R Excessive redness

O/R Pain

O/R Blisters

O/R Numbness

If you observe these signs, the application may be causing tissue damage.

Residents' Rights

Keep them covered.

When applying warm or cold applications, keep residents' bodies covered. Only expose the area that needs treatment. Doing this promotes dignity, and honors a resident's right to privacy.

For warm compresses, you may use a washcloth or a commercial warm compress. There are different types of commercial compresses available (Fig. 14-23). If these are provided, follow the package directions and the nurse's instructions.

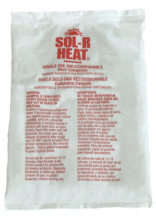

Fig. 14-23. *Disposable heat compresses are used only once and then discarded. The compress shown here must be squeezed to activate and then applied. It maintains heat for a certain amount of time, usually up to 20 minutes.* (REPRINTED WITH PERMISSION OF BRIGGS CORPORATION, 800-247-2343, WWW.BRIGGSCORP.COM)

Applying warm compresses

Equipment: washcloth or compress, plastic wrap, towel, basin, bath thermometer

1. Wash your hands.

2. Identify yourself by name. Identify the resident by name.

3. Explain procedure to the resident. Speak clearly, slowly, and directly. Maintain face-to-face contact whenever possible.

4. Provide for the resident's privacy with curtain, screen, or door.

5. Fill basin one-half to two-thirds full with hot water. Test water temperature with thermometer or your wrist. Ensure it is safe. Water temperature should be no more than 105°F. Have resident check water temperature. Adjust if necessary.

6. Soak the washcloth in the water and wring it out. Immediately apply it to the area needing

a warm compress. Note the time. Quickly cover the washcloth with plastic wrap and the towel to keep it warm (Fig. 14-24).

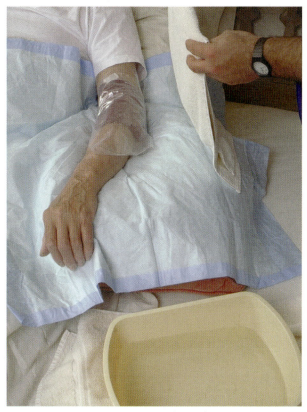

Fig. 14-24. *Cover compresses to keep them warm.*

7. Check the area every five minutes. Remove the compress if the area is red or numb or if the resident has pain or discomfort. Change the compress if cooling occurs. Remove the compress after 20 minutes.

8. Remove privacy measures. Make resident comfortable.

9. Place soiled towels in proper container.

10. Empty, rinse, and wipe basin. Return to proper storage. Discard plastic wrap.

11. Place call light within resident's reach.

12. Wash your hands.

13. Report any changes in resident to the nurse.

14. Document procedure using facility guidelines.

Administering warm soaks

Equipment: towel, basin, bath thermometer, bath blanket

1. Wash your hands.

2. Identify yourself by name. Identify the resident by name.

3. Explain procedure to the resident. Speak clearly, slowly, and directly. Maintain face-to-face contact whenever possible.

4. Provide for the resident's privacy with curtain, screen, or door.

5. Fill the basin half full of warm water. Test water temperature with thermometer or your wrist. Ensure it is safe. Water temperature should be no more than 105°F. Have resident check water temperature. Adjust if necessary.

6. Immerse the body part in the basin. Pad the edge of the basin with a towel if needed (Fig. 14-25). Use a bath blanket to cover the resident if needed for extra warmth.

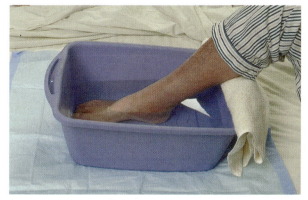

Fig. 14-25. *Pad the edge of the basin to make the resident more comfortable.*

7. Check water temperature every five minutes. Add hot water as needed to maintain the temperature. Never add water hotter than 105°F to avoid burns. To prevent burns, tell the resident not to add hot water. Observe the area for redness. Discontinue the soak if the resident has pain or discomfort.

8. Soak for 15-20 minutes, or as ordered.

9. Remove basin. Use the towel to dry resident.

10. Remove privacy measures. Make resident comfortable.

11. Place soiled towel in proper container.

12. Empty, rinse, and wipe basin. Return to proper storage. Discard plastic wrap.

13. Place call light within resident's reach.

14. Wash your hands.

15. Report any changes in resident to the nurse.

16. Document procedure using facility guidelines.

Applying an Aquamatic K-Pad ®

Equipment: K-Pad ® and control unit (Fig. 14-26), covering for pad, distilled water

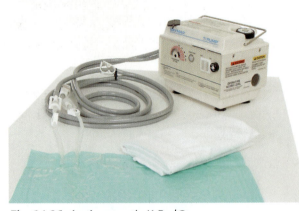

Fig. 14-26. *An Aquamatic K-Pad®.*

1. Wash your hands.

2. Identify yourself by name. Identify the resident by name.

3. Explain procedure to the resident. Speak clearly, slowly, and directly. Maintain face-to-face contact whenever possible.

4. Provide for the resident's privacy during procedure with curtain, screen, or door.

5. Place the control unit on the bedside table. Make sure cords are not frayed or damaged.

Check that tubing between pad and unit is intact.

6. Remove cover of control unit to check level of water. If it is low, fill it with distilled water to the fill line.

7. Put the cover of control unit back in place.

8. Plug unit in and turn pad on. Temperature should have been pre-set. If it was not, check with the nurse for proper temperature.

9. Place the pad in the cover. Do not pin the pad to the cover.

10. Uncover area to be treated. Place the covered pad. Note the time. Make sure the tubing is not hanging below the bed. It should be coiled on the bed.

11. Return and check area every five minutes. Remove the pad if the area is red or numb or if the resident reports pain or discomfort.

12. Check water level. Refill when necessary.

13. Remove pad after 20 minutes.

14. Remove privacy measures. Make resident comfortable.

15. Clean and store supplies.

16. Place call light within resident's reach.

17. Wash your hands.

18. Report any changes in resident to the nurse.

19. Document procedure using facility guidelines.

Another type of heat application is a **sitz bath**. This is a warm soak of the perineal area. Sitz baths clean perineal wounds and reduce inflammation and pain. Circulation in the perineal area is increased. Voiding may be stimulated by a sitz bath. Persons with perineal swelling (such as hemorrhoids) or perineal wounds (such as those that occur during childbirth) may be ordered to take sitz baths. Because the sitz bath causes increased blood flow to the pelvic area, blood flow to other parts of the body decreases. Residents may feel weak, faint, or dizzy after a sitz bath. Always wear gloves when helping with a sitz bath.

Assisting with a sitz bath

A disposable sitz bath fits on the toilet seat and is attached to a rubber bag containing warm water (Fig. 14-27).

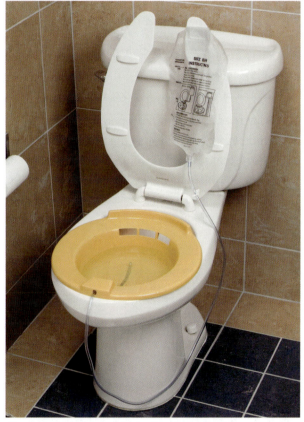

Fig. 14-27. *A disposable sitz bath.* (REPRINTED WITH PERMISSION OF BRIGGS CORPORATION, 800-247-2343, WWW.BRIGGSCORP.COM)

Equipment: disposable sitz bath, bath thermometer, towels, gloves

1. Wash your hands.

2. Identify yourself by name. Identify the resident by name.

3. Explain procedure to the resident. Speak clearly, slowly, and directly. Maintain face-to-face contact whenever possible.

4. Provide for the resident's privacy with curtain, screen, or door.

5. Put on gloves.

6. Fill the sitz bath two-thirds full with hot water. Place the disposable sitz bath on the toilet seat. Water temperature should be no more than 105°F. Check the water temperature using the bath thermometer. If having a sitz bath to help relieve pain and to stimulate circulation, the water temperature may need to be higher. Follow instructions in the care plan.

7. Help the resident undress and be seated on the sitz bath. A valve on the tubing connected to the bag allows the resident or you to fill the sitz bath again with hot water.

8. You may be required to stay with the resident during the bath for safety reasons. If you leave the room, check on the resident every five minutes to make sure he or she is not dizzy or weak. Stay with a resident who seems unsteady.

9. Help the resident out of the sitz bath in 20 minutes. Provide towels. Help with dressing if needed.

10. Make sure resident is comfortable.

11. Clean and store supplies.

12. Remove gloves.

13. Wash your hands.

14. Place call light within resident's reach.

15. Report any changes in resident to the nurse.

16. Document procedure using facility guidelines.

For applying ice packs, you may use a commercial cold pack. There are different types of commercial packs available (Fig. 14-28). If these are provided, follow the package directions and the nurse's instructions.

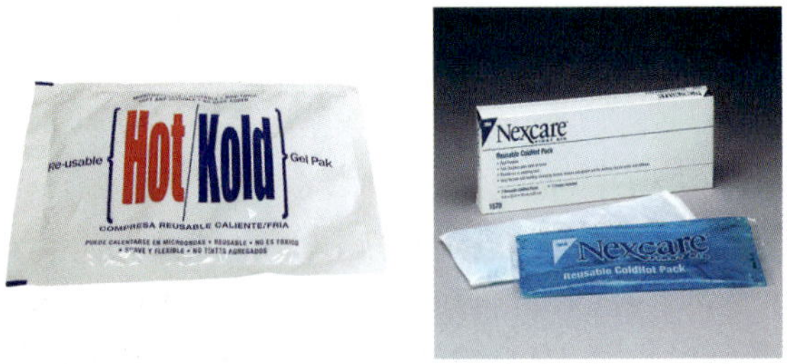

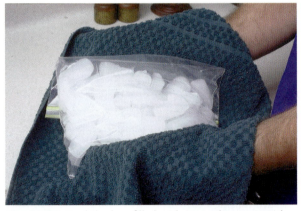

Fig. 14-28. *Some types of reusable packs may be used for heat or cold. They can be microwaved to heat or stored in the freezer for cold.* (REPRINTED WITH PERMISSION OF BRIGGS CORPORATION, 800-247-2343, WWW.BRIGGSCORP.COM)

Applying ice packs

Equipment: ice pack or sealable plastic bag and crushed ice, towel to cover pack or bag

1. Wash your hands.

2. Identify yourself by name. Identify the resident by name.

3. Explain procedure to the resident. Speak clearly, slowly, and directly. Maintain face-to-face contact whenever possible.

4. Provide for the resident's privacy with curtain, screen, or door.

5. Fill plastic bag or ice pack 1/2 to 2/3 full with crushed ice. Seal bag. Remove excess air. Cover bag or ice pack with towel (Fig. 14-29).

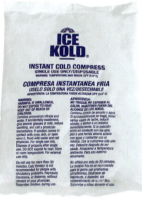

Fig. 14-29. *Seal the bag filled with ice and cover it with a towel.*

6. Apply bag to the area as ordered. Note the time. Use another towel to cover bag if it is too cold.

7. Check the area after ten minutes for blisters or pale, white, or gray skin. Stop treatment if resident reports numbness or pain.

8. Remove ice after 20 minutes or as ordered.

9. Remove privacy measures. Make resident comfortable.

10. Store ice pack. Place towel in proper container.

11. Place call light within resident's reach.

12. Wash your hands.

13. Report any changes in resident to the nurse.

14. Document procedure using facility guidelines.

You may use a washcloth dipped in cold water as a cold compress; you may also use a disposable or reusable compress (Fig. 14-30). Follow instructions on the package.

Fig. 14-30. *This type of cold compress is disposable. You squeeze it to activate and it will last up to 30 minutes. It remains flexible when activated.* (REPRINTED WITH PERMISSION OF BRIGGS CORPORATION, 800-247-2343, WWW.BRIGGSCORP.COM)

Applying cold compresses

Equipment: basin filled with water and ice, two washcloths, disposable bed protector, towels

1. Wash your hands.

2. Identify yourself by name. Identify the resident by name.

3. Explain procedure to the resident. Speak clearly, slowly, and directly. Maintain face-to-face contact whenever possible.

4. Provide for the resident's privacy with curtain, screen, or door.

5. Place bed protector under area to be treated. Rinse washcloth in basin and wring out (Fig. 14-31). Cover the area to be treated with a cloth sheet or towel. Apply cold washcloth to the area as directed. Change washcloths often to keep area cold.

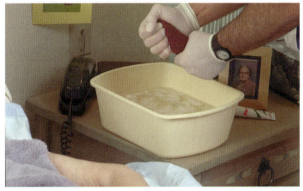

Fig. 14-31. Wring out the washcloth before applying it to the area to be treated.

6. Check the area after five minutes for blisters, pale, white, or gray skin. Stop treatment if resident complains of numbness or pain.

7. Remove compresses after 20 minutes or as ordered in the care plan. Give resident towels as needed to dry the area.

8. Remove privacy measures. Make resident comfortable.

9. Clean and store basin. Place towels in proper container.

10. Place call light within resident's reach.

11. Wash your hands.

12. Report any changes in resident to the nurse.

13. Document procedure using facility guidelines.

7. Explain how to apply non-sterile dressings and discuss sterile dressings

Sterile dressings cover open or draining wounds. A nurse changes these dressings. Non-sterile dressings are applied to dry, closed wounds that have less chance of infection. Nursing assistants may help with non-sterile dressing changes.

Changing a dry dressing using non-sterile technique

Equipment: package of square gauze dressings, adhesive tape, scissors, 2 pairs of gloves

1. Wash your hands.

2. Identify yourself by name. Identify the resident by name.

3. Explain procedure to the resident. Speak clearly, slowly, and directly. Maintain face-to-face contact whenever possible.

4. Provide for resident's privacy with curtain, screen, or door.

5. Cut pieces of tape long enough to secure the dressing. Hang tape on the edge of a table within reach. Open four-inch gauze square package without touching gauze. Place the open package on a flat surface.

6. Put on gloves.

7. Remove soiled dressing by gently peeling tape toward the wound. Lift dressing off the wound. Do not drag it over wound. Observe dressing for any odor or drainage. Notice color and size of the wound. Dispose of used dressing in proper container. Remove and dispose of gloves.

8. Put on new gloves. Touching only outer edges of new four-inch gauze, remove it from package. Apply it to wound. Tape gauze in place. Secure it firmly (Fig. 14-32).

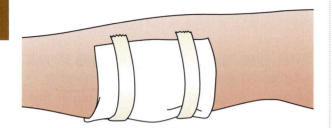

Fig. 14-32. Tape gauze in place to secure the dressing. Do not completely cover all areas of the dressing with tape.

9.   Remove and dispose of gloves properly.

10. Wash your hands.

11. Remove privacy measures. Make resident comfortable.

12. Place call light within resident's reach.

13. Report any changes in resident to the nurse.

14. Document procedure using facility guidelines.

Even though nursing assistants do not change sterile dressings, they can gather and store equipment and supplies, observe and report about the dressing site and they may be allowed to clean the equipment. Duties may also include properly positioning the resident, cutting the tape, and disposing of the soiled dressing. Supplies that may be needed for changing a sterile dressing include:

•   Special gauze has one side that has a shiny, non-stick surface, which will not stick to wounds when removed.

•   Abdominal pads (ABDs) are large, heavy gauze dressings that cover smaller gauze dressings and help keep them in place and provide absorbency.

•   Cotton bandages (sometimes called "Kerlix" or "Kling" bandages) can stretch and mold to a body part and help hold it in place; these are often used on bony areas, such as the knees and elbows.

•   Binders are stretchable pieces of fabric that can be fastened. They hold dressings in place and give support to surgical wounds. Binders can also reduce swelling and ease discomfort.

•   Medical-grade adhesive tape panels (sometimes called "Montgomery Straps") help keep frequently-changed dressings in place. The adhesive is not removed with each dressing change so that skin is less likely to become irritated.

When gathering sterile supplies, keep the following tips in mind:

•   If the wrapper on the supply is torn, it is no longer considered sterile and cannot be used.

•   The wrapper on the supply cannot be opened and closed again. Once a wrapper is opened, the supplies inside are no longer sterile.

•   If a wrapper is wet or has wrinkles or marks that indicate it was once wet, it is no longer considered sterile.

•   If the date on the supply shows it has expired, it is no longer considered sterile. Commercially prepared supplies are all dated. A sterile supply that has expired should not be used.

•   If you are unsure whether a wrapper is sterile or not, do not use it.

Sterile dressings cover open or draining wounds. Because of the way the wound and the skin around it may look, the resident may feel embarrassed about having others see the area. Promote the resident's comfort and dignity when assisting the nurse with a sterile dressing change by being professional and matter-of-fact. Do not show any discomfort, even if you are bothered by the appearance of the resident's skin.

Observing and documenting your observations are very important parts of your job. While you are assisting with changing a sterile dressing, observe for any changes in the wound, especially the following:

- Skin that has changed color
- Scab that has come off
- Bleeding
- Swelling
- Odor
- Drainage

8. Discuss guidelines for non-sterile bandages

Elastic, or non-sterile, bandages (sometimes called "ACE® bandages") are used to hold dressings in place, secure splints, and support and protect body parts. In addition, these bandages may decrease swelling that occurs with an injury (Fig. 14-33).

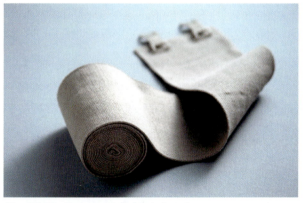

Fig. 14-33. *One type of elastic bandage.*

NAs may be required to assist with the use of an elastic bandage. Duties may include bringing the bandage to the resident, positioning the resident to apply the bandage, washing and storing the bandage, and documenting observations about the bandage. Some states allow NAs to apply and remove elastic bandages. Follow your facility's policies and the care plan regarding elastic bandages. If you are allowed to assist with these bandages, know the following safety guidelines.

Guidelines:
Elastic Bandages

G Keep the area to be wrapped clean and dry.

G Apply elastic bandages snugly enough to control bleeding and prevent movement of dressings. However, make sure that the body part is not wrapped too tightly, which can decrease circulation.

G Wrap the bandage evenly so that no part of the wrapped area is pinched.

G Do not tie the bandage because this cuts off circulation to the body part; the end is held in place with special clips or tape.

G Remove the bandage as often as indicated in the care plan.

G Check the bandage often because it can become wrinkled or loose, which causes it to lose effectiveness, and bunched-up, which causes pressure and possible discomfort.

G Check on the resident 15 minutes after the bandage is first applied to see if there are any signs of poor circulation. Signs and symptoms of poor circulation include:
- Swelling
- Bluish, or cyanotic, skin
- Shiny, tight skin
- Skin cold to touch
- Sores
- Numbness
- Tingling
- Pain or discomfort

Loosen the bandage if you note any signs of poor circulation, and notify the nurse immediately.

9. List care guidelines for a resident who is on an IV

IV stands for **intravenous**, or into a vein. A resident with an IV is receiving medication, nutrition, or fluids through a vein.

When a doctor prescribes an IV, a nurse inserts a needle or tube into a vein. This allows direct access to the bloodstream. Medication, nutrition, or fluids either drip from a bag suspended on a pole or are pumped by a portable pump through a tube and into the vein (Fig. 14-34). Some residents with chronic conditions have a permanent opening for IVs. This opening has been surgically created to allow easy access for IV fluids. Nursing assistants never insert or remove IV lines. You will not be responsible for care of the IV site. Your only responsibility for IV care is to report and document any observations of changes or problems with the IV.

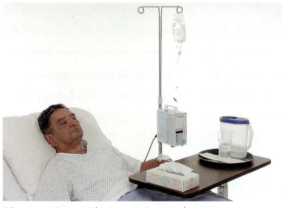

Fig. 14-34. *A resident receiving IV therapy.*

Observing and Reporting:
IVs

O/R The tube/needle falls out or is removed.

O/R The tubing disconnects.

O/R The dressing around the IV site is loose or not intact.

O/R Blood is present in the tubing or around the site of the IV.

O/R The site is swollen or discolored.

O/R The resident complains of pain.

O/R The bag is broken, or the level of fluid does not seem to decrease.

O/R The IV fluid is not dripping.

O/R The IV fluid is nearly gone.

O/R The pump beeps, indicating a problem.

O/R The pump is dropped.

As always, document your observations and the care provided. Do not get the IV site wet or lower the bag below the IV site. Never disconnect the IV from the pump or turn off a beeping alarm. Do not take a resident's blood pressure on an arm that has an IV. Having an IV in place makes some basic care procedures more difficult. Always be careful not to pull or catch on IV tubing when performing or assisting with care of residents with IVs.

Assisting in changing clothes for a resident who has an IV

Equipment: clean clothes

1. Wash your hands.

2. Identify yourself by name. Identify the resident by name.

3. Explain procedure to the resident. Speak clearly, slowly, and directly. Maintain face-to-face contact whenever possible.

4. Provide for resident's privacy with curtain, screen, or door.

5. If the bed is adjustable, adjust to a safe level, usually waist high. If the bed is movable, lock bed wheels.

6. Assist resident to sitting position with feet flat on the floor.

7. Have the resident remove the arm without the IV from clothing. Assist as necessary.

8. Help the resident gather the clothing on the arm with the IV. Carefully lift the clothing over the IV site and move it up the tubing toward the IV bag (Fig. 14-35).

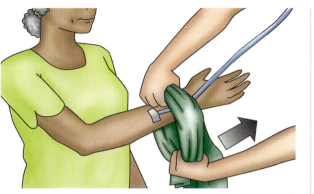

Fig. 14-35. Make sure clothing does not catch on tubing.

9. Lift the IV bag off its pole, keeping it higher than the IV site. Carefully slide the clothing over the bag. Place the bag back on the pole.

10. Set the used clothing aside to be placed with soiled laundry.

11. Gather the sleeve of the clean clothing.

12. Lift the IV bag off its pole and, keeping it higher than the IV site, carefully slide the clothing over the bag (Fig. 14-36). Place the IV bag back on the pole.

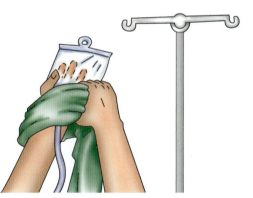

Fig. 14-36. Always keep the IV bag higher than the IV site.

13. Carefully move the clean clothing down the IV tubing, over the IV site, and onto the resident's arm.

14. Have the resident put his other arm in the clothing. Assist as necessary.

15. Check that the IV is dripping properly. Make sure none of the tubing is dislodged and the IV site dressing is in place.

16. Assist the resident with changing the rest of his clothing, as necessary.

17. Place soiled clothes in proper container.

18. Make resident comfortable. Make sure sheets are free from wrinkles and the bed free from crumbs.

19. Return bed to lowest position. Remove privacy measures.

20. Place call light within resident's reach.

21. Wash your hands.

22. Report any changes in resident to the nurse.

23. Document procedure using facility guidelines.

Special gowns with sleeves that snap and unsnap are available to lessen the risk of pulling out IVs.

Residents' Rights

IVs

Protect the rights of a resident with an IV by helping him or her be as independent as possible. Set up the area so the resident may still feed him- or herself, help with bathing and hair care, if able, etc. Ask the nurse how to transport the resident to the activities he or she wants to attend. Assure privacy for procedures by pulling the privacy curtain and closing the door.

10. Discuss oxygen therapy and explain related care guidelines

As you learned in Chapter 6, some residents may receive oxygen therapy. **Oxygen therapy** is the administration of oxygen to increase the supply of oxygen to the lungs. This increases the availability of oxygen to the body tissues. Oxygen therapy is often used to treat breathing difficulties and is prescribed by a doctor. Nursing assistants never stop, adjust, or administer oxygen.

Oxygen may be piped into a resident's room through a central system. It may be in tanks or produced by an oxygen concentrator. An **oxygen concentrator** is a box-like device that changes air in the room into air with more oxygen. Oxygen concentrators are quiet machines. They can be larger units or portable ones that can move or travel with the resident. Oxygen concentrators typically plug into wall outlets and are turned on and off by a switch. It may take a while for the oxygen concentrator to reach full power after it is turned on.

Some residents receive oxygen through a nasal cannula. A **nasal cannula** is a piece of plastic tubing that fits around the face and is secured by a strap that goes over the ears and around the back of the head. The face piece has two short prongs made of tubing. These prongs fit inside the nose, and oxygen is delivered through them. A respiratory therapist fits the cannula. The length of the prongs (usually no more than half an inch) is adjusted for the resident's comfort. The resident can talk and eat while wearing the cannula.

Residents who do not need concentrated oxygen all the time may use a face mask when they need oxygen. The face mask fits over the nose and mouth. It is secured by a strap that goes over the ears and around the back of the head. The mask should be checked to see that it fits snugly on the resident's face, but it should not pinch the face. It is difficult for a resident to talk when wearing an oxygen face mask. The mask must be removed for the resident to eat or drink anything.

Oxygen can be irritating to the nose and mouth. The strap of a nasal cannula or face mask can also cause irritation around the ears. Wash and dry skin carefully, and provide frequent mouth care. Offer the resident plenty of fluids. Report and document any irritation you observe.

Oxygen is a very dangerous fire hazard because it makes other things burn (supports combustion). Observe the safety guidelines for oxygen use found in Chapter 6.

Follow these guidelines for oxygen tanks, oxygen concentrators, and liquid oxygen:

Guidelines:
Oxygen Delivery Devices

For residents using oxygen tanks:

G   Take and record pulse and respirations before and after resident uses the oxygen tank to see if there are any changes.

G   The flow meter shows how much oxygen is flowing out to the resident at any time. It should be set at the amount stated on the care plan. If it is not, report this to the nurse. Do not adjust oxygen level.

G   Make sure the humidifying bottle has sterile water in it and is attached correctly . Wash the humidifying bottle according to the care plan or equipment supplier's instructions.

G   Change the nasal cannula when ordered. It will need to be changed when it is hard or cracked, at least once per week.

G   Make sure the oxygen tank is secured and will not tip over.

For residents using oxygen concentrators:

G   Take and record pulse and respirations before and after resident uses the oxygen concentrator to see if there are any changes.

G   The oxygen concentrator dial must be set at the same rate as indicated in the care plan. If it is not, report this to the nurse. Do not adjust oxygen level.

G   Check the humidifying bottle each time the device is used to see that it has sterile water in it and that it is screwed on tightly. Sterile water must be used, not tap water, because minerals in tap water may clog the tubing.

G   Make sure the concentrator is in a well-ventilated area, at least six inches from a wall. Because the air filter cleans the air going into the machine, brush it off daily to remove dust.

For residents using liquid oxygen:

G Turn off supply valves when the reservoir is not in use.

G Do not tip the reservoir on its side.

G Make sure the reservoir is not in a closet, cupboard, or other closed-in space.

G Do not cover the reservoir with bed linens or clothing.

G When lifting the reservoir, lift with two hands. Do not roll the reservoir or walk it on edge.

G Do not touch frosted parts of the equipment, because the cold can cause frostbite. Do not touch liquid oxygen; it can cause frostbite. Report if the reservoir is leaking.

Humidifiers

A humidifier is a device that puts moisture into the air. Residents who use oxygen equipment or who have breathing problems may use humidifiers. Making the air moist or humid can make them more comfortable.

There are different types of humidifiers; some humidifiers put warm moisture into the air and some put cool moisture into the air.

Follow the care plan's instructions for cleaning and care of a humidifier. Because pathogens grow in moist areas, the water tank of the humidifier should be washed often. Your other responsibilities may include adding water to the humidifier when needed, and possibly adding special tablets to prevent mineral buildup.

Chapter Review

1. List five vital signs that must be monitored.

2. What are the four sites for taking the body's temperature?

3. Which temperature site is considered to be the most accurate?

4. What is the most common site for monitoring the pulse? Where is it located?

5. List the normal pulse rate range for adults.

6. Why should respirations be counted immediately after measuring the pulse rate?

7. List the two parts of measuring blood pressure and briefly define both phases.

8. Define the following terms: hypertension, prehypertension, and hypotension.

9. List the two pieces of equipment normally used to monitor blood pressure.

10. How are blood pressure numbers written and recorded?

11. List 15 signs that may show that a resident is in pain.

12. List seven measures to reduce pain.

13. What are the benefits of warm applications? What are the benefits of cold applications?

14. What four signs should an NA watch for at the site of a warm or cold application?

15. What is the purpose of a sitz bath?

16. When are non-sterile dressings usually used?

17. What duties may a nursing assistant have regarding sterile dressings?

18. List six signs of poor circulation that an NA should observe for when an elastic bandage is applied.

19. What is a nursing assistant's responsibility with IV care?

20. List seven things to observe and report about a resident's IV.

21. What is an oxygen concentrator?

22. What is a nasal cannula?

23. Why is oxygen a dangerous fire hazard?

15
Nutrition and Hydration

1. Describe the importance of good nutrition

Good nutrition is very important. **Nutrition** is how the body uses food to maintain health. Bodies need a well-balanced diet with essential nutrients and plenty of fluids. This helps us grow new cells, maintain normal body function, and have energy for activities. Good nutrition in early life helps ensure good health later in life. For the ill or elderly, a well-balanced diet helps maintain muscles and skin tissues and prevent pressure sores. A good diet promotes healing of wounds. It also helps us cope with stress.

2. List the six basic nutrients and explain the USDA's MyPyramid

A **nutrient** is something found in food that provides energy, promotes growth and health and helps regulate metabolism. Metabolism is the physical and chemical process by which nutrients are broken down to be used by the body for energy and other needs. The body needs the following six nutrients for growth and development:

1. **Protein**. Proteins are part of every body cell. They are needed for tissue growth and repair. Proteins also supply energy for the body. Excess proteins are excreted by the kidneys or stored as body fat. Sources of protein include fish, seafood, poultry, meat, eggs, milk, cheese, nuts, nut butters, peas, dried beans or legumes, and soy products (tofu, tempeh, veggie burgers)

(Fig. 15-1). Whole grain cereals, pastas, rice, and breads contain some proteins, too.

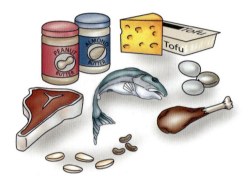

Fig. 15-1. Sources of protein.

2. **Carbohydrates**. Carbohydrates supply fuel for the body's energy needs. They supply extra protein and help the body use fat efficiently. Carbohydrates also provide fiber, which is necessary for bowel elimination. Carbohydrates can be divided into two basic types: complex and simple carbohydrates (Fig. 15-2). **Complex carbohydrates** are found in bread, cereal, potatoes, rice, pasta, vegetables, and fruits. **Simple carbohydrates** are found in sugars, sweets, syrups, and jellies. Simple carbohydrates do not have the same nutritional value that complex carbohydrates do.

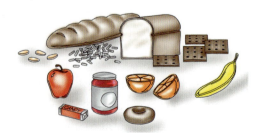

Fig. 15-2. Sources of carbohydrates.

3. **Fats**. Fat helps the body store energy. Body fat also provides insulation. It protects body organs. In addition, fats add flavor to food and are important for the absorption of certain vitamins. Excess fat in the diet is stored as fat in the body. Examples of fats are butter, margarine, salad dressings, oils, and animal fats in meats, dairy products, fowl, and fish (Fig. 15-3). Monounsaturated vegetable fats (including olive oil and canola oil) and polyunsaturated vegetable fats (including corn and safflower oils) are healthier. Saturated fats, including animal fats like butter, lard, bacon, and other fatty meats, are not as healthy. They should be limited in most diets.

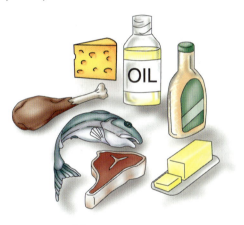

Fig. 15-3. Sources of fat.

4. **Vitamins**. Vitamins are substances the body needs to function. The body cannot make most vitamins; they can only be gotten from food. Vitamins A, D, E, and K are fat-soluble vitamins. This means they are carried and stored in body fat. Vitamins B and C are water-soluble vitamins that are broken down by water in our bodies. They cannot be stored in the body. They are eliminated in urine and feces.

5. **Minerals**. Minerals form and maintain body functions. They provide energy and control processes. Zinc, iron, calcium, and magnesium are examples of minerals. Minerals are found in many foods.

6. **Water**. One-half to two-thirds of our body weight is water. We need about 64 ounces, or eight glasses, of water or other fluids a day. Water is the most essential nutrient for life.

Without it, a person can only live a few days. Water helps in the digestion and absorption of food. It helps with waste elimination. Through perspiration, water also helps maintain normal body temperature. Keeping enough fluid in our bodies is necessary for good health (Fig. 15-4).

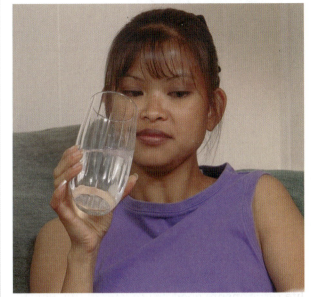

Fig. 15-4. Water is the most essential nutrient for life. Drinking plenty of water promotes good health.

The fluids we drink—water, juice, soda, coffee, tea, and milk—provide most of the water our bodies use. Some foods are also sources of water, including soup, celery, lettuce, apples, and peaches.

Most foods contain several nutrients, but no one food contains all the nutrients that are necessary to maintain a healthy body. That is why it is important to eat a daily diet that is well-balanced. There is not one single dietary plan that is right for everyone. People have different nutritional needs depending upon their age, gender, and activity level.

In 1980, the U.S. Department of Agriculture (USDA) developed the Food Guide Pyramid to help promote healthy eating practices. In 2005, in response to new scientific information about nutrition and health and new technology for support tools, MyPyramid was developed (Fig. 15-5). MyPyramid replaces the Food Guide Pyramid. MyPyramid is a personalized version of the

Food Guide Pyramid that offers individual plans based on age, gender, and activity level.

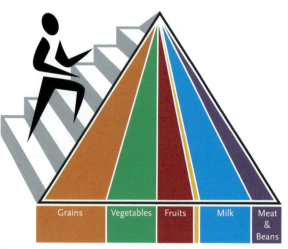

Fig. 15-5. *MyPyramid was developed to help promote healthy eating practices. It offers individual plans based on age, gender, and activity level.*

The Pyramid is made up of six bands of different widths and colors. Each color represents a food group—orange for grains, green for vegetables, maroon for fruits, yellow for oils, blue for milk, and purple for meat and beans. The different widths indicate that not all groups should make up an equal part of a healthy diet. The orange band, grains, is the widest, which means that grains should make up the highest proportion of the diet. The smaller bands, such as the purple band representing meat and beans, should make up a smaller part of the diet. The smallest band, the yellow one, represents oils. Oils contain essential fatty acids. However, this band is not emphasized because the body needs fats and oils in smaller quantities.

The bands of the Pyramid are wide at the bottom and narrow into a point at the top. This is a reminder that there are a great variety of foods that make up each group. Many choices are available to help meet the daily requirements. Foods that are nutrient-dense and low in fat and calories should form the "base" of a healthy diet. They are represented by the wide base of the Pyramid. Foods that are high in fat and sugar and have less nutritional value are at the narrow top. They should be eaten less often.

The new Pyramid also emphasizes the importance of physical activity, as represented by the figure climbing the stairs. Physical activity goes hand-in-hand with diet to make up an overall healthy lifestyle. The USDA recommends at least 30 minutes per day of vigorous activity for everyone. Sixty minutes or more is even better.

Grains: The grains group includes all foods made from wheat, rice, oats, corn, barley, and other grains. Examples are bread, pasta, oatmeal, breakfast cereals, tortillas, and grits. One slice of bread, one cup of ready-to-eat cereal, or ½ cup of cooked rice, pasta, or cooked cereal can be considered a one-ounce equivalent from the grains group.

At least half of all grains consumed should be whole grains. Words on food labels that ensure that grains are whole grains are: brown rice, wild rice, bulgur, oatmeal, whole-grain corn, whole oats, whole wheat, and whole rye.

Vegetables: The vegetable group includes all fresh, frozen, canned, and dried vegetables, and vegetable juices. One cup of raw or cooked vegetables or vegetable juice or two cups of raw leafy greens can be counted as one cup from the vegetable group. There are five subgroups within the vegetable group. They are organized by nutritional content. These are dark green vegetables, orange vegetables, dry beans and peas, starchy vegetables, and other vegetables. A variety of vegetables from these subgroups should be eaten every day. Dark green vegetables, orange vegetables, and dried beans and peas have the best nutritional content.

Vegetables are low in fat and calories and have no cholesterol (although sauces and seasonings may add fat, calories, and cholesterol). They are good sources of dietary fiber, potassium, vitamin A, vitamin E, and vitamin C.

Fruits: The fruit group includes all fresh, frozen, canned, and dried fruits, and fruit juices. One cup of fruit or 100 percent fruit juice or ½ cup of dried fruit can be counted as one cup from the fruit group. Most choices should be whole or cut-up fruit rather than juice for the additional dietary fiber provided.

Fruits, like vegetables, are naturally low in fat, sodium, and calories and have no cholesterol. They are important sources of dietary fiber and many nutrients, including folic acid and vitamin C.

Milk: The milk group includes all fluid milk products and foods made from milk that retain their calcium content, such as yogurt and cheese. Foods made from milk that have little to no calcium, such as cream cheese, cream, and butter, are not part of the group. Most milk group choices should be fat-free or low-fat (Fig. 15-6). One cup of milk or yogurt, 1½ ounces of natural cheese, or two ounces of processed cheese can be counted as one cup from the milk group.

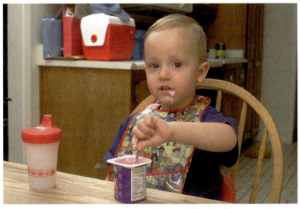

Fig. 15-6. *Low-fat yogurt is a good source of calcium.*

Foods in the milk group provide nutrients that are vital for the health and maintenance of your body. These nutrients include calcium, potassium, vitamin D, and protein. Calcium is used for building bones and teeth and in maintaining bone mass. Milk products are the primary source of calcium in American diets.

Meat and Beans: One ounce of lean meat, poultry, or fish; one egg; one tablespoon of peanut butter; ¼ cup cooked dry beans; or ½ ounce of nuts or seeds can be counted as a one ounce equivalent from the meat and beans group. Dry beans and peas can be included as part of this

group or as part of the vegetable group. If meat is eaten regularly, dry beans and peas should be included with vegetables. If not, they should be included as part of this group.

Most meat and poultry choices should be lean or low-fat. Diets that are high in saturated fats raise "bad" cholesterol levels in the blood. Fish, nuts, and seeds contain healthy oils. These foods are a good choice instead of meat or poultry. Some nuts and seeds (flax, walnuts) are excellent sources of essential fatty acids. These acids may reduce the risk of cardiovascular disease. Some (sunflower seeds, almonds, hazelnuts) are good sources of vitamin E.

Vegetarians get enough protein from this group as long as the variety and amounts of foods selected are adequate. Protein sources for vegetarians from this group include eggs (for ovo-vegetarians), beans, nuts, nut butters, peas, and soy products (tofu, tempeh, veggie burgers).

Oils: Oils include fats that are liquid at room temperature, such as canola, corn, olive, soybean, and sunflower oil (Fig. 15-7). Some foods are naturally high in oils, like nuts, olives, some fish, and avocados. Foods that are mainly oil include mayonnaise, certain salad dressings, and soft margarine.

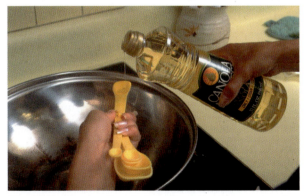

Fig. 15-7. *Canola oil and olive oil are healthier types of oils to use in cooking and baking.*

Most of the fats you eat should be polyunsaturated (PUFA) or monounsaturated (MUFA) fats. Oils are the major source of MUFAs and PUFAs in the diet. PUFAs contain some fatty acids that are necessary for health. These are called "essential fatty acids." Most Americans consume enough oil in the foods they eat, such as nuts, fish, cooking oil, and salad dressings.

Activity: Physical activity and nutrition work together for better health. Being active increases the amount of calories burned. As people age, their metabolism slows. Maintaining energy balance requires moving more and eating less. For health benefits, physical activity should be moderate or vigorous and add up to at least 30 minutes a day. For more information on MyPyramid, visit mypyramid.gov.

Because older adults have different nutritional needs, Tufts University developed a version of MyPyramid that is specifically designed for older adults. Due to slower metabolism and less activity, the elderly need to eat less to maintain body weight. Although calories can be reduced, daily needs for most nutrients do not decrease. The "Modified MyPyramid for Older Adults" has a narrower base to reflect a decrease in energy needs. It emphasizes nutrient-dense foods, fiber, and water. Dietary supplements may be appropriate for many older people. For more information on the "Modified MyPyramid for Older Adults," visit nutrition.tufts.edu.

3. Identify nutritional problems of the elderly or ill

Aging and illness can lead to emotional and physical problems that affect the intake of food. For example, people who are lonely or who suffer from illnesses that affect their ability to chew and swallow may have little interest in food. Weaker hands and arms due to paralysis or tremors make it hard to eat. People with illnesses that affect their ability to chew and swallow may not want to eat. In addition, people who are ill are often fatigued, nauseated, or in pain, which contributes to poor fluid and food intake. Other problems that affect nutritional intake include the following:

- Metabolism slows. Muscles weaken and lose tone, and body movement slows. Reduced activity or exercise affects appetite.

- A loss of vision may affect the way food looks, which can decrease appetite.

- Weakened senses of smell and taste affect appetite. Medication may impair these senses (Fig. 15-8).

- Less saliva production affects chewing and swallowing.

- Dentures, tooth loss, or poor dental health make chewing difficult.

- Digestion takes longer and is less efficient.

- Certain medications or limited activity cause constipation. Constipation often interferes with appetite. Fiber, fluids, and exercise can improve this common problem.

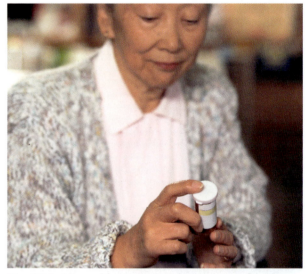

Fig. 15-8. *Many elderly people take a variety of medications, which can affect the way food smells and tastes.*

Unintended weight loss is a serious problem for the elderly. Weight loss can mean that the resident has a serious medical condition. It can lead to skin breakdown, which leads to pressure sores. It is very important to report any weight loss, no matter how small. If a resident has diabetes, chronic obstructive pulmonary disease, cancer, HIV, or other diseases, he is at a greater risk for malnutrition. (See Chapter 18 for more information on these diseases.)

Observing and Reporting:
Unintended Weight Loss

Report any of these to the nurse:

O/R Resident needs help eating or drinking

O/R Resident eats less than 70% of meals/snacks served

O/R Resident has mouth pain

O/R Resident has dentures that do not fit

O/R Resident has difficulty chewing or swallowing

O/R Resident coughs or chokes while eating

O/R Resident is sad, has crying spells, or withdraws from others

O/R Resident is confused, wanders, or paces

Guidelines:
Preventing Unintended Weight Loss

G Report observations and warning signs to the nurse.

G Encourage residents to eat. Talk about food served in a positive tone of voice, using positive words (Fig. 15-9).

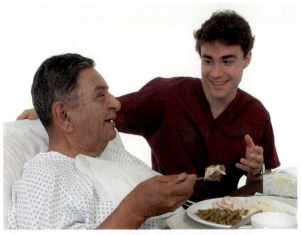

Fig. 15-9. Be social, friendly, and positive while helping residents with eating. This helps promote appetite and prevent weight loss.

G Honor residents' food likes and dislikes.

G Offer different kinds of foods and beverages.

G Help residents who have trouble feeding themselves.

G Food should look, taste, and smell good. The person may have a poor sense of taste and smell.

G Season foods to residents' preferences.

G Allow enough time for residents to finish eating.

G Tell the nurse if residents have trouble using utensils.

G Record the meal/snack intake.

G Give oral care before and after meals.

G Position residents sitting upright for feeding.

G If a resident has had a loss of appetite and/or seems sad, ask about it.

Care must be taken in meal planning to ensure good nutrition for the elderly and ill. Many illnesses require restrictions in fluids, proteins, certain minerals, or calories. Conditions that make eating or swallowing difficult include the following:

- Stroke, or CVA, which can cause facial weakness and paralysis

- Nerve and muscle damage from head and neck cancer

- Multiple sclerosis

- Parkinson's disease

- Alzheimer's disease

You will learn more about these diseases in Chapters 18 and 19. If a resident has trouble swallowing, soft foods and liquids that have been thickened may be easier to swallow. Thickening improves the ability to control fluid in the mouth and throat. Thickened liquids include milk shakes, pureed foods, sherbet, gelatin, thin hot cereal, cream soups, and fruit juices that have been frozen to a slushy consistency. You will learn more about swallowing problems and thickened liquids later in the chapter.

When the digestive system does not function properly, hyperalimentation, or **total parenteral nutrition (TPN)** may be necessary. With TPN a solution of nutrients is administered directly into the bloodstream. It bypasses the digestive system.

When a person is unable to swallow, he or she may be fed through a tube. A **nasogastric tube** is inserted into the nose, past the throat, and down into the stomach. A tube can also be placed through the skin directly into the stomach. This is called a **percutaneous endoscopic gastrostomy (PEG) tube**. The opening in the stomach and abdomen is called a **gastrostomy** (Fig. 15-10). Tube feedings are used when residents cannot swallow but can digest food. Conditions that may prevent residents from swallowing include coma, cancer, stroke, refusal to eat, or extreme weakness. Remember that residents have to the right to refuse treatment, which includes insertion of tubes.

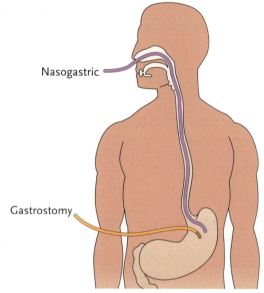

Fig. 15-10. *Nasogastric tubes are inserted through the nose, and PEG tubes are inserted through the skin directly into the stomach.*

Nursing assistants are not responsible for inserting tubes, doing the feeding, or cleaning the tubes. You may be assigned to take the person's temperature or assemble equipment and supplies and hand them to the nurse. You may need to position the resident. You may also discard or clean and store used equipment and supplies. In addition, you should observe, report, and document any observation of changes in the resident or problems with the feeding. Make sure the tubing is not coiled or kinked or resting underneath the resident.

Observing and Reporting: Tube Feedings

Report any of these to the nurse:

- Redness or drainage around the opening
- Skin sores or bruises
- Cyanotic skin
- Resident complaints of pain or nausea
- Choking
- Tube falls out
- Problems with equipment
- Feeding pump alarm sounds (report to the nurse immediately)

4. Describe factors that influence food preferences

Culture, ethnicity, income, education, religion, and geography all affect ideas about nutrition. Food preferences may be formed by what you ate as a child, by what tastes good, or by personal beliefs about what should be eaten (Fig. 15-11). Some people choose not to eat any animals or animal products, such as steak, chicken, butter, or eggs. These people are vegetarians or vegans.

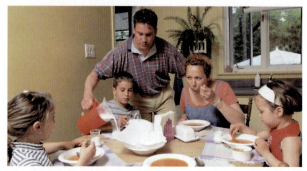

Fig. 15-11. *Food likes and dislikes are influenced by what you ate as a child.*

The region or culture you grow up in often influences your food preference. For example, people from the southwestern United States may like spicy foods. "Southern cooking" may include fried foods, like fried chicken or fried okra. Ethnic groups often share common foods. These may be eaten at certain times of the year or all the time. Religious beliefs affect diet, too. For example, some Muslims and Jewish people do not eat any pork. Mormons may not drink alcohol, tea, or coffee.

Food preferences may change while a resident is living at a facility. Just as you may decide that you like some foods for a time and then change your mind, so may residents. Whatever your residents' food preferences may be, respect them. Do not make fun of personal preferences. If you notice that certain food is not being eaten—no matter how small the amount—report it to the nurse.

Residents' Rights

Food Choices

Residents have the legal right to make choices about their food. They can choose what kind of food they want to eat and they can refuse the food and drink being offered. You must honor a resident's personal beliefs and preferences about selecting and avoiding specific foods. Although residents have the right to refuse, it is best to ask questions when they do. Communication is the key to understanding why a resident refuses something. For example, if a resident refuses his dinner, ask if there is something wrong with the food. He may tell you he is Jewish and cannot eat a pork chop because it's not kosher. Respond to requests for different food in a pleasant way. Explain that you will report to the nurse and will get him another meal as quickly as possible. Remove the tray and take it to the dietician or dietary department so that an alternative may be offered.

5. Explain the role of the dietary department

The dietary department is responsible for planning meals for all residents. Residents have different nutritional needs. When planning meals, the dietary department considers these needs,

along with individual likes and dislikes. Meals must be balanced to provide proper nutrition, and the food has to be prepared in a way that each resident can manage it. Food must also look appealing. The dietary department must follow strict infection prevention procedures when preparing food.

The dietary department also makes **diet cards** (Fig. 15-12). Diet cards list the resident's name and information about special diets, allergies, likes and dislikes, and other instructions.

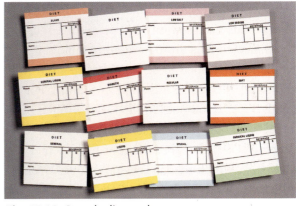

Fig. 15-12. Sample diet cards. (REPRINTED WITH PERMISSION OF BRIGGS CORPORATION, 800-247-2343, WWW.BRIGGSCORP.COM)

6. Explain special diets

A doctor sometimes places residents who are ill on special diets. These diets are known as **therapeutic**, **modified**, or **special diets**. Certain nutrients or fluids may be restricted or eliminated. Some medications may also interact with certain foods, which then must be restricted. Residents who do not eat enough may be placed on a special supplementary diet. Diets are also prescribed for weight control and food allergies. Several types of modified diets are available for different illnesses. Some residents may be on a combination of restricted diets. The care plan should specify any special diet the resident is on. It should also explain any eating problems that a resident may have and how the resident's eating habits can be improved (Fig. 15-13). Never modify a resident's diet yourself. Therapeutic diets can only be prescribed by doctors and planned by dietitians. Follow the resident's diet plan without making judgments. Report observations to the nurse. Examples of special diets are listed below.

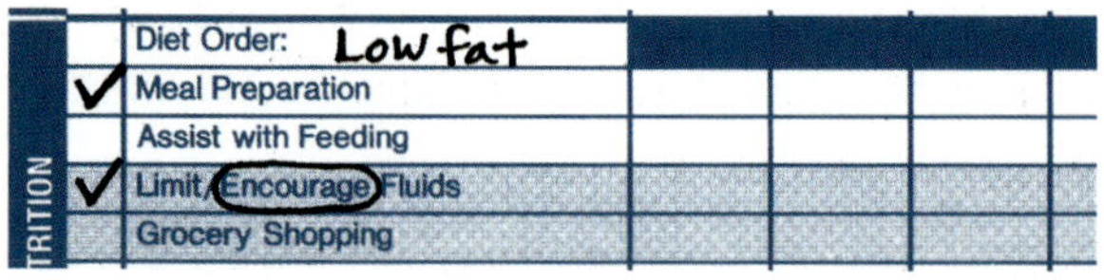

Fig. 15-13. *The care plan specifies special diets or dietary restrictions.*

Low-Sodium Diet: Residents with high blood pressure, heart disease, kidney disease, or fluid retention may be placed on a low-sodium diet. Many foods have sodium, but people are most familiar with it as an ingredient in table salt. Salt is the first food to be restricted in a low-sodium diet because it is high in sodium. For residents on a low-sodium diet, salt will not be used. Salt shakers or packets will not be on the diet tray. Common abbreviations for this diet are "Low Na," which means low sodium or "NAS," which stands for "No Added Salt."

Fluid-Restricted Diets: The fluid consumed through food and fluids must equal the fluid that leaves the body through perspiration, stool, urine, and expiration. This is **fluid balance**. When fluid intake is greater than fluid output, body tissues become swollen with fluid. In addition, people with severe heart disease and kidney disease may have trouble processing fluid. To prevent further damage, doctors may restrict fluid intake. For residents on fluid restriction, you will need to measure and document exact amounts of fluid intake and report excesses to the nurse. Do not offer additional fluids or foods that count as fluids, such as ice cream, puddings, gelatin, etc. If the resident complains of thirst or requests fluids, tell the nurse. A common abbreviation for this diet is "RF," which stands for "Restrict Fluids." You will learn more about intake and output later in this chapter.

High-Potassium Diets (K+): Some residents are on **diuretics**, which are medications that reduce fluid volume, or on blood pressure medications. These residents may be excreting so much fluid that their bodies could be depleted of potassium. Other residents may be placed on a high-potassium diet for different reasons.

Foods high in potassium include bananas, grapefruit, oranges, orange juice, prune juice, prunes, dried apricots, figs, raisins, dates, cantaloupes, tomatoes, potatoes with skins, sweet potatoes and yams, winter squash, legumes, avocados, and unsalted nuts. "K+" is the common abbreviation for this diet.

Low-Protein Diet: In addition to restricted intake of fluids, sodium, and potassium, people who have kidney disease may also be on low-protein diets. Protein is restricted because it breaks down into compounds that may further damage the kidneys. The extent of the restrictions depends on the stage of the disease and if the resident is on dialysis.

Exchange lists show foods that can be exchanged for one another on a meal plan. They are used extensively in special diets for people with diabetes. Exchange lists have also been developed for residents on diets modified for protein, potassium, and sodium.

Low-Fat/Low-Cholesterol Diet: People who have high levels of cholesterol in their blood are at risk for heart attacks and heart disease. People with gallbladder disease, diseases that interfere with fat digestion, and liver disease are also placed on low-fat/low-cholesterol diets.

Low-fat/low-cholesterol diets permit skim milk, low-fat cottage cheese, fish, white meat of turkey and chicken, veal, and vegetable fats (especially monounsaturated fats such as olive, canola, and peanut oils) (Fig. 16-26).

Residents may be advised to limit their diets in the following ways:

- Eat lean cuts of meat including lamb, beef, and pork, and eat these only three times a week.

- Limit egg yolks to three or four per week (including eggs used in baking).

- Avoid organ meats, shellfish, fatty meats, cream, butter, lard, meat drippings, coconut and palm oils, and desserts and soups made with whole milk.

- Avoid fried foods and sweets.

People who have gallbladder disease or other digestive problems may be placed on a diet that restricts all fats. A common abbreviation for this diet is "Low-Fat/Low-Chol."

Modified Calorie Diet: Some residents may need to reduce calories to lose weight or prevent weight gain. Other residents may need to increase calories because of malnutrition, surgery, illness, or fever. Residents with certain conditions need more protein to promote growth and repair of tissue and regulation of body functions. Common abbreviations for this diet are "Low-Cal" or "High-Cal."

Nutritional Supplements

Illness often causes residents to need extra nutrients, as well as additional calories. Sometimes a resident will be advised by his doctor or dietician to add a high-nutrition supplement to the regular or modified diet. Usually this is done to encourage weight gain or the intake of proteins, vitamins, or minerals.

Nutritional supplements may come in a powdered or liquid form. Supplements may be pre-mixed and ready to consume. Some powdered supplements need to be mixed with a liquid before being taken; the care plan will include instructions on how much liquid to add. When preparing supplements, make sure the supplement is mixed thoroughly.

Make sure the resident takes the supplement at the ordered time. Residents who are ill, tired, or in pain may not have much of an appetite. It may take a long time for him or her to drink a large glass of a thick liquid. Be patient and encouraging. If a resident does not want to drink the supplement, do not insist that he do so, but do report this to the nurse.

Bland Diet: Gastric and duodenal ulcers can be irritated by foods that produce or increase levels of acid in the stomach. People who have ulcers usually know the foods that cause them discomfort. Doctors will probably advise them to avoid these foods as well as the following: alcohol; beverages containing caffeine, such as coffee, tea, and soft drinks; citrus juices; spicy foods; and spicy seasonings such as black pepper, cayenne, and chili pepper. Three meals or more a day are usually advised. If alcohol is allowed, it should be drunk with meals.

Dietary Management of Diabetes. People with diabetes must be very careful about what they eat (Fig. 15-14). Calories and carbohydrates are carefully controlled in the diets of diabetic residents. Protein and fats are also regulated. The foods and the amounts are determined by nutritional and energy needs. A dietitian and the resident will make up a meal plan, taking into account the person's health status, activity levels, and lifestyle. It will include all the right types and amounts of food for each day. The resident uses exchange lists, or lists of similar foods that can substitute for one another, to make up a menu. Using meal plans and exchange lists, a person with diabetes can control his diet while still making food choices.

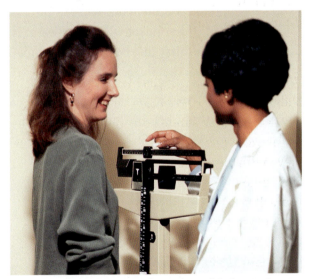

Fig. 15-14. *Diabetics must be very careful about what they eat. They should also keep their weight in a healthy range. Dietitians will help diabetics manage their illness.*

Sample Exchange List

Following the meal plan for how many servings of each type of food to eat, the person chooses specific foods and determines serving sizes using the exchange lists.

Exchange List Sample Items

Starch list: 1 slice of bread, ½ bagel, ½ cup cereal, ½ cup pasta, ½ cup rice, 1 baked potato, 3 cups popcorn, 15-20 fat-free potato chips

Milk list: 1 cup milk (skim, 1%, 2%, or whole, depending on other dietary guidelines), ¾ cup yogurt

Fruit list: ½ cup unsweetened applesauce, 1 small banana, ½ cup orange juice, 2 tablespoons raisins, 1 small orange, ½ cup canned pears

Vegetable list: ½ cup cooked vegetables or vegetable juice, 1 cup raw vegetables (not included are corn, potatoes, and peas, which are on the starch exchange list instead)

Meat list: 1 ounce meat, fish, poultry, or cheese, 1 egg, or ½ cup dried beans

Fat list: 1 teaspoon margarine or butter, 2 teaspoons peanut butter, 2 tablespoons sour cream, 1 teaspoon mayonnaise, 10 peanuts

To keep their blood glucose levels near normal, diabetic residents must eat the right amount of the right type of food at the right time. They must eat all that is served. Encourage them to do so. Do not offer other foods without the nurse's approval. If a resident will not eat what is directed, or if you think that he or she is not following the diet, tell the nurse.

Diabetics should avoid foods that are high in sugar, such as candy, because sugary foods can cause problems with insulin balance. Foods and drinks high in sugar include candy, ice cream, cakes, cookies, jellies, jams, fruits canned in heavy syrup, soft drinks, and alcoholic beverages. Many foods are high in sugar that do not appear to be so, such as canned vegetables, many breakfast cereals, and ketchup.

A diabetic's meal tray may have artificial sweetener, low-calorie jelly, and maple syrup. When serving coffee or tea to a diabetic resident, use artificial sweeteners rather than sugar. The common abbreviations for this diet on a diet card are "NCS," which stands for "No Concentrated Sweets" or the amount of calories followed by the abbreviation "ADA," which stands for American Diabetic Association. See Chapter 18 for more information on diabetes.

Low-Residue (Low-Fiber) Diet: This diet decreases the amount of fiber, whole grains, raw fruits and vegetables, seeds, and other foods, such as dairy and coffee. The low-residue diet is used for people with bowel disturbances.

High-Residue (High-Fiber) Diet: High-residue diets increase the intake of fiber and whole grains, such as whole grain cereals, bread, and raw fruits and vegetables. This diet helps with problems such as constipation and bowel disorders.

Diets may also be modified in consistency:

Liquid Diet: A liquid diet is usually ordered for a short time due to a medical condition or before or after a test or surgery. It is ordered when a resident needs to keep the intestinal tract free of food. A liquid diet consists of foods that are in a liquid state at body temperature. Liquid diets are usually ordered as "clear" or "full." A clear liquid diet includes clear juices, broth, gelatin, and popsicles. A full liquid diet includes all the liquids served on a clear liquid diet with the addition of cream soups, milk, and ice cream.

Soft Diet and Mechanical Soft Diet. The soft diet is soft in texture and consists of soft or chopped foods that are easier to chew and swallow. Foods that are hard to chew and swallow, such as raw fruits and vegetables and some meats, will be restricted. High-fiber foods, fried foods, and spicy foods may also be limited to help with digestion. Doctors order this diet for residents who have trouble chewing and swallowing due to dental problems or other medical conditions. It is also ordered for people who are making the transition from a liquid diet to a regular diet.

The mechanical soft diet consists of chopped or blended foods that are easier to chew and swallow. Foods are prepared with blenders, food processors, or cutting utensils. Unlike the soft diet, the mechanical soft diet does not limit spices, fat, and fiber. Only the texture of foods is changed. For example, meats and poultry can be ground and moistened with sauces or water to ease swallowing. This diet is used for people recovering from surgery or who have difficulty chewing and swallowing.

Pureed Diet: To **puree** a food means to chop, blend, or grind it into a thick paste of baby food consistency. The food should be thick enough to hold its form in the mouth. This diet does not require a person to chew his or her food. A pureed diet is often used for people who have trouble chewing and/or swallowing more tex- tured foods.

Some special diets are based on a person's reli- gious, moral, or other beliefs:

- Many Jewish people eat kosher foods. They do not eat pork or shellfish, and do not eat meat products at the same meal with dairy products. Kosher food is food prepared ac- cording to Jewish dietary laws.

- Many Muslims do not eat pork or shellfish. They may not drink alcohol. Muslims may have regular periods of fasting. Fasting means not eating food or eating very little food.

- Some Catholics do not eat meat on Fridays.

- Some people are vegetarians. **Vegetarians** do not eat meat, fish, or poultry. They may or may not eat eggs and dairy products. Vegans are vegetarians who do not eat or use any animal products, including milk, cheese, other dairy items, eggs, wool, silk, and leather. Reasons that a person may be a vegetarian include the following:

  - Health issues
  - Religious issues
  - Dislike of meat
  - Compassion for animals
  - Belief in non-violence
  - Financial issues

7. Explain thickened liquids and identify three basic thickened consistencies

Residents with swallowing problems may be restricted to consuming only thickened liquids. Thickening improves the ability to control fluid in the mouth and throat. A doctor orders the necessary thickness after the resident has been evaluated by a speech therapist.

Special products are used for thickening. Some beverages arrive already thickened from the dietary department. In other facilities, the thick- ening agent is added on the nursing unit before serving. If thickening is ordered, it must be used with all liquids. You need to know what thick- ened liquids mean. Do not offer these residents regular liquids. Do not offer water, water pitch- ers, or any beverages to a resident who must have thickened liquids. Follow the directions for each resident as ordered. Three basic thickened consistencies are:

1. **Nectar Thick**: This consistency is thicker than water. It is the thickness of a thick juice, such as a pear nectar or tomato juice. A resident can drink this from a cup.

2. **Honey Thick**: This consistency has the thick- ness of honey. It will pour very slowly. A resident will usually use a spoon to consume it.

3. **Pudding Thick**: With this consistency, the liquids have become semi-solid, much like pudding. A spoon should stand up straight in the glass when put into the middle of the drink. A resident must consume these liq- uids with a spoon.

8. Describe how to make dining enjoyable for residents

Mealtime is often an important part of a resi- dent's day. Not only is it the time for getting proper nourishment, but it is also a time for socializing, which has a positive effect on eating.

It can help prevent weight loss, dehydration, and malnutrition. It can also prevent loneliness and boredom.

Promoting healthy eating is an important part of your job. Mealtime should be a pleasant time. Use the following tips to help promote appetites and to make dining enjoyable:

Guidelines:
Promoting Appetites

G Check the environment. The temperature should be comfortable. Address any odors. Keep noise level low. Television sets should be off. Do not shout or raise your voice. Do not bang plates or cups. Some facilities play quiet music while residents are dining.

G Assist residents with grooming and hygiene tasks before dining, as needed.

G Help residents wash hands before eating.

G Give oral care before eating.

G Offer a trip to the bathroom or help with toileting before eating.

G Encourage the use of dentures, glasses, and hearing aids. If these are damaged, notify the nurse.

G Properly position residents for eating. Usually, the proper position is upright, at a 90-degree angle. This helps prevent swallowing problems. If residents use a wheelchair, make sure they are sitting at a table that is the right height. Most facilities have adjustable tables for wheelchairs. Residents who use "geri-chairs"—reclining chairs on wheels—should be upright, not reclined, while eating (Fig. 15-15).

G Seat residents next to their friends or people with like interests. Encourage conversation.

G Serve food at the correct temperature.

G Plates and trays should look appetizing.

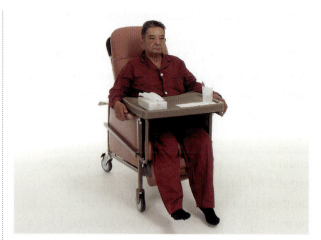

Fig. 15-15. *Residents should be positioned upright before eating. Residents seated in geriatric chairs, or geri-chairs, like the one shown here, also need to be sitting upright.*

G Give the resident proper eating tools. Use adaptive utensils if needed (Fig. 15-16).

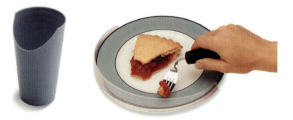

Fig. 15-16. *Cups with lids to avoid spills and utensils with thick handles that are easier to hold are two examples of adaptive devices that help with eating and drinking.*
(PHOTOS COURTESY OF NORTH COAST MEDICAL, INC., 800-821-9319, WWW.NCMEDICAL.COM)

G Be cheerful, positive, and helpful. Make conversation if the resident wishes.

G Give more food when requested.

9. Explain how to serve meal trays and assist with eating

Food may be served on trays or carried to residents from the kitchen. To make sure that food is served at the right temperature you will have to work quickly. You do not want to make residents wait for their food. Serve all residents who are sitting together at one table before serving another table. Residents will then be able to eat together and not have to watch others eat.

Before you begin serving or helping residents, wash your hands. As you learned earlier in this textbook, it is very important to identify residents before serving a meal tray. Feeding a resident the wrong food can cause serious problems, even death. Identify each resident before placing food in front of him or her.

Before you deliver trays or plates, check them closely. Make sure that you have the correct resident and the correct food and beverages for that person. Trays and plates should also be closely checked for added sugar and salt packets (Fig. 15-17). Be aware of residents who are on special diets. Watch for foods in residents' rooms or in the dining room that are not permitted by their doctors. Report any problems to the nurse.

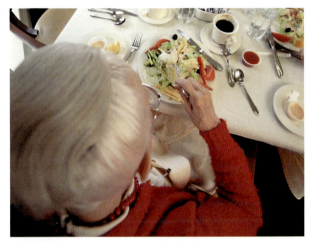

Fig. 15-17. *Observe residents' plates carefully to make sure they are receiving the correct food.*

Before helping a resident to eat, prepare the food by following these steps. Only do what the resident cannot do for himself.

- Remove the food and drink if it is on a tray and set it out on the table.

- Cut food into small, bite-sized portions. Only cut meat and vegetables when necessary. If you know residents need their food cut, cut it before bringing it to the table. This promotes dignity.

- Open milk or juice cartons. Open and insert a straw if the resident uses one. Place straws in the container using the paper wrapper;

do not touch them directly with your fingers. Some residents may not be able to use straws due to swallowing problems. This should be noted on their diet cards, and no straws should be on the tray. Residents may want you to pour the beverage into a cup. Do so if the resident wishes.

- Butter roll, bread, and vegetables as the resident likes.

- Open any condiment packets. Offer to season food as resident likes, including pureed food.

Residents will need different levels of help with eating. Some residents will not need any help. Other residents will only need help setting up; they may only need help opening cartons and cutting and seasoning their food. Once that is done, they can feed themselves. If this is the case, check in with these residents from time to time to see if they need anything else.

Other residents will be completely unable to feed themselves, and it will be your job to feed them. Residents who must be fed are often embarrassed and depressed about their dependence on another person. Be sensitive to this. Give privacy while the resident is eating. Do not rush him or her through the meal.

Only give assistance as specified, when necessary, or when the resident requests it. Encourage residents to do what they can. For example, if a resident can hold and use a napkin, she should. If she can hold and eat finger foods, offer them. There are devices that help residents eat more independently (see Fig. 15-16 on previous page). More adaptive devices are shown in Chapter 21.

Mealtime involves more than eating. It is a chance for social interaction. Residents look forward to their interaction with you and with others. It may be the highlight of their day. To avoid weight loss and dehydration, you must do all that you can to increase food and drink intake. Cheerful company and conversation can greatly increase how much a resident eats and drinks.

Fewer digestive problems may occur. They also have a positive effect on residents' attitudes. The reverse is also true. Negative attitudes and poor communication can decrease how much a resident consumes. Do not make negative comments, such as, "I don't know how you can eat this" or, "This looks awful." Do not judge a resident's food preferences.

Guidelines:
Assisting a Resident with Eating

G Never treat the resident like a child. This is embarrassing and disrespectful. It is hard for many people to accept help with feeding. Be supportive and encouraging.

G Sit at a resident's eye level. Resident should be sitting upright, at a 90-degree angle. Make eye contact with the resident.

G If the resident wishes, allow time for prayer.

G Verify that you have the right resident. Check the diet card against the resident's ID photo or bracelet. Ask the resident to state his name. Check that the diet on the tray is correct and matches the diet card.

G Test the temperature of the food by putting your hand over the dish to sense the heat. Do not touch food to test its temperature. If you think the food is too hot, do not blow on it to cool it. Offer other food to give it time to cool.

G Cut foods and pour liquids as needed.

G Identify the foods and fluids that are in front of the resident. Call pureed foods by the correct name. For example, ask, "Would you like green beans?" rather than referring to it as "some green stuff."

G Ask the resident which food he prefers to eat first. Allow him to make the choice, even if he wants to eat dessert first.

G Do not mix foods unless the resident requests it.

G Do not rush the meal. Allow time for the resident to chew and swallow each bite. Be relaxed.

G Be social and friendly. Make simple conversation if the resident wishes to do so (Fig. 15-18). Try not to ask questions that require long answers. Use appropriate topics, such as the news, weather, the resident's life, things the resident enjoys, and food preferences. Say positive things about the food being served, such as, "This smells really good," and, "The [type of food] looks so fresh."

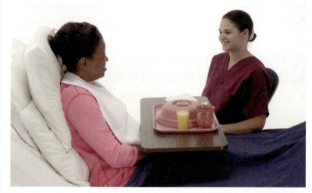

Fig. 15-18. Be friendly and social while helping residents with eating. Encourage them to do whatever they can for themselves.

G Give the resident your full attention while he or she is eating. Do not talk to other staff members while helping residents eat.

G Alternate offering food and drink. Alternating cold and hot foods or bland foods and sweets can help increase appetite.

G If the resident wants a different food from what is being served, inform the dietitian so that an alternative may be offered.

Residents' Rights

Clothing Protectors

Residents have the right to refuse to wear a clothing protector (Fig. 15-19). Offer a clothing protector, but do not insist that a resident wear one. Respect the resident's wishes. In addition, use the term "clothing protector" instead of "bib." This promotes residents' dignity and avoids treating them like children.

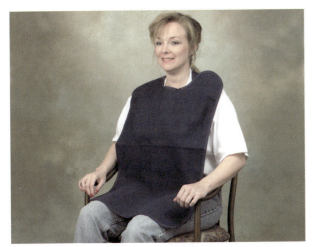

Fig. 15-19. *Residents have the right to choose whether or not to use a clothing protector. Respect each resident's decision.* (REPRINTED WITH PERMISSION OF BRIGGS CORPORATION, 800-247-2343, WWW.BRIGGSCORP.COM)

Feeding a resident who cannot feed self

Equipment: meal tray, clothing protector, 1-2 wash-cloths or wipes

1. Wash your hands.

2. Identify yourself by name. Identify the resident by name.

3. Explain procedure to the resident. Speak clearly, slowly, and directly. Maintain face-to-face contact whenever possible.

4. Pick up diet card and ask resident to state his or her name. Verify that resident has received the right tray.

5. Raise the head of the bed. Make sure resident is in an upright sitting position (at a 90-degree angle).

6. Adjust bed height to where you will be to able to sit at resident's eye level. Lock bed wheels.

7. Help resident to clean hands with hand wipes if resident cannot do it on her own.

8. Place meal tray where it can be easily seen by the resident, such as on the overbed table.

9. Help resident to put on clothing protector, if desired.

10. Sit facing resident at the resident's eye level (Fig. 15-20). Sit on the stronger side if the resident has one-sided weakness.

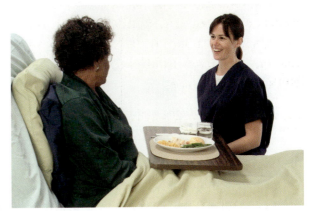

Fig. 15-20. *The resident should be sitting upright and you should be sitting at her eye level.*

11. Tell the resident what foods are on tray and ask what resident would like to eat first.

12. Offer the food in bite-sized pieces, telling the resident the content of each bite of food offered (Fig. 15-21). Alternate types of food, allowing for resident's preferences. Do not feed all of one type before offering another type. Report any swallowing problems to the nurse immediately.

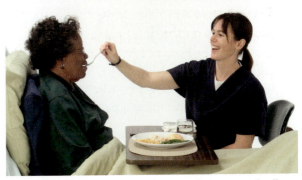

Fig. 15-21. *Offer the food in bite-sized pieces, and tell resident the content of each bite of food.*

13. Offer drink of beverage to resident throughout the meal.

14. Make sure resident's mouth is empty before next bite or sip.

15. Talk with resident during meal (Fig. 15-22).

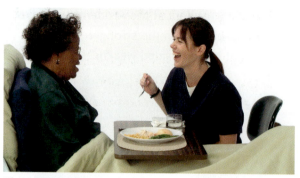

Fig. 15-22. Talking with the resident makes mealtime more enjoyable and helps promote appetite.

16. Use washcloths or wipes to wipe food from resident's mouth and hands as needed during the meal. Wipe again at the end of the meal (Fig. 15-23).

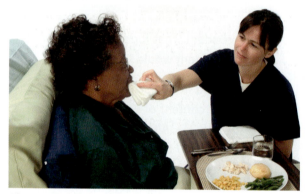

Fig. 15-23. Wiping food from the mouth during the meal helps to maintain the resident's dignity.

17. Remove clothing protector if used. Dispose of protector in proper container.

18. Remove food tray. Check for eyeglasses, dentures, or any personal items before removing tray. Place tray in proper area.

19. Make resident comfortable. Make sure sheets are free from wrinkles and the bed free from crumbs.

20. Return bed to lowest position. Remove privacy measures.

21. Place call light within resident's reach.

22. Wash your hands.

23. Report any changes in resident to the nurse.

24. Document procedure using facility guidelines.

Food trays and plates should also be observed after the meal. It is important to observe food trays and plates after a meal. This helps to identify residents with poor appetites. It may also signal illness, a problem, such as dentures that do not fit properly, or a change in food preferences.

10. Describe how to assist residents with special needs

Residents with specific diseases or conditions, such as stroke, Parkinson's disease, Alzheimer's disease or other dementias, head trauma, blindness, or confusion may need special assistance when eating. Follow these techniques for helping residents with special needs:

Guidelines:
Dining Techniques

G Residents with the diseases or conditions listed above may benefit from physical and verbal cues. The hand-over-hand approach is an example of physical cuing. If a resident can help lift the utensils, put your hand over his to help with eating. After the spoon is in the resident's hand, place your hand over the resident's hand. Help the resident in getting some food on the spoon. Steer the spoon from the food to the mouth and back. This promotes independence (Fig. 15-24).

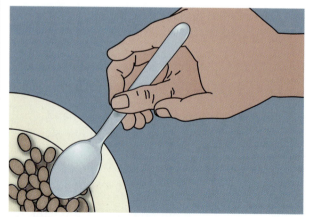

Fig. 15-24. The hand-over-hand approach is used when a resident can help by lifting utensils. It helps promote independence.

G Verbal cues must be short and clear and prompt the resident to do something. Give verbal cues one at a time. Wait until the resident has finished one task before asking him or her to do another. Examples of appropriate verbal cues include the following:

- "Pick up your spoon."
- "Put some carrots on your spoon."
- "Raise the spoon to your lips."
- "Open your mouth."
- "Place the spoon in your mouth."
- "Close your mouth."
- "Take the spoon out of your mouth."
- "Chew."
- "Swallow."
- "Drink some water."

G Use assistive devices such as utensils with built-up handle grips, plate guards, and drinking cups. These are ordered for specific residents and should be included on the meal tray.

G For visually-impaired residents, use the face of an imaginary clock to explain the position of what is in front of them (Fig. 15-25).

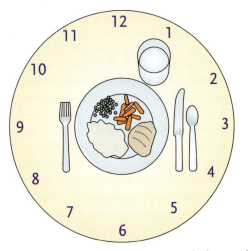

Fig. 15-25. Use the face of an imaginary clock to explain the position of food to visually-impaired residents.

G For residents who have had a stroke and have a paralyzed or weaker side, place food in the unaffected, or stronger, side of the mouth.

Make sure food is swallowed before offering another bite.

G If a resident has "blind spots," place food in the resident's field of vision (Fig. 15-26). The nurse will determine a resident's field of vision.

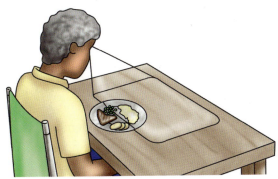

Fig. 15-26. A resident who has had a stroke may have a limited field of vision. The nurse will determine the resident's field of vision. Make sure the resident can see what you place in front of him.

G Tremors or shaking make it very difficult for a person to eat. For residents who have Parkinson's disease, tremors or shaking can make it very difficult to eat. Help by using physical cues. Place food and drinks close so that the resident can easily reach them. Use assistive devices as needed.

G If a resident has poor sitting balance, seat him or her in a regular dining room chair with armrests, rather than in a wheelchair. Proper position in chair means hips at a 90-degree angle, knees flexed, and feet and arms fully supported. Push the chair under the table. Place forearms on the table. If a resident tends to lean to one side, ask him or her to keep elbows on the table.

G If a resident has poor neck control, a neck brace may be used to stabilize the head. Use assistive devices as needed. If resident is in a geri-chair, a wedge cushion behind the head and shoulders may be used.

G If the resident bites down on utensils, ask him to open his mouth. Do not pull the utensil out of the mouth. Wait until the jaw relaxes.

Nutrition and Hydration

G If the resident pockets food in his cheeks, ask him to chew and swallow the food. Touch the side of his cheek. Ask him to use his tongue to get the food. Using your fingers on the cheek (near the lower jaw), gently push food toward teeth.

G If the resident holds food in his mouth, ask him to chew and swallow the food. You may need to trigger swallowing. To do this, gently press down on the tongue when taking the spoon out of the mouth. You can also try to gently press down on the top of his head with your hand. Make sure the resident has swallowed the food before offering more.

> **Residents' Rights**
>
> **Residents with Special Needs**
>
> Residents have the right to be treated with dignity and as adults. They have the right to self-determination. This means, in part, that they should be given the opportunity to choose and state their preferences for care and services. For example, a blind resident may want to feed herself without using utensils. This may not look dignified to others, but it is the resident's choice.

11. Define "dysphagia" and identify signs and symptoms of swallowing problems

Residents may have conditions that make eating or swallowing difficult. Dysphagia means difficulty in swallowing. A stroke, or CVA, can cause weakness on one side of the body and paralysis. Nerve and muscle damage from head and neck cancer, multiple sclerosis, Parkinson's or Alzheimer's disease may also be present. If a resident has difficulty swallowing, they will probably eat soft foods and drink thickened liquids. A straw or special cup will help make swallowing easier.

You need to be able to recognize and report signs that a resident has a swallowing problem.

If you notice any of the following signs and symptoms of swallowing problems, notify the nurse immediately:

- Coughing during or after meals
- Choking during meals
- Dribbling saliva, food, or fluid from the mouth
- Food residue inside the mouth or cheeks during and after meals
- Gurgling sound in voice during or after meals or loss of voice
- Slow eating
- Avoidance of eating
- Spitting out pieces of food
- Several swallows needed per mouthful
- Frequent throat clearing during and after meals
- Watering eyes when eating or drinking
- Food or fluid coming up into the nose
- Visible effort to swallow
- Shorter or more rapid breathing while eating or drinking
- Difficulty chewing food
- Difficulty swallowing medications

Swallowing problems put residents at high risk for choking on food or drink. Inhaling food or drink into the lungs is called aspiration. Aspiration can cause pneumonia or death. Alert the nurse immediately if any problems occur while feeding. Follow these guidelines to help prevent aspiration:

Guidelines:
Preventing Aspiration

G Position residents properly in a straight, upright position when eating or drinking. Do not try to feed residents in a reclining position.

G Offer small pieces or spoonfuls of food.

G Do not rush the eating process; feed the resident slowly.

G   Place food in the unaffected, or stronger, side of the mouth.

G   Make sure the resident has swallowed and that the mouth is empty before offering another bite of food or sip of drink.

G   If possible, keep residents in the upright position for about 30 minutes after eating and drinking.

12. Explain intake and output (I&O)

To maintain health, the body must take in a certain amount of fluid each day. Fluid comes in the form of liquids you drink and is also found in semi-liquid foods like gelatin, soup, ice cream, pudding, and yogurt. Generally, a healthy person needs to take in from 64 to 96 ounces (oz.) of fluid each day. The fluid a person consumes is called **intake**, or **input**. When a person's intake is not in a healthy range, he or she can become dehydrated. Dehydration is a serious medical condition that requires immediate attention. More information on dehydration is in the next learning objective.

All fluid taken in each day cannot remain in the body. It must be eliminated as **output**. Output includes urine, feces (including diarrhea), and vomitus. It also includes perspiration and moisture in the air we exhale. If a person's intake exceeds his or her output, fluid builds up in body tissues. This fluid retention can cause medical problems and discomfort.

Fluid balance is maintaining equal input and output, or taking in and eliminating equal amounts of fluid. Most people do this naturally. But some residents must have their intake and output, or I&O, monitored and recorded. To do this, you will need to measure and document all fluids the resident takes by mouth, as well as all urine and vomitus the resident produces. This is recorded on an Intake/Output (I&O) sheet (Fig. 15-27).

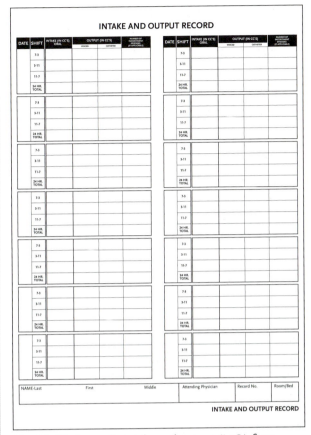

Fig. 15-27. *A sample intake and output (I&O) form.*

Fluids are usually measured in milliliters (mL or ml). Ounces (oz.) are often converted to milliliters. To convert ounces to milliliters, multiply by 30. For example, you serve Mrs. Wyant a glass of milk. You know the glass holds six ounces. She finishes most but not all of the milk. You guess that she drank four ounces. What was her input? To convert ounces to milliliters, multiply four by 30. The answer is 120 milliliters (mL or ml). You would document "120 mL milk" on your input sheet.

Conversions

A milliliter (mL or ml) is a unit of measure equal to one cubic centimeter (cc). Follow your facility's policies on whether to document using "mL" or "cc".

1 oz. = 30 mL or 30 cc

2 oz. = 60 mL

3 oz. = 90 mL

4 oz. = 120 mL	
5 oz. = 150 mL	
6 oz. = 180 mL	
7 oz. = 210 mL	
8 oz. = 240 mL	
¼ cup = 2 oz. = 60 mL	
½ cup = 4 oz. = 120 mL	
1 cup = 8 oz. = 240 mL	

Before beginning, explain to the resident that you need to keep track of his intake. Ask the resident to let you know when he drinks something (if it is not something you served to him) and how much it was.

Measuring and recording intake and output

Monitoring fluid balance begins with measuring intake.

Equipment: I&O sheet, graduate (measuring container) (Fig. 15-28), pen and paper to record your findings

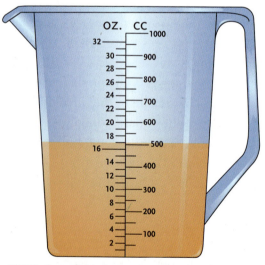

Fig. 15-28. *A graduate is a measuring container.*

1. Wash your hands.

2. Identify yourself by name. Identify the resident by name.

3. Explain procedure to the resident. Speak clearly, slowly, and directly. Maintain face-to-face contact whenever possible.

4. Provide for resident's privacy with curtain, screen, or door.

5. Using the graduate, measure how much fluid a resident is served. Note the amount on paper.

6. When resident has finished a meal or snack, measure any leftover fluids. Note this amount on paper.

7. Subtract the leftover amount from the amount served. If you have measured in ounces, convert to milliliters (mL) by multiplying by 30.

8. Document amount of fluid consumed (in mL) in input column on I&O sheet. Record the time and what fluid was taken. Report anything unusual that was observed, such as the resident refusing to drink, drinking very little, feeling nauseated, etc.

9. Wash your hands.

Measuring output is the other half of monitoring fluid balance.

Equipment: I&O sheet, graduate, gloves, pen and paper

1. Wash your hands.

2. Put on gloves before handling bedpan/urinal.

3. Pour the contents of the bedpan or urinal into measuring container. Do not spill or splash any of the urine.

4. Measure the amount of urine. Keep container level (Fig. 15-29).

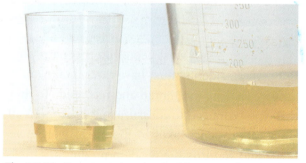

Fig. 15-29. *Keep container level while measuring output.*

5. After measuring urine, empty measuring container into toilet. Do not splash.

6. Rinse measuring container and pour rinse water into toilet. Clean container using facility guidelines.

7. Rinse bedpan/urinal. Pour rinse water into toilet. Use approved disinfectant.

8. Return bedpan/urinal and measuring container to proper storage.

9. Remove and dispose of gloves.

10. Wash hands before recording output.

11. Document the time and amount of urine in output column on sheet. For example: 3:45 p.m. 200 mL urine. To measure vomitus, pour from basin into measuring container, then discard in the toilet. If resident vomits on the bed or floor, estimate the amount. Document emesis and amount on the I&O sheet.

12. Report any changes in resident to the nurse.

All facilities keep track of how much food and liquid a resident consumes. The method varies. Some facilities use a percentage method, for example: "R" Refused = 0% No food eaten; "P" Poor = 25% Very little food eaten; "F" Fair = 50% Half of the food eaten; "G" Good = 75% Most of the food eaten; and "A" All = 100% Entire meal eaten.

Other facilities may document the percentage of specific foods eaten—protein, carbohydrates, fats, etc. Your instructor will explain your facility's documentation. Follow your facility's policy and document food intake very carefully and accurately. Report to the charge nurse if a resident eats less than 70% of his or her meal.

13. Identify ways to assist residents in maintaining fluid balance

Most residents should be encouraged to drink at least 64 ounces, or eight glasses, of water or other fluids a day. Remember that water is essential for life. Proper fluid intake is important.

It helps prevent constipation and urinary incontinence. Without enough fluid, urine becomes concentrated. More concentrated urine creates a higher risk for infection. Proper fluid intake also helps to dilute wastes and flush out the urinary system. It may even help prevent confusion.

The sense of thirst can lessen as people age. Infection, fever, diarrhea, and some medications will also increase the need for fluid intake. Remind elderly residents to drink fluids often (Fig. 15-30). However, some residents will have an order to force fluids (FF) or restrict fluids (RF) because of medical conditions. **Force fluids** means to encourage the resident to drink more fluids. **Restrict fluids** means the person is allowed to drink, but must limit the daily amount to a level set by the doctor. When a resident has a restrict fluids order, you cannot give the resident any extra fluids or a water pitcher unless the nurse approves it. Make sure you know which residents have these orders.

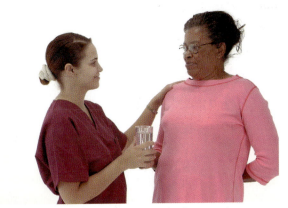

Fig. 15-30. *Encourage residents to drink every time you see them.*

The abbreviation "NPO " stands for "Nothing by Mouth." This means that a resident is not allowed to have anything to eat or drink. Some residents have such a severe problem with swallowing that it is unsafe to give them anything by mouth. These types of residents will receive nutrition through a feeding tube or intravenously. Some residents may be NPO for a short time before a medical test or surgery. You need to know this abbreviation. Never offer any food or drink to a resident with this order, not even water.

Dehydration occurs when a person does not have enough fluid in the body. Dehydration is a serious condition and is a major problem among the elderly. People can become dehydrated if they do not drink enough or if they have diarrhea or are vomiting. Preventing dehydration is very important.

Observing and Reporting:
Dehydration

Report any of the following immediately:

O/R Resident drinks less than six 8-ounce glasses of liquid per day

O/R Resident drinks little or no fluids at meals

O/R Resident needs help drinking from a cup or glass

O/R Resident has trouble swallowing liquids

O/R Resident has frequent vomiting, diarrhea, or fever

O/R Resident is easily confused or tired

Report if resident has any of the following:

O/R Dry mouth

O/R Cracked lips

O/R Sunken eyes

O/R Dark urine

O/R Strong-smelling urine

O/R Weight loss

Guidelines:
Preventing Dehydration

G Report observations and warning signs to the nurse immediately.

G Encourage residents to drink every time you see them.

G Offer fresh water or other fluids often. Be aware that residents have different preferences. Some may not like water and prefer other types of beverages, such as juice, soda, tea, or milk. Report to the nurse if the resident tells you he does not like the fluids being served. Offer drinks that the resident enjoys. Some residents do not want ice in their drinks. Honor this preference.

G Record fluid intake and output.

G Ice chips, frozen flavored ice sticks, and gelatin are also forms of liquids. Offer them often. Do not offer ice chips or sticks if a resident has a swallowing problem.

G If appropriate, offer sips of liquid between bites of food at meals and snacks.

G Make sure pitcher and cup are near enough and light enough for the resident to lift (Fig. 15-31).

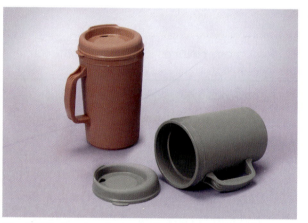

Fig. 15-31. *Insulated cups and pitchers can help keep drinks cold or warm, depending on the drink and the resident's preference. However, as with all glasses and cups, they must be light enough for the resident to be able to lift them.* (REPRINTED WITH PERMISSION OF BRIGGS CORPORATION, 800-247-2343, WWW.BRIGGSCORP.COM)

G Offer assistance if resident cannot drink without help. Use adaptive cups as needed.

Serving fresh water

Equipment: water pitcher, ice scoop, glass, straw, gloves

1. Wash your hands.

2. Identify yourself by name. Identify the resident by name.

3. Put on gloves.

4. Scoop ice into water pitcher. Add fresh water.

5. Use and store ice scoop properly. Do not allow ice to touch your hand and fall back into container. Place scoop in proper receptacle after each use.

6. Take pitcher to resident.

7. Pour glass of water for resident. Leave pitcher and glass at the bedside.

8. Make sure that pitcher and glass are light enough for resident to lift. Leave a straw if the resident desires.

9. Place call light within resident's reach.

10. Remove gloves.

11. Wash your hands.

Residents' Rights

Fluid Intake

As you have learned, offering fresh fluids often helps prevent dehydration, and helps keep residents healthy. Encourage, but do not force, fluids. Ask residents which beverages they prefer and arrange for those to be available. Respond to drink requests from residents, unless there is a doctor's order restricting fluid intake. If this is the case, inform the resident about the order, and report the request to the nurse. If fluid intake is increased, offer additional trips to the bathroom and promote privacy. If urine is being measured, do it with the door closed.

Fluid overload occurs when the body cannot handle the amount of fluid consumed. This condition often affects people with heart or kidney disease.

Observing and Reporting:
Fluid Overload

Report any of the following to the nurse:

O/R Swelling/edema of extremities (ankles, feet, fingers, hands); **edema** is swelling caused by excess fluid in body tissues

O/R Weight gain (daily weight gain of one to two pounds)

O/R Decreased urine output

O/R Shortness of breath

O/R Increased heart rate

O/R Skin that appears tight, smooth, and shiny

Chapter Review

1. How does a well-balanced diet help the ill and the elderly?

2. List the six basic nutrients and identify which nutrient is the most essential for life.

3. Identify what each of the six colored bands of MyPyramid stand for. Which color band is the smallest and why?

4. How much activity per day does MyPyramid recommend?

5. How can vegetarians fulfill requirements of the meat and beans group?

6. List four problems that may affect an elderly person's nutritional intake.

7. Why is it important for an NA to report any weight loss, no matter how small?

8. Describe ten ways that an NA can help prevent unintended weight loss.

9. What are two ways a resident may be fed if he has a digestive system that does not function properly or he cannot swallow?

10. List three factors that influence food preferences.

11. What information do diet cards contain?

12. What is the first food to be restricted in a low-sodium diet?

13. Why might a resident be placed on a low-fat/low-cholesterol diet?

14. List four things that are carefully regulated in a diabetic diet.

15. What is the difference between a clear liquid diet and a full liquid diet?

16. How is the mechanical soft diet different from the soft diet?

17. List five reasons that a person may choose to be a vegetarian.

18. How can thickened liquids help a person with swallowing problems?

19. In addition to eating, what does mealtime involve?

20. How should a resident be positioned for eating?

21. How can being cheerful and positive while a resident eats affect the amount of food consumed?

22. How can a nursing assistant verify that she has the correct resident for the meal tray that she is serving?

23. How should a nursing assistant test the temperature of food?

24. Give two examples of appropriate topics for a nursing assistant to discuss with a resident during mealtime.

25. What should the nursing assistant do if a resident wants a different food from what is being served?

26. Should a nursing assistant insist that a resident wear a clothing protector if he does not want to wear one? Why or why not?

27. When feeding a resident, how should the bed height be adjusted?

28. How does giving verbal cues assist a resident with eating?

29. When assisting a resident who is visually-impaired, how should the nursing assistant explain the position of food and objects in front of the resident?

30. To which side of the mouth should food be directed if a resident has a weaker side—the weaker (affected) or stronger (unaffected) side?

31. What is the medical term that means "difficulty in swallowing?"

32. List 12 signs and symptoms of swallowing problems that should be reported to the nurse.

33. Describe five ways to help prevent aspiration.

34. How many ounces of fluid does a healthy person need each day?

35. What is fluid balance?

36. How many milliliters (mL) equal one ounce (oz.)?

37. What counts as output?

38. What does the abbreviation "NPO" stand for? What does it mean for a resident?

39. List five signs that a nursing assistant should report immediately about dehydration.

40. Describe six ways that a nursing assistant can help prevent dehydration.

41. List four signs that a nursing assistant should report about fluid overload.

16

Urinary Elimination

1. List qualities of urine and identify signs and symptoms about urine to report

Urination, also known as micturition or voiding, is the act of passing urine from the bladder through the urethra to the outside of the body. Urine is made up of water and waste products filtered from the blood by the kidneys. Normal urine output varies with age and the amount and type of liquids consumed. Adults should produce about 1200 to 1500 mL of urine per day, although elderly adults may produce less.

Urine is normally pale yellow to amber in color (Fig. 16-1). However, there are many factors that can cause urine to be an abnormal color, such as medications, certain foods or food dyes, and vitamins and supplements. For example, beets can make urine appear pink or red, and B vitamins can make urine very bright yellow. Unusual urine color can also be a sign of illness.

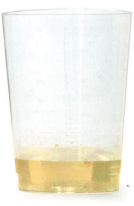

Fig. 16-1. *Urine is normally light or pale yellow in color. It should be clear, not cloudy.*

Normal urine should be clear or transparent when freshly voided and should have a faint smell. Urine that is cloudy or murky or that smells bad or fruity can be a sign of infection or illness. If you observe these signs, report to the nurse right away.

Observing and Reporting:
Urine

Report any of these to the nurse:

- O/R Cloudy urine

- O/R Dark or rust-colored urine

- O/R Strong-, offensive-, or fruity-smelling urine

- O/R Pain, burning, or pressure when urinating

- O/R Blood, pus, mucus, or discharge in urine

- O/R Protein or glucose in urine (you will learn more about these things later in the chapter)

- O/R Urinary incontinence (the inability to control the bladder, which leads to an involuntary loss of urine)

2. List factors affecting urination and demonstrate how to assist with elimination

There are many factors that can affect normal urination, including the following:

Normal changes of aging: The ability of the kidneys to filter blood decreases. The bladder muscle tone weakens. The bladder is not able to hold the same amount of urine as it did when people were younger. Elderly people may need to urinate more frequently. Many awaken several times during the night to urinate. The bladder may not empty completely, causing susceptibility to infection.

To help promote normal urination, offer frequent trips to the bathroom or bedpans and urinals. The best position for women to have normal urination is sitting. For men, it is standing. Avoid the supine (lying on the back) position if possible because in this position, a person cannot put pressure on the bladder. This works against gravity. Follow a toileting schedule for residents if there is one.

Assist with perineal care, when necessary. Promote proper hygiene to help prevent infection; always wipe from front to back. Help resident to wash hands after urinating.

Psychological factors: A lack of privacy, new environments, stress, anxiety, and depression can all affect urination. To promote normal urination, it is very important to provide plenty of privacy for elimination. Close the bathroom door if residents are in the bathroom. If the resident needs to use a bedpan or urinal, pull the privacy curtain and close the door. Do not rush or interrupt residents when they are in the bathroom. Report signs of depression and anxiety (Chapter 20), as well as any changes in output.

Fluid intake: As you learned in the last chapter, the sense of thirst lessens as a person ages. When a person drinks fewer fluids, urinary output decreases, and dehydration may result. Some beverages, such as those containing alcohol and caffeine, increase urine output.

To promote normal urination, encourage residents to drink fluids often. Remember that a healthy person needs to take in from 64 to 96 ounces of fluid each day (Fig. 16-2). Provide fresh water and juices often. Beverages that are high in vitamin C are especially good for pre-

venting urinary tract infections. Follow any fluid restrictions.

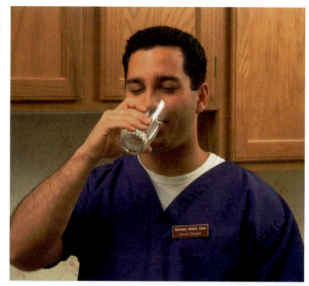

Fig. 16-2. *Drinking plenty of fluids is important to promoting a healthy urinary system.*

Medications: Medications can affect urinary output. For example, a resident who is taking diuretics (medications that reduce fluid in the body) will frequently need to urinate. To promote normal urination, offer a trip to the bathroom, or a bedpan or urinal often. Encourage fluid intake. Report any changes in output or discoloration of urine to the nurse.

Disorders: Many disorders and illnesses affect urination, such as bladder disease, infections, arthritis, congestive heart disease, neurological diseases, and diabetes. You will learn more about these diseases in Chapter 18.

Assisting with Elimination

Residents who cannot get out of bed to go to the bathroom may be given a bedpan, a fracture pan, or a urinal. A **fracture pan** is a bedpan that is flatter than the regular bedpan. It is used for residents who cannot assist with raising their hips onto a regular bedpan (Fig. 16-3). Women will generally use a bedpan for urination and bowel movements. Men will generally use a urinal for urination and a bedpan for a bowel movement (Fig. 16-4).

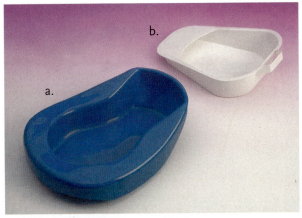

Fig. 16-3. *a) Standard pan and b) fracture pan.*

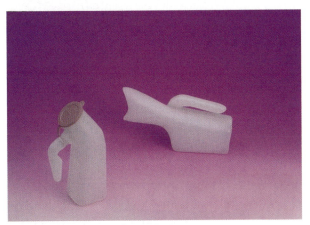

Fig. 16-4. *Two types of urinals.*

Elimination equipment should be rinsed with a facility-approved disinfectant after each use. It is usually kept in the bathroom between uses. Residents who share bathrooms may need to have urinals and bedpans labeled. Follow your facility's policy for storage. Never place this equipment on an overbed table or on top of a side table.

Some residents are able to get out of bed, but may still need help walking to the bathroom and using the toilet. Others who are able to get out of bed but cannot walk to the bathroom may use a portable commode. A **portable commode** is a chair with a toilet seat and a removable container underneath (Fig. 16-5). Toilets can be fitted with raised seats to make it easier for residents to get up and down (Fig. 16-6). Hand rails can also be installed next to the toilet. Observe and report if these assistive devices are needed but not present. When residents need assistance

to get to the bathroom or use the commode, offer to help often. This can avoid accidents and embarrassment.

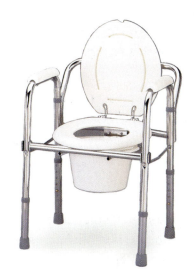

Fig. 16-5. *A portable commode.* (PHOTO COURTESY OF NOVA ORTHO MED, INC.)

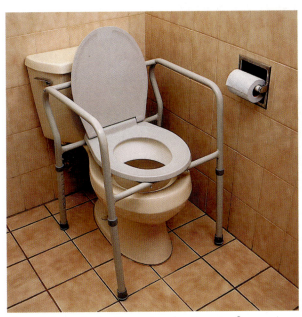

Fig. 16-6. *A raised toilet seat makes it easier for a resident to get up and down.* (PHOTO COURTESY OF NORTH COAST MEDICAL, INC., WWW.NCMEDICAL.COM, 800-821-9319)

Wastes such as urine and feces can carry infection. Always dispose of wastes in the toilet, and be careful not to spill or splash the wastes. Always wear gloves when handling bedpans, urinals, or basins that contain wastes, including dirty bath water. Wash these containers thoroughly with an approved disinfectant. Rinse and dry them and return them to storage.

Rights with Elimination

Residents have the right to privacy and to be treated with dignity. Remember that residents may be embarrassed about needing assistance with bodily functions. Always be professional when giving assistance. Provide as much privacy as possible.

Treat residents as adults. Be aware of the language you use when assisting with toileting needs. Do not use childish words. Use the proper terms for bodily functions. Although it is important that the resident understand the words that are used, some non-medical words for bodily functions sound crude and unprofessional.

Assisting a resident with the use of a bedpan

Equipment: bedpan, bedpan cover, protective pad or sheet, bath blanket, toilet paper, disposable washcloths or wipes, soap, towel, 2 pairs of gloves

1. Wash your hands.

2. Identify yourself by name. Identify the resident by name.

3. Explain procedure to the resident. Speak clearly, slowly, and directly. Maintain face-to-face contact whenever possible.

4. Provide for resident's privacy with curtain, screen, or door.

5. Adjust bed to a safe working level, usually waist high. Before placing bedpan, lower the head of the bed. Lock bed wheels.

6. Put on gloves.

7. Cover the resident with the bath blanket. Ask him to hold it while you pull down the top covers underneath. Do not expose more of the resident than you have to.

8. Place a protective pad under the resident's buttocks and hips. To do this, have the resident roll toward you. If the resident cannot do this, you must turn the resident toward you (see Chapter 10). Be sure resident cannot roll off the bed. Move to the empty side of bed. Place the protective pad on the area

where the resident will lie on his back. The side of protective pad nearest the resident should be fanfolded (folded several times into pleats) (Fig. 16-7).

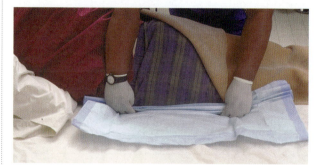

Fig. 16-7. Fanfold the bed protector near the resident's back.

Ask the resident to roll onto his back, or roll him as you did before. Unfold the rest of protective pad so it completely covers the area under and around the resident's hips. (Fig. 16-8)

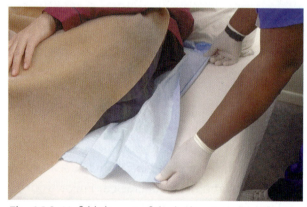

Fig. 16-8. Unfold the rest of the bed protector so it completely covers area under and around the resident's hips.

9. Ask the resident to remove undergarments or help him do so.

10. Place bedpan near his hips in the correct position. **Standard bedpan** should be positioned with the wider end aligned with the resident's buttocks. **Fracture pan** should be positioned with handle toward foot of bed.

11. If resident is able, ask him to raise hips by pushing with feet and hands at the count of three (Fig. 16-9). Slide the bedpan under his hips.

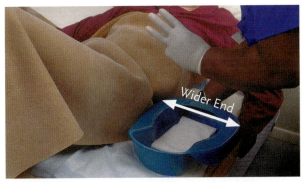

Fig. 16-9. On the count of three, slide the bedpan under the resident's hips. The wider end of bedpan should be aligned with the resident's buttocks.

If the resident cannot do this himself, place your arm under the small of his back and tell him to push with his heels and hands on your signal as you raise his hips (Fig. 16-10). Place the bedpan underneath the resident.

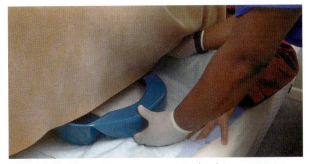

Fig. 16-10. If a resident cannot raise his hips, you can raise his hips while he pushes with his heels and hands.

If a resident cannot help you in any way, keep the bed flat and roll the resident onto the far side. Slip the bedpan under the hips and gently roll the resident back onto the bedpan, keeping the bedpan centered underneath.

12. Remove and discard gloves. Wash your hands.

13. Raise the head of the bed. Prop the resident into a semi-sitting position using pillows.

14. Check the bedpan to be certain it is in the correct position. Make sure the blanket is still covering the resident. Place toilet tissue and washcloths or wipes within resident's reach. Ask resident to clean his hands with the hand wipe when finished, if he is able.

15. Place the call light within resident's reach. Ask resident to signal when done. Leave the room.

16. When called by the resident, return and put on clean gloves.

17. Lower the head of the bed. Make sure resident is still covered. Do not overexpose the resident.

18. Remove bedpan carefully and cover bedpan.

19. Provide perineal care if assistance is needed. For female residents, wipe from the front to the back. Dry the perineal area with a towel. Help the resident put on undergarment. Place the towel in a hamper or bag, and discard disposable supplies.

20. Take bedpan to the bathroom. Empty the bedpan carefully into the toilet unless a specimen is needed. Note color, odor, and consistency of contents before flushing. If you notice anything unusual about the stool or urine (for example, the presence of blood), do not discard it. You will need to inform the nurse.

21. Turn the faucet on with a paper towel. Rinse the bedpan with cold water first and empty it into the toilet. Place bedpan in proper area for cleaning or clean it according to facility policy.

22. Remove and discard gloves.

23. Wash your hands.

24. Make resident comfortable. Remove bath blanket and cover resident.

25. Return bed to lowest position. Remove privacy measures.

26. Place call light within resident's reach.

27. Report any changes in resident to the nurse.

28. Document procedure using facility guidelines.

Assisting a male resident with a urinal

Equipment: urinal, protective pad or sheet, wash-cloths or wipes, 2 pairs of gloves

1. Wash your hands.

2. Identify yourself by name. Identify the resident by name.

3. Explain procedure to the resident. Speak clearly, slowly, and directly. Maintain face-to-face contact whenever possible.

4. Provide for resident's privacy with curtain, screen, or door.

5. Adjust bed to a safe working level, usually waist high. Lock bed wheels.

6. Put on gloves.

7. Place a protective pad under the resident's buttocks and hips, as in earlier procedure.

8. Hand the urinal to the resident. If the resident is not able to help himself, place urinal between his legs and position penis inside the urinal (Fig. 16-11). Replace covers.

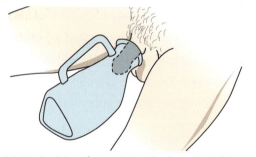

Fig. 16-11. *Position the penis inside the urinal if the resident cannot do it himself.*

9. Remove and discard gloves. Wash your hands.

10. Place wipes within resident's reach. Ask the resident to clean his hands with the hand wipe when finished, if he is able. Leave call light within reach while resident is using urinal. Ask resident to signal when done. Leave the room.

11. When called by the resident, return and put on clean gloves.

12. Remove urinal or have resident hand it to you. Empty contents into toilet unless specimen is needed or the urine is being measured for intake/output monitoring. Note color, odor, and qualities (for example, cloudiness) of contents before flushing.

13. Turn the faucet on with a paper towel. Rinse the urinal with cold water first and empty it into the toilet. Place urinal in proper area for cleaning or clean it according to facility policy.

14. Remove and discard gloves.

15. Wash your hands.

16. Make resident comfortable.

17. Return bed to lowest position. Remove privacy measures.

18. Place call light within resident's reach.

19. Report any changes in resident to the nurse.

20. Document procedure using facility guidelines.

Assisting a resident to use a portable commode or toilet

Equipment: portable commode with basin, toilet paper, washcloths or wipes, gloves

1. Wash your hands.

2. Identify yourself by name. Identify the resident by name.

3. Explain procedure to the resident. Speak clearly, slowly, and directly. Maintain face-to-face contact whenever possible.

4. Provide for resident's privacy with curtain, screen, or door.

5. Help resident out of bed and to the portable commode or bathroom. Make sure resident is wearing non-skid shoes and that the laces are tied.

6. If needed, help resident remove clothing and sit comfortably on toilet seat. Put toilet tissue within reach.

7. Provide privacy. Leave call light within reach while resident is using commode. Ask resident to signal when done. Leave the room.

8. When called by resident, return and apply gloves.

9. Give perineal care if help is needed. Wipe female residents from front to back.

10. Help resident to wash hands after using commode. Dispose of soiled washcloth or wipes properly.

11. Help resident back to bed. Make resident comfortable. Make sure sheets are free from wrinkles and the bed free from crumbs.

12. Remove waste container. Empty into toilet. Note color, odor, and consistency of contents.

13. Rinse container. Pour rinse water into toilet. Place container in proper area for cleaning or clean it according to facility policy.

14. Remove and dispose of gloves properly.

15. Wash your hands.

16. Return bed to lowest position. Remove privacy measures.

17. Place call light within resident's reach.

18. Report any changes in resident to the nurse.

19. Document procedure using facility guidelines.

3. Describe common diseases and disorders of the urinary system

Urinary Incontinence

When people cannot control the muscles of the bowels or bladder, they are said to be incontinent. Urinary incontinence is the inability to control the bladder, which leads to an involuntary loss of urine. Incontinence can occur in residents who are confined to bed, ill, elderly, paralyzed, or who have circulatory or nervous system diseases or injuries. There are different types of incontinence, including the following:

- Stress incontinence is the loss of urine due to an increase in intra-abdominal pressure, for example, when sneezing, laughing, or coughing.

- Urge incontinence is involuntary voiding from an abrupt urge to void.

- Mixed incontinence is a combination of both urge incontinence and stress incontinence.

- Functional incontinence is urine loss caused by things outside the urinary tract.

- Overflow incontinence is loss of urine due to overflow or over-distention of the bladder.

Incontinence is *not* a normal part of aging. Always report incontinence. It may be a sign or symptom of an illness. Urinary incontinence is a major risk factor for pressure sores. Cleanliness and good skin care are important for residents who are incontinent. Keep residents clean and dry. In addition, follow these guidelines:

Guidelines:
Urinary Incontinence

G Offer a bedpan, urinal, commode or trip to the bathroom often.

G Follow toileting schedules.

G Answer call lights and requests for assistance immediately.

G Rules for documenting incontinence have changed. The Minimum Data Set (MDS) counts any time a resident's skin or anything touching a resident's skin (pad, brief, or underwear) is wet from urine as an episode of incontinence. This is true even if it is a small amount of urine. This is important to help prevent pressure sores. Document carefully and accurately.

G   Urine is very irritating to the skin. It should be washed off immediately and completely. Keep residents clean, dry, and free from odor. Observe the skin carefully when bathing and giving perineal care.

G   Incontinent residents who are bedbound should have a plastic, latex, or disposable sheet placed under them to protect the bed. Place a draw sheet over it to absorb moisture and protect the skin.

G   Disposable incontinence pads or briefs for adults are available. They keep body wastes away from the skin (Fig. 16-12). Change wet briefs immediately. Never refer to an incontinence brief or pad as a "diaper." Residents are not children. This is disrespectful.

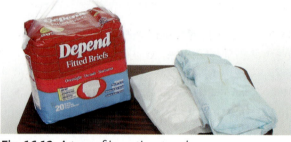

Fig. 16-12. A type of incontinent pad.

G   Residents who are incontinent need reassurance and understanding. Be professional and kind when dealing with incontinence.

Providing perineal care for an incontinent resident

Equipment: 2 clean protective pads, 4 washcloths or wipes, 1 towel, gloves, basin with warm water, soap, bath blanket, bath thermometer

1. Wash your hands.

2. Identify yourself by name. Identify the resident by name.

3. Explain procedure to the resident. Speak clearly, slowly, and directly. Maintain face-to-face contact whenever possible.

4. Provide for resident's privacy with curtain, screen, or door.

5. Adjust bed to a safe level, usually waist high. Lock bed wheels.

6. Lower head of the bed. Position resident lying flat on his or her back.

7. Test water temperature with thermometer or your wrist to ensure safety. Water temperature should be 105°F. Have resident check water temperature. Adjust if necessary.

8. Put on gloves.

9. Cover resident with bath blanket. Move top linens to foot of bed.

10. Remove soiled protective pad from under resident by turning resident on his side, away from you. (See procedure "Turning a resident" in Chapter 10.) Roll soiled pad into itself with wet side in/dry side out.

11. Place clean protective pad under his or her buttocks.

12. Return resident to lying on his back.

13. Expose perineal area only; avoid overexposure of the resident. Clean the perineal area.

    For a female resident: Wash the perineum with soap and water from **front to back**. Use single strokes (Fig. 16-13). Do not wash from the back to the front. This may cause infection. Use a clean area of washcloth or clean washcloth for each stroke. First wipe the center of the perineum, then each side. Spread the labia majora, the outside folds of perineal skin that protect the urinary meatus and the vaginal opening. Wipe from front to back on each side. Rinse the area in the same way. Dry entire perineal area. Move from front to back, using a blotting motion with towel. Ask resident to turn on her side. Wash, rinse, and dry buttocks and anal area. Cleanse the anal area without contaminating the perineal area.

Urinary Elimination

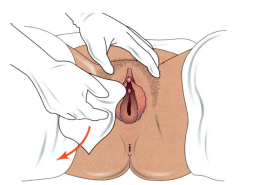

Fig. 16-13. Using single strokes, wipe from front to back when cleaning.

For a male resident: If the resident is uncircumcised, retract the foreskin. Gently push skin towards the base of penis.

Hold the penis by the shaft. Wash in a circular motion from the tip down to the base (Fig. 16-14). Use a clean area of washcloth or clean washcloth for each stroke. Rinse the penis. If the resident is uncircumcised, gently return foreskin to its normal position. Then wash the scrotum and groin. Rinse and pat dry. Ask the resident to turn on his side. Wash, rinse, and dry buttocks and anal area. Cleanse the anal area without contaminating the perineal area.

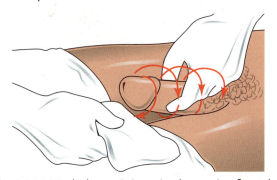

Fig. 16-14. Wash the penis in a circular motion from the tip down to the base.

14. Turn resident on his side away from you. Remove the wet protective pad after drying buttocks.

15. Place a dry protective pad under the resident.

16. Reposition the resident and make the resident comfortable.

17. Replace top covers and remove bath blanket.

18. Place soiled linens, clothing and protective pads in proper containers.

19. Empty, rinse, and wipe basin. Return to proper storage.

20. Remove and dispose of gloves properly.

21. Wash your hands.

22. Return bed to lowest position. Remove privacy measures.

23. Place call light within resident's reach.

24. Report any changes in resident to the nurse.

25. Document procedure using facility guidelines.

Urinary Tract Infection (UTI)

Urinary tract infection (UTI) causes inflammation of the bladder and the ureters. This results in painful burning during urination and the frequent feeling of needing to urinate. UTI or **cystitis**, also inflammation of the bladder, may be caused by a bacterial infection. Certain situations, such as being bedbound, can cause urine to stay in the bladder too long. This provides an ideal environment for bacteria to grow.

Cystitis is more common in women because the urethra is much shorter in women (three to four inches) than in men (seven to eight inches). Bacteria can reach a woman's bladder more easily. To avoid infection, women should wipe the perineal area from front to back after bladder and bowel elimination.

Guidelines:
Preventing UTIs

G   Encourage residents to wipe from front to back after elimination (Fig. 16-15). When you give perineal care, make sure you do this too.

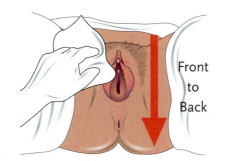

Fig. 16-15. *After elimination, wipe from front to back to prevent infection.*

G   Give careful perineal care when changing incontinence briefs.

G   Encourage plenty of fluids. Drinking plenty of fluids helps prevent UTIs. Drinking cranberry and blueberry juice acidifies urine, which helps to prevent infection. Vitamin C also has this effect.

G   Offer bedpan or a trip to the toilet at least every two hours. Answer call lights promptly.

G   Taking showers, rather than baths, helps prevent UTIs.

G   Report cloudy, dark, or foul-smelling urine, or if a resident urinates often and in small amounts.

Calculi

Calculi, or kidney stones, form when urine crystallizes in the kidneys. Kidney stones can block the kidneys and ureters, causing severe pain. Kidney stones can be caused by some of the same conditions that cause cystitis. They can also be the result of a vitamin deficiency, mineral imbalance, structural abnormalities of the urinary tract, or infection.

Symptoms of calculi may not be felt until they begin to move down the ureter, causing pain. Symptoms include the following:

- Abdominal pain

- Flank or back pain

- Groin pain

- Burning during urination, painful urination

- Frequent urination

- Blood in the urine

- Nausea, vomiting

- Chills, fever

Urine straining is the process of pouring all urine through a fine filter to catch any particles. This is done to detect the presence of calculi that can develop in the urinary tract. Kidney stones can be as small as grains of sand or as large as golf balls. If any stones are found, they are saved and then sent to a laboratory for examination.

If straining urine is listed on your assignment sheet, you will first collect a routine urine specimen (see more information later in the chapter). Then you will go into the bathroom and pour the specimen through a strainer or a 4x4-inch piece of gauze into a specimen container. Any stones that are found are wrapped in the filter and are placed in the specimen container to go to the lab.

Treatment of calculi includes drinking plenty of water to produce greater quantities of urine. Pain relievers may be ordered. Kidney stones usually pass on their own, but if they do not, surgery may be required.

Nephritis

Nephritis is an inflammation of the kidneys. Symptoms include a decrease in urine output, rusty-colored urine, and a burning feeling during urination. A person with nephritis often has a swollen face, eyelids, and hands because she is retaining fluid. Children and young adults usually recover without problems. Older people can develop a chronic form of nephritis.

Renovascular Hypertension

Renovascular hypertension is a condition in which a blockage of arteries in the kidneys causes high blood pressure. Medications may be used to help control blood pressure. Further treatment may include surgery. You will learn more about hypertension and its symptoms, treatment, and related care in Chapter 18.

Chronic Kidney Failure or Chronic Renal Failure

Chronic kidney failure, or **chronic renal failure**, occurs because the kidneys become unable to eliminate certain waste products from the body. This disease can develop as the result of chronic urinary tract infections, nephritis, or diabetes. Excessive salt in the diet can also cause damage to the kidneys. Over time, the disease becomes worse. Symptoms include the following:

* High blood pressure
* Decreased urine output or no urine output
* Darkly colored urine
* Anemia
* Nausea, vomiting
* Loss of appetite
* Weight changes
* Fatigue and weakness
* Headaches
* Difficulty sleeping
* Back pain
* Edema
* Stool that is bloody or black

Kidney dialysis, an artificial means of removing the body's waste products, can improve and extend life for several years. Residents will be on fluid restrictions of different degrees. Chronic kidney failure can progress to end-stage kidney disease, which is fatal without kidney dialysis or a kidney transplant.

4. Describe guidelines for urinary catheter care

Some residents you care for may have a urinary catheter. A catheter is a thin tube inserted into the body that is used to drain fluids or inject fluids. A urinary catheter is used to drain urine from the bladder. A **straight catheter** does not remain inside the person. It is removed immediately after urine is drained. An **indwelling catheter** remains inside the bladder for a period of time (Fig. 16-16). The urine drains into a bag. Nursing assistants do not insert, remove, or irrigate catheters. You may be asked to provide daily care for the catheter, cleaning the area around the urethral opening and emptying the drainage bag.

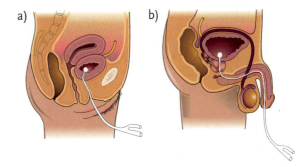

Fig. 16-16. *a) An indwelling catheter (female). b) An indwelling catheter (male).*

An external, or **condom catheter** (also called a Texas catheter), has an attachment on the end that fits onto the penis (Fig. 16-17). The attachment is fastened with tape. The external catheter is changed daily or as needed.

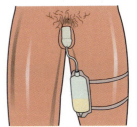

Fig. 16-17. *An external or condom catheter.*

Guidelines:
Catheters

G The drainage bag must always be kept lower than the hips or bladder. Urine must never flow from the bag or tubing back into the bladder. This can cause infection.

G Keep the drainage bag off the floor.

G Tubing should be kept as straight as possible and should not be kinked. Kinks, twists, or pressure on the tubing (such as from the resident sitting or lying on the tubing) can prevent urine from draining.

G The genital area must be kept clean to prevent infection. Because the catheter goes all the way into the bladder, bacteria can enter the bladder more easily. Daily care of the genital area is especially important.

Observing and Reporting:
Catheters

Report any of these to the nurse:

O/R Blood in the urine or any other unusual appearance of the urine

O/R Catheter bag does not fill after several hours

O/R Catheter bag fills suddenly

O/R Catheter is not in place

O/R Urine leaks from the catheter

O/R Resident reports pain or pressure

O/R Odor

Providing catheter care

Equipment: bath blanket, protective pad, bath basin, soap, bath thermometer, 2-4 washcloths or wipes, 1 towel, gloves

1. Wash your hands.

2. Identify yourself by name. Identify the resident by name.

3. Explain procedure to the resident. Speak clearly, slowly, and directly. Maintain face-to-face contact whenever possible.

4. Provide for resident's privacy with curtain, screen, or door.

5. Adjust bed to a safe working level, usually waist high. Lock bed wheels.

6. Lower head of bed. Position resident lying flat on his back.

7. Remove or fold back top bedding. Keep resident covered with bath blanket.

8. Test water temperature with thermometer or your wrist and ensure it is safe. Water temperature should be 105° F. Have resident check water temperature. Adjust if necessary.

9. Put on gloves.

10. Ask the resident to flex his knees and raise the buttocks off the bed by pushing against the mattress with his feet. Place clean protective pad under his buttocks.

11. Expose only the area necessary to clean the catheter; avoid overexposure of resident.

12. Place towel or pad under catheter tubing before washing.

13. Apply soap to wet washcloth. Clean area around meatus. Use a clean area of the washcloth for each stroke.

14. Hold catheter near meatus to avoid tugging the catheter.

15. Clean at least four inches of catheter nearest meatus. Move in only one direction, away from meatus. Use a clean area of the cloth for each stroke.

16. Dip a clean washcloth in the water. Rinse area around meatus, using a clean area of washcloth for each stroke.

17. Dip a clean washcloth in the water. Rinse at least four inches of catheter nearest

meatus. Move in only one direction, away from meatus (Fig. 16-18). Use a clean area of the cloth for each stroke.

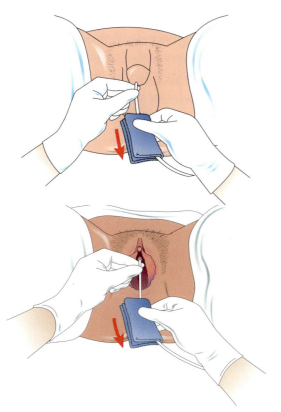

Fig. 16-18. *Hold the catheter near the meatus, so that you do not tug it. Moving in only one direction, away from meatus, helps prevent infection.*

18. Remove towel or pad from under catheter tubing. Replace top covers and remove bath blanket.

19. Dispose of linen in proper containers.

20. Empty, rinse, and wipe basin. Return to proper storage.

21. Remove and dispose of gloves.

22. Wash your hands.

23. Return bed to lowest position. Remove privacy measures.

24. Place call light within resident's reach.

25. Report any changes in resident to the nurse.

26. Document procedure using facility guidelines.

Urinary Catheters

Protect privacy when a resident has a urinary catheter. Keep the tubing and bag covered. Close doors and pull privacy screens when giving catheter care.

Emptying the catheter drainage bag

Equipment: graduate (measuring container), alcohol wipes, paper towels, gloves

1. Wash your hands.

2. Identify yourself by name. Identify the resident by name.

3. Explain procedure to the resident. Speak clearly, slowly, and directly. Maintain face-to-face contact whenever possible.

4. Provide for resident's privacy with curtain, screen, or door.

5. Put on gloves.

6. Place paper towel on the floor under the drainage bag. Place measuring container on the paper towel.

7. Open the drain or spout on the bag. Allow urine to flow out of the bag into the measuring container (Fig. 16-19). Do not let spout touch the measuring container.

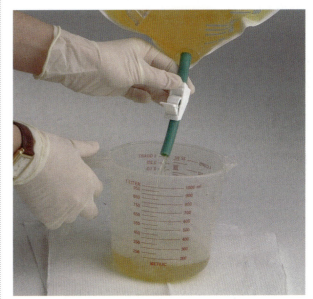

Fig. 16-19. *Keep the spout from touching the graduate while draining urine.*

8. When urine has drained, close spout. Using alcohol wipe, clean the drain spout. Replace the drain in its holder on the bag.

9. Note the amount and the appearance of the urine. Empty into toilet.

10. Clean and store measuring container.

11. Remove and dispose of gloves.

12. Wash your hands.

13. Document procedure and amount of urine.

Applying a condom catheter

Equipment: condom catheter and collection bag, catheter tape, gloves, plastic bag, bath blanket, supplies for perineal care

1. Wash your hands.

2. Identify yourself by name. Identify the resident by name.

3. Explain procedure to the resident. Speak clearly, slowly, and directly. Maintain face-to-face contact whenever possible.

4. Provide for resident's privacy with curtain, screen, or door.

5. Adjust bed to a safe level, usually waist high. Lock bed wheels.

6. Lower head of bed. Position resident lying flat on his back.

7. Remove or fold back top bedding. Keep resident covered with bath blanket.

8. Put on gloves.

9. Adjust bath blanket to expose only genital area.

10. If condom catheter is present, gently remove it. Place it in the plastic bag.

11. Help as necessary with perineal care.

12. Attach collection bag to leg.

13. Move pubic hair away from the penis so it does not get rolled into the condom.

14. Hold penis firmly. Place condom at tip of penis and roll towards base of penis. Leave space between the drainage tip and glans of penis to prevent irritation. If resident is not circumcised, be sure that foreskin is in normal position.

15. Gently secure condom to penis with tape provided (Fig. 16-20).

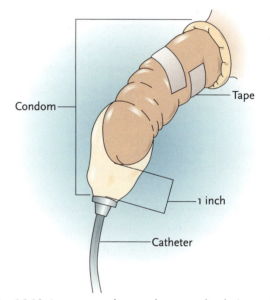

Condom — Tape — 1 inch — Catheter

Fig. 16-20. Leave enough room between the drainage tip and the glans of the penis to prevent irritation.

16. Connect catheter tip to drainage tubing. Make sure tubing is not twisted or kinked.

17. Discard used supplies in plastic bag. Place soiled clothing and linens in proper containers. Clean and store supplies.

18. Remove and dispose of your gloves.

19. Wash your hands.

20. Make resident comfortable. Make sure sheets are free from wrinkles and the bed free from crumbs.

21. Return bed to lowest position. Remove privacy measures.

22. Place call light within resident's reach.

23. Report any changes in resident to the nurse.

24. Document procedure using facility guidelines.

You may be asked to collect a urine specimen from a resident who is wearing a catheter. If the nurse requests you do this, and it is within your scope of practice, you will disconnect the tubing from the drainage bag. Allow the specimen to drip directly into the specimen container. If the resident's input and output are being monitored, measure the amount of urine collected. Collecting a specimen this way may take some time. Do not collect a urine sample from the drainage bag unless ordered to do so.

5. Identify types of urine specimens that are collected

You may be asked to collect a specimen from a resident. A **specimen** is a sample that is used for analysis in order to try to make a diagnosis. Different types of specimens are used for different tests.

There are factors to consider when collecting specimens. Body wastes and elimination needs are very private matters for most people. Having another person handle body wastes may make residents embarrassed and uncomfortable. Be sensitive to this, and be empathetic. Think about how difficult this may be for the resident. When collecting specimens, behave professionally and matter-of-factly. If you feel that this is an unpleasant task, do not make it known. Do not make faces or frown. Do not use words that let the resident know you are uncomfortable. Remaining professional when collecting specimens can help put residents at ease.

Urine specimens may be routine, clean catch (mid-stream), or 24-hour. A **routine urine specimen** is collected anytime the resident voids. The resident will void into a bedpan, uri-

nal, commode, or "hat." A **"hat"** is a plastic collection container sometimes put into a toilet to collect and measure urine or stool (Fig. 16-21). Some residents will be able to collect their own urine specimens. Others will need your help. Be sure to explain exactly how the specimen must be collected (Fig. 16-22).

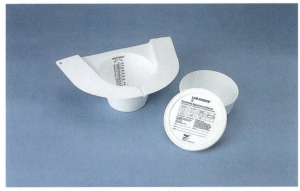

Fig. 16-21. A "hat" is a container that is placed under the toilet seat to collect and measure urine or stool. Hats should be labeled and must be cleaned after each use.

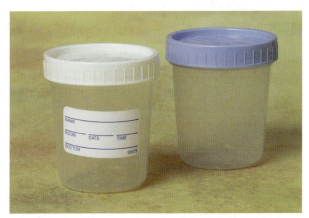

Fig. 16-22. Specimens must always be labeled with the resident's name, room number, the date, and the time, before being taken to the lab. (REPRINTED WITH PERMISSION OF BRIGGS CORPORATION, 800-247-2343, WWW.BRIGGSCORP.COM)

Collecting a routine urine specimen

Equipment: urine specimen container and lid, label (labeled with resident's name, room number, date and time), gloves, bedpan or urinal (if resident cannot use a portable commode or toilet), "hat" for toilet (if resident can get to the bathroom), 2 plastic bags, washcloth, towel, paper towel, supplies for perineal care, lab slip, if required

1. Wash your hands.

2. Identify yourself by name. Identify the resident by name.

3. Explain procedure to the resident. Speak clearly, slowly, and directly. Maintain face-to-face contact whenever possible.

4. Provide for resident's privacy with curtain, screen, or door.

5. Put on gloves.

6. Help the resident to the bathroom or commode, or offer the bedpan or urinal.

7. Have resident void into "hat," urinal, or bedpan. Ask the resident not to put toilet paper in with the sample. Provide a plastic bag to discard toilet paper.

8. After urination, help as necessary with perineal care. Help resident wash his or her hands. Make the resident comfortable.

9. Take bedpan, urinal, or commode pail to the bathroom.

10. Pour urine into the specimen container. Specimen container should be at least half full.

11. Cover the urine container with its lid. Do not touch the inside of container. Wipe off the outside with a paper towel.

12. Place the container in a plastic bag.

13. If using a bedpan or urinal, discard extra urine. Rinse and clean equipment. Store.

14. Remove and dispose of gloves.

15. Wash your hands.

16. Return bed to lowest position if adjusted. Remove privacy measures.

17. Place call light within resident's reach.

18. Report any changes in resident to the nurse.

19. Take specimen and lab slip to proper area. Document procedure using facility guidelines. Note amount and characteristics of urine.

Residents' Rights

Specimens

When collecting specimens, first explain how you will be collecting the specimen. Do this in private, keeping your voice low. Close the door to the bathroom or bedroom and pull the privacy curtain. Be discreet when removing the specimen from the room.

The **clean catch specimen** is called "midstream" because the first and last urine are not included in the sample. Its purpose is to determine the presence of bacteria in the urine.

Collecting a clean catch (mid-stream) urine specimen

Equipment: specimen kit with container and lid, label (labeled with resident's name, room number, date and time), cleansing solution, gauze or towelettes, gloves, bedpan or urinal (if resident cannot use a portable commode or toilet), plastic bag, washcloth, paper towel, towel, supplies for perineal care, lab slip, if required

1. Wash your hands.

2. Identify yourself by name. Identify the resident by name.

3. Explain procedure to the resident. Speak clearly, slowly, and directly. Maintain face-to-face contact whenever possible.

4. Provide for resident's privacy with curtain, screen, or door.

5. Put on gloves.

6. Open the specimen kit. Do not touch the inside of the container or lid.

7. If the resident cannot clean his or her perineal area, you will need to do it. Using the towelettes or gauze and cleansing solution, clean the area around the meatus. **For females**, separate the labia. Wipe from front to back along one side. Discard towelette/gauze. With a new towelette or gauze, wipe from front to back along the other side.

Using a new towelette or gauze, wipe down the middle.

For males, clean the head of the penis. Use circular motions with the towelettes or gauze. Clean thoroughly. Change towelettes/gauze after each circular motion. Discard after use. If the man is uncircumcised, gently pull back the foreskin of the penis before cleaning. Hold it back during urination. Make sure it is pulled back down after collecting the specimen.

8. Ask the resident to urinate into the bedpan, urinal, or toilet, and to stop before urination is complete.

9. Place the container under the urine stream. Have the resident start urinating again. Fill the container at least half full. Have the resident finish urinating in bedpan, urinal, or toilet.

10. Cover the urine container with its lid. Do not touch the inside of container. Wipe off the outside with a paper towel.

11. Place the container in a plastic bag.

12. If using a bedpan or urinal, discard extra urine. Rinse and clean equipment. Store.

13. After urination, assist as necessary with perineal care.

14. Remove and dispose of gloves.

15. Wash your hands. Help resident wash his or her hands.

16. Make resident comfortable. Make sure sheets are free from wrinkles and the bed free from crumbs.

17. Return bed to lowest position if adjusted. Remove privacy measures.

18. Place call light within resident's reach.

19. Report any changes in resident to the nurse.

20. Take specimen and lab slip to proper area. Document procedure using facility guide-lines. Note amount and characteristics of urine.

A **24-hour urine specimen** tests for certain chemicals and hormones by collecting all the urine voided by a resident in a 24-hour period. Usually the collection begins at 7:00 a.m. and runs until 7:00 a.m. the next day. When beginning a 24-hour urine specimen collection, the resident must void and discard the first urine so that the collection begins with an empty bladder. All urine must be collected and stored properly. If any is accidentally thrown away or improperly stored, the collection will have to be done over again.

Collecting a 24-hour urine specimen

Equipment: 24-hour specimen container with lid, bedpan or urinal (for residents confined to bed), "hat" for toilet (if resident can get to the bathroom), plastic bag, gloves, washcloth, towel, supplies for perineal care, sign to alert other team members that a 24-hour urine specimen is being collected, lab slip, if required

1. Wash your hands.

2. Identify yourself by name. Identify the resident by name.

3. Explain procedure to the resident. Speak clearly, slowly, and directly. Maintain face-to-face contact whenever possible. Emphasize that all urine must be saved.

4. Provide for resident's privacy with curtain, screen, or door.

5. Place a sign on the resident's bed to let all care team members know that a 24-hour specimen is being collected. Sign may read "Save all urine for 24-hour specimen."

6. When starting the collection, have the resident completely empty the bladder. Discard the urine. Note the exact time of this voiding. The collection will run until the same time the next day (Fig. 16-23).

INTAKE-OUTPUT RECORD

Resident/Patient Name		Room No.	
	FLUID INTAKE	URINE	EMESIS or DRAINAGE

7:00 A.M. to 3:00 P.M.

8-Hour Total		

3:00 P.M. to 11:00 P.M.

8-Hour Total		

11:00 P.M. to 7 A.M.

8-Hour Total		

Form 3039 © Briggs, Des Moines, IA 50306 PRINTED IN U.S.A. R404

DON'T BREAK THE LAW   Save   1-800-247-2343
MAKE THE CALL   13%   www.BriggsCorp.com
savings on buying vs. copying

Fig. 16-23. *One type of form to record urine output over 24 hours.* (REPRINTED WITH PERMISSION OF BRIGGS CORPORATION, 800-247-2343, WWW.BRIGGSCORP.COM)

7. Label the container. Write resident's name, room number, and dates and times the collection period began and ended.

8. Put on gloves each time the resident voids.

9. Pour urine from bedpan, urinal, or toilet attachment into the container. Container may be stored on ice when not used. The ice will keep the specimen cool. Follow facility policy.

10. After each voiding, help as necessary with perineal care. Help the resident wash his or her hands.

11. Clean equipment according to facility policy, after each voiding.

12. Remove gloves.

13. Wash your hands.

14. After the last void of the 24-hour period, add the urine to the specimen container. Remove the sign.

15. Place container in plastic bag.

16. Remove and dispose of gloves.

17. Wash your hands.

18. Make resident comfortable. Make sure sheets are free from wrinkles and the bed free from crumbs.

19. Return bed to lowest position if adjusted. Remove privacy measures.

20. Place call light within resident's reach.

21. Report any changes in resident to the nurse.

22. Take specimen and lab slip to proper area. Document procedure using facility guidelines. Make sure to include the time of the last void of the 24-hour collection period.

6. Explain types of tests performed on urine

Different types of tests can be used to detect different things in urine. Your facility may use dip strips to test for such things as pH level, glucose, ketones, blood, and specific gravity. These strips, called reagent strips, have different sections that change color when they react with urine (Fig. 16-24).

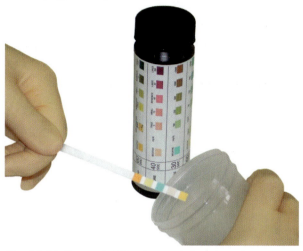

Fig. 16-24. *Reagent strips change color when they react with urine. The color is then compared to a color chart to determine levels of each chemical factor.* (PHOTO COURTESY OF LW SCIENTIFIC, INC., WWW.LWSCIENTIFIC.COM, 800-726-7345)

Testing pH levels: The term "pH" means "parts Hydrogen." The pH scale ranges from 0 to 14, and the lower the number, the more acidic the fluid. The higher the number, the more alkaline the fluid. Normal pH range for urine is 4.6–8.0. A disruption of pH may be due to medication, food, or illness.

Testing for glucose and ketones: In diabetes mellitus, commonly called diabetes, the pancreas does not produce enough insulin (see Chapter 18). Insulin is the substance the body needs to convert glucose, or natural sugar, into energy. Without insulin to process glucose, these sugars collect in the blood. Some sugar appears in the urine.

Diabetics may also have ketones in the urine. Ketones are produced when the body burns fat for energy or fuel. Ketones are produced when there is not enough insulin to help the body use sugar for energy. Without enough insulin, glucose builds up in the blood. Since the body cannot use glucose for energy, it breaks down fat instead. When this occurs, ketones form in the blood and spill into the urine.

In addition to strip testing, a double-voided (also called "fresh-fractional") urine specimen may be used to test for glucose. A double-voided specimen is a urine specimen that is collected after first emptying the bladder and then waiting until another specimen can be collected. This may be ordered because testing urine that has been in the bladder for some time may not accurately reflect the amount of glucose present. With a double-voided specimen, after the person has voided, he is encouraged to drink fluids. Then approximately 30 minutes later, a second (double-voided) specimen is collected and tested.

Testing for blood: Blood should not be present in normal urine. Conditions like illness and disease can cause blood to appear in urine. Some blood is hidden, or occult, which can be detected by testing the urine.

Specific gravity: A urine specific gravity (also called urine density) test is performed to measure the concentration of particles in the urine. The test evaluates the body's water balance and urine concentration by showing how the urine compares to water. Normal values range from 1.002 to 1.028. The test usually requires a clean-catch urine specimen.

Testing urine with reagent strips

Equipment: urine specimen as ordered, reagent strip, gloves

1. Wash your hands.

2. Put on gloves.

3. Take a strip from the bottle and recap bottle. Close it tightly.

4. Dip the strip into the specimen.

5. Follow manufacturer's instructions for when to remove strip. Remove strip at correct time.

6. Follow manufacturer's instructions for how long to wait after removing strip. After proper time has passed, compare strip with color

chart on bottle. Do not touch bottle with strip.

7. Read results.

8. Discard used items. Discard specimen in the toilet.

9. Remove and dispose of gloves.

10. Wash your hands.

11. Document procedure using facility guidelines.

7. Explain guidelines for assisting with bladder retraining

Injury, illness, or inactivity may cause a loss of normal bladder function. Residents may need help in re-establishing regular routine and normal function. Problems with elimination can be embarrassing or difficult to discuss. Be sensitive to this. Always be professional when handling incontinence or helping to re-establish routines. It is hard enough for residents to handle incontinence without having to worry about your reactions. Never show anger or frustration toward residents who are incontinent.

Guidelines:
Bladder Retraining

G Follow Standard Precautions. Wear gloves when handling body wastes.

G Explain the bladder training schedule to the resident. Follow the schedule carefully.

G Keep a record of the resident's bladder habits. When you see a pattern of elimination, you can predict when the resident will need a bedpan or a trip to the bathroom.

G Offer a commode or a trip to the bathroom before beginning long procedures (Fig. 16-25).

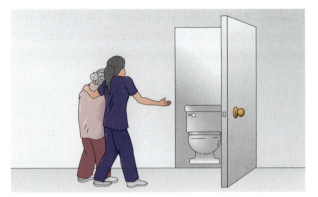

Fig. 16-25. *Offer regular trips to the bathroom.*

G Encourage the resident to drink plenty of fluids. Do this even if urinary incontinence is a problem. About 30 minutes after fluids are taken, offer a trip to the bathroom or a bedpan or urinal.

G Answer call lights promptly. Residents cannot wait long when the urge to go to the bathroom occurs. Leave call lights within reach (Fig. 16-26).

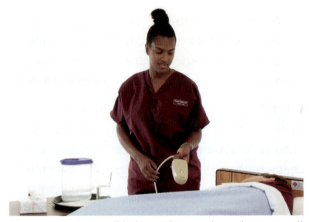

Fig. 16-26. *Leave call lights within reach, and answer call lights promptly.*

G Provide privacy for elimination—both in the bed and in the bathroom.

G If a resident has trouble urinating, try running water in the sink. Have him or her lean forward slightly. This puts pressure on the bladder.

G Do not rush the resident during voiding.

G Help residents with good perineal care. Urine is irritating to the skin, and giving good care helps prevents skin breakdown and promotes proper hygiene. Carefully observe for skin changes.

G   Discard wastes according to facility rules.

G   Discard clothing protectors and incontinence briefs properly. Some facilities require double bagging these items. This stops odors from collecting.

G   Some facilities use washable bed pads or briefs. Follow Standard Precautions when rinsing before placing these items in the laundry.

G   Keep an accurate record of urination. This includes episodes of incontinence.

G   Offer positive words for successes or for attempts to control bladder. However, do not talk to residents as if they are children. Keep your voice low and do not draw attention to any aspect of retraining.

G   Never show frustration or anger toward residents who are incontinent. The problem is out of their control. Your negative reactions will only make things worse. Be positive.

When the resident is incontinent or cannot toilet when asked, be positive. Never make the resident feel like a failure. Praise and encouragement are essential for a successful program. Some residents will always be incontinent. Be patient. Offer these persons extra care and attention. Skin breakdown may lead to pressure sores without proper care. Always report changes in skin.

Chapter Review

1.   What is the normal color of urine?

2.   List five things to observe and report to the nurse about urine.

3.   What is the best position for women to have normal urination? What is the best position for men?

4.   Briefly describe four factors that affect urination and how to promote normal urination.

5.   In what direction should a person be wiped during perineal care?

6.   What will women who are unable to get out of bed use for urination? What will men use?

7.   What is a fracture pan and when it is used?

8.   How should a standard bedpan be positioned under a resident? How should a fracture pan be positioned under a resident?

9.   List and define five types of incontinence.

10.   Is urinary incontinence a normal part of aging?

11.   Why should a nursing assistant never refer to an incontinence brief as a "diaper?"

12.   What are four ways that nursing assistants can help prevent urinary tract infections?

13.   Why should the catheter drainage bag always be kept lower than the hips or the bladder?

14.   Why should catheter tubing be kept as straight as possible?

15.   List five signs and symptoms to report to the nurse about catheters.

16.   What is a clean catch urine specimen?

17.   How can nursing assistants help reduce discomfort and embarrassment when assisting with specimen collection?

18.   What is the normal pH range for urine?

19.   List four things reagent strips can test for in urine.

20.   Why do incontinent residents need good perineal care?

21.   About how long after fluids are taken should you offer to take a resident to the bathroom?

22.   Out of the list of guidelines for bladder retraining, list two that help promote dignity.

17

Bowel Elimination

1. List qualities of stools and identify signs and symptoms to report about stool

Defecation, or bowel elimination, is the act of passing feces from the large intestine out of the body through the anus. Feces, also called stool or bowel movements, are semi-solid material made up of water, solid waste material, bacteria, and mucus. The number of bowel movements a person has varies with age and with the amount and type of foods consumed.

Stool is normally brown, soft, and formed in a tubular shape from its passage through the colon. However, food, medications, and supplements, as well as illness, can cause a change in the normal color of stool. For example, iron supplements can cause stool to appear black. Red food coloring, beets, and tomato juice can make stool red.

Observing and Reporting:
Stool

Report any of these to the nurse:

°/ᴿ Whitish, black, red, or hard stools

°/ᴿ Liquid stools (diarrhea)

°/ᴿ Constipation (the inability to have a bowel movement)

°/ᴿ Flatulence

°/ᴿ Pain when having a bowel movement

°/ᴿ Blood, pus, mucus, or discharge in stool

°/ᴿ Fecal/anal incontinence (inability to control the bowels, leading to involuntary passage of stool)

2. List factors affecting bowel elimination

There are many factors that can affect normal bowel elimination, including the following:

Normal changes of aging: As a person ages, peristalsis slows. **Peristalsis** refers to the involuntary contractions that move food through the gastrointestinal system. Digestion takes longer and is less efficient. Proteins, vitamins, and minerals are not absorbed as well. Decreased saliva production affects the ability to chew and swallow, as does tooth loss. Medication use and dulled sense of taste may result in poor appetite.

To help promote normal bowel elimination, encourage fluids and nutritious, appealing meals. Dentures should fit properly and be cleaned regularly. Give regular oral care. Help make mealtimes enjoyable. Residents who have trouble chewing and swallowing are at risk of choking. Provide plenty of fluids with meals and cut food into smaller pieces if ordered. Follow a toileting schedule for residents if there is one.

Promote proper hygiene and assist with perineal care, when necessary. Residents who have anal incontinence or diarrhea must be kept clean and dry. To prevent infection, always wipe from front to back. It is important to help resident to wash hands after having bowel movements.

Psychological factors: Stress, anger, fear, and depression all affect gastrointestinal function. Stress, anger, and fear can increase peristalsis and elimination, while depression may decrease it. A lack of privacy can greatly affect elimination, too.

To promote normal bowel elimination, it is very important to provide plenty of privacy. Close the bathroom door if residents are in the bathroom. If the resident needs to use a bedpan, pull the privacy curtain and close the door. Do not rush or interrupt residents when they are in the bathroom. Report signs of depression (Chapter 20), as well as any changes in frequency of elimination.

Food and fluids: What a person consumes greatly affects bowel elimination. Fiber intake improves bowel elimination. Foods high in fiber include fruits, whole grains, and raw vegetables (Fig. 17-1). Some high-fiber foods cause flatulence, or gas, which can aid elimination, but can also cause discomfort. Foods that may cause gas include the following:

- Beans
- Fruits (e.g., pears, apples, peaches)
- Whole grains
- Vegetables (e.g., broccoli, cabbage, onions, asparagus)
- Dairy products
- Carbonated drinks

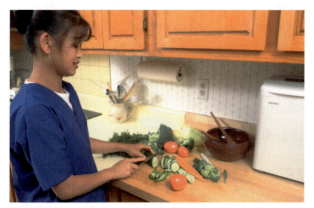

Fig. 17-1. *Raw fruits and vegetables are high in fiber, which helps with bowel elimination.*

Some foods can cause constipation, such as foods high in animal fats (dairy products, meats, and eggs) or foods high in refined sugar but low in fiber. Inadequate fluid intake not only contributes to dehydration, but also can cause constipation.

To promote normal bowel elimination, residents should eat a diet that contains fiber and drink plenty of fluids to help prevent constipation. Offer drinks to residents every time you see them, as long as they are not on fluid restrictions. Remember that a healthy person needs from 64 to 96 ounces of fluid each day.

Physical activity: Regular physical activity helps bowel elimination (Fig. 17-2). It strengthens abdominal and pelvic muscles, which helps peristalsis. Immobility and a lack of exercise weakens these muscles and may slow elimination.

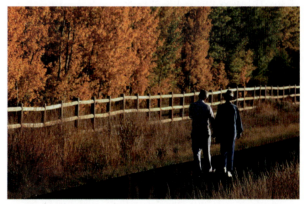

Fig. 17-2. *Regular exercise and activity is important for promoting normal bowel elimination.*

To promote normal bowel elimination, encourage regular activity and assist as needed. Try to make it fun. A walk can be a chore or it can be the highlight of the day.

Personal habits: The time of day that bowel movements occur varies from person to person. For example, one person may have a bowel movement early in the day, while another has one in the early afternoon. Another person may have a few bowel movements throughout the day. This depends on the person, his habits, and the amount of food and drink consumed. Elimination usually occurs after meals.

The position of the body affects elimination. A person who is supine (flat on his back) will have the most trouble with bowel elimination. It is almost impossible to contract muscles in this position.

To promote normal bowel elimination, allow residents to have an opportunity to have a bowel movement at the time of day that is normal for them. The best position for elimination is squatting and leaning forward. If the person cannot get out of bed, raise the head of the bed for elimination. That way, the resident does not have to work against gravity.

Medications: Medications affect the bowel elimination. Laxatives are used to cause bowel movements and may cause excessive elimination. Other medications, such as pain relievers, can slow elimination. Antibiotics may cause diarrhea. To promote normal bowel elimination, offer a trip to the bathroom or a bedpan often. Report any changes in appearance or frequency of bowel elimination.

Disorders and illnesses affect bowel elimination. You will learn more about these in the next Learning Objective.

3. Describe common diseases and disorders of the gastrointestinal system

Constipation

Constipation is the inability to eliminate stool (have a bowel movement), or the difficult and painful elimination of a hard, dry stool. Constipation occurs when the feces move too slowly through the intestine as the result of decreased fluid intake, poor diet, inactivity, medications, aging, certain diseases, or ignoring the urge to eliminate. Signs of constipation include abdominal swelling, gas, irritability, and record of no recent bowel movement.

Treatment often includes increasing the amount of fiber eaten and fluids consumed, increasing the activity level, and possibly medication.

An enema or suppository may be ordered to help with constipation. An **enema** is a specific amount of water, with or without an additive, that is introduced into the colon to eliminate stool. A **suppository** is a medication given rectally to cause a bowel movement.

Fecal Impaction

A **fecal impaction** is a hard stool that is stuck in the rectum and cannot be expelled. It results from unrelieved constipation. Symptoms include no stool for several days, oozing of liquid stool, cramping, abdominal swelling, and rectal pain. When an impaction occurs, a nurse or doctor will insert one or two gloved fingers into the rectum and break the mass into fragments so that it can be passed. Prevention of fecal impactions often includes the same measures as those used for preventing constipation, i.e. high-fiber diet, plenty of fluids, an increase in activity level, and possibly medication.

Hemorrhoids

Hemorrhoids are enlarged veins in the rectum that may also be visible outside the anus. Hemorrhoids can develop from an increase in pressure in the lower rectum due to straining during bowel movements. Chronic constipation, obesity, pregnancy, and sitting for long periods of time on the toilet are other causes. Signs and symptoms include rectal itching, burning, pain, and bleeding. Treatment may include medications, compresses, and sitz baths. Surgery may be necessary to correct hemorrhoids. When cleaning the anal area, be very careful to avoid causing pain and bleeding from hemorrhoids.

Diarrhea

Diarrhea is the frequent elimination of liquid or semi-liquid feces. Abdominal cramps, urgency, nausea, and vomiting can accompany diarrhea, depending on the cause. Bacterial and viral infections, microorganisms in food and water, irritating foods, and certain medications can cause diarrhea. Treatment usually involves medication and a change of diet. A diet of bananas, rice, apples, and tea/toast (BRAT diet) is often recommended.

Anal/Fecal Incontinence

Anal, or fecal, incontinence is the inability to control the bowels, leading to involuntary passage of stool. Common causes are constipation, muscle and nerve damage, loss of storage capacity in the rectum, and diarrhea. Treatment includes a change in diet, medication, bowel training, or surgery.

Flatulence

Flatulence, also called flatus or gas, is air in the intestine that is passed through the rectum, which can result in cramping or abdominal pain. Flatulence may have any of the following causes:

- Swallowing air while eating

- Eating high-fiber foods

- Eating foods that a person cannot tolerate, for example, when a person who has lactose intolerance eats dairy products (**Lactose intolerance** is the inability to digest lactose, a type of sugar found in milk and other dairy products. It is caused by a deficiency of lactase enzyme.)

- Antibiotics

- **Colitis**, or irritable bowel syndrome, which is a chronic form of stomach upset that gets worse from stress

- **Malabsorption**, which means that the body cannot absorb or digest a particular nutrient properly; it is often accompanied by diarrhea

Excessive flatulence, depending on the cause, is often treated with change of diet, medication, and reducing the amount of air swallowed. A return-flow enema (also called a "Harris flush") may be ordered to expel the flatus.

Heartburn

Heartburn is the result of a weakening of the sphincter muscle, which joins the esophagus and the stomach. When healthy, this muscle prevents the leaking of stomach acid and other contents back into the esophagus. Stomach acid causes a burning sensation, commonly called heartburn, in the esophagus. If heartburn occurs frequently and remains untreated, it can cause scarring or **ulceration**.

Gastroesophageal Reflux Disease

Gastroesophageal reflux disease, commonly referred to as **GERD**, is a chronic condition in which the liquid contents of the stomach back up into the esophagus. The liquid can inflame and damage the lining of the esophagus. It can cause bleeding or ulcers. In addition, scars from tissue damage can narrow the esophagus and make swallowing difficult.

Heartburn is the most common symptom of GERD. Heartburn and GERD must be reported to the nurse. These conditions are usually treated with medications. Serving the evening meal three to four hours before bedtime may help. The resident should not lie down until at least two to three hours after eating. Provide residents with an extra pillow so the body is more upright during sleep. Serving the largest meal of the day at lunchtime, serving several meals of small portions throughout the day, and reducing fast foods, fatty foods, and spicy foods may also help.

Peptic Ulcers

Peptic ulcers are raw sores in the stomach or the small intestine. A dull or gnawing pain occurs one to three hours after eating, accompanied by belching or vomiting. Food, antacids, and medications temporarily relieve the pain. Ulcers are caused by excessive acid production. Residents with peptic ulcers should avoid smoking and drinking too much alcohol and caffeine, which increase the production of gastric acid.

A bland diet may be ordered (Chapter 15). Peptic ulcers may cause bleeding. Feces, or bowel movements, may appear black and tarry because of the bleeding.

Ulcerative Colitis and Colitis

Ulcerative colitis is a chronic inflammatory disease of the large intestine. Symptoms include cramping, diarrhea, pain occurring to one side of the lower abdomen, rectal bleeding, and loss of appetite. Ulcerative colitis is a serious illness that can cause intestinal bleeding and death if left untreated. Medications can relieve symptoms, but they cannot cure ulcerative colitis. Surgical treatment may include a **colostomy**, which is the diversion of waste to an artificial opening (**stoma**) through the abdomen. All bowels are diverted through the stoma instead of the anus. See later in this chapter for more information on colostomy care.

Colitis, or irritable bowel syndrome, has symptoms similar to but milder than those of ulcerative colitis. Diet and/or medication can usually control colitis.

Colorectal Cancer

Colorectal cancer, also known as colon cancer, is cancer of the gastrointestinal tract. Signs and symptoms include changes in normal bowel patterns, cramps, abdominal pain, and rectal bleeding. Colorectal cancer must be treated with surgery. See Chapter 18 for more information on cancer.

4. Discuss how enemas are given

An enema is putting fluid into the colon in order to eliminate stool or feces. Enemas may be given prior to surgery or a medical test, or when a person cannot eliminate stool on his or her own. Depending upon the state and facility in which you work, you may be trained to give enemas. If you are allowed to give enemas, make sure to follow policies and procedures. Discuss any questions you may have with the nurse before giving an enema.

Doctors will write an enema order. Cleansing enemas include tap water enemas (TWE) and saline (salt water) enemas. A tap water enema uses approximately 500-1000 mL of water from a faucet, and a saline enema contains the same amount of water, but with two teaspoons of salt added. A soapsuds or soap solution enema (SSE) is another type of cleansing enema. This enema has 500-1000 mL of water with 5 mL of mild castile soap added.

A commercially-prepared enema (commercial enema) usually has 120 mL solution and may have additives. These enemas come prepackaged and do not require mixing (Fig. 17-3). An oil retention enema has a type of oil in it to soften the stool to allow it to pass more easily. It is often used when a person has been constipated for a long time, resulting in a stool that is very hard, or when a person has a fecal impaction.

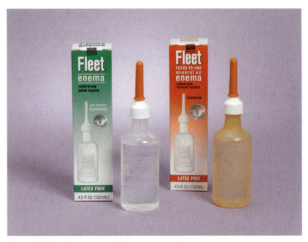

Fig. 17-3. *Commercially prepared enemas may come with additives, such as saline (on the left) and mineral oil (on the right).* (REPRINTED WITH PERMISSION OF BRIGGS CORPORATION, 800-247-2343, WWW.BRIGGSCORP.COM)

Equipment used for giving cleansing enemas includes an IV pole, the enema solution, tubing and a clamp. Commercially-prepared enemas do not require an IV pole, tubing, or clamp, because they are prepackaged and pre-mixed.

Guidelines:
Enemas

G   Keep the bedpan nearby or make sure that the bathroom is vacant before assisting with an enema.

G   The resident will be placed in Sims' (left side-lying) position (Fig. 17-4). Positioning on the left side means that the water does not have to flow against gravity.

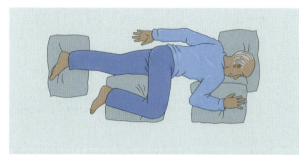

Fig. 17-4. *The Sims' position (left side-lying position) is the proper position in which to place a resident for an enema.*

G   The enema solution should be warm, not hot or cold.

G   The enema bag should not be raised to more than the height listed in the care plan.

G   The tip of the tubing should be lubricated with lubricating jelly, if not already pre-lubricated.

G   Unclamp the tube and allow a small amount of solution run through the tubing. Then re-clamp the tube. This gets rid of the air before it is inserted (the air could cause cramping).

G   The solution should flow in slowly; the resident will be less likely to have cramps.

G   Hold the enema tubing in place while giving the enema. Stop immediately if the resident has pain or if you feel resistance. Report to the nurse if this happens.

G   The resident should take slow deep breaths when taking an enema to help hold the solution longer.

G   Report any of the following to the nurse:

• Resident could not tolerate enema because of cramping.

• The enema had no results.

• The amount of stool was very small.

• Stool was hard, streaked with red, very dark or black.

Giving a cleansing enema

Equipment: 2 pair of gloves, bath blanket, IV pole, enema solution, tubing and clamp, bed protector, bedpan, lubricating jelly, bath thermometer, tape measure, toilet paper, 2 washcloths, robe, non-skid footwear

1. Wash your hands.

2. Identify yourself by name. Identify the resident by name.

3. Explain procedure to the resident. Speak clearly, slowly, and directly. Maintain face-to-face contact whenever possible.

4. Provide for resident's privacy with curtain, screen, or door.

5. Adjust bed to a safe level, usually waist high. Lock bed wheels.

6. If the bed has side rails, raise side rail on far side of bed. Lower side rail nearest you.

7. Help resident into left-sided Sims' position. Cover with a bath blanket.

8. Place the IV pole beside the bed. Raise the side rail.

9. Clamp the enema tube. Prepare the enema solution. Fill bag with 500-1000 mL of warm water (105° F), and mix the solution.

10. Unclamp the tube. Let a small amount of solution run through the tubing. Re-clamp the tube.

11. Hang the bag on IV pole. The bottom of the enema bag should not be more than 12 inches above the resident's anus (Fig. 17-5).

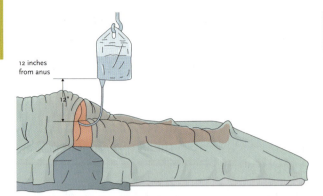

12 inches from anus

12"

Fig. 17-5. *Bottom of the bag should not be more than 12 inches above the anus.*

12. Put on gloves.

13. Lower the side rail. Uncover resident enough to expose anus only.

14. Place bed protector under resident. Place bedpan close to resident's body.

15. Lubricate tip of tubing with lubricating jelly.

16. Ask the resident to breathe deeply. This relieves cramps during procedure.

17. Place one hand on the upper buttock. Lift to expose the anus (Fig. 17-6). Ask the resident to take a deep breath and exhale. Using other hand, gently insert the tip of the tubing two to four inches into the rectum. Stop immediately if you feel resistance or if the resident complains of pain. If this happens, clamp the tube. Tell the nurse immediately.

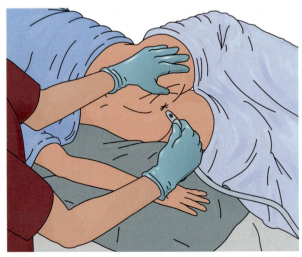

Fig. 17-6. *Lift the upper buttock to expose the anus. Ask the resident to take a deep breath before inserting the tubing.*

18. Unclamp the tubing. Allow the solution to flow slowly into the rectum. Ask resident to take slow, deep breaths. If resident complains of cramping, clamp the tubing and stop for a couple of minutes. Encourage him or her to take as much of the solution as possible.

19. Clamp the tubing when the solution is almost gone. Remove the tip from the rectum. Place the tip into the enema bag. Do not contaminate yourself, resident, or bed linens.

20. Ask the resident to hold the solution inside as long as possible.

21. Help resident to use bedpan, commode, or get to the bathroom. If the resident uses a commode or bathroom, apply robe and non-skid footwear. Lower the bed to its lowest position before the resident gets up.

22. Place toilet tissue and washcloths or wipes within resident's reach. Ask the resident to clean his hands with the hand wipe when finished, if he is able. If the resident is using the bathroom, ask him not to flush the toilet when finished.

23. Place the call light within resident's reach. Ask resident to signal when done. Leave the room.

24. Discard disposable equipment. Clean area.

25. Remove gloves. Wash your hands.

26. When called by the resident, return and put on clean gloves. Assist with perineal care as needed.

27. Take bedpan to the bathroom. Empty the bedpan carefully into the toilet. Note color, odor, and consistency of contents before flushing. If resident used toilet, check toilet contents.

28. Turn the faucet on with a paper towel. Rinse the bedpan with cold water first and empty it into the toilet. Place bedpan in proper area for cleaning or clean it according to facility policy.

29. Remove and discard gloves.

30. Wash your hands.

31. Make resident comfortable. Remove bath blanket and cover resident.

32. Return bed to lowest position. Remove privacy measures.

33. Place call light within resident's reach.

34. Report any changes in resident to the nurse.

35. Document procedure using facility guidelines.

Giving a commercial enema

Equipment: 2 pairs of gloves, bath blanket, standard or oil retention commercial enema kit, bed protector, bedpan, lubricating jelly, washcloths or wipes, toilet tissue, robe, non-skid footwear

1. Wash your hands.

2. Identify yourself by name. Identify the resident by name.

3. Explain procedure to the resident. Speak clearly, slowly, and directly. Maintain face-to-face contact whenever possible.

4. Provide for resident's privacy with curtain, screen, or door.

5. Adjust bed to a safe level, usually waist high. Lock bed wheels.

6. If the bed has side rails, raise side rail on far side of bed. Lower side rail nearest you.

7. Help resident into left-sided Sims' position. Cover with a bath blanket.

8. Put on gloves.

9. Lower the side rail. Uncover resident enough to expose anus only.

10. Place bed protector under resident. Place bedpan close to resident's body.

11. Lubricate tip of bottle with lubricating jelly.

12. Ask resident to breathe deeply to relieve cramps during procedure.

13. Place one hand on the upper buttock. Lift to expose the anus. Ask the resident to take a deep breath and exhale. Using other hand, gently insert the tip of the tubing about one and a half inches into the rectum. Stop if you feel resistance or if the resident complains of pain. Tell the nurse immediately.

14. Slowly squeeze and roll the enema container so that the solution runs inside the resident. Only release pressure after removing tip from the rectum.

15. When tip is removed, place bottle inside the box upside-down (Fig. 17-7).

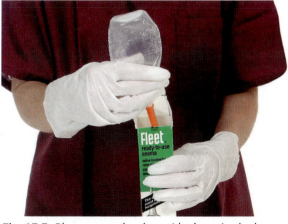

Fig. 17-7. Place enema bottle upside-down in the box.

16. Ask the resident to hold the solution inside as long as possible.

17. Help resident to use bedpan, commode, or get to the bathroom. If the resident uses a commode or bathroom, apply robe and non-skid footwear. Lower the bed to its lowest position before the resident gets up.

18. Place toilet tissue and washcloths or wipes within resident's reach. Ask the resident to clean his hands with the hand wipe when finished, if he is able. If the resident is using the bathroom, ask him not to flush the toilet when finished.

19. Place the call light within resident's reach. Ask resident to signal when done. Leave the room.

20. Discard disposable equipment. Clean area.

21. Remove gloves. Wash your hands.

22. When called by the resident, return and put on clean gloves. Assist with perineal care as needed.

23. Take bedpan to the bathroom. Empty the bedpan carefully into the toilet. Note color, odor, and consistency of contents before flushing. If resident used toilet, check toilet contents.

24. Turn the faucet on with a paper towel. Rinse the bedpan with cold water first and empty it into the toilet. Place bedpan in proper area for cleaning or clean it according to facility policy.

25. Remove and discard gloves.

26. Wash your hands.

27. Make resident comfortable. Remove bath blanket and cover resident.

28. Return bed to lowest position. Remove privacy measures.

29. Place call light within resident's reach.

30. Report any changes in resident to the nurse.

31. Document procedure using facility guidelines.

5. Demonstrate how to collect a stool specimen

Stool (feces) specimens are collected so that the stool can be tested for blood, pathogens, and other things, such as worms or amebas. Worms and amebas can be detected with an ova and parasites test. If the specimen is to be examined for ova and parasites, take it to the lab immediately. This examination must be made while the stool is still warm.

If the resident uses a bedpan or portable commode for elimination, you will take the stool specimen from there. If the resident uses the toilet, you will use a hat for collection. When collecting a stool specimen, ask the resident not to get urine or tissue in the sample because they can ruin the sample.

Collecting a stool specimen

Equipment: specimen container and lid, label (labeled with resident's name, room number, date, and time), 2 tongue blades, 2 pairs of gloves, bedpan (if resident cannot use portable commode or toilet), "hat" for toilet (if resident uses toilet or commode), 2 plastic bags, toilet tissue, washcloth or towel, supplies for perineal care, lab slip, if required

Ask the resident to let you know when he can have a bowel movement. Be ready to collect the specimen.

1. Wash your hands.

2. Identify yourself by name. Identify the resident by name.

3. Explain procedure to the resident. Speak clearly, slowly, and directly. Maintain face-to-face contact whenever possible.

4. Provide for resident's privacy with curtain, screen, or door.

5. Put on gloves.

6. When the resident is ready to move bowels, ask him not to urinate at the same time and

not to put toilet paper in with the sample. Provide a plastic bag for toilet paper.

7. Fit hat to toilet or commode, or provide resident with bedpan. Ask the resident to signal when he is finished with the bowel movement. Make sure call light is within reach and leave the room.

8. When called by resident, return and help with perineal care, if needed. Help resident wash his hands.

9. Remove and dispose of gloves.

10. Wash your hands.

11. Put on clean gloves.

12. Using the two tongue blades, take about two tablespoons of stool, and put it in the container. Cover it tightly.

13. Place the container in a plastic bag.

14. Wrap the tongue blades in toilet paper and throw them away. Empty the bedpan or container into the toilet. Rinse and clean equipment. Store.

15. Remove and dispose of gloves.

16. Wash your hands.

17. Return bed to lowest position if adjusted. Remove privacy measures.

18. Place call light within resident's reach.

19. Report any changes in resident to the nurse.

20. Take specimen and lab slip to proper area. Document procedure using facility guidelines. Note amount and characteristics of stool.

6. Explain occult blood testing

Occult blood testing is performed to detect blood in stool. **Occult** means something that is hidden or difficult to see or observe. Hidden, or occult, blood in stool may be an indication of colorectal cancer, or of other illnesses.

The Hemoccult® fecal occult blood test helps to detect blood in stool. Stool specimens may be sent to the laboratory for this test; however, you may be asked to perform this test at your facility, if you are trained and allowed to do so.

Testing a stool specimen for occult blood

Equipment: labeled stool specimen, Hemoccult® test kit (Fig. 17-8) or other ordered test kit (Fig. 17-9), 1 or 2 tongue blades, paper towel, plastic bag, gloves

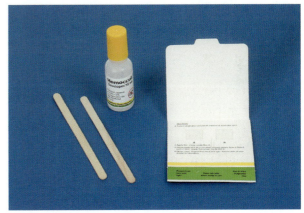

Fig. 17-8. *A Hemoccult® test kit.*

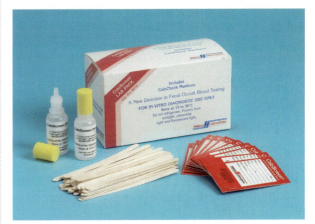

Fig. 17-9. *This is another type of screening test for occult blood. Use the test that is ordered at your facility.* (REPRINTED WITH PERMISSION OF BRIGGS CORPORATION, 800-247-2343, WWW.BRIGGSCORP.COM)

1. Wash your hands.

2. Put on gloves.

3. Open the test card.

4. Pick up a tongue blade. Get small amount of stool from specimen container.

5. Using tongue blade, smear a small amount of stool onto Box A of test card (Fig. 17-10).

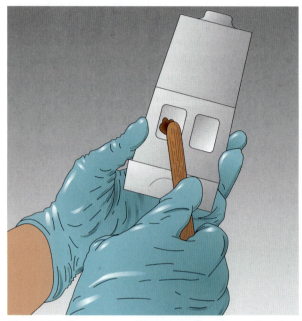

Fig. 17-10. *Smear a small amount of stool onto Box A.*

6. Flip tongue blade, or use a new tongue blade. Get some stool from another part of specimen. Smear small amount of stool onto Box B of test card.

7. Close the test card. Turn over to other side.

8. Open the flap, and open the developer. Apply developer to each box. Follow manufacturer's instructions.

9. Wait the amount of time listed in instructions, usually between 10 and 60 seconds.

10. Watch the squares for any color changes. Record color changes. Follow instructions.

11. Place tongue blade and test packet in plastic bag, and dispose of plastic bag properly.

12. Remove and dispose of gloves.

13. Wash your hands.

14. Document procedure using facility guidelines.

7. Define the term "ostomy" and list care guidelines

An **ostomy** is an operation to create an opening from an area inside the body to the outside. The terms "colostomy" and "ileostomy" refer to the surgical removal of a portion of the intestines. It may be necessary due to bowel disease, cancer, or trauma. In a resident with one of these ostomies, the end of the intestine is brought out of the body through an artificial opening in the abdomen. This opening is called a stoma. Stool, or feces, are eliminated through the ostomy rather than through the anus. (When an ureter is opened to abdomen for urine to be eliminated, it is called a **ureterostomy**.)

The terms "colostomy" and "ileostomy" indicate what part of the intestine was removed and the type of stool that will be eliminated. In a colostomy, stool will generally be semi-solid. With an **ileostomy**, stool may be liquid and irritating to the skin.

Residents who have had an ostomy wear a disposable bag or pouch that fits over the stoma to collect the feces (Fig. 17-11). The bag is attached to the skin by adhesive. A belt may also be used to secure it.

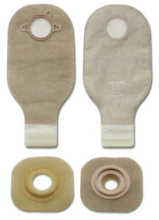

Fig. 17-11. *The top of this photo shows the front and back of one type of drainage pouch for an ostomy. An example of a skin barrier is at the bottom of the photo.*
(PHOTOS COURTESY OF HOLLISTER INCORPORATED, LIBERTYVILLE, ILLINOIS)

Many people manage the ostomy appliance by themselves. You should receive training before you provide this care. Use the following general guidelines if you are providing ostomy care.

Guidelines:
Ostomies

G Make certain that the resident receives good skin care and hygiene. The ostomy bag should be emptied and cleaned or replaced whenever a stool is eliminated.

G Always wear gloves and wash hands carefully when providing ostomy care. Follow Standard Precautions.

G Teach proper handwashing techniques to residents with ostomies.

G Skin barriers protect the skin around the stoma from irritation of the waste products and/or the adhesive material that is used to secure the pouch to the body. Barriers may come in the form of a powder, gel, ring, paste, wafer, or square.

G Residents who have an ileostomy may experience food blockage. A food blockage is a large amount of undigested food, usually high-fiber food, that collects in the small intestine and blocks the passage of stool. Food blockages can occur if the resident eats large amounts of foods that are high-fiber and/or if the resident does not chew the food well. Follow the diet instructions in the care plan and the nurse's instructions for assisting with feeding.

G Many residents with ostomies feel they have lost control of a basic bodily function. They may be embarrassed or angry about the ostomy. Be sensitive and supportive when working with these residents. Always provide privacy for ostomy care.

Caring for an ostomy

Equipment: bedpan, disposable bed protector, bath blanket, clean ostomy bag and belt/appliance, toilet paper or gauze squares, basin of warm water, soap or cleanser, washcloth, skin cream as ordered, 2 towels, plastic disposable bag, gloves

1. Wash your hands.

2. Identify yourself by name. Identify the resident by name.

3. Explain procedure to the resident. Speak clearly, slowly, and directly. Maintain face-to-face contact whenever possible.

4. Provide for resident's privacy with curtain, screen, or door.

5. Adjust bed to a safe level, usually waist high. Lock bed wheels.

6. Place bed protector under resident. Cover resident with a bath blanket. Pull down the top sheet and blankets. Only expose ostomy site. Offer resident a towel to keep clothing dry.

7. Put on gloves.

8. Remove ostomy bag carefully. Place it in plastic bag. Note the color, odor, consistency, and amount of stool in the bag.

9. Wipe the area around the stoma with toilet paper or gauze squares. Discard paper/gauze in plastic bag.

10. Using a washcloth and warm soapy water, wash the area in one direction, away from the stoma (Fig. 17-12). Pat dry with another towel. Apply cream as ordered.

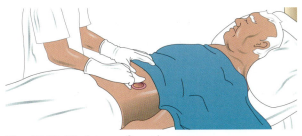

Fig. 17-12. *Wash away from the stoma.*

11. Place the clean ostomy appliance on resident. Make sure the bottom of the bag is clamped.

12. Remove disposable bed protector and discard. Place soiled linens in proper container.

13. Remove bag and bedpan. Discard bag in proper container. Empty bedpan into toilet.

14. Rinse bedpan and pour rinse water into toilet. Place container in proper area for cleaning or clean it according to facility policy.

15. Remove and dispose of gloves.

16. Wash your hands.

17. Make resident comfortable. Make sure sheets are free from wrinkles and the bed free from crumbs.

18. Return bed to lowest position. Remove privacy measures.

19. Place call light within resident's reach.

20. Report any changes in resident to the nurse. Report if stoma is very red or blue, or if swelling or bleeding is present.

21. Document procedure using facility guidelines.

8. Explain guidelines for assisting with bowel retraining

Residents who have had a disruption in their bowel routines from illness, injury, or inactivity may need help to re-establish a regular routine and normal function. To assist with bowel retraining, the doctor may order suppositories, laxatives, stool softeners, or enemas. Remember that bowel elimination issues may be difficult to discuss. Be sensitive to this and promote residents' privacy. Be professional when assisting residents with bowel retraining.

Residents' Rights

Bowel Retraining

Residents who have problems controlling their bowels need to be treated with dignity. Think about how you might feel in the same situation. For example, if a resident has a bowel movement in her bed, she probably feels extremely embarrassed about this and the fact that you have to clean her and change the sheets. You can help the resident keep her dignity by being kind and supportive. The resident has the right to privacy. Do not violate that by discussing her accident in a public area.

Guidelines:
Bowel Retraining

G Follow Standard Precautions. Wear gloves when handling body wastes.

G Explain the bowel training schedule to the resident. Follow the schedule carefully.

G Keep a record of the resident's bowel habits. When you see a pattern of elimination, you can predict when the resident will need a bedpan or a trip to the bathroom.

G Encourage the resident to drink plenty of fluids.

G Encourage the resident to eat foods that are high in fiber. Encourage residents to follow special diets, as ordered. Chapter 15 has more information on diet and nutrition.

G Answer call lights promptly. Leave call lights within reach.

G Provide privacy—both in the bed and in the bathroom.

G Do not rush the resident during elimination.

G Help residents with good perineal care. This prevents skin breakdown and promotes proper hygiene. Carefully watch for skin changes.

G Discard wastes according to facility rules.

G Discard clothing protectors and incontinence briefs properly.

G Some facilities use washable bed pads or briefs. Follow Standard Precautions when placing these items in the laundry.

G Keep an accurate record of elimination.

G Praise successes or attempts to control bowels. However, do not talk to residents as if they are children. Keep your voice low and do not draw attention to any aspect of bowel retraining.

G Never show frustration or anger toward residents who are incontinent or have "accidents." The problem is out of their control. Your negative reactions will only make things worse. Be positive.

Chapter Review

1. How does stool normally appear?

2. List five things to observe and report to the nurse about stool.

3. What is the best position for bowel elimination? What should be done if a person cannot get out of bed for defecation?

4. Briefly describe four factors that affect bowel elimination and how to promote normal defecation.

5. List three possible treatments for constipation.

6. List three signs of a fecal impaction.

7. List three causes of diarrhea.

8. What is gastroesophageal reflux disease (GERD)?

9. What are two things that people with peptic ulcers should avoid?

10. What are three symptoms of colorectal cancer?

11. List the equipment used for giving cleansing enemas.

12. In what position must the resident be placed for an enema?

13. What should the nursing assistant do if a resident feels pain or if the nursing assistant feels resistance while giving an enema?

14. What two things should not be included in a stool specimen?

15. If a stool specimen needs to be tested for ova and parasites, what should be done immediately and why?

16. What may occult blood in stool indicate?

17. What are three reasons that a resident may need a colostomy or ileostomy?

18. How often should an ostomy bag be emptied?

19. List 10 guidelines for bowel retraining.

18

Common Chronic and Acute Conditions

Residents in long-term care may have many different diseases and conditions. Diseases and conditions are either acute or chronic. An acute illness or condition means an illness has severe symptoms that last a relatively short time. It is usually treated immediately. A chronic illness is long-term or long-lasting. Symptoms are managed and are usually less severe from day to day, although there may be short periods of severity. The person may need to be hospitalized to stabilize the disease. This textbook describes diseases or conditions according to the body system in which they are located. You first learned about these body systems in Chapter 9:

- Integumentary
- Musculoskeletal
- Nervous
- Cardiovascular or circulatory
- Respiratory
- Endocrine
- Reproductive
- Immune and Lymphatic

The list above is only a partial list; you learned about common diseases of the urinary and gastrointestinal systems in Chapters 16 and 17.

If you think of the body system under which a disease is classified, the signs and symptoms will be easier to remember.

1. Describe common diseases and disorders of the integumentary system

Pressure sores, a common disorder of the integumentary system, are covered in Chapter 13. Burns are covered in Chapter 7.

Scabies

Scabies is a skin condition caused by a tiny mite called *Sarcoptes scabiei*. The mite burrows into the skin, where it lays eggs. Scabies is contagious and is spread through direct contact with an infected person. It can spread quickly in crowded places, such as long-term care facilities and child care facilities. Signs and symptoms of scabies include intense itching and a skin rash that may look like thin burrow tracks. These tracks typically appear in the folds of the skin.

Treatment of scabies involves medications, often in the form of prescription creams and lotions (Chapter 13 has information on applying lotions). Oral medications may be used, too, if the person does not respond to the creams and/or lotions.

Shingles

Shingles, also called herpes zoster, is a skin rash caused by the varicella-zoster virus (VZV), which is the same virus that causes chickenpox. (Herpes zoster is not the same virus that causes the sexually transmitted disease.) Any person who has had chickenpox is at risk for developing shingles. After having chickenpox, the virus remains in the body, where it usually does not cause problems. However, it can reappear later in life and cause shingles.

Initial signs and symptoms of shingles include pain, tingling, or itching in an area, which later develops into a rash of fluid-filled blisters that is similar to chickenpox (Fig. 18-1). The rash usually goes away within two to four weeks.

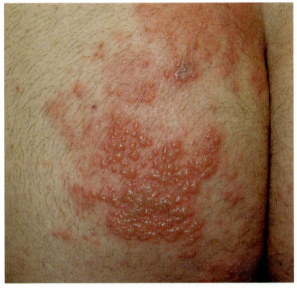

Fig. 18-1. *Shingles in blister form.* (PHOTO COURTESY OF DR. JERE MAMMINO, DO)

Shingles cannot be transmitted to other people. However, if a person has never had chickenpox, he may acquire chickenpox from a person who has active shingles (when the rash is in the blister phase). The risk of getting shingles increases as a person ages. People with immune systems weakened by diseases such as cancer and HIV are at greater risk of getting shingles.

Keeping the rash covered, especially while it is in blister form, is important. The rash should not be scratched or touched, and the person should wash her hands often.

Shingles is treated with medication, which should be started as soon as possible. A vaccine for the varicella-zoster virus (VZV) was approved by the Food and Drug Administration (FDA) in 2006 to give to people 60 years or older who have had chickenpox.

Wounds

A **wound** is a type of injury to the skin. Wounds are classified as either open or closed. Open wounds can be categorized in the following ways: incisions, lacerations, abrasions, and puncture wounds. Incisions are caused by a knife or razor, such as a cut made during surgery with a surgical instrument. Lacerations are irregular wounds caused by ripping or blunt trauma, such as tearing of skin during childbirth. Abrasions are wounds in which the top layer of skin is scraped or worn off, often by coming into moving contact with a rough surface. Puncture wounds are breaks in the skin caused by a nail or a needle.

Closed wounds can be contusions (bruises) or hemotomas. Contusions are caused by blunt force trauma that damages tissue under the skin. Hemotomas are caused by damage to a blood vessel that causes blood to collect under the skin.

Wounds are examined and cleaned with various solutions, such as tap water, sterile saline, or antiseptic solution. Bleeding may need to be stopped. Dressings, bandages, sutures, staples, or special strips or glue may need to be applied.

Dermatitis

Dermatitis is a general term that refers to an **inflammation**, or swelling, of the skin. There are different types of dermatitis, including atopic dermatitis, also known as eczema, and stasis dermatitis. Dermatitis usually involves swollen, reddened, irritated, and itchy skin.

Eczema commonly occurs along with allergies, including asthma or chronic hay fever. Physical and mental stressors may also cause eczema, and it may be inherited. Eczema usually begins in childhood and may not be as severe later in life. Symptoms include dry, itchy, and inflamed skin, usually on the cheeks, arms, and legs, although it can cover other parts of the body. Symptoms improve and worsen at various times. Atopic dermatitis is not contagious.

Special lotions are used to treat this condition. Further measures to help cracked skin may be prescribed, such as wet dressings. Antihistamines may help intense itching.

Stasis dermatitis is a skin condition that commonly affects the lower legs and ankles. The condition occurs due to a build up of fluid under the skin. This build-up causes problems with circulation, and poor circulation results in skin that is fragile and poorly nourished. Stasis dermatitis can also lead to severe skin problems such as open ulcers and wounds.

Early signs of stasis dermatitis include a rash, a scaly, red area, and itching. Other signs are: swelling of the legs, ankles, or other areas; thin, tissue-like skin; darkening skin at ankles or legs; thickening skin at ankles or legs; signs of skin irritation; and leg pain. Report any of these signs to the nurse.

Treatment of stasis dermatitis includes surgery for varicose veins and medications, such as diuretics, to reduce fluid in the body. Stockings and shoes should fit properly and not be too tight. The resident may need to keep his feet elevated, and he should not cross his legs. You may need to apply special elastic stockings to help promote circulation. The person may be on a low-sodium diet.

Fungal Infections

Mushrooms, mold, and yeasts (Candida) are all examples of fungi. Some types of fungi, such as Candida, normally live in and on the body, in such places as the skin and in the vagina and intestines. However, sometimes normal balances of fungi can change, resulting in fungal infections, such as athlete's foot or vaginal yeast infections. Tinea, often referred to as "ringworm," is another example of a fungal infection (Fig. 18-2). These imbalances that result in infections can be caused by a weakened immune system or by taking antibiotics.

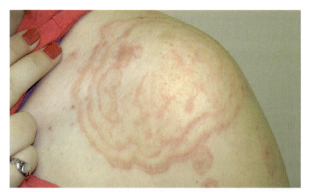

Fig. 18-2. *Tinea is a fungal infection that causes red, ring-like patches to appear on the upper body, hands and/or feet.* (PHOTO COURTESY OF DR. JERE MAMMINO, DO)

Fungi can be difficult to kill. Treatment generally consists of applying antifungal drugs directly on the infection, such as the skin, inside the mouth, or in the vagina. Medication may also need to be taken orally or injected if the infection is more serious.

Residents' Rights

Diseases and Disorders

Respect the privacy of residents who are ill. Do not discuss their condition where you can be overheard. Do not make negative comments or show negative facial reactions to unpleasant symptoms, such as vomiting, or to conditions like skin disorders.

2. Describe common diseases and disorders of the musculoskeletal system

Arthritis

Arthritis is a general term that refers to inflammation, or swelling, of the joints. It causes stiffness, pain, and decreased mobility. Arthritis may be the result of aging, injury, or an **autoimmune illness**. During an autoimmune illness, the body's immune system attacks normal tissue in the body. There are several types of arthritis.

Osteoarthritis is a common type of arthritis that affects the elderly. It may occur with aging or as the result of joint injury. Hips and knees, which are weight-bearing joints, are usually affected. Joints of the fingers, thumbs, and spine can also be affected. Pain and stiffness seem to increase in cold or damp weather.

Rheumatoid arthritis can affect people of all ages. Joints become red, swollen, and very painful (Fig. 18-3). Movement is eventually restricted. Fever, fatigue, and weight loss are also symptoms. Rheumatoid arthritis usually affects the smaller joints first, then progresses to larger ones. The heart, lungs, eyes, kidneys, and skin may also be affected.

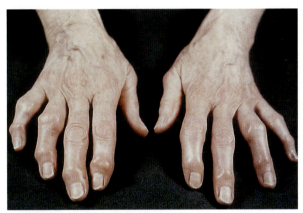

Fig. 18-3. *Rheumatoid arthritis.* (PHOTO COURTESY OF FREDERICK MILLER, MD)

Arthritis is generally treated with some or all of the following:

- Anti-inflammatory medications such as aspirin or ibuprofen
- Local applications of heat to reduce swelling and pain
- Range of motion exercises (Chapter 21)
- Regular exercise and/or activity routine
- Diet to reduce weight or maintain strength

Guidelines:
Caring for Residents with Arthritis

G   Watch for stomach irritation or heartburn caused by aspirin or ibuprofen. Some residents cannot take these medications. Report signs of stomach irritation or heartburn immediately.

G   Encourage activity. Gentle activity can help reduce the effects of arthritis. Follow care plan instructions carefully. Use canes or other walking aids as needed.

G   Adapt activities of daily living (ADLs) to allow independence. Many devices are available to help residents to bathe, dress, and feed themselves even when they have arthritis (Chapter 21).

G   Choose clothing that is easy to put on and fasten. Encourage use of handrails and safety bars in the bathroom. Special utensils make it easier for residents to feed themselves (Fig. 18-4).

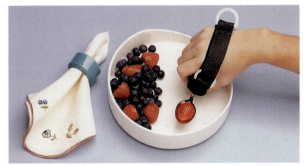

Fig. 18-4. *Special equipment can help a person with arthritis be independent.* (PHOTO COURTESY OF NORTH COAST MEDICAL, INC., WWW.NCMEDICAL.COM, 800-821-9319)

G   Treat each resident as an individual. Arthritis is very common among elderly residents. Do not assume that each resident has the same symptoms and needs the same care.

G   Help maintain resident's self-esteem by encouraging self-care. Have a positive attitude. Listen to the resident's feelings. You can help him or her remain independent for as long as possible.

Osteoporosis

Osteoporosis is a disease that causes bones to become porous and brittle. Brittle bones can break easily. Weakness in the bones may be due to age, lack of hormones, lack of calcium in bones, alcohol consumption, or lack of exercise.

Osteoporosis is more common in women after menopause. Menopause is the stopping of menstrual periods. Extra calcium and regular exercise can help prevent osteoporosis. Signs and symptoms of osteoporosis include low back pain, stooped posture, and becoming shorter over time (Fig. 18-5).

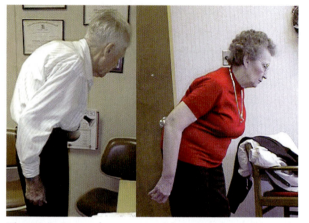

Fig. 18-5. *Stooped posture, or "dowager's hump" is a common sign of osteoporosis.* (PHOTOS COURTESY OF JEFFREY T. BEHR, MD)

To prevent or slow osteoporosis, encourage residents to walk and do other light exercise, as ordered. Exercise can strengthen bones as well as muscles. Nursing assistants must move residents with osteoporosis very carefully. Medication, calcium, and fluoride supplements are used to treat osteoporosis.

Fractures

Fractures are broken bones caused by accidents or by osteoporosis. A **closed fracture** is a broken bone that does not break the skin. An **open fracture**, also known as a compound fracture, is a broken bone that penetrates the skin. An open fracture carries a high risk of infection and usually requires immediate surgery.

Preventing falls, which can lead to fractures, is very important. Fractures of arms, elbows, legs, and hips are the most common. Signs and symptoms of a fracture are pain, swelling, bruising, changes in skin color at the site, and limited movement.

When bones are fractured, they must be placed in alignment so the body can heal. The body can grow new bone tissue and fuse the sections of fractured bone together. The bone must be unable to move for this healing to occur. This is often accomplished by the use of a cast.

Two common types of casts are made of plaster and fiberglass. Plaster casts take longer to dry, up to one to two days. Fiberglass casts dry quickly. A cast must be completely dry before a person can bear weight on it. As a cast dries, it gives off heat. This heat must escape or it will burn the skin. Never cover a cast with any material until it has completely dried.

Guidelines:
Caring for a Resident who has a Cast

G Do not cover a cast until it is dry. Follow instructions with position changes. Assist the resident to change positions as ordered; this allows the cast to dry evenly. Place the cast on pillows. A hard surface alters the shape of the cast. Use the palms of the hands to lift the cast. Fingers will dent it, and dents will cause pressure on the resident's skin.

G Elevate the extremity that is in a cast. This helps stop swelling (Fig. 18-6). If the resident is in bed, elevate the arm or leg slightly above the level of the heart.

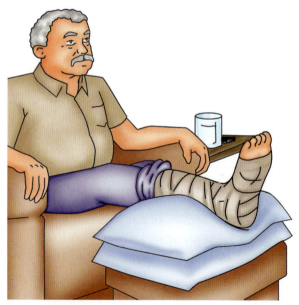

Fig. 18-6. *To help stop swelling, elevate the extremity that is in a cast.*

G   Observe the affected extremity for swelling, redness, pale or blue-tinged skin, cast tightness or pressure, sores, skin that feels hot or cold, pain, burning, numbness or tingling, drainage, bleeding, or odor. Compare to the extremity that does not have a cast. Report any of these to the nurse, along with any signs of infection, such as fever or chills.

G   Protect the skin from the rough edges of the cast. The stocking that lines the inside of the cast can be pulled up and over the edges and secured with tape. Tell the nurse if cast edges irritate the resident's skin.

G   Keep the cast dry. Wet casts lose their shape. Keep the cast clean.

G   Do not insert or allow the resident to insert anything inside the cast, even when skin itches. Pointed or blunt objects may injure dry and fragile skin. Skin can become infected under the cast.

G   Tell the nurse prior to moving or exercising if pain medication is needed. Help with range of motion exercises as ordered. Allow plenty of time for movement. Assist resident with cane, walker, or crutches as needed.

G   Use bed cradles as needed.

Hip Fractures

Weakened bones make hip fractures more common (Fig. 18-7). A sudden fall can result in a fractured hip that takes months to heal. Preventing falls is very important. Hip fractures can also occur because of weakened bones that fracture and cause a fall. A hip fracture is a serious condition. The elderly heal slowly. They are also at risk for secondary illnesses and disabilities.

Most fractured hips need surgery. Total hip replacement is surgery that replaces the head of the long bone of the leg (femur) where it joins the hip. This surgery is often performed for the following reasons:

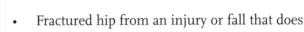

Fig. 18-7. *An illustration of a fractured hip.*

- Fractured hip from an injury or fall that does not heal properly

- Weakened hip due to aging

- Hip is painful and stiff because the joint is weak and the bones are no longer strong enough to bear the person's weight

After the surgery, the person cannot stand on that leg while the hip heals. A physical therapist will assist after surgery. The goals of care include slowly strengthening the hip muscles and getting the resident walking on that leg.

Be familiar with the resident's care plan. It will state when the resident may begin putting weight on the hip. It will also give instructions on how much the resident is able to do. It is important to help with personal care and using assistive devices, such as walkers or canes.

Guidelines:
Caring for Residents Recovering from Hip Replacements

G   Keep often-used items, such as medications, telephone, tissues, call light, and water, within easy reach. Avoid placing items in high places.

G   Dress starting with the affected side first.

G Never rush the resident. Use praise and encouragement often. Do this even for small tasks.

G Ask the nurse to give pain medication prior to moving and positioning if needed.

G Have the resident sit to do tasks if allowed. This saves energy.

G Follow the care plan exactly, even if the resident wants to do more. Follow orders for weight-bearing. An order may be written as partial weight bearing (PWB) or non-weight bearing (NWB). **Partial weight bearing** means the resident is able to support some weight on one or both legs. **Non-weight bearing** means the resident is unable to support any weight on one or both legs. **Full weight bearing** (FWB) means that one or both legs can bear 100 percent of the body weight on a step. Assist resident as needed with cane, walker, or crutches.

G Never perform range of motion exercises on a leg on the side of a hip replacement unless directed by the nurse.

G Caution the resident not to sit with his or her legs crossed or turn toes inward. The hip cannot be bent or flexed more than 90 degrees. It cannot be turned inward or outward (Fig. 18-8).

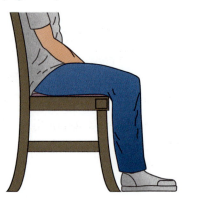

Fig. 18-8. The hip must maintain a 90-degree angle in the sitting position.

G When preparing to transfer the resident from the bed, a pillow should be used between the thighs to keep the legs separated. The head

of the bed can be raised to allow the resident to move her legs over the side of the bed with the thighs still separated. It is better to transfer from the bed on the side where the unaffected hip is so that the strong side leads in standing, pivoting, and sitting.

G With chair or toilet transfers, the operative leg/knee should be straightened. The strong leg should stand first (with a walker or crutches) before bringing the foot of the affected leg back to the walking position.

Observing and Reporting:
Hip Replacement

Report any of these to the nurse:

O/R If the incision or area around it is red, draining, bleeding, or warm

O/R An increase in pain

O/R Numbness or tingling

O/R Abnormal vital signs, especially change in temperature

O/R If the resident cannot use equipment properly and safely

O/R If the resident is not following doctor's orders for activity and exercise

O/R Any problems with appetite

O/R Increasing strength and improving ability to walk

A cast or traction may also be used to immobilize a fractured hip. Traction helps to immobilize a fractured bone, relieve pressure, and lessen muscle spasms due to injury. A resident in traction will require special care.

If traction is used, the traction assembly must never be disconnected. Keep the weights off the floor and do not add or remove weights. Keep the resident in good alignment. Good skin care and repositioning according to the care plan are essential for all residents who are immobilized. Skin will rapidly deteriorate over pressure points. Perform range of motion exercises as directed. Report to the nurse if the resident complains of pain, numbness or tingling, or burning. Report if swelling, redness, bleeding or sores are present.

Knee Replacement

Knee replacement is the surgical insertion of a prosthetic knee. A **prosthesis** is a device that replaces a body part that is missing or deformed because of an accident, injury, illness, or birth defect. It is used to improve a person's ability to function and/or to improve appearance. Knee replacement surgery is performed to relieve pain. It also restores motion to a knee damaged by injury or arthritis. It can help stabilize a knee that buckles or gives out repeatedly.

Care is similar to that for the hip replacement, but the recovery time is much shorter. These residents have more ability to care for themselves.

Guidelines:
Caring for Residents Recovering from Knee Replacements

G   To prevent blood clots, apply special stockings as ordered. One type is a compression stocking. It is a plastic, air-filled, sleeve-like device that is applied to the legs and hooked to a machine. This machine inflates and deflates on its own. It acts in the same way that the muscles usually do under normal circumstances. The sleeves are normally applied after surgery while the resident is in bed. Anti-embolic stockings are another type of special stocking. They aid circulation. See later in the chapter for more information on this type of stocking.

G   Perform ankle pumps as ordered. These are simple exercises that promote circulation to the legs. Ankle pumps are done by raising the toes and feet toward the ceiling and lowering them again.

G   Encourage fluids, especially cranberry and orange juices, which contain vitamin C, to prevent urinary tract infections (UTIs).

G   Assist with deep breathing exercises as ordered.

G   Continuous passive motion (CPM) may be ordered after a knee replacement. This is a treatment method using a machine to constantly move the knee through a range of motion (Fig. 18-9). The person does not have to actively help; the machine does the work. CPM can help speed recovery. The goal is to decrease stiffness, increase range of motion and promote healing. The nurse or physical therapist will set the rate and position the resident. You may be asked to stay with the resident while the machine is turned on.

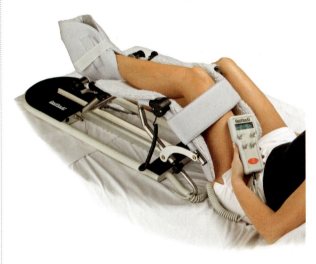

Fig. 18-9. *One type of CPM machine.* (PHOTO COURTESY OF THE MEDCOM GROUP, LTD., 800-231-4276, WWW.MEDCOMGROUP.COM)

G   Ask the nurse to give pain medication prior to moving and positioning if needed.

G   Report to the nurse if you notice redness, swelling, heat, or deep tenderness in one or both calves.

Muscular Dystrophy (MD)

Muscular dystrophy (MD) refers to several progressive diseases that cause a variety of physical disabilities due to muscle weakness. MD is an inherited disease. It causes a gradual wasting of muscle, weakness, and deformity. The muscles of the hands are impaired, and there may be twitching of the hand and arm muscles. Legs may be weak and stiff. The person may be in a wheelchair.

Most forms of MD are present at birth or become apparent during childhood. Many forms of MD are very slow to progress. Often people with MD can live to middle or even late adulthood.

In the early stages of this disease, help with ADLs or range of motion exercises. In the more advanced stages, help with skin care and positioning and perform ADLs for the resident.

Amputation

Amputation is the removal of some or all of a body part, usually a foot, hand, arm or leg. Amputation may be the result of an injury or disease. After amputation, some people feel that the limb is still there. They may feel pain in the part that has been amputated. This is called "**phantom sensation.**" It may last for a short time or for several years. The pain or sensation, which is caused by remaining nerve endings, is real. It should not be ignored or ridiculed.

Residents who have had a body part amputated must make many physical, psychological, social, and occupational adjustments. Be supportive. When a body part has been amputated, day-to-day activities may be limited. A resident will need special care to help him adjust to these changes. When the condition is new, a physical and/or occupational therapist may work with the resident.

Assist residents in performing their ADLs. Follow the care plan for care of the prosthesis and the stump. See Chapter 21 for more information on prosthetics and related care.

Complementary or Alternative Health Practices

Many people now use complementary or alternative health practices. **Complementary medicine** refers to treatments that are used in addition to the con-

ventional treatments prescribed by a doctor. **Alternative medicine** refers to practices and treatments used instead of conventional methods. Your residents may use any of the following:

- Chiropractic medicine concentrates on the spine and musculoskeletal system. Chiropractors believe that a misaligned spine can interfere with the body's proper function. Chiropractors do not use drugs or surgery; they use hands-on manipulations, also called adjustments, of the spine or other joints. They also teach exercises and provide nutrition and other health counseling.

  Heat, cold, and muscle stimulation are used to improve function. Chiropractors are frequently consulted for back, neck, and joint pain, as well as for headaches.

- Massage therapy manipulates soft body tissues with touch and pressure and is used to reduce stress and to promote relaxation and pain relief.

- Acupuncture is a very old Chinese healing technique used to restore health, relieve pain, or treat other conditions. Very fine needles are inserted into specific points on the body.

- Homeopathy involves giving small doses of a substance to stimulate the body's ability to heal itself. If given in large doses, the substance would produce symptoms of an illness or the illness itself.

- Herbs and other dietary supplements may be taken for prevention as well as treatment of diseases or conditions. If you know that a resident is taking herbs or supplements, report this to the nurse as some can cause serious problems if taken with certain medications.

If residents are using complementary or alternative medicine, do not make judgments about their treatment or discuss your opinions. Do not make recommendations about these methods. If you have concerns, talk to the charge nurse.

3. Describe common diseases and disorders of the nervous system

Chapter 19 has information on dementia and Alzheimer's disease. Dementia and Alzheimer's disease are common disorders of the nervous system.

CVA or Stroke

As you learned in Chapters 4 and 7, the medical term for a stroke is a cerebrovascular accident, or CVA. CVA, or stroke, is caused when the blood supply to the brain is cut off suddenly by a clot or a ruptured blood vessel. Without blood, part of the brain gets no oxygen. This causes brain cells to die. Brain tissue is further damaged by leaking blood, clots, and swelling. These cause pressure on surrounding areas of healthy tissue. Strokes can be mild or severe.

Afterward, a resident may experience paralysis, weakness, inability to speak or understand words, trouble swallowing, and loss of bowel or bladder control. Review Chapter 4 for a more comprehensive list of how a CVA may affect a person.

The two sides of the brain control different functions. Symptoms that a person experiences depend on which side of the brain the CVA affected. Weaknesses on the right side show that the left side of the brain was affected. Weaknesses on the left side show that the right side of the brain was affected.

If the stroke was mild, the resident may experience few, if any, of complications. Physical therapy may help regain physical abilities. Speech and occupational therapy can also help a person learn to communicate and perform ADLs again.

Guidelines:
Residents Recovering from Stroke

G   Residents with paralysis, weakness, or loss of movement will usually have physical or occupational therapy. You may be asked to assist residents in performing exercises. Range of motion exercises will help strengthen muscles and keep joints mobile. Residents may also perform leg exercises to aid circulation. Safety is always important when post-CVA residents are exercising.

G   Never refer to the weaker side as the "bad side." Do not talk about the "bad" leg or arm. Use the terms "weaker" or "involved" to refer to the side with paralysis or paresis.

G   Residents with speech loss or communication problems may receive speech therapy. You may be asked to help. This includes helping residents recognize written words, as well as helping them to speak. Speech therapists will also evaluate a resident's swallowing ability. They will decide if therapy or thickened liquids are needed.

G   Use verbal and nonverbal communication to express your positive attitude. Let the resident know you have confidence in his or her abilities through smiles, touches, and gestures. Gestures and pointing can also help you convey information or allow the resident to speak to you. More ideas for communicating with residents recovering from stroke are listed in Chapter 4.

G   Experiencing confusion or memory loss is upsetting. People often cry for no apparent reason after suffering a stroke. Be patient and understanding. Your positive attitude will be important. Keeping a routine may help residents feel more secure.

G   Encourage independence and self-esteem. Let the resident do things for him- or herself whenever possible, even if you could do a better or faster job. Make tasks less difficult for the resident to do. Appreciate and acknowledge residents' efforts to do things for themselves even when they are unsuccessful. Praise even the smallest successes to build confidence.

G   Always check on the resident's body alignment. Sometimes an arm or leg can be caught and the resident is unaware.

G   Pay special attention to skin care and observe for changes in the skin if a resident is unable to move.

G If residents have a loss of touch or sensation, check for potentially harmful situations (for example, heat and sharp objects). If residents are unable to sense or move a part of the body, assist with changing positions to prevent pressure sores.

G Adapt procedures when caring for residents with one-sided paralysis or weakness. Carefully assist with shaving, grooming, and bathing. Diminished sensation or paralysis causes lack of awareness about such things as water temperature and sharpness of razors. Take care so that injury does not occur.

When assisting with transfers or walking, remember the following:

G Always use a gait belt for safety.

G Stand on the weaker side. Support the weaker (involved) side.

G Lead with the stronger (uninvolved) side (Fig. 18-10).

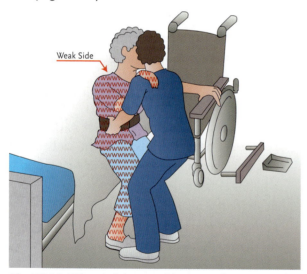

Weak Side

Fig. 18-10. When helping a resident transfer, support the weak side while leading with the stronger side.

When assisting with dressing, remember the following:

G Dress the weaker side first. Place the weaker arm or leg into the clothing first. This prevents unnecessary bending and stretching of the limb. Undress the stronger side first,

and then remove the weaker arm or leg from clothing to prevent the limb from being stretched and twisted.

G Use assistive equipment to help the resident dress himself (see Chapters 13 and 21). Encourage self-care.

When assisting with eating, remember the following:

G Place food in the resident's field of vision.

G Use assistive devices such as silverware with built-up handle grips, plate guards, and drinking cups.

G Watch for signs of choking.

G Serve soft foods if swallowing is difficult.

G Always place food in the unaffected, or non-paralyzed, side of the mouth.

G Make sure food is swallowed before offering more bites.

Home Care Focus

Monitoring the home safety of clients who have had a stroke is essential. Clients who are unsteady, weak, or confused are at risk of falling. Clients with loss of sensation are at risk of burning themselves in the bathroom or at the stove. Some safety tips include:

• Remove any hazards from the home, including unnecessary clutter or throw rugs.

• Unplug appliances like toasters and coffee makers when not in use.

• Check the refrigerator and cabinets for spoiled food. A stroke may impair the senses of smell and taste.

• Report any suspected safety hazards to your supervisor.

See Chapters 4 and 7 for more information on CVA.

Parkinson's Disease

Parkinson's disease is a progressive disease. It causes a section of the brain to degenerate, and it affects the muscles, causing them to become stiff. In addition, it causes stooped posture and a shuffling gait, or walk. It can also cause pill-rolling. This is a circular movement of the tips of the thumb and the index finger when brought together, which looks like rolling a pill. Tremors or shaking make it hard for a person to perform ADLs such as eating and bathing. A person with Parkinson's may have a mask-like facial expression.

Guidelines:
Parkinson's Disease

G Residents are at a high risk for falls. Protect residents from any unsafe areas and conditions.

G Help with ADLs as needed.

G Assist with range of motion exercises exactly as ordered to prevent contractures and to strengthen muscles (Fig. 18-11).

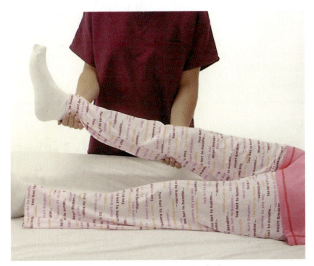

Fig. 18-11. Range of motion exercises help prevent contractures, strengthen muscles, and increase circulation.

G Encourage self-care. Be patient with self-care and communication. Allow the resident time to do and say things. Listen.

Multiple Sclerosis (MS)

Multiple sclerosis (MS) is a progressive disease that affects the central nervous system. When a person has MS, the protective covering for the nerves, spinal cord, and white matter of the brain breaks down over time. Without this covering, or sheath, nerves cannot send messages to and from the brain in a normal way.

Residents with MS have varying abilities. Multiple sclerosis is usually diagnosed when a person is in his or her early twenties to thirties. It progresses slowly and unpredictably. Symptoms include blurred vision, fatigue, tremors, poor balance, and trouble walking. Weakness, numbness, tingling, incontinence, and behavior changes are also symptoms. MS can cause blindness, contractures, and loss of function in the arms and legs (Fig. 18-12).

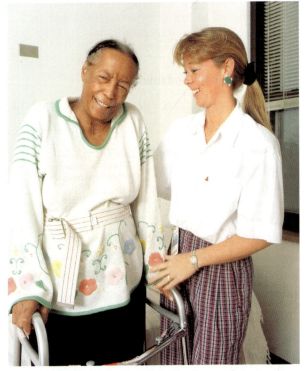

Fig. 18-12. MS is an unpredictable disease that causes varying symptoms and impairments. MS can cause a range of problems, including fatigue, poor balance, and trouble walking.

Guidelines:
Multiple Sclerosis

G Assist with ADLs as needed.

G Be patient with self-care and movement.

G Allow enough time for tasks. Offer rest periods as necessary.

G   Give resident plenty of time to communicate. People with MS may have trouble forming their thoughts. Be patient. Do not rush him or her.

G   Prevent falls, which may due to a lack of coordination, fatigue, or vision problems.

G   Stress can worsen the effects of MS. Be calm. Listen to residents when they want to talk.

G   Encourage a healthy diet with plenty of fluids.

G   Give excellent skin care to prevent pressure sores.

G   Assist with range of motion exercises exactly as ordered to prevent contractures and to strengthen muscles.

Head and Spinal Cord Injuries

Diving, sports injuries, falls, car and motorcycle accidents, industrial accidents, war, and criminal violence are common causes of injuries. Problems from these injuries range from mild confusion or memory loss to coma, paralysis, and death.

Head injuries can cause permanent brain damage. Residents who have had a head injury may have the following problems: mental retardation; personality changes; breathing problems; seizures; coma; memory loss; loss of consciousness; paresis; and paralysis. Paresis is paralysis, or loss of ability, that affects only part of the body. Often, paresis describes a weakness or loss of ability on one side of the body.

The effects of spinal cord injuries depend on the force of impact and the location of the injury. The higher the injury, the greater the loss of function is. People with spinal cord injuries may have **paraplegia**, or loss of function of lower body and legs. These injuries may also cause **quadriplegia**, in which the person is then unable to use his legs, trunk, and arms (Fig. 18-13).

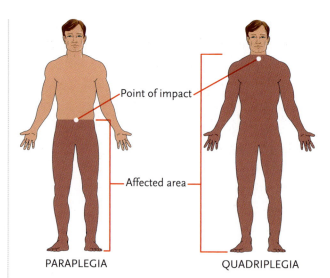

Point of impact

Affected area

PARAPLEGIA   QUADRIPLEGIA

Fig. 18-13. *Loss of function depends on where the spine is injured.*

Rehabilitation is needed for residents with spinal cord injuries. It will help them maintain muscle function and to live as independently as possible. Residents will need emotional support as they adjust to their disability. Their specific needs will vary.

Guidelines:
Head or Spinal Cord Injury

G   Give emotional support, as well as physical help. Frustration and anger may surface as residents with these injuries deal with the reality of their lives. Do not take it personally.

G   Be patient with all care.

G   Safety is very important. Be very careful that residents do not fall or burn themselves. Because these residents have no sensation, they are unable to feel a burn.

G   Be patient with self-care. Allow as much independence as possible with ADLs.

G   Give good skin care. It is needed to prevent pressure sores when mobility is limited.

G   Assist residents to change positions at least every two hours to prevent pressure sores. Be gentle when turning and repositioning.

G   Perform passive range of motion exercises exactly as ordered to prevent contractures and to strengthen muscles.

G   Immobility leads to constipation. Encourage fluids and a high-fiber diet, if ordered.

G   Loss of control of urination may lead to the need for a urinary catheter. Urinary tract infections are common. Encourage a high intake of fluids and give extra catheter care as needed.

G   Lack of activity leads to poor circulation and fatigue. Offer rest periods as necessary. You may be directed to use special stockings to help increase circulation.

G   Difficulty coughing and shallow breathing can lead to pneumonia. Encourage deep breathing exercises as ordered.

G   Male residents may have involuntary erections, which may cause them to feel embarrassed. These are not deliberate. Provide for privacy and be sensitive to this.

G   Assist with bowel and bladder training if needed.

Epilepsy

Epilepsy is an illness of the brain that causes seizures. Epileptic seizures can be mild tremors, brief blackouts, or violent convulsions lasting several minutes. The cause of most cases of epilepsy is unknown. Excessive alcohol use, substance abuse, brain tumors, or injuries may be factors.

During a seizure, the main goal of the caregiver is to make the resident safe. Moving furniture away can help prevent injury. A pillow can be placed under the resident's head. Do not try to restrain the resident or force anything between his teeth because you could be bitten. Notice the time a seizure begins so that you can report the length of the seizure.

Vision Impairment

You first learned about vision impairment in Chapter 4. Vision impairment can affect people of all ages. Some vision impairment causes people to wear corrective lenses, such as eyeglasses or contact lenses (Figs. 18-14 and 18-15). Some people need eyeglasses all the time. Others only need them to read or for things such as driving that require seeing distant objects.

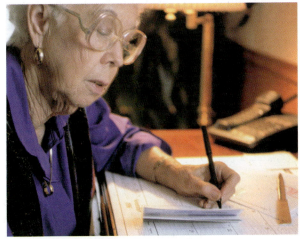

Fig. 18-14. Nearsightedness (the ability to see objects nearby better than objects in the distance) and farsightedness (the ability to see objects in the distance better than objects nearby) are often corrected by the use of eyeglasses.

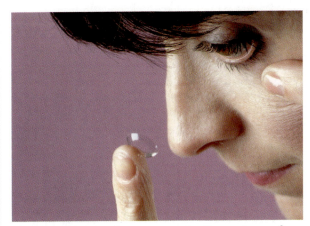

Fig. 18-15. Contact lenses are made of many types of plastic. Some can be worn and disposed of daily. Others are worn for longer periods.

People over the age of 40 are at risk for developing certain serious vision problems. These include cataracts, glaucoma, and blindness. When a **cataract** develops, the lens of the eye becomes cloudy. This prevents light from entering the eye (Fig. 18-16). Vision blurs and dims initially. All vision is eventually lost. This disease can occur in one or both eyes. It is corrected with surgery, in which a permanent lens is usually implanted.

Glaucoma is a disease that causes the pressure in the eye to increase. This eventually damages the retina and the optic nerve. It causes blindness. Glaucoma can occur suddenly, causing severe pain, nausea, and vomiting. It can also occur gradually. Symptoms include blurred vision, tunnel vision, and blue-green halos around lights. Glaucoma is treated with medication and sometimes surgery.

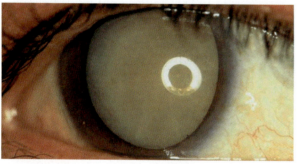

Fig. 18-16. When a cataract develops, the lens of the eye becomes cloudy. This prevents light from entering the eye.

Braille

For residents who are visually impaired, books on tape, large-print books, and Braille books are available. Braille is a system of writing for the blind using raised dots, which was developed by Louis Braille (1809-1852). Each letter is represented as a raised pattern that can be read by touching with the fingers (Fig. 18-17). Reading Braille takes a long time and requires special training.

hello	help
yes	no

Fig. 18-17. Examples of words in Braille.

See Chapter 4 for information on assisting residents with vision and hearing impairments.

4. Describe common diseases and disorders of the cardiovascular system

Hypertension (HTN) or High Blood Pressure

When blood pressure is consistently 140/90 or higher, a person is diagnosed as having hypertension, or high blood pressure. If blood pressure is between 120/80 and 139/89 mmHg, it is called prehypertension. This means that the person does not have high blood pressure now but is likely to develop it in the future.

Hypertension may be caused by **atherosclerosis**, or a hardening and narrowing of the blood vessels (Fig. 18-18). It can also result from kidney disease, tumors of the adrenal gland, and complications of pregnancy. Hypertension can develop in persons of any age.

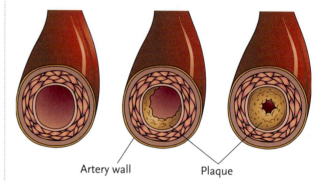

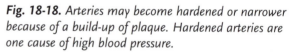
Artery wall   Plaque

Fig. 18-18. Arteries may become hardened or narrower because of a build-up of plaque. Hardened arteries are one cause of high blood pressure.

Signs and symptoms of high blood pressure are not always obvious. This is especially true in the early stages. Often it is only discovered when a blood pressure measurement is taken. Persons with the disease may complain of headaches, blurred vision, and dizziness.

Guidelines:
Hypertension

G   High blood pressure can lead to serious conditions such as CVA, heart attack, kidney disease, or blindness. Treatment to control it is vital. Residents may take diuretics or medication that lowers cholesterol. Diuretics are drugs that reduce fluid in the body.

G Residents may also have a prescribed exercise program or be on a low-fat, low-sodium diet. You may need to take blood pressure measurements often. You can also help by encouraging residents to follow their diet and exercise programs.

Coronary Artery Disease (CAD)

Coronary artery disease occurs when the blood vessels in the coronary arteries narrow. This lowers the supply of blood to the heart muscle and deprives it of oxygen and nutrients. Over time, as fatty deposits block the artery, the muscle that was supplied by the blood vessel dies. CAD can lead to heart attack or stroke.

The heart muscle that is not getting enough oxygen causes chest pain, pressure, or discomfort, called **angina pectoris**. The heart needs more oxygen during exercise, stress, excitement, or a heavy meal. In CAD, narrow blood vessels prevent the extra blood with oxygen from getting to the heart (Fig. 18-19).

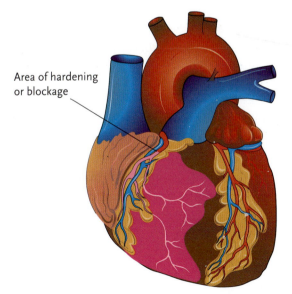

Area of hardening or blockage

Fig. 18-19. Angina pectoris results from the heart not getting enough oxygen.

The pain of angina pectoris is usually described as pressure or tightness in the left side or the center of the chest behind the sternum or breast-

bone. Some people have pain extending down the inside of the left arm or to the neck and left side of the jaw. A person suffering from angina pectoris may perspire or look pale. The person may feel dizzy and have trouble breathing.

Risk factors for getting CAD include increasing age, gender (men are more likely to get CAD than women), family history of heart disease, tobacco use, high cholesterol, high blood pressure, lack of activity, obesity, and diabetes.

Guidelines:
Angina Pectoris

G Rest is extremely important. Rest reduces the heart's need for extra oxygen. It helps the blood flow return to normal, often within three to fifteen minutes.

G Medication is also needed to relax the walls of the coronary arteries. This allows them to open and get more blood to the heart. This medication, **nitroglycerin**, is a small tablet that the resident places under the tongue. There it dissolves and is rapidly absorbed. Residents with angina pectoris may keep nitroglycerin on hand to use as soon as symptoms arise. Nursing assistants are not allowed to give any medication unless they have had special training. Tell the nurse if a resident needs help taking the medication. Nitroglycerin is also available as a patch. Do not remove the patch. Tell the nurse immediately if the patch comes off. Nitroglycerin may also come in the form of a spray that the resident sprays onto or under the tongue.

G Residents may also need to avoid heavy meals, overeating, intense exercise, and cold or hot and humid weather.

Myocardial Infarction (MI) or Heart Attack

When blood flow to the heart muscle is blocked, oxygen and nutrients fail to reach cells in that region (Fig. 18-20). Waste products are not removed and the muscle cells die. This is called a

myocardial infarction, or MI, or heart attack. The area of dead tissue may be large or small, depending on the artery involved. A myocardial infarction is an emergency that can result in serious heart damage or death. See Chapter 7 for warning signs of an MI.

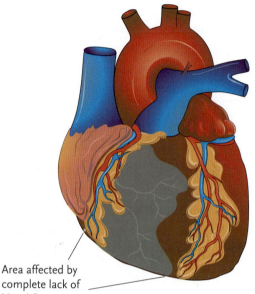

Area affected by complete lack of blood flow

Fig. 18-20. A heart attack occurs when the blood flow to the heart or a portion of the heart is cut off.

Guidelines:
Myocardial Infarction

G Generally, residents who have had an MI will be placed on a regular exercise program.

G Residents may be on a diet that is low in fat and cholesterol and/or a low-sodium diet.

G Medications may be used to regulate heart rate and blood pressure.

G Quitting smoking will be encouraged.

G A stress management program may be started to help reduce stress levels.

G Residents recovering from a heart attack may need to avoid exposure to cold temperatures.

Congestive Heart Failure (CHF)

Coronary artery disease, myocardial infarction, high blood pressure, or other disorders may damage the heart. When the heart muscle has been severely damaged, it fails to pump effectively. Blood backs up into the heart instead of circulating. This is called **congestive heart failure**, or CHF. It can occur on one or both sides of the heart.

Signs and symptoms of congestive heart failure include the following:

- Trouble breathing; coughing or gurgling with breathing

- Dizziness, confusion, and fainting

- Pale or blue skin

- Low blood pressure

- Swelling of the feet and ankles (edema)

- Bulging veins in the neck

- Weight gain

Guidelines:
CHF

G Although CHF is a serious illness, it can be treated and controlled. Medications can strengthen the heart muscle and improve its pumping.

G Medications help remove excess fluids. This means more trips to the bathroom. Answer call lights promptly. Keep a portable commode nearby if the resident is weak and has trouble getting out of bed and walking to the bathroom. Assist resident as needed.

G A low-sodium diet or fluid restrictions may be prescribed.

G A weakened heart may make it hard for residents to walk, carry items, or climb stairs. Limited activity or bedrest may be prescribed. Allow for a period of rest after an activity.

G Intake and output of fluids may need to be measured (see Chapter 15).

G   Resident may be weighed daily at the same time to watch for weight gain from fluid retention.

G   Elastic leg stockings may be used to reduce swelling in feet and ankles.

G   Range of motion exercises improve muscle tone when activity and exercise are limited.

G   Extra pillows may help residents who have trouble breathing. Keeping the head of the bed elevated may also help with breathing.

G   Help with personal care and ADLs as needed.

A common side effect of medications for CHF is dizziness. This may result from a lack of potassium. High-potassium foods and drinks such as bananas or raisins, orange juice, or other citrus juices can help. These foods should be eaten as a preventive measure as well. Follow the instructions in the care plan.

Peripheral Vascular Disease (PVD)

Peripheral vascular disease (PVD) is a disease in which the legs, feet, arms, or hands do not have enough blood circulation. This is due to fatty deposits in the blood vessels that harden over time. The legs, feet, arms, and hands feel cool or cold. Nail beds and/or feet become ashen or blue. Swelling occurs in the hands and feet. Ulcers of the legs and feet may develop and can become infected. Pain may be very severe when walking; however, it is usually relieved with rest.

Some changes in health may lead to inactivity. A lack of mobility may contribute to PVD. For some cases of poor circulation to legs and feet, elastic stockings are ordered. These stockings help prevent swelling and blood clots and aid circulation. These stockings are called "anti-embolic hose" or "elastic stockings." They need to be put on before the resident gets out of bed. Follow manufacturer's instructions and illustrations on how to put on stockings.

Putting elastic stockings on a resident

Equipment: elastic stockings

1. Wash your hands.

2. Identify yourself by name. Identify resident by name.

3. Explain procedure to resident. Speak clearly, slowly, and directly. Maintain face-to-face contact whenever possible.

4. Provide for resident's privacy with curtain, screen, or door.

5. With resident lying down, remove his or her socks, shoes, or slippers, and expose one leg.

6. Turn stocking inside out at least to heel area (Fig. 18-21).

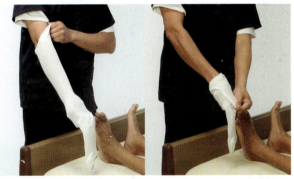

Fig. 18-21. Turning the stocking inside out allows stocking to roll on gently.

7. Gently place the foot of the stocking over toes, foot, and heel (Fig. 18-22). Make sure the heel is in the right place (heel of foot should be in heel of stocking).

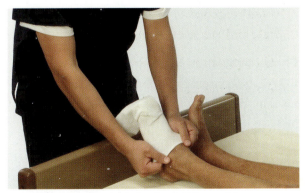

Fig. 18-22. Gently place the foot of the stocking over toes, foot, and heel. Promote the resident's comfort and safety by avoiding force and over-extension of joints.

Common Chronic and Acute Conditions

8. Gently pull the top of stocking over foot, heel, and leg.

9. Make sure there are no twists or wrinkles in stocking after it is applied (Fig. 18-23). It must fit smoothly.

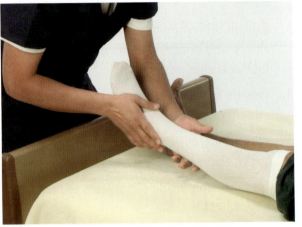

Fig. 18-23. Make stocking smooth. Twists or wrinkles cause the stocking to be too tight, which reduces circulation.

10. Repeat for the other leg.

11. Place call light within resident's reach.

12. Wash your hands.

13. Report any changes in resident to nurse.

14. Document procedure using facility guidelines.

5. Describe common diseases and disorders of the respiratory system

Chronic Obstructive Pulmonary Disease (COPD)

Chronic obstructive pulmonary disease, or **COPD**, is a chronic disease. This means the resident may live for years with it but never be cured. Residents with COPD have trouble breathing, especially in getting air out of the lungs. There are two chronic lung diseases that are grouped under COPD: chronic bronchitis and emphysema.

Bronchitis is an irritation and inflammation of the lining of the bronchi. Chronic bronchitis is a form of bronchitis that is usually caused by cigarette smoking. Symptoms include persistent coughing that brings up sputum (phlegm) and mucus. Breathlessness and wheezing may be present. Treatment includes stopping smoking and possibly medications.

Emphysema is a chronic disease of the lungs that usually results from chronic bronchitis and cigarette smoking. People with emphysema have trouble breathing. Other symptoms are coughing, breathlessness, and a fast heartbeat. There is no cure for emphysema. Treatment includes managing symptoms and pain. Oxygen therapy may be ordered, as well as medications. Quitting smoking is very important.

Over time, a resident with either of these lung disorders becomes chronically ill and weakened. There is a high risk for acute lung infections, such as pneumonia. **Pneumonia** is an illness that can be caused by a bacterial, viral, or fungal infection. Acute inflammation occurs in lung tissue. The affected person develops a high fever, chills, cough, greenish or yellow sputum, chest pains, and rapid pulse. Treatment includes antibiotics, along with plenty of fluids. Recovery from pneumonia may take longer for older adults and persons with chronic illnesses.

When the lungs and brain do not get enough oxygen, all body systems are affected. Residents may have a constant fear of not being able to breathe. This can cause them to sit upright to improve their ability to expand the lungs. These residents can have poor appetites. They usually do not get enough sleep. All of this can add to feelings of weakness and poor health. They may feel they have lost control of their bodies, and particularly their breathing. They may fear suffocation.

Residents with COPD may experience the following symptoms:

• Chronic cough or wheeze

• Difficulty breathing, especially when inhaling and exhaling deeply

- Shortness of breath, especially during physical effort

- Pale or cyanotic skin or reddish-purple skin

- Confusion

- General state of weakness

- Difficulty completing meals due to shortness of breath

- Fear and anxiety

Guidelines:
Caring for Residents with COPD

G Colds or viruses can make residents very ill quickly. Always observe and report signs of symptoms getting worse.

G Help residents sit upright or lean forward. Offer pillows for support (Fig. 18-24).

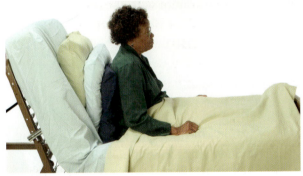

Fig. 18-24. *It helps residents with COPD to sit upright and lean forward slightly.*

G Offer plenty of fluids and small, frequent meals.

G Encourage a well-balanced diet.

G Keep oxygen supply available as ordered.

G Being unable to breathe or fearing suffocation is very frightening. Be calm, reassuring, and supportive.

G Use good infection control, especially with handwashing by the resident and the disposal of used tissues.

G Encourage as much independence with ADLs as possible.

G Remind residents to avoid situations where they may be exposed to infections, especially colds and the flu. Ensure that residents always have help ready, especially in case of a breathing crisis.

G Encourage pursed-lip breathing. Pursed-lip breathing is placing the lips as if kissing and taking controlled breaths. A nurse should teach residents how to do this type of breathing.

G Encourage residents to save energy for important tasks. Encourage residents to rest during tasks.

Observing and Reporting:
COPD

Report any of the following to the nurse:

O/R Temperature over 101°F

O/R Changes in breathing patterns, including shortness of breath

O/R Changes in color or consistency of lung secretions

O/R Changes in mental state or personality

O/R Refusal to take medications as ordered

O/R Excessive weight loss

O/R Increasing dependence upon caregivers and family

Asthma

Asthma is a chronic inflammatory disease. It occurs when the respiratory system is hyper-reactive (that is, reacts quickly and strongly) to irritants, infection, cold air, or to allergens such as pollen and dust. Exercise and stress can also bring on asthma attacks. The bronchi become irritated. They constrict, making it difficult to breathe. As a response to irritation and inflammation, the mucous membrane produces thick mucus. This further inhibits respiration. As a result, air is trapped in the lungs, causing coughing and wheezing (Fig. 18-25).

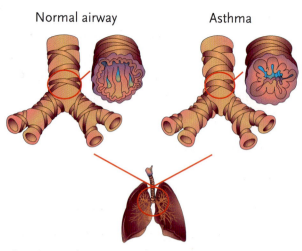

Normal airway   Asthma

Fig. 18-25. *When a person has asthma, air passages in the lungs become inflamed and swollen.*

The exact cause of asthma is unknown. It may be caused by a combination of factors, such as family history and certain environmental exposures. Treatment for asthma includes medications that are given directly into the lungs using sprays or inhalers (Fig. 18-26). Residents with asthma should avoid triggers that bring on asthma attacks, such as allergens, smoke, strong odors, and strenuous exercise.

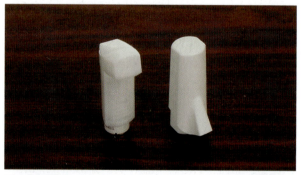

Fig. 18-26. *People with asthma should carry their inhalers with them at all times.*

Bronchiectasis

Bronchiectasis is a condition in which the bronchial tubes are abnormally enlarged. A person may have it in childhood or may acquire it later in life as a result of chronic infections and inflammation. Cystic fibrosis is a common cause of bronchiectasis. This abnormal state of the bronchial tubes is permanent. Bronchiec-

tasis causes chronic coughing, which produces thick white or green sputum. A person with this disorder may have recurrent pneumonia and weight loss.

Treatment of bronchiectasis includes controlling infections and preventing complications. Antibiotics may be prescribed. Postural drainage may be ordered to eliminate fluid from the lungs. Postural drainage involves using different body positions to drain mucus from the lungs or to loosen it so that it can be coughed up.

Upper Respiratory Infection (URI)

Upper respiratory infection (URI) is commonly called a cold. It is the result of a bacterial or viral infection of the nose, sinuses, and throat. Symptoms usually include nasal discharge, sneezing, sore throat, fever, and fatigue. For most people, it can be dealt with by the body's immune system with the help of rest and extra fluids. Antibiotics may be required if the infection is bacterial.

Lung Cancer

Lung cancer is the development of abnormal cells or tumors in the lungs. Symptoms of lung cancer include chronic cough, shortness of breath, and bloody sputum. You will learn more about cancer and treatment later in the chapter.

Tuberculosis (TB)

Tuberculosis (TB) is a highly contagious lung disease. Symptoms include coughing, low-grade fever, shortness of breath, weight loss, and fatigue. Chapter 5 includes more information about tuberculosis, care guidelines, and treatment.

For residents with TB, you may need to collect a sputum specimen. Sputum is thick mucus coughed up from the lungs. It is not the same as saliva, which comes from the mouth. People with colds or respiratory illnesses may cough up large amounts of sputum. Sputum specimens may help diagnose respiratory problems, illness, or evaluate the effects of medication.

Early morning is the best time to collect sputum. The resident should cough up the sputum and spit it directly into the specimen container. Because sputum may be infectious, do not let the resident cough on you. Standing behind the resident during the collection process may prevent sputum from coming into contact with you. Wear the proper PPE when collecting sputum. The required PPE is gloves and, sometimes, a mask. Follow Standard Precautions. Make sure that both your hands and the specimen container are clean before beginning this procedure.

Collecting a sputum specimen

Equipment: specimen container and lid with label (labeled with resident's name, room number, date and time), tissues, plastic bag, gloves, mask

1. Wash your hands.

2. Identify yourself by name. Identify resident by name.

3. Explain procedure to resident. Speak clearly, slowly, and directly. Maintain face-to-face contact whenever possible.

4. Provide for resident's privacy with curtain, screen, or door.

5. Put on mask and gloves. If the resident has known or suspected TB or another infectious disease, wear a mask when collecting a sputum specimen. Coughing is one way TB droplets can enter the air. Stand behind the resident if the resident can hold the specimen container by himself.

6. Ask the resident to cough deeply, so that sputum comes up from the lungs. To prevent the spread of infectious material, give the resident tissues to cover his or her mouth. Ask the resident to spit the sputum into the container.

7. When you have obtained a good sample (about two tablespoons of sputum), cover the container tightly. Wipe any sputum off the outside of the container with tissues. Discard the tissues. Put the container in the plastic bag and seal the bag.

8. Remove and dispose of gloves and mask.

9. Wash your hands.

10. Place call light within resident's reach.

11. Report any changes in resident to the nurse.

12. Document procedure using facility guidelines.

6. Describe common diseases and disorders of the endocrine system

Diabetes

In **diabetes mellitus**, commonly called diabetes, the pancreas does not produce enough or properly use insulin. **Insulin** is a hormone that converts **glucose**, or natural sugar, into energy for the body. Without insulin to process glucose, these sugars collect in the blood. This causes problems with circulation and can damage vital organs.

Diabetes is common in people with a family history of the illness, in the elderly, and in people who are obese. Two major types of diabetes are:

1. **Type 1 diabetes** is usually diagnosed in children and young adults. It was formerly known as juvenile diabetes because it most often appears before age 20. However, a person can develop Type 1 diabetes up to age 40. In Type 1 diabetes, the body does not produce enough insulin. The condition will continue throughout a person's life. Type 1 diabetes is treated with insulin and a special diet.

2. **Type 2 diabetes**, also known as adult-onset diabetes, is the most common form of diabetes.

In Type 2 diabetes, either the body does not produce enough insulin, or the body fails to properly use insulin. This is known as "insulin resistance." Type 2 diabetes usually develops slowly and is the milder form of diabetes. It typically develops after age 35. The risk of getting this type increases with age. However, the number of children with Type 2 diabetes is growing rapidly. Type 2 diabetes often occurs in obese people or those with a family history of the disease. Type 2 diabetes can usually be controlled with diet and/or oral medications.

Pre-diabetes occurs when a person's blood glucose levels are above normal but not high enough for a diagnosis of Type 2 diabetes. Research indicates that some damage to the body, especially to the heart and circulatory system, may already be occurring during pre-diabetes.

Pregnant women who have never had diabetes before but who have high blood sugar (glucose) levels during pregnancy are said to have **gestational diabetes**.

People with diabetes mellitus may have these signs and symptoms (Fig. 18-27):

- Excessive thirst

- Extreme hunger

- Frequent urination

- Weight loss

- High levels of blood sugar

- Sugar in the urine

- Sudden vision changes

- Tingling or numbness in hands or feet

- Feeling very tired much of the time

- Very dry skin

- Sores that are slow to heal

- More infections than usual

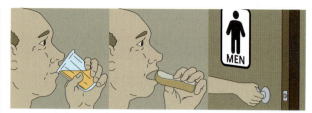

Fig. 18-27. Increased thirst, hunger, and urination are all symptoms of diabetes.

Diabetes can lead to further complications:

- Changes in the circulatory system can cause heart attack and stroke, reduced circulation, poor wound healing, and kidney and nerve damage.

- Damage to the eyes can cause vision loss and blindness.

- Poor circulation and impaired wound healing may cause leg and foot ulcers, infected wounds, and gangrene. Gangrene can lead to amputation.

- Insulin reaction and diabetic ketoacidosis can be serious complications of diabetes. See Chapter 7 for signs and symptoms of each.

Diabetes must be carefully controlled to prevent complications and severe illness. When working with people with diabetes, follow care plan instructions carefully.

Guidelines:
Diabetes

G Follow diet instructions exactly. The intake of carbohydrates, including breads, potatoes, grains, pasta, and sugars, must be regulated. Meals must be eaten at the same time each day. The resident must eat all that is served. If a resident will not eat what is served, or if you suspect that he or she is not following the diet, tell the nurse. More information on diabetic diets is found in Chapter 15.

G Encourage the resident to follow his or her exercise program. A regular exercise program is important. This may include 30 to 60 minutes of activity on most days of the week. Exercise affects how quickly bodies use food. Exercise also improves circulation. Exercise may include walking or other active exercise (Fig. 18-28). It may also include passive range of motion exercises. Help with exercises as necessary. Be positive and try to make it fun and appealing.

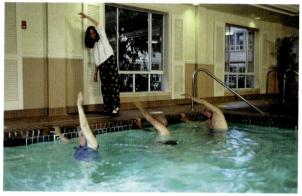

Fig. 18-28. *Exercise is very important for diabetic residents. It helps to increase circulation and maintain a healthy weight.*

G Observe the resident's management of insulin. Doses are calculated exactly. They are given at the same time each day. Nursing assistants should know when residents take insulin and when their meals should be served. There must be a balance between the insulin level and food intake. Unless you have had special training, you will not inject insulin.

G Perform urine and blood tests only as directed (Fig. 18-29). A fingerstick blood glucose test is one type of blood test that may be used to check blood sugar. This is a simple test that is performed by quickly piercing the fingertip, then placing the blood on a chemically active disposable strip. The strip will indicate the result. Sometimes the care plan will specify a daily blood or urine test for insulin levels. Not all states allow you to do this. Know your state's rules. Your facility will train you if you need to do these tests. Perform tests only as directed and allowed.

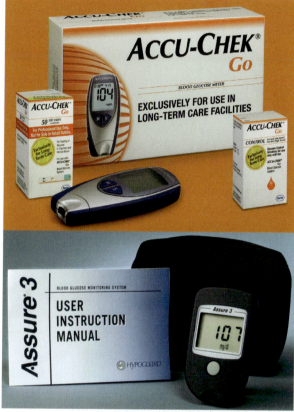

Fig. 18-29. *There are different types of equipment to measure glucose levels in the blood.* (REPRINTED WITH PERMISSION OF BRIGGS CORPORATION, 800-247-2343, WWW.BRIGGSCORP.COM)

G Perform foot care as directed. Diabetics have poor circulation. Because of this, even a small sore on the leg or foot can grow into a large wound. It can require amputation. Careful foot care, including regular, daily inspection, is vital. The goals of diabetic foot care are to check for irritation or sores, to promote blood circulation, and to prevent infection (Fig. 18-30).

G Encourage diabetics to wear comfortable, well-fitting leather shoes that do not hurt their feet. Leather shoes breathe and help to prevent build-up of moisture. To avoid injuries to the feet, diabetics should never go barefoot. Cotton socks are best to absorb sweat. You should never trim or clip any resident's toenails, but especially not a diabetic's toenails. Only a nurse or doctor should do this.

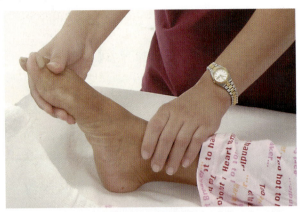

Fig. 18-30. Observe the legs and feet carefully when giving care. Poor circulation can increase the risk of infection and the loss of toes, feet, or legs to gangrene.

Observing and Reporting:
Diabetes

Report any of these to the nurse:

- O/R Skin breakdown
- O/R Change in appetite (person overeating or not eating enough)
- O/R Increased thirst
- O/R Change in urine output
- O/R Nausea or vomiting
- O/R Weight changes
- O/R Change in mental status
- O/R Irritability
- O/R Nervousness or anxiety
- O/R Feeling faint or dizzy
- O/R Visual changes
- O/R Change in mobility
- O/R Change in sensation
- O/R Sweet or fruity breath
- O/R Numbness or tingling in arms or legs

Providing foot care for the diabetic resident

Equipment: basin of warm water (water temperature should be no more than 105° F), mild soap, washcloth, soft towel, lotion, cotton socks, shoes or slippers, gloves

Support the foot and ankle throughout procedure.

1. Wash your hands.

2. Identify yourself by name. Identify resident by name.

3. Explain procedure to resident. Speak clearly, slowly, and directly. Maintain face-to-face contact whenever possible.

4. Provide for resident's privacy with curtain, screen, or door.

5. Put on gloves.

6. Using the washcloth and soap, wash the feet gently. Rinse with the warm water.

7. Pat the feet dry gently, wiping between the toes.

8. Starting at the toes and working up to the ankles, gently rub lotion into the feet with circular strokes. Your goal is to increase circulation, so take several minutes on each foot. Do not put lotion between the toes.

9. Observe the feet, ankles, and legs for dry skin, irritation, blisters, redness, sores, corns, discoloration, or swelling.

10. Help resident put on socks and shoes or slippers.

11. Put soiled linens in appropriate container. Pour water into the toilet. Clean and store basin and supplies.

12. Remove and dispose of gloves.

13. Wash your hands.

14. Place call light within resident's reach.

15. Report any changes in resident to the nurse.

16. Document procedure using facility guidelines.

Hyperthyroidism

When the thyroid produces too much thyroid hormone, the cells burn too much food. Weight loss, nervousness, and hyperactivity occur. This condition is called **hyperthyroidism**. Hyperthyroidism is usually treated with medication. Occasionally, part of the thyroid is surgically removed.

Hypothyroidism

When the thyroid produces too little thyroid hormone, body processes slow down. Weight gain and physical and mental sluggishness result. This condition is called **hypothyroidism**. Hypothyroidism is sometimes treated with medication.

7. Describe common diseases and disorders of the reproductive system

Sexually Transmitted Diseases (STDs) and Infections (STIs)

Sexually transmitted diseases (STDs), also called venereal diseases, are diseases passed through sexual contact with an infected person. This contact includes sexual intercourse, contact of the mouth with the genitals or anus, and contact of the hands to the genitals. A person may be infected, and may potentially infect others, without showing signs of the disease. This is called a **sexually transmitted infection (STI)**.

Using latex condoms during sexual contact can reduce the chances of being infected with or passing on some STDs and STIs. The human immunodeficiency virus (HIV), acquired immune deficiency syndrome (AIDS), and some kinds of hepatitis can be sexually transmitted. (HIV/AIDS is discussed in detail in the next learning objective.) STDs are very common. They can cause serious health problems. Residents may be unaware of or embarrassed by symptoms of an STD.

Chlamydia infection is caused by organisms in the mucous membranes of the reproductive tract. Chlamydia can cause serious infection, including pelvic inflammatory disease (PID) in women. PID can cause sterility. Signs of chlamydia infection are yellow or white discharge from the penis or vagina and burning with urination. It is treated with antibiotics.

Syphilis can be treated effectively in the early stages, but if left untreated, it can cause brain damage, mental illness, and even death. Babies born to mothers with syphilis may be born blind or with other serious birth defects. Syphilis is easier to detect in men than in women. This is due to open sores called **chancres** that form on the penis soon after infection.

The chancres are painless and can go unnoticed. If untreated, the infection spreads to the heart, brain, and other vital organs. Common symptoms at this stage include rash, sore throat, or fever. When detected, syphilis can be treated with penicillin or other antibiotics. The sooner it is treated, the better the chances of preventing long-term damage and avoiding infection of others.

Gonorrhea, like syphilis, can be treated with antibiotics and is easier to detect in men than in women. If untreated, gonorrhea can cause sterility in both men and women. Most women with gonorrhea show no early symptoms. This makes it easy for women to spread the disease. Men with gonorrhea will often show a greenish or yellowish discharge from the penis within a week after infection. Burning with urination is another common symptom in men.

Herpes simplex 2, unlike the other STDs discussed here, is caused by a virus. It cannot be treated with antibiotics. Once infected with the herpes virus, a person cannot be cured. The person may have repeated outbreaks of the disease for the rest of his or her life. A herpes outbreak includes burning, painful, red sores on the genitals. These heal in about two weeks. The sores are infectious, but a person with herpes virus can also spread the infection when sores are not present.

Some people infected with herpes never have repeated outbreaks. The later episodes may not be as painful as the first outbreak. Antiviral drugs can help people stay symptom-free longer. Babies born to women infected with herpes simplex 2 can be infected during birth. Pregnant women experiencing a herpes outbreak are usually delivered by cesarean section, or C-section.

Benign Prostatic Hypertrophy

Benign prostatic hypertrophy is a disorder that occurs in men as they age. The prostate becomes enlarged and causes pressure on the urethra. The pressure leads to frequent urination, dribbling of urine, and difficulty in starting the flow of urine. Urinary retention (urine remaining in the bladder) may also occur, causing urinary tract infection. Urine can also back up into the ureters and kidneys, causing damage to these organs. Benign prostatic hypertrophy can be treated with medications or surgery. A test is also available to screen for cancer of the prostate. As men age, they are at increased risk for prostate cancer. Prostate cancer is usually slow-growing and responsive to treatment if detected early.

Vaginitis

Vaginitis is an infection of the vagina. It may be caused by a bacteria, protozoa (one-celled animals), or fungus (yeast). It may also be caused by hormonal changes after menopause. Women who have vaginitis have a white vaginal discharge, accompanied by itching and burning. Report these symptoms to the nurse. Treatment of vaginitis includes oral medications, as well as vaginal gels or creams.

Douches

Putting a solution into the vagina in order to cleanse the vagina, introduce medication to treat an infection or condition, or to relieve

discomfort is called a "**douche**" or a "vaginal irrigation." After the solution is inserted, it is immediately returned out of the vagina.

If you are trained to do so, and depending upon the rules in your state and at your facility, you may be allowed to assist with or give a douche. If trained and allowed to give a douche, follow these guidelines:

Guidelines:
Vaginal Douche

G   Provide plenty of privacy for this procedure. Pull the curtain and close the door.

G   Wear gloves while assisting with this procedure.

G   The woman will be placed in the dorsal recumbent position (Fig. 18-31).

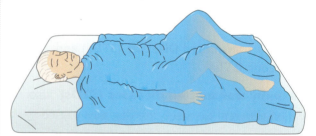

Fig. 18-31. The dorsal recumbent position is when the person is flat on her back with her knees flexed and slightly separated. The feet are flat on bed.

G   Inspect the nozzle or tip of the douche for any breaks, cracks, or rough edges before use. This helps prevent injury to the vagina. If you observe any problems with the nozzle, do not use it, and notify the nurse.

G   Clean the container, tubing, and nozzle before using to prevent infection. Reusable equipment should be washed with hot, soapy water after use.

G   Follow the care plan's instructions to make sure the douche solution is at the right temperature.

G   If using a commercially-prepared douche, follow instructions on the package.

G   Allow some of the solution to run through the tubing to remove air before the tubing is inserted.

G   Do not force the nozzle of the douche into the vagina if you meet resistance. If you are unable to insert the nozzle, stop and notify the nurse.

G   The same amount of douche solution should return as was put into the vagina. The solution should be the same color as before it was inserted. It should be clear with a mild odor.

G   Report any of the following to the nurse:

- Fatigue

- Pain

- Anything unusual about the returned douche solution: amount; color (pink or streaked with red); odor; presence of material, such as mucus or particles

8. Describe common diseases and disorders of the immune and lymphatic systems

HIV and AIDS

Acquired immune deficiency syndrome, or **AIDS**, is an illness caused by the human immunodeficiency virus, or HIV. HIV attacks the body's immune system and gradually disables it. Eventually the HIV-infected person has less resistance to other infections. Death may be the result of these infections. HIV is a sexually-transmitted disease. It is also spread through infected blood, infected needles, or to a fetus from an infected mother.

In general, HIV affects the body in stages. The first stage involves symptoms similar to the flu, with fever, muscle aches, cough, and fatigue. These are symptoms of the immune system fighting the infection. As the infection worsens, the immune system overreacts. It attacks not only the virus, but also normal tissue.

When the virus weakens the immune system in later stages, a group of problems may appear. These include opportunistic infections, tumors, and central nervous system symptoms. These would not occur if the immune system were healthy. This stage of the disease is known as AIDS.

In the late stages of AIDS, damage to the central nervous system may cause memory loss, poor coordination, paralysis, and confusion. These symptoms together are known as **AIDS dementia complex**.

The following are signs and symptoms of HIV infection and AIDS:

- Appetite loss

- Involuntary weight loss of 10 pounds or more

- Vague, flu-like symptoms, including fever, cough, weakness, and severe or constant fatigue

- Night sweats

- Swollen lymph nodes in the neck, underarms, or groin

- Severe diarrhea

- Dry cough

- Skin rashes

- Painful white spots in the mouth or on the tongue

- Cold sores or fever blisters on the lips and flat, white ulcers on a reddened base in the mouth

- Cauliflower-like warts (caused by the human papilloma virus) on the skin and in the mouth

- Inflamed and bleeding gums

- Low resistance to infection, particularly pneumonia, but also tuberculosis, herpes, bacterial infections, and hepatitis

- Bruising that does not go away

- **Kaposi's sarcoma**, a rare form of skin cancer that appears as purple or red skin lesions (Fig. 18-32)

- AIDS dementia complex

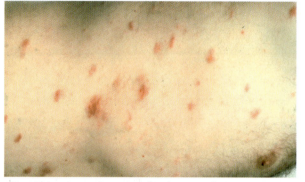

Fig. 18-32. *A purple or red skin lesion called Kaposi's sarcoma can be a sign of AIDS.*

Opportunistic infections, such as pneumonia, tuberculosis, or hepatitis, invade the body when the immune system is weak and cannot defend itself. These illnesses worsen AIDS. They further weaken the immune system. It is difficult to treat these infections. Generally, over time, a person develops a resistance to some antibiotics. These infections often cause death in people with AIDS.

People with HIV are treated with drugs that slow the progress of the disease but do not cure it. The medicines must be taken at precise times. They have many unpleasant side effects. For some people, the medications work less well than for others. Other aspects of HIV treatment are relief of symptoms and prevention and treatment of infection.

Behaviors that put people at high risk for HIV/AIDS infection include the following:

- Sharing drug needles

- Having unprotected sex (not using latex condoms during sexual contact)

- Sexual contact with many partners

- Any sexual activity that involves exchange of body fluids with a partner who has not tested negative for HIV or who has had many sexual partners. Be aware that it may

take six months after contact with the virus for an HIV test to show positive results.

Ways to protect against the spread of HIV and AIDS include the following:

- Never share needles for injections of any type of drug.

- Practice safer sex. Use latex condoms during sexual contact.

- Stay in a monogamous relationship with a partner who has tested negative for HIV. Being monogamous means having only one sexual partner.

- Practice abstinence. Abstinence means not having sexual contact with anyone.

- Get tested if you think you may have been infected with HIV. It can take up to six months from the time you are infected for the antibodies to be detected in your blood. Get re-tested periodically if necessary. It is especially important that pregnant women get tested.

- Follow Standard Precautions at work to protect yourself.

Residents' Rights

Handshakes and Hugs

Understanding the facts about HIV/AIDS is important. This will help you not to feel afraid of a person with this disease. A handshake or a hug cannot spread the AIDS virus. The disease cannot be transmitted by telephones, doorknobs, tables, chairs, toilets, mosquitoes, or by breathing the same air as an infected person. Spend time with residents who have HIV/AIDS. They need the same thoughtful, personal attention you give to all your residents.

Guidelines:
HIV/AIDS

G   People with poor immune systems are more sensitive to infections. Wash your hands often. Follow Standard Precautions. Keep everything clean.

G   Involuntary weight loss occurs in almost all people who develop AIDS. High-protein, high-calorie, and high-nutrient meals can help maintain a healthy weight.

G Some people with HIV/AIDS lose their appetites and have difficulty eating. These residents should be encouraged to relax before meals and to eat in a pleasant setting. Familiar and favorite foods should be served. Report appetite loss or difficulty eating to the nurse. If appetite loss continues to be a problem, the doctor may prescribe an appetite stimulant.

G Residents with infections of the mouth may need food that is low in acid and neither cold nor hot. Spicy seasonings should not be used. Soft or pureed foods may be easier to swallow. Liquid meals and fortified drinks may help ease the pain of chewing. Warm salt water or other rinses may ease the pain of mouth sores. Good mouth care is vital.

G Someone who has nausea or vomiting should eat small, frequent meals, if possible. The person should eat slowly. The person should avoid high-fat and spicy foods, and eat a soft, bland diet. When nausea and vomiting persist, liquids and salty foods should be encouraged. Residents should eat small, frequent meals and drink fluids in between meals. Care must be taken to maintain proper intake of fluids.

G Residents with mild diarrhea may need frequent small meals that are low in fat, fiber, and milk products. If diarrhea is severe, the doctor may order a "BRAT" diet (a diet of bananas, rice, apples, and toast). This diet is helpful for short-term use.

G Diarrhea rapidly depletes the body of fluids. Fluid replacement is necessary. Good rehydration fluids include water, juice, soda, and broth. Caffeinated drinks should be avoided.

G **Neuropathy**, or numbness, tingling, and pain in the feet and legs is usually treated with medication. Going barefoot or wearing loose, soft slippers may be helpful. If blan-

kets cause pain, a bed cradle can keep sheets and blankets from resting on legs and feet (Fig. 18-33).

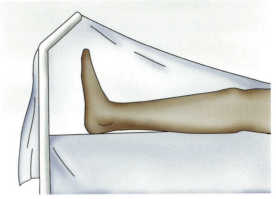

Fig. 18-33. *A bed cradle help keep covers from resting on the feet.*

G Residents with HIV/AIDS may have anxiety and depression. They often suffer the judgments of family, friends, and society. Some people blame them for their illness. People with HIV/AIDS may have tremendous stress. They may feel uncertainty about their illness, health care, and finances. They may also have lost people in their social support network of friends and family. Residents with this disease need support from others. This may come from family, friends, religious and community groups, and support groups, as well as the care team. Treat all your residents with respect. Help give the emotional support they need.

G Withdrawal, apathy, avoidance of tasks, and mental slowness are early symptoms of HIV infection. Medications may also cause side effects of this type. AIDS dementia complex may cause further mental symptoms. There may also be muscle weakness and loss of muscle control, making falls a risk. Residents will need a safe environment and close supervision in their ADLs.

The right to confidentiality is especially important to people with HIV/AIDS. Others may pass judgment on people with this disease. A person with HIV/AIDS cannot be fired because of the disease. However, a healthcare worker with

HIV/AIDS may be reassigned to job duties with a lower risk of transmitting the disease.

HIV testing requires consent. This means no one can test you for HIV unless you agree. HIV test results are confidential. They cannot be shared with a person's family, friends, or employer without his or her consent. If you are HIV-positive, you might want to tell your supervisor. Your tasks can be adjusted to avoid putting you at high risk for exposure to other infections. Everyone has a right to privacy about his or her health status. Never discuss a resident's status with anyone.

Home Care Focus

When working in the home, it is extremely important to carefully follow guidelines for safe food preparation and storage when working with a resident who has HIV/AIDS. Food-borne illnesses caused by improperly cooking or storing food can cause death for someone with HIV/AIDS. (See Chapter 28 for safe food handling practices.) Wash your hands frequently. Keep everything clean, especially countertops, cutting boards, and knives after they have been used to cut meat. Thaw food in the refrigerator, and wash and cook foods thoroughly. When storing food, keep cold foods cold and hot foods hot. Use small containers that seal tightly. Check expiration dates, and remember "when in doubt, throw it out."

Cancer

Cancer is a general term used to describe many types of malignant tumors. A **tumor** is a group of abnormally growing cells. **Benign tumors** are considered non-cancerous. They usually grow slowly in local areas. **Malignant tumors** are cancerous. They grow rapidly and invade surrounding tissues.

Cancer invades local tissue, and can spread to other parts of the body. When it spreads from the site where it first appeared, it can affect other body systems. In general, treatment is more difficult and cancer is more deadly after this has occurred. Cancer often appears first in the breast, colon, rectum, uterus, prostate, lungs, or skin.

There is no known cure for cancer, but some treatments are effective. They are discussed later in the chapter.

Risk factors for cancer include the following:

- Tobacco use
- Exposure to sunlight (Fig. 18-34)
- Excessive alcohol use
- Exposure to some chemicals and industrial agents
- Some food additives
- Radiation
- Poor nutrition
- Lack of physical activity

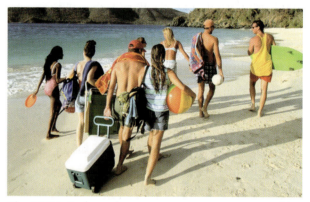

Fig. 18-34. *Prolonged sun exposure puts a person at risk for skin cancer.*

When diagnosed early, cancer can often be treated and controlled. The American Cancer Society has identified some warning signs of cancer:

- Unexplained weight loss
- Fever
- Fatigue
- Pain
- Skin changes
- Change in bowel or bladder habits
- Sores that do not heal
- Unusual bleeding or discharge
- Thickening or lump in the breast or other part of the body

Common Chronic and Acute Conditions

- Indigestion or difficulty swallowing
- Recent change in a wart or mole
- Nagging cough or hoarseness

People with cancer can live longer and sometimes recover if they are treated early. Often these treatments are combined.

Surgery is the first line of defense against most forms of cancer. It is the key treatment for malignant tumors of the skin, breast, bladder, colon, rectum, stomach, and muscle. Surgeons remove as much of the tumor as they can to keep cancer from spreading.

Chemotherapy refers to medications given to fight cancer. Some drugs destroy cancer cells and limit the rate of cell growth. However, many of these drugs are toxic to the body. They kill healthy cells as well as cancer cells. Chemotherapy can have severe side effects, including nausea, vomiting, diarrhea, hair loss, and decreased resistance to infection.

Radiation therapy directs radiation to a limited area to kill cancer cells. However, other normal or healthy cells in its path are also destroyed (Fig. 18-35). By controlling cell growth, radiation can reduce pain. Radiation can cause the same side effects as chemotherapy. The skin of the area that is exposed to radiation may become sore, irritated, and sometimes burned.

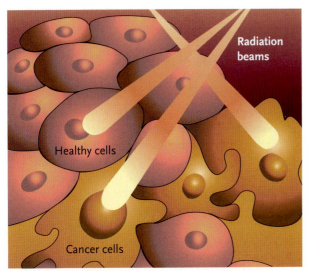

Fig. 18-35. *Radiation is targeted at cancer cells, but it also destroys some healthy cells in its path.*

Guidelines:
Cancer

G Each case is different. Cancer is a general term. It refers to many separate situations. Residents may live many years or only several months. Treatment affects each person differently. Do not make assumptions about a resident's condition.

G Residents may want to talk or may avoid talking. Respect each resident's needs. Listen if a resident wants to share feelings or experiences with you. However, never push a resident to talk. Be honest. Never say, "Everything will be okay." Be sensitive. Remember that cancer is a disease, and we do not know its cause. Have a positive attitude. Focus on concrete details; for example, comment if a resident seems stronger, or mention that the sun is shining outside.

G Good nutrition is important for residents with cancer. Follow the care plan carefully. Residents frequently have poor appetites. Encourage a variety of nutritious foods. Liquid nutrition supplements may be used in addition to, not in place of, meals. If nausea or swallowing is a problem, foods such as soups, gelatin, or starches may appeal to the resident. Use plastic utensils for a resident receiving chemotherapy. It makes food taste better. Silver utensils cause a bitter taste.

G Cancer can cause great pain, especially in the late stages. Watch for signs of pain. Report them to the nurse. Help with comfort measures, such as repositioning and providing conversation, music, or reading materials (Fig. 18-36). Report if pain seems to be uncontrolled.

G Offer back rubs to provide comfort and increase circulation. For residents who spend many hours in bed, moving to a chair for some period of time may improve comfort as well. Residents who are very weak or immobile need to be repositioned every two hours.

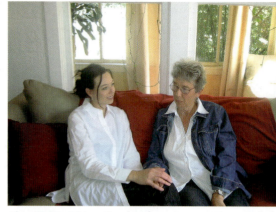

Fig. 18-36. Distractions such as conversation can help a resident with cancer deal with pain.

G Use lotion regularly on dry or delicate skin. Do not apply lotion to areas receiving radiation therapy. Do not remove any markings that are used in radiation therapy. Follow any special skin care orders (for example: no hot or cold packs, no soap or cosmetics, no tight stockings).

G Help residents brush and floss teeth regularly. Medications, nausea, vomiting, or mouth infections may cause pain and a bad taste in the mouth. You can help ease discomfort by using a soft-bristled toothbrush, rinsing with baking soda and water, or using a prescribed rinse. Do not use a commercial mouthwash if it has alcohol in it. Alcohol can further irritate a resident's mouth. For residents with mouth sores, using oral swabs, rather than toothbrushes, may be preferable. The swabs can be dipped in a rinse and gently wiped across the gums. Mouth sores can make oral care very painful; be very gentle when giving residents oral care.

G People with cancer may have a low self-image because they are weak and their appearance has changed. For example, hair loss is a common side effect of chemotherapy. Be sensitive. Provide help with grooming if it is desired. Your concern and interest can help improve self-image.

G It may help a person with cancer to think of something else for a while. Pursue other top-

ics. Get to know what interests your residents have. As always, report any signs of depression immediately.

G If visitors help cheer your resident, encourage them. Do not intrude. If some times of day are better than others, suggest this. Support groups exist for people with cancer. Check with the nurse for groups in your area.

G Having a family member with cancer can be very difficult. Be alert to needs that are not being met or stresses created by the illness.

Observing and Reporting:
Cancer

Report any of these to the nurse:

O/R Increased weakness or fatigue

O/R Weight loss

O/R Nausea, vomiting, or diarrhea

O/R Changes in appetite

O/R Fainting

O/R Signs of depression (see Chapter 20)

O/R Confusion

O/R Blood in stool or urine

O/R Change in mental status

O/R Changes in skin

O/R New lumps, sores, or rashes

O/R Increase in pain, or unrelieved pain

Mastectomy

A **mastectomy** is the surgical removal of all or part of the breast and sometimes other surrounding tissue. This operation is usually performed because of a tumor. After a mastectomy, the care plan may include arm exercises for the side of the body on which the surgery was performed. The goal of arm exercises is to strengthen the arm and chest muscles and reduce swelling in the arm and underarm. Exercises may include raising the arm, opening and closing the hand, and bending and straightening the elbow. The resident should wear loose, comfortable clothing while doing any arm exercises. Follow the care plan and the nurse's instructions regarding care after a mastectomy. Instructions may include keeping the arm on the affected side raised on pillows to decrease swelling. The resident may use a sling to keep the arm elevated. In addition, deep breathing exercises may be ordered.

9. Identify community resources for residents who are ill

Numerous services and support groups are available for people who are ill and their families or caregivers. These resources can help them through difficult times and help solve problems. Social service agencies, hospitals, hospice programs, churches, and synagogues offer many resources. These include meal services, transportation to doctors' offices or hospitals, counseling, and support groups.

For cancer, visit the American Cancer Society online at cancer.org, or call the local or state chapter. The National Association of Area Agencies on Aging, n4a.org, operates the Eldercare Locator, which is a free national service that links older adults and caregivers to aging information and resources in their own communities.

Depending on the community, many resources and services may be available for people with HIV/AIDS. These may include counseling, meal services, access to experimental drugs, and any number of other services. Look in the phone book or on the Internet for resources available in your area. Speak to the nurse if you feel a resident with HIV/AIDS needs more help. A social worker or another member of the care team may be able to coordinate services for residents with HIV/AIDS.

Chapter Review

1. What is an acute illness? What is a chronic illness?

2. What are signs and symptoms of scabies? How is scabies spread?

3. What causes shingles?

4. Briefly define these categories of open wounds: incisions, lacerations, abrasions, and puncture wounds.

5. What is dermatitis and how does it generally look?

6. What can cause fungal infections?

7. What causes arthritis?

8. What health problems can anti-inflammatory medications cause?

9. What can happen to bones when they are brittle?

10. What can a nursing assistant do to prevent or slow osteoporosis?

11. Why should casts not be covered until they are dry?

12. What type of surface can a cast be placed on?

13. Why should extremities in casts be elevated?

14. Why is a hip fracture a serious condition for an elderly person?

15. A person recovering from a hip replacement should not sit at an angle less than how many degrees?

16. When dressing a person who has just had a hip replacement, which side should be dressed first: the affected/weaker side or the unaffected/stronger side?

17. Which of the following medical orders mean that a person can bear some weight on one or both legs: partial weight bearing (PWB), non-weight bearing (NWB), or full weight bearing (FWB)?

18. How can traction help fractured bones?

19. List reasons that knee replacements are performed.

20. List three physical problems that muscular dystrophy can cause.

21. What is phantom sensation? Is it real?

22. What is complementary medicine? What is alternative medicine?

23. What causes a CVA (stroke)?

24. What terms should an NA use to refer to the weaker side of a person who has had a stroke?

25. When helping a resident who has had a stroke with transfers or walking, on which side should an NA stand—the weaker or stronger?

26. When dressing a resident with a one-sided weakness, which side should an NA dress first?

27. In which side of the mouth should food be placed if a resident has a one-sided weakness?

28. Why may people with Parkinson's disease have trouble eating and bathing themselves?

29. List six care guidelines for a person with multiple sclerosis.

30. List 10 care guidelines for a person with a head or spinal cord injury.

31. What should a nursing assistant NOT do when a resident is having a seizure?

32. What is hypertension? What does prehypertension mean?

33. List two care guidelines for a resident who has high blood pressure.

34. List three care guidelines for a resident with angina pectoris.

35. List two care guidelines for a resident recovering from a myocardial infarction.

36. List seven care guidelines for a resident who has congestive heart failure.

37. What are two ways that elastic stockings can benefit a person?

38. What are some effects of having chronic obstructive pulmonary disease (COPD)?

39. List four care guidelines for a resident who has COPD.

40. What are two causes of emphysema?

41. How is asthma treated?

42. How is bronchiectasis treated?

43. What is sputum?

44. When is the best time of day to collect a sputum specimen?

45. Briefly describe the two major types of diabetes.

46. Why is good foot care especially important for a resident with diabetes?

47. List eight signs or symptoms of diabetes that a nursing assistant needs to report.

48. What two things are true of a diabetic resident's diet?

49. What are three types of sexual contact that can transmit STDs and STIs?

50. Why are antibiotics not used to treat herpes simplex 2?

51. What are three signs and symptoms that should be reported when giving a douche?

52. How is HIV spread?

53. List four ways to protect against the spread of HIV/AIDS.

54. Because people who have HIV/AIDS are sensitive to infections, what should the nursing assistant do?

55. Is it possible to get AIDS by breathing the same air as an infected person?

56. What are some things that should be done when a person with HIV/AIDS loses his or her appetite and has difficulty eating?

57. What is a tumor? Which kind of tumor is considered non-cancerous? Which kind is considered cancerous?

58. List the risk factors for cancer.

59. What are the side effects of chemotherapy and radiation?

60. For each of these topics in the care guidelines for a resident with cancer, list one way that a nursing assistant can help: individuality of each case; communication; nutrition; pain control; comfort; skin care; oral care; and self-image.

61. List ten signs and symptoms that a nursing assistant should observe and report about cancer.

19

Confusion, Dementia, and Alzheimer's Disease

1. Describe normal changes of aging in the brain

As we age, we may lose some of our ability to think logically and quickly. This ability is called **cognition**. When we lose some of this ability we are said to have **cognitive impairment**. How much ability is lost depends on the individual. Cognitive impairment affects concentration and memory. Elderly residents may lose their memories of recent events, which can be frustrating for them. You can help by encouraging them to make lists of things to remember and writing down names, events and phone numbers.

Other normal changes of aging in the brain include slower reaction time, difficulty finding or using the right words, and sleeping less.

2. Discuss confusion and delirium

Confusion is the inability to think clearly. A confused person has trouble focusing his attention and may feel disoriented. Confusion interferes with the ability to make decisions. Personality may change. The person may not know his name, the date, other people, or where he is. A confused person may be angry, depressed, or irritable.

Confusion may come on suddenly or gradually and can be temporary or permanent. Confusion is more common in the elderly. It may occur when a person is in the hospital. Some causes of confusion include the following:

- Low blood sugar
- Head trauma or head injury
- Dehydration
- Nutritional problems
- Fever
- Sudden drop in body temperature
- Lack of oxygen
- Medications
- Infections
- Brain tumor
- Illness
- Loss of sleep
- Seizures

Guidelines:
Confusion

G Do not leave a confused resident alone.

G Stay calm. Provide a quiet environment.

G Speak in a lower tone of voice. Speak clearly and slowly.

G Introduce yourself each time you see the resident.

G Remind the resident of his or her location, name, and the date. A calendar can help.

G Explain what you are going to do, using simple instructions.

G Do not rush the resident.

G Talk to confused residents about plans for the day. Keeping a routine may help.

G Encourage the use of glasses and hearing aids. Make sure they are clean and are not damaged.

G Promote self-care and independence.

G Report observations to the nurse.

Delirium is a state of severe confusion that occurs suddenly; it is usually temporary. Possible causes include infections, disease, fluid imbalances, and poor nutrition. Drugs and alcohol may also cause delirium. Symptoms include the following:

- Agitation
- Anger
- Depression
- Irritability
- Disorientation
- Trouble focusing
- Problems with speech
- Changes in sensation and perception
- Changes in consciousness
- Decrease in short-term memory

Report these signs to the nurse. The goal of treatment is to control or reverse the cause. Emergency care may be needed, as well as a stay in a hospital.

Tip

Confusion and Delirium

When communicating with a person who is confused or disoriented, keep your voice low. Do not raise your voice or shout. Use the person's name,

and speak clearly in simple sentences. Use facial expressions and body language to aid in understanding. Reduce distractions in the environment by taking action, such as turning down the TV. Be gentle and try to decrease fears.

3. Describe dementia and define related terms

Dementia is a general term that refers to a serious loss of mental abilities such as thinking, remembering, reasoning, and communicating. As dementia advances, these losses make it difficult to perform ADLs such as eating, bathing, dressing, and toileting. Dementia is not a normal part of aging (Fig. 19-1).

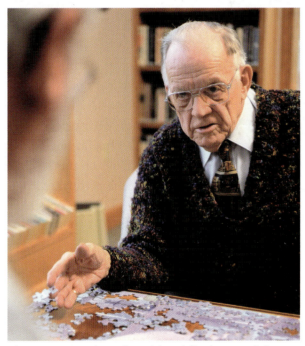

Fig. 19-1. Some loss of cognitive ability is normal; however, dementia is not a normal part of aging.

Here are some terms that are related to dementia:

Progressive: Once they begin, progressive diseases advance. They tend to spread to other parts of the body and affect many body functions.

Degenerative: Degenerative diseases get continually worse. They eventually cause a breakdown of body systems. They cause a greater and greater loss of mental and physical health and abilities. Degenerative diseases can cause death.

Onset: The onset of a disease is the time the signs and symptoms begin.

Irreversible: An irreversible disease or condition cannot be cured. Someone with irreversible dementia (like Alzheimer's) will either die from the disease or die with the disease.

The following are a few of the common causes of dementia:

- Alzheimer's disease

- Multi-infarct or vascular dementia (a series of strokes causing damage to the brain)

- Lewy body dementia

- Parkinson's disease

- Huntington's disease

A diagnosis of dementia involves getting a patient's medical history and having a physical examination, as well as a neurological exam. Blood tests and imaging tests (CT or MRI scan, for example), may be ordered. Electroencephalography (EEG), a test using electrodes on the scalp to trace brain wave activity, may be performed. Diagnosis is a process of ruling out other possible diseases that mimic symptoms of dementia.

4. Describe Alzheimer's disease and identify its stages

Alzheimer's disease (AD) is the most common cause of dementia in the elderly. The Alzheimer's Association (alzheimers.org) estimates that as many as 5.2 million people in the U.S. are living with Alzheimer's, and one in eight persons age 65 and over has Alzheimer's disease. Women are more likely than men to have Alzheimer's disease and dementia. The risk of getting AD increases with age, but it is not a normal part of aging.

Alzheimer's disease is a progressive, degenerative, and irreversible disease. AD causes tangled

nerve fibers and protein deposits to form in the brain. They eventually cause dementia. There is no known cause of AD, and there is no cure. Diagnosis is difficult, involving many physical and mental tests to rule out other causes. However, the only sure way to determine AD at this time is by autopsy. The length time it takes AD to progress from onset to death varies greatly. It may take anywhere from three to 20 years.

Symptoms of AD appear gradually and generally begin with memory loss. As the disease progresses the symptoms get worse. People with AD may get disoriented. They may be confused about time and place. Communication problems are common, and the ability to read, write, speak, or understand may be lost. Mood swings occur and behavior changes. Aggressiveness, wandering, and withdrawal are all part of AD. AD progresses to complete loss of all ability to care for oneself. The person eventually requires constant care.

Each person with Alzheimer's disease will show different signs at different times. For example, one resident with Alzheimer's may be able to read, but cannot use the phone or recall her address. Another may have lost the ability to read, but can still do simple math. Skills a person has used often over a lifetime are usually kept longer. Thus some people with Alzheimer's can play an instrument with some help long after they have lost much of their memory (Fig. 19-2).

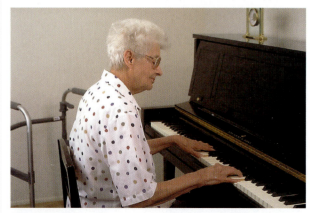

Fig. 19-2. *Even when a person loses much of her memory, she may still keep skills she has used her whole life.*

Encourage residents with AD to do ADLs. Help them keep their minds and bodies as active as possible. Working, socializing, reading, problem solving, and exercising should all be encouraged (Fig. 19-3). Having residents with AD do as much as possible for themselves may even help slow the progression of the disease. Look for tasks that are challenging but not frustrating. Help your residents succeed in doing them.

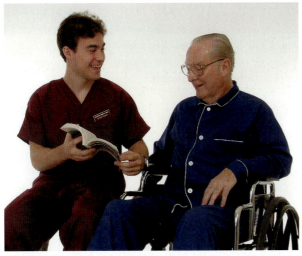

Fig. 19-3. *Encourage reading and thinking activities for residents with AD.*

Alzheimer's disease generally progresses in three stages:

Stage I

- Recent (short-term) memory loss

- Disorientation to time

- Lack of interest in doing things, including work, dressing, recreation

- Inability to concentrate

- Mood swings

- Irritability

- Petulance, or peevish, ill-humored, and rude behavior

- Tendency to blame others

- Carelessness in personal habits

- Poor judgment

Stage II

- Increased memory loss, may forget family members and friends

- Slurred speech

- Difficulty finding right word, finishing thoughts, or following directions

- Tendency to make statements that are illogical

- Inability to read, write, or do math

- Inability to care for self or perform ADLs without assistance

- Incontinence

- Dulled senses (for example, cannot distinguish between hot and cold)

- Restlessness, wandering, and/or agitation (increase of these in the evening is called "sundowning")

- Sleep problems

- Lack of impulse control (for example, swears excessively or is sexually aggressive or rude)

- Obsessive repetition of movements, words, or behavior

- Temper tantrums

- Hallucinations or delusions

Stage III

- Total disorientation to time, place, and person

- Apathy

- Total dependence on others for care

- Total incontinence

- Inability to speak or communicate, except for grunting, groaning, or screaming

- Total immobility/confined to bed

- Inability to recognize family or self

- Increased sleep disturbances

- Difficulty swallowing, which produces risk of choking

- Seizures

- Coma

- Death

5. Identify personal attitudes helpful in caring for residents with Alzheimer's disease

These attitudes will help you give the best possible care to your residents with AD:

Do not take things personally. Alzheimer's disease is a devastating mental and physical disorder. It affects everyone who surrounds and cares for the one with AD. People with Alzheimer's disease do not have control over their words and actions. They may often be unaware of what they say or do. If a resident with Alzheimer's does not know you, does not do what you say, ignores you, accuses you, or insults you, remember that it is the disease acting, not the person.

Put yourself in their shoes. Think about what it would be like to have Alzheimer's disease. Imagine being unable to do ADLs and being dependent on others for care. Think how frustrating it would be to have no memory of recent events or to be unable find words for what you want to say. Assume that people with AD have insight and are aware of the changes in their abilities. Treat residents with AD with dignity and respect.

Work with the symptoms and behaviors you see. Each person with Alzheimer's disease is an individual. People with AD will not all show the same symptoms at the same times (Fig. 19-4). Each resident will do some things that others will never do. The best plan is to work with what you see each day. For example, an Alzheimer's resident may want to go for a walk one day, when the day before he did not want to go to the bathroom without help. If it is allowed, try to go for a walk with him. Notice and report changes in behavior, mood, and independence.

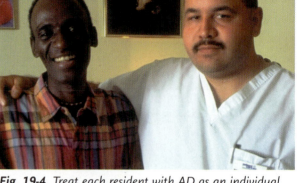

Fig. 19-4. *Treat each resident with AD as an individual. They will not have the same symptoms at the same time; work with symptoms you see.*

Work as a team. Always report and document your observations. Symptoms and behavior change daily. Observing and reporting carefully to all team members, as well as listening to others' reports, can help the team to develop solutions. For example, a resident with AD may refuse to eat her meals. You might discover that if you sit next to her and eat something while she has food in front of her, she will also eat. You may also notice that she always eats her bite-sized sandwiches. This is important to report to the team, and can help the team provide better nutrition for the resident. You are in a great position to give details about your residents. Being with residents often allows you be an expert on each case. Make the most of this opportunity. Residents with AD may not be able to recognize or distinguish between aides, nurses, or administrators. Be prepared to help when needed.

Take care of yourself. Caring for someone with dementia can be both physically and emotionally exhausting, as well as incredibly stressful. Take care of yourself so you can continue giving the best care (Fig. 19-5). Be aware of your body's signals to slow down, rest, or eat better. Your feelings are real; you have a right to them. Use your mistakes as learning experiences. Unmanaged stress can cause physical and emotional problems. Talk to your supervisor if you need help addressing stress or would like to find support groups in your area. See Chapter 31 for more information on handling stress.

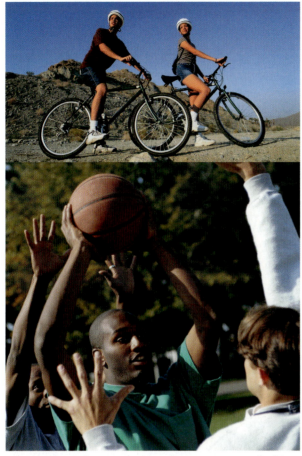

Fig. 19-5. Regular exercise is an important part of taking care of yourself.

Work with family members. Family members can be a wonderful resource. They can help you learn more about your resident. They also give stability and comfort to the resident with Alzheimer's. Build relationships with family members. Keep the lines of communication open.

Remember the goals of the care plan. Along with practical tasks you will perform, the care plan will also call for maintaining residents' dignity and self-esteem. Help them to be independent.

6. List strategies for better communication with residents with Alzheimer's disease

Some general communication guidelines for residents with AD include the following:

- Always approach from the front, and do not startle the resident.

- Determine how close the resident wants you to be.

- If possible, communicate in a calm place with little background noise and distraction.

- Always identify yourself, and use the resident's name.

- Speak slowly, using a lower tone of voice than normal. This is calming and easier to understand.

In addition, communication with residents with AD can be helped by using these techniques for specific situations:

If the resident is frightened or anxious:

- Try to keep him or her calm. Speak slowly in a low, calm voice. Find a room with little background noise and distraction. Get rid of noise and distractions, such as televisions or radios (Fig. 19-6).

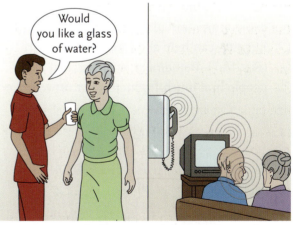

Fig. 19-6. Try to find a room with little background noise and distraction when communicating with residents with AD.

- Try to see and hear yourself as they might. Always describe what you are going to do.

- Use simple words and short sentences. If doing a procedure or helping with self-care, list steps one at a time.

- Check your body language. Make sure you are not tense or hurried.

If the resident forgets or shows memory loss:

- Repeat yourself. Use the same words if you need to repeat an instruction or question. However, you may be using a word the resident does not understand, such as "tired." Try other words like "nap," "lie down," "rest," etc.

- Repetition can also be soothing for a resident with Alzheimer's. Many residents with AD will repeat words, phrases, questions, or actions. This is called **perseveration**. If your resident perseverates, do not try to stop him. Answer his questions, using the same words each time, until he stops.

- Keep messages simple. Break complex tasks into smaller, simpler ones.

If the resident has trouble finding words or names:

- Suggest a word that sounds correct. If this upsets the resident, learn from it. Try not to correct a resident who uses an incorrect word. As words (written and spoken) become more difficult, smiling, touching, and hugging can help show love and concern (Fig. 19-7). Remember, however, that some people find touch frightening or unwelcome.

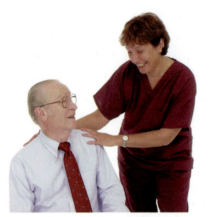

Fig. 19-7. Touch, smiles, hugs, and laughter will be understood longer, even after a resident's speaking abilities decline.

If the resident seems not to understand basic instructions or questions:

- Ask the resident to repeat your words.

- Use short words and sentences, and allow time to answer.

- Note the communication methods that are effective. Use them.

- Watch for nonverbal cues as the ability to talk lessens. Observe body language—eyes, hands, and face.

- Use signs, pictures, gestures, or written words. Use pictures, such as a drawing of a toilet on the bathroom door. Use gestures, such as holding up a shirt when you want to help your resident dress. Combine verbal and nonverbal communication. For example, saying "Let's get dressed now," as you hold up clothes.

If the resident wants to say something but cannot:

- Ask him or her to point, gesture, or act it out.

- If the resident is upset but cannot explain why, offer comfort with a hug or a smile, or try to distract. Verbal communication may be frustrating.

If the resident does not remember how to perform basic tasks:

- Break each activity into simple steps. For instance, "Let's go for a walk. Stand up. Put on your sweater. First the right arm..." Always encourage the person to do what he can.

If the resident insists on doing something that is unsafe or not allowed:

- Try to limit the times you say "don't." Instead, redirect activities toward something else.

If the resident hallucinates (sees or hears things that are not really happening), is paranoid or accusing:

- Do not take it personally.

- Try to redirect behavior or ignore it. Attention span is limited. This behavior often passes quickly.

If the resident is depressed or lonely:

- Take time, one-on-one, to ask how he or she is feeling. Really listen.

- Try to involve the resident in activities.

- Always report signs of depression to the nurse. You will learn more about depression in Chapter 20.

If the resident is verbally abusive, or uses bad language:

- Remember it is the dementia speaking and not the person. Try to ignore the language, and redirect attention to something else (Fig. 19-8).

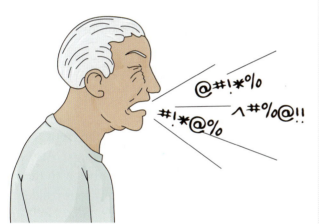

Fig. 19-8. If a resident with AD says something abusive or uses bad language, try to ignore it and redirect interest. Remember that it is the disease talking.

If the resident has lost most verbal skills:

- Use nonverbal skills. As speaking abilities decline, people with AD will still understand touch, smiles, and laughter for much longer. Remember that some people do not like to be touched. Approach touching slowly. Be gentle. Softly touch the hand or place your arm around the resident. A hug or a kiss on the hand or cheek can show affection and caring. A smile can say you want to help.

- Even after verbal skills are lost, signs, labels, and gestures can reach people with dementia.

- Assume people with AD can understand more than they can express. Never talk about them as though they were not there.

7. Explain general principles that will help assist residents with personal care

Use the same procedures for personal care and ADLs for residents with Alzheimer's disease as you would with other residents. However, there are some guidelines to keep in mind when assisting these residents. Three general principles will help you give the best care:

1. Develop a routine and stick to it. Being consistent is important for residents who are confused and easily upset.

2. Promote self-care. Help your residents to care for themselves as much as possible. This will help them cope with this difficult disease.

3. Take good care of yourself, both mentally and physically. This will help you give the best care.

8. List and describe interventions for problems with common activities of daily living (ADLs)

As Alzheimer's disease worsens, residents will have trouble doing their ADLs. By knowing interventions, you can provide better care. An **intervention** means a way to change an action or development.

Problems with Incontinence

- Encourage fluids. Never withhold or discourage fluids because a resident is incontinent. If you notice the resident is not drinking fluids, tell the nurse.

- Note when the resident is incontinent over two to three days. Check him or her every 30 minutes. This can help determine "bathroom times." Take the resident to the bathroom just before his or her "bathroom time."

- Take the resident to the bathroom before and after meals and just before bed.

- Make sure the resident actually urinates before getting off the toilet.

- Mark the restroom with a sign or a picture. This is a reminder of where it is and to use it.

- Family or friends may be upset by their loved one's incontinence. Be matter-of-fact about cleaning after episodes of incontinence. Do not show any disgust or irritation.

- For incontinence during the night, observe toilet patterns for two to three nights to try to determine nighttime bathroom times.

- Make sure there is enough light in the bathroom and on the way there.

- Put lids on trash cans, waste baskets, or other containers if the resident urinates in them.

Problems with Bathing

- Schedule bathing when the resident is least agitated. Be organized so the bath can be quick. Give sponge baths if the resident resists a shower or tub bath.

- Prepare the resident before bathing. Hand him or her the supplies (washcloth, soap, shampoo, towels). This serves as a visual aid.

- Take a walk with the resident down the hall. Stop at the tub or shower room, rather than asking directly about the bath.

- Make sure the bathroom is well-lit and is at a comfortable temperature.

- Provide privacy during the bath.

- Be calm and quiet when bathing. Keep the process simple.

- Be sensitive when talking to your resident about bathing (Fig. 19-9).

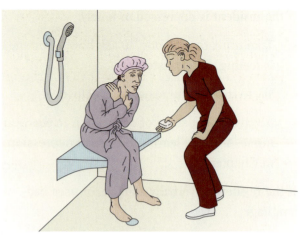

Fig. 19-9. *When a resident has AD, she may be frightened or not understand what you are trying to do. Stay calm. Gently explain what you are trying to do.*

- Give the resident a washcloth to hold. This can distract him or her while you finish the bath.

- Be safe. Always follow safety precautions. Ensure safety by using non-slip mats, tub seats, and hand-holds.

- Be flexible about when you bathe. Your resident may not always be in the mood. Also, be aware that not everyone bathes with the same frequency. Understand if your resident does not want to bathe.

- Be relaxed. Allow the resident to enjoy the bath. Offer encouragement and praise.

- Let the resident do as much as possible during the bath.

- While bathing, check the skin regularly for signs of irritation.

Problems with Dressing

- Show the resident clothing to put on. This brings up the idea of dressing.

- Avoid delays or interruptions while dressing.

- Provide privacy. Close doors and curtains. Dress the resident in the resident's room.

- Encourage the resident to pick clothes to wear. Simplify this by giving just a few choices. Make sure the clothing is clean and appropriate. Lay out clothes in the order in which they are put on (Fig. 19-10). Choose clothes that are simple to put on. Some people with Alzheimer's disease make a habit of layering clothing regardless of the weather.

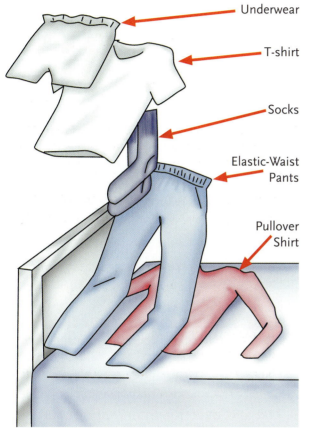

Fig. 19-10. Lay out clothes in the order in which they should be put on.

- Break the task down into simple steps. Introduce one step at a time. Do not rush the resident.

- Use a friendly, calm voice when speaking.

- Praise and encourage the resident at each step.

Residents' Rights

Rights with Alzheimer's Disease

Protect the privacy rights of residents with AD by keeping them dressed or covered with a sheet when in bed. Residents may not be aware that they are exposed. Do not discuss their personal information with others. Allow residents with AD to make the decisions they are able to make, such as what shirt to wear or where to sit to eat.

Problems with Eating

Food may not interest a resident with Alzheimer's disease at all. It may be of great interest, but a resident may only want to eat a few types of food. In either case, a resident with AD is at risk for malnutrition. Nutritious food intake should be encouraged. The following are ideas for improving eating habits:

- Have meals at regular, consistent times each day. You may need to remind the resident that it is mealtime. Serve familiar foods. Foods should look and smell appetizing.

- Make sure there is adequate lighting.

- Keep noise and distractions low during meals.

- Keep the task of eating simple. If restlessness prevents getting through an entire meal, try smaller, more frequent meals. Finger foods (foods that are easy to pick up with the fingers) may be easier to eat and can allow eating while moving around. They allow residents to choose the food they want to eat. Examples of finger foods that may be good to serve are sandwiches cut into fourths, chicken nuggets or small pieces of cooked boneless chicken, fish sticks, cheese cubes, halved hard-boiled eggs, and fresh fruit and soft vegetables cut into bite-sized pieces.

- Do not serve steaming or very hot foods or drinks.

- Use dishes without a pattern. White usually works best. Use a simple place setting with a single eating utensil. Remove other items from the table (Fig. 19-11).

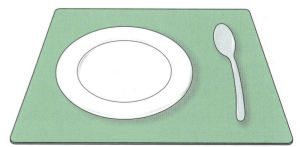

Fig. 19-11. Simple place settings with white plates on a solid-colored placemat may help avoid confusion and distraction during eating.

- Put only one item of food on the plate at a time. Multiple kinds of food on a plate or a tray may be overwhelming.

- Residents with AD may not understand how to eat or use utensils. Give simple, clear instructions. Help the resident taste a sample of the meal first. To get him to eat, place a spoon to the lips. This will encourage the resident to open his mouth. Ask him to open his mouth.

- Guide the resident through the meal. Provide simple instructions. Offer regular drinks of water, juice, and other fluids to avoid dehydration.

- Use adaptive equipment, such as special spoons and bowls, as needed.

- If a resident needs to be fed, do so slowly. Give small pieces of food.

- Make mealtimes simple and relaxed. Allow time for eating. Give the resident time to swallow before each bite or drink.

- Seat residents with AD with others at small tables. This encourages socializing.

- Observe for eating or swallowing problems. Report them to the nurse as soon as possible.

- Observe and report changes or problems in eating habits.

In addition, use the following tips when caring for residents with AD:

- Help with grooming. Help the people in your care feel attractive and dignified.

- Prevent infections. Follow Standard Precautions.

- Observe the resident's physical health. Report any potential problems. People with dementia may not notice their own health problems.

- Maintain a daily exercise routine.

- Maintain self-esteem. Encourage independence in ADLs.

- Share in fun activities, looking at pictures, talking, and reminiscing.

- Reward positive and independent behavior with smiles, hugs, warm touches, and thanks (Fig. 19-12).

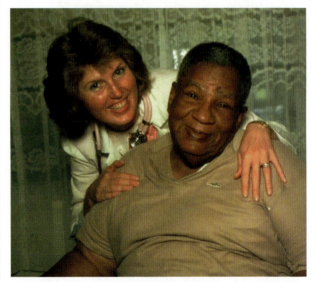

Fig. 19-12. *Reward positive behavior with warm touches, smiles, and thanks.*

9. List and describe interventions for common difficult behaviors related to Alzheimer's disease

Below are some common difficult behaviors that you may face with Alzheimer's residents. Remember that each resident is different. Work with each person as an individual. Report behavior in detail to the nurse.

Agitation: A resident who is excited, restless, or troubled is said to be **agitated**. Situations that lead to agitation are **triggers**. Triggers may include change of routine or caregiver, new or frustrating experiences, or even television. Responses that may help calm a person who is agitated include the following:

- Try to remove triggers. Keep routine constant and avoid frustration (Fig. 19-13).

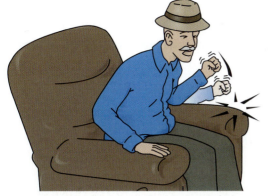

Fig. 19-13. *Nonverbal clues, such as facial expressions or body language, can warn you of increasing agitation. Take steps early to calm down a resident who is becoming agitated.*

- Focus on a soothing, familiar activity, such as sorting things or looking at pictures.

- Stay calm. Use a low, soothing voice to speak to and reassure the resident.

- An arm around the shoulder, patting, or stroking may soothe some residents.

Sundowning: When a person gets restless and agitated in the late afternoon, evening, or night, it is called **sundowning**. Sundowning may be caused by hunger or fatigue, a change in routine or caregiver, or any new or frustrating situation. These are some effective responses to sundowning:

- Remove triggers. Give snacks or encourage rest.

- Avoid stressful situations during this time. Limit activities, appointments, trips, and visits.

- Play soft music.

- Set a bedtime routine and keep it.

- Recognize when sundowning occurs. Plan a calming activity just before.

- Remove caffeine from the diet.

- Give a soothing back massage.

- Distract the resident with a simple, calm activity like looking at a magazine.

- Maintain a daily exercise routine.

Catastrophic Reactions: When a person with AD overreacts to something in an unreasonable way it is called a **catastrophic reaction**. It may be triggered by any of the following:

- Fatigue

- Change of routine, environment, or caregiver

- Overstimulation (too much noise or activity)

- Difficult choices or tasks

- Physical pain

- Hunger

- Need for toileting

You can respond to catastrophic reactions as you would to agitation or sundowning. For example, remove triggers. Help the resident focus on a soothing activity.

Violent Behavior. A resident who attacks, hits, or threatens someone is violent. Violence may be triggered by many situations. These include frustration, overstimulation, or a change in routine, environment, or caregiver. The following are appropriate responses to violent residents:

- Block blows but never hit back (Fig. 19-14).

- Step out of reach.

- Call for help if needed.

- Do not leave resident alone.

- Try to remove triggers.

- Use techniques to calm residents as you would for agitation or sundowning.

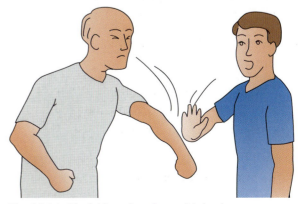

Fig. 19-14. *Block blows but do not hit back.*

Pacing and Wandering: A resident who walks back and forth in the same area is **pacing**. A resident who walks aimlessly around the facility or the facility grounds is **wandering**. Pacing and wandering may have some of the following causes:

- Restlessness

- Hunger

- Disorientation

- Need for toileting

- Constipation

- Pain

- Forgetting how or where to sit down

- Too much daytime napping

- Need for exercise

Remove causes when you can. For example, give nutritious snacks, encourage an exercise routine, and maintain a toileting schedule. If residents pace and wander, let them do so in a safe and secure (locked) area where you can keep an eye on them (Fig. 19-15). Suggest another activity, such as going for a walk together.

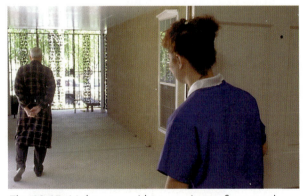

Fig. 19-15. *Make sure residents are in a safe, secured area if they pace or wander.*

Marking rooms with signs or pictures may prevent residents from wandering into areas where they should not go (Fig. 19-16). Bed, body, or door alarms can be used in beds or on wheelchairs, chairs, or doors. They help by alerting staff with an alarm when confused or demented residents attempt to leave the bed or chair or open a door. They also help prevent falls and decrease the need for side rails. If a resident is ordered to have a body alarm (bed or chair), make sure it is on the resident and turned on.

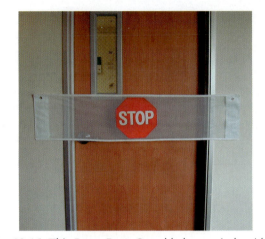

Fig. 19-16. *This Posey Door Guard helps remind residents with dementia not to exit or enter a restricted area.*
(REPRINTED WITH PERMISSION OF BRIGGS CORPORATION, 800-247-2343, WWW.BRIGGSCORP.COM)

If a resident wanders away from the protected area, or **elopes**, notify the nurse immediately. Follow the facility's policies and procedures for missing residents.

Hallucinations or Delusions: A resident who sees things that are not there is having **hallucinations** (Fig 19-17). A resident who believes things that are not true is having **delusions** (Fig. 19-18). You can respond to hallucinations and delusions in the following ways:

- Ignore harmless hallucinations and delusions.

- Reassure a resident who seems agitated or worried.

- Do not argue with a resident who is imagining things. The feelings are real to him or her. Do not tell the resident that you can see or hear his or her hallucinations. Redirect resident to other activities or thoughts.

- Be calm. Reassure resident that you are there to help.

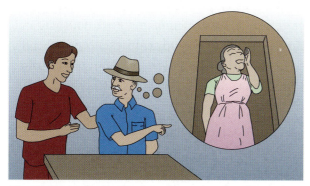

Fig. 19-17. *Hallucinating is seeing or hearing things that are not really there. For example, a resident may think he is hearing his mother calling him to dinner. You know that his mother died 20 years ago, but to him this is very real.*

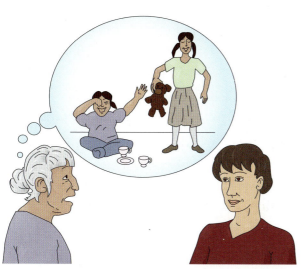

Fig. 19-18. *A delusion is a belief in something that is not true, or is out of touch with reality. For example, a resident thinks that her long-deceased sister is stealing from her room, like she did when they were young.*

Depression: When residents become withdrawn, have no energy, or do not eat or do things they used to enjoy, they may be depressed. Chapter 20 has more information on depression and its symptoms. Depression may have many causes, including the following:

- Loss of independence

- Inability to cope

- Feelings of failure, fear

- Reality of facing a progressive, degenerative illness

- Chemical imbalance

You can respond to depression in a number of ways:

- Report signs of depression to the nurse immediately. It is an illness that can be treated with medication.

- Encourage independence, self-care, and activity.

- Talk about moods and feelings if the resident wishes. Be a good listener.

- Encourage social interaction.

Perseveration or Repetitive Phrasing: A resident who repeats a word, phrase, question, or activity over and over is perseverating. Repeating a word or phrase is also called **repetitive phrasing**. Such behavior may be caused by several factors, such as disorientation or confusion. Respond to this with patience. Do not try to silence or stop the resident. Answer questions each time they are asked. Use the same words each time.

Disruptiveness: Disruptive behavior is anything that disturbs others, such as yelling, banging on furniture, slamming doors, etc. Often this behavior is triggered by a wish for attention, by pain or constipation, or by frustration. When a resident is being disruptive, gain his attention. Be calm and friendly, and try to find out why the behavior is occurring. Gently direct the resident to a more private area, if possible. Ask the resident about it, if possible. There may be a physical reason, such as pain or discomfort.

The following are appropriate ways to help prevent or respond to disruptive behavior:

- Notice and praise improvements in the resident's behavior. Be tactful and sensitive when you do this. Avoid treating the resident like a child.

- Tell the resident about any changes in schedules, routines, or the environment in advance. Involve the resident in developing routine activities and schedules, if possible.

- Encourage the resident to join in independent activities that are safe (for example, folding towels). This helps the resident feel in charge. It can prevent feelings of powerlessness. Independence is power.

- Help the resident find ways to cope. Focus on positive activities he or she may still be able to do, such as knitting, crocheting, crafts, etc. This can provide a diversion.

Inappropriate Social Behavior: Inappropriate social behavior may be cursing, name-calling, or other unpleasant behavior. As with violent or disruptive behavior, there may be many reasons why a resident is behaving in this way. Try not to take it personally. The resident may only be reacting to frustration or other stress, not to you. Remain calm and be reassuring. Try to find out what caused the behavior (for example, too much noise, too many people, too much stress, pain, or discomfort). If possible, gently direct the resident to a private area if he or she is disturbing others. Respond positively to any appropriate behavior. Report any physical abuse or serious verbal abuse to the nurse.

Inappropriate Sexual Behavior: Inappropriate sexual behavior, such as removing clothes or touching one's own genitals, can be embarrassing or uncomfortable to those who see it. Be matter-of-fact when dealing with such behavior. Do not over-react, as this may reinforce the behavior. Be sensitive to the nature of the problem. Is the behavior actually intentional? Is it consistent? Try to distract the resident. If this does not work, gently direct him or her to a private area. Tell the nurse. A resident may be reacting to a need for physical stimulation or affection. Consider other ways to provide physical stimulation. Try backrubs, a soft doll or stuffed animal to cuddle, comforting blankets, pieces of cloth, or physical touch that is appropriate.

Pillaging and Hoarding: Pillaging is taking things that belong to someone else. A person with dementia may honestly think something belongs to him, even when it clearly does not. **Hoarding** is collecting and putting things away in a guarded way. Pillaging and hoarding should

not be considered stealing. A person with Alzheimer's disease cannot and does not steal. Stealing is planned and requires a conscious effort. In most cases, the person with AD is only collecting something that catches his attention.

It is common for those with AD to wander in and out of rooms collecting things. They may carry these objects around for a while, and then leave them in other places. This is not intentional. People with AD will often take their own things and leave them in another room, not knowing what they are doing. You can help lessen problems by doing the following:

- Label all personal belongings with the resident's name and room number. This way there is no confusion about what belongs to whom.

- Place a label, symbol, or object on the resident's door. This helps the resident find his or her own room.

- Do not tell family that their loved one is "stealing" from others.

- Prepare the family so they are not upset when they find items that do not belong to their family member.

- Ask the family to tell staff if they notice strange items in the room.

- Regularly check areas where residents store items. They may store uneaten food in these places. Provide a rummage drawer—a drawer with items that are safe for the resident to take with him or her.

Safety in the Home for a Person with AD

A nurse should assess a home's safety before a home health aide visits a client with Alzheimer's. She will indicate changes that need to be made. Examples include using gates on stairways, putting locks on certain doors, and removing clutter. When the client's condition changes, report this to your supervisor. Another visit will be made to reassess the home and make further changes. In general, follow these safety guidelines:

For disoriented clients:

- Use signs to mark rooms, including stop signs on rooms that should not be entered.
- Use calendars and other reminders of day, date, and location.
- Put bells on the door to indicate when someone is coming or going.
- Keep pictures and familiar objects around.
- Put stickers or brightly colored tape on glass doors, large windows, or glass furniture

For clients who wander:

- Use locks on doors. These can be installed lower or higher than usual, so the client will not see them.
- Install alarms that sound when exit doors are opened.
- Have clients wear identification. Sew labels into clothes.
- Alert neighbors that client may wander. Show them a recent photo of the client. Keep a recent photo handy, as well as a piece of clothing the client has worn. These can help police and police dogs track a client who has wandered away.

For clients who pace:

- Remove clutter and throw rugs.
- Do not rearrange furniture.
- Do not wax floors.
- Be sure shoes and slippers fit and have non-slip soles.

For clients who have difficulty walking:

- Keep areas well lit, even at night.
- Block access to stairs with a gate.
- Clear walkways of electrical cords and clutter.

General tips:

- Keep medications and other chemicals out of reach.
- Display emergency numbers, including poison control, and home address near the phone.
- Use red tape around radiators or heating vents to prevent burns.
- Check refrigerator and potential "hiding places" for spoiled food.
- Prevent kitchen accidents by removing knobs on stove, unplugging toasters and other small appliances, and supervising kitchen visits.

10. Describe creative therapies for residents with Alzheimer's disease

Although Alzheimer's cannot be cured, there are many ways to improve the quality of life for residents with AD.

Reality orientation involves the use of calendars, clocks, signs, and lists to help residents remember who and where they are. It is useful in early stages of AD when residents are confused but not totally disoriented. In later stages, reality orientation may only frustrate residents.

Example: Each day when you go into Mrs. Elkin's room, you show her the calendar and point out what day of the week it is. On the calendar or another piece of paper, list all the things you will do today, for example, take a shower, eat lunch, and go for a walk. When you speak to her, call her by her name: Mrs. Elkin. When helping with tasks, explain why you do things as you do. For example, "We use a shower chair in the shower so you don't have to stand up for so long, Mrs. Elkin."

Benefits: Using the calendar, making lists, and using names frequently all help your resident stay in touch with the world around her. This will help her feel more in control of her life. It will also allow her to do as much as possible for herself. Explaining what you do and why you do it as you assist her will make her feel more like a participant in her care and less like an invalid.

Validation therapy means letting residents believe they live in the past or in imaginary circumstances. **Validating** means giving value to or approving. When using validation therapy, make no attempt to reorient the resident to actual circumstances. Explore the resident's beliefs. Do not argue with him or her. Validating can give comfort and reduce agitation. It is useful in cases of moderate to severe disorientation.

Example: Mr. Baldwin tells you he does not want to eat lunch today because he is going out to a restaurant with his wife. You know his wife has been dead for many years and that Mr. Baldwin can no longer eat out. Instead of telling him that he is not going out to eat, you ask what restaurant he is going to and what he will have. You suggest that he eat a good lunch now because sometimes the service is slow in restaurants (Fig. 19-19).

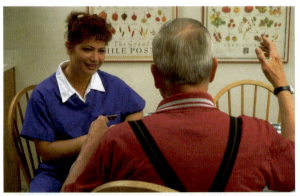

Fig. 19-19. *Validation therapy accepts a resident's fantasies without attempting to reorient him to reality.*

Benefits: By "playing along" with Mr. Baldwin's fantasy, you let him know that you take him seriously. You do not think of him as a crazy person or a child who does not know what is happening in his own life. You also learn more about your resident. He used to enjoy eating out in restaurants. He liked to order certain dishes. Eating out is something he probably associates with being with his wife. These things can help you give Mr. Baldwin better care in the future.

Reminiscence therapy involves encouraging residents to remember and talk about the past. Explore memories by asking about details. Focus on a time of life that was pleasant. Work through feelings about a hard time in the past. It is useful in many stages of AD, but especially with moderate to severe confusion.

Example: Mr. Benton, an 82-year-old man with Alzheimer's, fought in World War II. In his room are many mementos of the war. He has pictures of his war buddies, a medal he was given, and more. You ask him to tell you where he was sent in the war. He tells you about being in the Pacific. You ask him more detailed questions. Eventually he tells you a lot: the friends he made in the service, why he was given the

medal, times he was scared, and how much he missed his wife and daughter (Fig. 19-20).

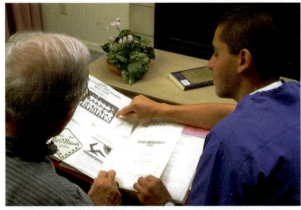

Fig. 19-20. *Reminiscence therapy encourages a resident to remember and talk about his past.*

Benefits: By asking questions about Mr. Benton's experiences in the war, you show an interest in him as a person, not just as a resident. You let him show you that he is a person who was competent, social, responsible, and brave. This boosts his self-esteem. You also learn that Mr. Benton cared very much for his wife and daughter. He probably would enjoy more visits from his daughter, which you can pass along to the nurse.

Activity therapy uses activities the resident enjoys to prevent boredom and frustration. These activities also promote self-esteem. Help the resident take walks, listen to music, read, or do other things he or she enjoys (Fig. 19-21). Activities may be done in groups or one-on-one. Activity therapy is useful in most stages of AD.

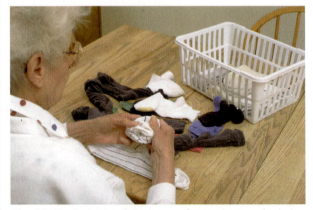

Fig. 19-21. *Activities that are not frustrating can be helpful for residents with AD. They promote mental exercise.*

Example: Mrs. Hoebel, a 70-year-old woman with AD, was a librarian for almost 45 years. She loves books and reading, but she cannot read much anymore. You bring in books that are filled with pictures. She sits with the books, sorting them and turning pages and looking at pictures.

Benefits: Mrs. Hoebel can enjoy an activity that always brought her pleasure. She feels competent, because she is sorting books and looking at books, which are tasks she can handle. You show her that you care about her by taking the time to show an interest in her past. She will associate positive feelings with you. That will make caring for her much easier.

Tip

Music Therapy

Music therapy involves using music to accomplish specific goals, such as managing stress and improving mood and cognition. This type of therapy has been used with Alzheimer's patients with success, although studies are still being performed. Music is a form of sensory stimulation. Hearing familiar songs can cause a response in people with dementia who do not respond well or do not respond at all to other treatments. Music therapists, who are trained health professionals, perform music therapy.

11. Discuss how Alzheimer's disease may affect the family

Alzheimer's disease requires the person's family to make difficult adjustments.

The disease progresses at different rates, and people with AD will need more care as the disease progresses. Eventually all people with AD need continuous care. How well the family is able to cope with the effects of the disease depends, in part, on the family's emotional and financial resources.

A person with AD may be living alone, which can cause the family to worry about the person's health and safety. Financial resources may be limited, which adds to stress levels. Finding money needed to pay expenses of home care or adult daycare can be difficult. Families do not know what goes on when no one is in the home. They may be afraid that the person is not caring for him- or herself, may not take medications properly, could wander away, or cause a fire.

A person with AD may be living with the family, which can cause stress and other emotional difficulties for all involved. It is difficult to care for a person with Alzheimer's. The household schedule has to change; family members will lose the freedom to come and go as they please. Family members must monitor the loved one's activities and provide constant care. They may lose sleep, as well as lose time to do their own activities and time to relax.

Alzheimer's introduces other stressors, too. It is very difficult to watch a loved one's personality change, and his or her health and abilities deteriorate. It is also hard to switch roles—to go from being a child who was once cared for by the parent to being the one caring for the parent.

Families may make the decision to place a loved one with AD into a long-term care facility for any number of reasons. They may have safety concerns, or may not be able to care for the person at home. The family may not be able to handle the issues that AD causes, such as the problem behaviors, or the inability to perform personal care. The person with AD may not want his or her family to do the needed personal care. There may be no available family caregiver.

After making the decision to place a person with AD in a long-term care facility, family members usually feel guilty, even if they know that placement is necessary. The person with AD may be angry and unable to understand the decision. Families worry about mistreatment, and are sensitive to being judged by others. They also feel loss and a change in the relationship with their family member.

Family members are making emotional adjustments, just as residents are. They may be experiencing frustration, fear, sadness, anger, loneliness, and depression. It is important for families to be able to express their feelings. Refer to Chapter 8 to learn ways to respond to emotional needs of families. Be sensitive to the big adjustments your residents and their families are making. Refer them to your supervisor if help is needed.

12. Identify community resources available to people with Alzheimer's disease and their families

There are many resources, such as organizations, books, counseling, and support groups, available for people with Alzheimer's disease and their families. The Alzheimer's Association has a helpline that is available 24 hours a day, seven days at week for information, referral, and support. The number is 800-272-3900, or visit the website at alz.org. The National Institute on Aging has information and resources available at their Alzheimer's Disease Education and Referral (ADEAR) Center website, or by calling 800-438-4380. Counseling, support groups, and healthcare professionals can also be of assistance. Support groups are often helpful because many people in the group are experiencing the same kinds of emotions and problems. People often feel that it is helpful to know that they are not alone in what they are going through. People in support groups often share tips and ideas for care and interventions for problems, which can be beneficial. Inform the nurse if you think residents and/or their families could benefit from a list of community resources.

Chapter Review

1. What does cognitive impairment affect?

2. How can confusion affect a person?

3. Define the term "delirium" and list five causes.

4. What is dementia?

5. Alzheimer's disease is a progressive, degenerative, and irreversible disease. What does this mean?

6. What type of skills does a person with Alzheimer's disease usually retain?

7. What can nursing assistants encourage residents to do that may help slow the progression of AD?

8. Helpful personal attitudes when working with residents who have AD are described in Learning Objective 5. They are:

    *   Do not take things personally.

    *   Put yourself in their shoes.

    *   Work with the symptoms and behaviors you see.

    *   Work as a team.

    *   Take care of yourself.

    *   Work with family members.

    *   Remember the goals of the care plan.

    List one example of what an NA can do to express each attitude.

9. Possible communication challenges for residents with AD are listed in Learning Objective 6. They include challenges with a resident who may:

    *   Be frightened or anxious

    *   Forget or show memory loss

    *   Have trouble finding words or names

    *   Seem not to understand basic questions or instructions

    *   Want to say something but cannot

    *   Not remember how to perform basic tasks

    *   Insist on doing something that is unsafe or not allowed

- Hallucinate, or be paranoid or accusing

- Be depressed or lonely

- Be verbally abusive, or use bad language

- Have lost most verbal skills

For each communication challenge, list one tip that may help.

10. List three general principles that will assist residents with personal care.

11. List four interventions for each of the following topics: incontinence, bathing, dressing, and eating.

12. For each of the following common difficult behaviors seen in residents with AD, list one intervention: agitation; pacing and wandering; hallucinations or delusions; sundowning; catastrophic reactions; depression; perseveration; violent behavior; disruptiveness; inappropriate social behavior; inappropriate sexual behavior; and pillaging and hoarding.

13. Describe these four creative therapies for AD: reality orientation, validation therapy, reminiscence therapy, and activity therapy.

14. What difficulties might families of people who have AD face?

15. List two community resources that may help a person who has AD.

20

Mental Health and Mental Illness

1. Identify seven characteristics of mental health

Mental health is the normal functioning of emotional and intellectual abilities. Traits of a person who is mentally healthy include the abilities to:

- Get along with others (Fig. 20-1)

- Adapt to change

- Care for self and others

- Give and accept love

- Deal with situations that cause anxiety, disappointment, and frustration

- Take responsibility for decisions, feelings, and actions

- Control and fulfill desires and impulses appropriately

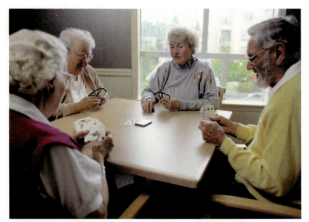

Fig. 20-1. The ability to interact well with other people is a characteristic of mental health.

2. Identify four causes of mental illness

While it involves the emotions and mental functions, **mental illness** is a disease. It is like any physical disease. It produces signs and symptoms and affects the body's ability to function. It responds to proper treatment and care. Mental illness disrupts a person's ability to function at a normal level in the family, home, or community. It often causes inappropriate behavior. Some signs and symptoms of mental illness are confusion, disorientation, agitation, and anxiety.

However, signs and symptoms like those of mental illness can also occur when mental illness is not present. A personal crisis, temporary physical changes in the brain, side effects or interactions from medications, and severe change in the environment may cause a **situation response**. In a situation response, the signs and symptoms are temporary.

Mental illness can be caused or made worse by chronic stress from any of these conditions:

1. **Physical factors**: Illness, disability, or aging can cause stress that may lead to mental illness. Substance abuse or a chemical imbalance can also cause mental illness. Self-respect and self-worth are the building blocks of mental health. They are challenged when ill or disabled people have difficulty with their activities of daily living (ADLs). They may fear the future. They may worry about their dependence on others.

2. **Environmental factors**: Weak interpersonal or family relationships, or traumatic early life experiences (such as being abused as a child) can lead to mental illness.

3. **Heredity**: Mental illness can occur repeatedly in some families. This may be due to inherited traits or family influence.

4. **Stress**: People can tolerate different levels of stress. People have different ways of handling stress. When the amount of stress is too great, a person may not be able to cope with it, and mental illness may arise.

3. Distinguish between fact and fallacy concerning mental illness

A **fallacy** is a false belief. The greatest fallacy about mental illness is that people who are mentally ill can control it. Mentally ill people cannot simply choose to be well. Mental illness is a disease like any other. Mentally healthy people are able to control their emotions and actions. Mentally ill people may not have this control. Knowing mental illness is a disease helps you work with mentally ill residents.

Fact and Fallacy

Fact: Mental illness is a disease like any physical illness. People with mental illness cannot control their illness.

Fallacy: People with mental illness can control their illness. They can choose to be well.

Mental Retardation and Mental Illness

Sometimes people confuse the terms "mental retardation" and "mental illness." They are not the same. Mental retardation is a developmental disability that causes below-average mental functioning. It may affect a person's ability to care for himself, as well as to live independently. Mental retardation is not a type of mental illness. Here are some ways that it differs from mental illness:

- Mental retardation is a permanent condition; mental illness can be temporary.

- Mental retardation is present at birth or emerges in childhood. Mental illness may occur any time during a person's life.

- Mental retardation affects mental ability. Mental illness may or may not affect mental ability.

- There is no cure for mental retardation, although persons who are mentally retarded can be helped. Many mental illnesses can be cured with treatment, such as medications and therapy.

Mental retardation and mental illness are different conditions; however, persons who have either condition need emotional support, as well as care and treatment.

4. Explain the connection between mental and physical wellness

Mental health is important to physical health. Reducing stress can help prevent some physical illnesses (Fig. 20-2). It can help people cope if illness or disability occur. Mental health can help protect and improve physical health. The reverse is also true. Physical illness or disability can cause or worsen mental illness. The stress these conditions create takes a toll on mental health.

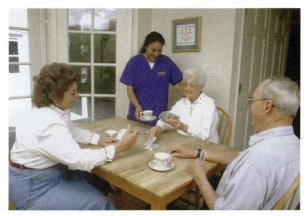

Fig. 20-2. Social interaction can promote mental and physical health.

5. List guidelines for communicating with mentally ill residents

Different types of mental illness will affect how well residents communicate. Treat each resident as an individual. Tailor your approach to the situation. Use these guidelines to communicate with residents who are mentally ill (Fig. 20-3).

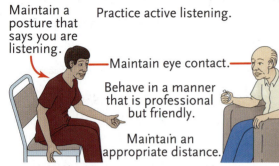

Maintain a posture that says you are listening.

Practice active listening.

Maintain eye contact.

Behave in a manner that is professional but friendly.

Maintain an appropriate distance.

Fig. 20-3. *Practice good communication skills with mentally ill residents.*

Guidelines:
Mental Illness

G   Do not talk to adults as if they are children.

G   Use simple, clear statements and a normal tone of voice.

G   Be sure that what you say and how you say it show respect and concern.

G   Sit or stand at a normal distance from the resident. Be aware of your body language.

G   Be honest and direct, as you would with any resident.

G   Avoid arguments.

G   Maintain eye contact.

G   Listen carefully.

6. Identify and define common defense mechanisms

Defense mechanisms are unconscious behaviors used to release tension or cope with stress. They help to block uncomfortable or threatening feelings. All people use them at times. However, people who are mentally ill use them to a greater degree. Overuse of these mechanisms keeps people from understanding their emotional

problems and actions. If a person is unable to recognize problems, he or she will not address them, and the problems may get worse. Common defense mechanisms include:

Denial: Completely rejecting the thought or feeling—"I'm not upset with you!"

Projection: Seeing feelings in others that are really one's own—"My teacher hates me."

Displacement: Transferring a strong negative feeling to a safer situation—for example, an unhappy employee cannot yell at his boss for fear of losing his job so he later yells at his wife.

Rationalization: Making excuses to justify a situation—for example, after stealing something, saying "Everybody does it."

Repression: Blocking painful thoughts or feelings from the mind—for example, not remembering sexual abuse.

Regression: Going back to an old, usually immature behavior—for example, throwing a temper tantrum as an adult.

7. Describe the symptoms of anxiety, depression, and schizophrenia

There are many degrees of mental illness, from mild to severe. A person with severe mental illness may lose touch with reality and become unable to communicate or make decisions. Some people with mild mental illness, however, seem to function normally, although they may sometimes become overwhelmed by stress or overly emotional. Many signs of mental illness are simply extreme behaviors most people experience some of the time. Being able to recognize such behavior may make it easier to understand the mentally ill.

Anxiety-related Disorders: **Anxiety** is uneasiness or fear, often about a situation or condition. When a mentally healthy person feels anxiety, he or she usually knows the cause. The anxiety fades once the cause is removed. A mentally ill person may feel anxiety all the time. He or she may not know the reason for feeling anxious. Physical signs and symptoms of anxiety-related disorders include shakiness, muscle aches, sweating, cold and clammy hands, dizziness, fatigue, racing heart, cold or hot flashes, a choking or smothering sensation, and a dry mouth (Fig. 20-4).

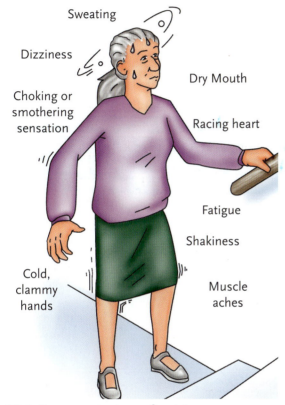

Fig. 20-4. *Common symptoms of anxiety.*

Sweating

Dizziness

Choking or smothering sensation

Cold, clammy hands

Dry Mouth

Racing heart

Fatigue

Shakiness

Muscle aches

Phobias are an intense form of anxiety. Many people are very afraid of certain things or situations. Examples include a fear of dogs or of flying. For a mentally ill person, a phobia is a disabling terror. It keeps the person from participating in normal activities. For example, the fear of being in a confined space, **claustrophobia**, may make using an elevator a terrifying task.

Other anxiety-related disorders include **panic disorder**, in which a person is terrified for no known reason. **Obsessive compulsive disorder** is obsessive behavior a person uses to cope

with anxiety. For example, a person may wash his hands over and over as a way of dealing with anxiety. Anxiety-related disorders may also be caused by a traumatic experience. This type of anxiety is known as **post-traumatic stress disorder**.

Depression: Clinical depression is a serious mental illness. It may cause intense mental, emotional, and physical pain and disability. Depression also makes other illnesses worse. If untreated, it may result in suicide. The National Institute of Mental Health lists depression as one of the most common links with suicide in older adults.

Clinical depression is not a normal reaction to stress. Sadness is only one sign of this illness. Not all people who have depression complain of sadness or appear sad. Other common symptoms of clinical depression include (Fig. 20-5):

- Pain, including headaches, abdominal pain, and other body aches
- Low energy or fatigue
- **Apathy**, or lack of interest in activities
- Irritability
- Anxiety
- Loss of appetite or overeating
- Problems with sexual functioning and desire
- Sleeplessness, difficulty sleeping, or excessive sleeping
- Lack of attention to basic personal care tasks (e.g. bathing, combing hair, changing clothes)
- Intense feelings of despair
- Guilt
- Difficulty concentrating
- Withdrawal and isolation
- Repeated thoughts of suicide and death

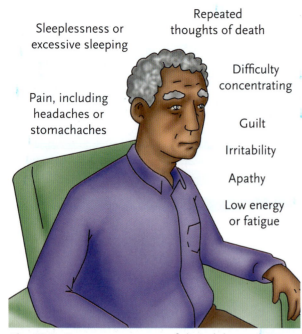

Sleeplessness or excessive sleeping

Repeated thoughts of death

Difficulty concentrating

Pain, including headaches or stomachaches

Guilt

Irritability

Apathy

Low energy or fatigue

Fig. 20-5. *Common symptoms of clinical depression.*

Depression can occur along with other illnesses. Cancer, HIV or AIDS, Alzheimer's disease, diabetes, and heart attack are among the illnesses often associated with depression. Depression is very common among the elderly.

There are different types and degrees of depression. **Major depression** may cause a person to lose interest in everything he once cared about. **Manic depression**, or **bipolar disorder**, causes a person to swing from deep depression to extreme activity. These manic episodes include high energy, little sleep, big speeches, rapidly changing moods, high self-esteem, overspending, and poor judgment.

People cannot overcome depression through sheer will. Depression is an illness like any other illness. It can be treated successfully. People who suffer from depression need compassion and support. Know the symptoms so that you can recognize the beginning or worsening of depression. Any suicide threat should be taken seriously and reported immediately. It should not be regarded as an attempt to get attention.

Schizophrenia: Despite popular belief, schizophrenia does not mean "split personality."

Schizophrenia is a brain disorder that affects a person's ability to think and communicate clearly. It also affects the ability to manage emotions, make decisions, and understand reality. It affects a person's ability to interact with other people. Treatment makes it possible for many people to lead relatively normal lives.

Some of the signs of schizophrenia are easy to see (Fig. 20-6). Hallucinations are illusions a person sees or hears. A person may see someone or something that is not really there, or hear a conversation that is not real. Delusions are persistent false beliefs. For example, a person may believe that other people are reading his thoughts. **Paranoid schizophrenia** is a form of the disease that centers mainly on hallucinations and delusions. Not all hallucinations or delusions are related to schizophrenia, though.

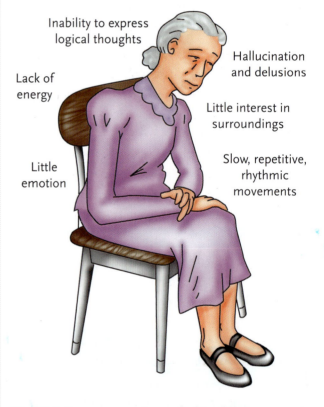

Inability to express logical thoughts

Lack of energy

Little emotion

Hallucination and delusions

Little interest in surroundings

Slow, repetitive, rhythmic movements

Fig. 20-6. *Common symptoms of schizophrenia.*

Other symptoms of schizophrenia include disorganized thinking and speech. This makes a person unable to express logical thoughts.

Disorganized behavior means a person moves slowly, repeating gestures or movements. People with schizophrenia may also show less emotion, have less interest in their environment, and lack energy.

8. Explain how mental illness is treated

It is extremely important to remember that mental illness can be treated. Medication and psychotherapy are common treatment methods. Medication is widely used for several diseases and can have a very positive effect. These drugs affect the brain and have been successful in treating the symptoms and behaviors of many people with mental disorders. Medication may allow mentally ill people to function more completely. Medication used to treat mental illness must be taken properly to promote benefits and reduce side effects. You may be assigned to observe residents taking their medications.

Psychotherapy is a method of treating mental illness that involves talking about one's problems with mental health professionals. Individuals, groups, couples, or families meet with trained, licensed professionals to work on their problems. Therapists work with their clients to identify problems and causes. They use different techniques to help clients learn more about themselves and to teach them new ways to handle problems and be more in control of their lives.

There are other methods of treating mental illness that are not as widely used as medication and psychotherapy. Electroconvulsive (shock) treatment (EST) causes seizures by applying electrical impulses to the brain. It is used for the treatment of depression and other mental illnesses. Many people do not approve of EST. It is generally used only when other treatments have not been successful.

Psychosurgery is brain surgery that is performed to improve chronic mental disorders. There are new techniques being developed and used that have less risk than older methods.

Residents' Rights
Mental Illness

Residents have the right to participate in the planning of their care. They also have the right to have their medical and personal records handled confidentially. A resident with a history of mental illness has the right to go to his care plan meetings, and state his or her preferences for care and treatment. He or she also has the right to refuse care and treatment. The fact that the resident has a mental illness is confidential information. Do not share this information with anyone.

9. Explain your role in caring for residents who are mentally ill

Personal care of residents who are mentally ill is like care of any resident. The care plan and your assignment sheet will tell you what to do. You will also have some special responsibilities, as described in these guidelines:

Guidelines:
Mentally Ill Residents

G Observe residents carefully for changes in condition or abilities. Document and report your observations.

G Support the resident and his or her family and friends. Coping with mental illness can be very frustrating. Your positive, professional attitude encourages the resident and the family. If you need help coping with stress of caring for someone who is mentally ill, speak to the nurse.

G Encourage residents to do as much as possible for themselves. Progress may be very slow. Be patient, supportive, and positive.

Home Care Focus

When working in the home, remember that a stable home environment is important in managing many forms of mental illness. By assisting the family with meeting their basic needs, you help the recovery process. This is true even if your care is not physically directed to the recovering person. For example, knowing that their children are being well cared for can greatly assist persons being treated for depression. You may be assigned to provide the following services:

- Food shopping, meal planning, and preparation

- Housecleaning and laundry

- Assistance with ADLs and personal care such as bathing

- Caring for children and other family members

If assisting in a client's home, help preserve the client's role and authority in the family. Remember that you are not replacing the client. You are only filling in until the client is well enough to resume his or her role in the family.

10. Identify important observations that should be made and reported

Carefully observe your residents. Report the facts of your observations, but do not draw conclusions about the cause of the behavior. Include what you saw or heard, how long it lasted, and how often it occurred.

Observing and Reporting:
Mentally Ill Residents

- O/R Changes in ability

- O/R Positive or negative mood changes, especially withdrawal (Fig. 20-7)

- O/R Behavior changes, including changes in personality, extreme behavior, and behavior that does not seem to fit the situation

- O/R Comments, including jokes, about hurting self or others

- O/R Failure to take medicine or improper use of medicine

- O/R Real or imagined physical symptoms

- O/R Events, situations, or people that upset or excite residents

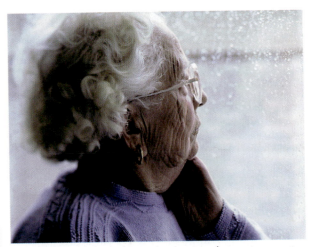

Fig. 20-7. *Withdrawal is an important change to report.*

11. List the signs of substance abuse

Substance abuse is the repeated use of legal or illegal drugs, cigarettes, or alcohol in a way that is harmful to oneself or others. The harm caused by substance abuse may come in many forms: damage to the abuser's health; legal problems; and damage to the abuser's relationships with family and friends. Chemical dependency is more severe, and may involve needing greater amounts of the drug and having symptoms, even when not using it. Chemical dependency is a disease. It affects a person physically, mentally, and emotionally. Like many other diseases, chemical dependency can develop at any age. It is treatable but frequently requires diagnosis and care by specialists. Treatment is not as simple as just stopping the drug.

A substance need not be illegal for it to be abused (Fig. 20-8). Alcohol and cigarettes are legal for adults, but are often abused. Over-the-counter medications, including diet aids and decongestants, can be addictive and harmful. Even substances such as paint or glue are sometimes abused, causing injury and death.

You may be in a position to observe signs of substance abuse in residents. Report these signs to the nurse. You can report your observations without accusing anyone. Simply report what you see, not what you think the cause may be.

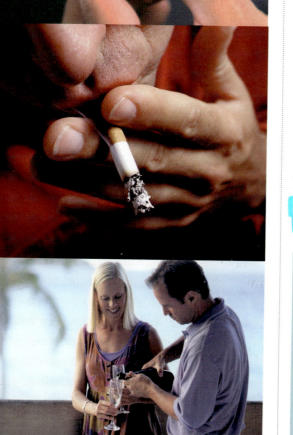

Fig. 20-8. Prescription drugs, cigarettes, and alcohol are examples of legal substances that may be abused.

Observing and Reporting:
Substance Abuse

- ^O/_R Changes in personality, moodiness, strange behavior, disruption of routines
- ^O/_R Irritability

- ^O/_R Changes in appearance (red eyes, dilated pupils, weight loss)
- ^O/_R Odor of cigarettes, liquor, or other substances on breath or clothes
- ^O/_R Reduced sense of smell
- ^O/_R Unexplained changes in vital signs
- ^O/_R Loss of appetite
- ^O/_R Inability to function normally
- ^O/_R Need for money
- ^O/_R Confusion/forgetfulness
- ^O/_R Blackouts or memory loss
- ^O/_R Frequent accidents
- ^O/_R Problems with family/friends

It is important to know that some of the same signs listed above may also indicate other problems. Depression, dementia, medication issues or medical conditions can also produce many of these same symptoms.

Residents' Rights

Rights with Alcohol

Most residents in long-term care facilities are adults and have the legal right to drink alcohol. However, there are instances when alcohol is not allowed. A doctor may have written an order for a resident not to drink alcohol. A facility may have policies against any alcohol being consumed, which would have been known and agreed to by potential residents before admission.

If a doctor has not written an order stating that a resident may not have alcohol and the facility has no rules against it, a resident may drink alcohol. If a resident is allowed to do so and enjoys having an alcoholic beverage, do not make judgments. Do not gossip about it with other residents or staff members. However, if you know that a resident should not be drinking alcohol, report this to the nurse.

Chapter Review

1. Give one example of behavior that demonstrates each of the seven characteristics of mental health in Learning Objective 1.

2. What are four possible causes of mental illness?

3. What is the most common fallacy about mental illness?

4. How does mental health affect physical health?

5. List six guidelines for communicating with a resident who is mentally ill.

6. What are defense mechanisms?

7. List three signs and symptoms of each of these mental illnesses: anxiety, depression, and schizophrenia.

8. What are the most common treatments for mental illness?

9. List three care guidelines for mentally ill residents.

10. List five important observations to make about mentally ill residents.

11. List four legal substances than can be abused.

12. List ten signs and symptoms of substance abuse.

21 Rehabilitation and Restorative Care

1. Discuss rehabilitation and restorative care

When a resident loses some ability to function due to illness or injury, rehabilitation may be ordered. **Rehabilitation** is care that is managed by professionals to help to restore a person to the highest possible level of functioning. It involves helping residents move from illness, disability, and dependence toward health, ability, and independence. Rehabilitation involves all parts of the person's disability, including physical (e.g. eating, elimination) and psychosocial (e.g. independence, self-esteem), needs.

Goals of a rehabilitative program include the following:

- To help a resident regain function or recover from illness

- To develop and promote a resident's independence

- To allow a resident to feel in control of his or her life

- To help a resident accept or adapt to the limitations of a disability

Rehabilitation will be used for many of your residents, particularly those who have suffered a stroke, accident, or trauma. Restorative care usually follows rehabilitation. The goal is to keep the resident at the level achieved by rehabilitative services.

Both rehabilitation and restorative care take a team approach (Fig. 21-1). The physician and nurses will establish goals of care. This includes promoting independence in activities of daily living (ADLs) and restoring health to optimal condition. The physical therapist, occupational therapist, or speech language pathologist will work with the resident to help restore or adapt specific abilities. Social workers or other counselors may see the resident to help promote attitudes of independence and acceptance. The effects of the illness or injury cannot always be reversed. Social workers and counselors help people adjust to trauma and loss.

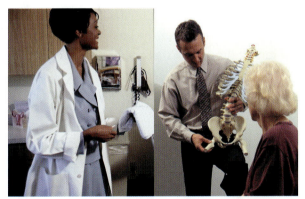

Fig. 21-1. *A team of specialists, including doctors, physical therapists, and other kinds of therapists, helps residents with rehabilitation.*

Because you spend many hours with these residents, you are a very important part of the team. You play a critical role in helping residents recover and regain independence. When assisting with restorative care, these guidelines are critical to your residents' progress:

Guidelines:
Restorative Care

G Be patient. Progress may be slow, and it will seem slower to you and to your residents if you are impatient. Your residents must do as much as possible for themselves. Encourage independence and self-care, regardless of how long it takes or how poorly they are able to do it. The more patient you are, the easier it will be for them to regain abilities and confidence.

G Be positive and supportive. A positive attitude can set the tone for success. Family members, friends, and residents will take cues from you. If you are encouraging and positive, you help create an atmosphere for successful rehabilitation.

G Focus on small tasks and small accomplishments. For example, getting dressed may seem overwhelming to some residents. Break the task down into smaller steps. Today's goal might be putting on a shirt without buttoning it. Next week the goal could be buttoning the shirt if that seems manageable. When the resident can put the shirt on without help, congratulate him. Take everything one step at a time.

G Recognize that setbacks occur. Progress occurs at different rates. Sometimes a resident can do something one day but cannot do it the next. Reassure residents that setbacks are normal. However, document any decline in a resident's abilities.

G Be sensitive to the resident's needs. Some residents may need more encouragement than others. Some may be embarrassed by encouragement. Get to know your residents. Understand what motivates them. Adapt your encouragement to fit each person's personality.

G Encourage independence. A resident's independence may help his or her ability to be active in the process of rehabilitation. Independence improves self-image and attitude. It also helps speed recovery.

G Involve residents in their care. Residents who feel involved and valued may be more motivated to work hard in rehabilitation. Fears may be eased by including family and friends in the rehabilitation program. A team approach is inspiring.

Residents' Rights

Call Lights

Residents may need help often, and not just while in rehabilitation and restorative care. It is never acceptable to unplug a resident's call light, no matter how often he or she uses it, or how demanding the resident is. Staff must respond kindly and promptly to call lights every time they are used. This response can even save lives.

Observing and Reporting:
Restorative Care

O/R Any increase or decrease in abilities (for example, "Yesterday Mr. Martinez used the portable commode without help. Today he asked for the bedpan.")

O/R Any change in attitude or motivation, positive or negative

O/R Any change in general health, such as changes in skin condition, appetite, energy level, or general appearance

O/R Signs of depression or mood changes

Rehabilitation and restorative care is one of the great joys of working as a caregiver. Enjoy seeing residents progress toward independence or recovery. Take pride in your contributions to their improving health.

Tip

Rehabilitation

Residents receiving rehabilitation and restorative care services have been ill or injured and are likely to feel tired, afraid, depressed, or be in pain. Help them feel safe and secure by being kind, patient, and helpful. For example, if therapy schedule interferes with mealtimes, collect the resident's meal and/or reheat it cheerfully if needed. A resident who is frightened may benefit from an unrushed conversation. If a resident says she is in pain, talk to the nurse. Take action to help her. Offer comfort measures, such as a back rub.

2. Describe the importance of promoting independence and list ways exercise improves health

Maintaining independence is vital during and after rehabilitation and restorative services. When an active and independent person is dependent, physical and mental problems may result. The body becomes less mobile and the mind is less focused. Studies show that the more active a person is, the better the mind and body work.

Exercise is important for improving and maintaining physical and mental health. Inactivity and immobility can result in loss of self-esteem, depression, pneumonia, urinary tract infection, constipation, blood clots, and dulling of the senses. People who are in bed for long periods of time are more likely to develop muscle atrophy or contractures. When atrophy occurs, the muscle wastes away, decreases in size, and becomes weak. When a contracture develops, the muscle shortens, becomes inflexible, and "freezes" in position. This can cause permanent disability of the limb.

A lack of mobility may cause other problems as well. Immobility reduces the amount of blood that circulates to the skin. Residents who have restricted mobility have an increased risk for pressure sores. In addition, a lack of mobility

can also cause problems with independence and self-esteem.

The staff's job is to keep residents as active as possible—whether they are bedbound or are able to get out of bed and walk (ambulate). Regular ambulation and exercise help improve the following:

- Quality and health of the skin
- Circulation
- Strength
- Sleep and relaxation
- Mood
- Self-esteem
- Appetite
- Elimination
- Blood flow
- Oxygen level

Promoting social interactions and thinking abilities is important, too. Most facilities have activities geared to residents' ages and abilities. Social involvement should be encouraged. When possible, nursing assistants should join in activities with residents. This promotes independence. It also gives NAs a chance to observe residents' abilities.

Basic Exercise Principles

It is important to get a doctor's approval before starting a new exercise or activity program. It is not safe to exercise with certain heart conditions. Exercising with high blood pressure can be risky. Caution must be used after surgery. It is also necessary to limit exercise with unstable bones, in the case of fractures or osteoporosis, and with extreme breathing problems.

Warming up should be done before doing any other exercises. This consists of light exercise, such as walking. The warm-up begins to increase heart rate and breathing. It helps prevent injury. Some people like to stretch at the beginning of their workout. Stretching should not be done until the muscles are warm.

Cool-down exercises are done to slowly lower the heart rate. They return other body functions to normal. Suddenly ending an exercise session without cooling down can cause blood to pool in the large leg muscles. This may cause dizziness or even fainting. It is good to stretch after the cool-down, while the muscles are still warm. Stretching keeps muscles flexible and helps them relax.

3. Describe assistive devices and equipment

Many devices are available to help people who are recovering from or adapting to a physical condition. You first learned about assistive or adaptive equipment in Chapter 2. This equipment helps residents perform their ADLs. Each adaptive device is made to support a particular disability. Raised seating, for example, makes it simpler for a resident with weak legs to stand.

Personal care equipment includes long-handled brushes and combs. Plate guards prevent food from being pushed off the plate and make it easier to scoop food onto utensils. Reachers can help put on underwear or pants. A sock aid can pull on socks, and a long-handled shoehorn assists in putting shoes on without bending. Long-handled sponges help with bathing.

Supportive devices, such as canes, walkers, and crutches, are used to assist residents with ambulation (see Chapter 10). Safety devices, such as shower chairs and gait or transfer belts, help prevent accidents. Safety bars/grab bars are often installed in and near the tub and toilet to give the resident something to hold on to while changing position. The items shown in Fig. 21-2 can be useful as residents relearn old skills or adapt to new limitations.

Tip

Walking Aids

Residents using new ambulatory aids, such as canes, walkers, boots, crutches, etc. are likely to be off-balance. Stay close by to be sure they are using these appliances safely. Observe residents for signs of dizziness. To avoid falls, clear pathways, and wipe up spills immediately.

Tip

Trapeze

A trapeze is a triangular piece of equipment that hangs over the head of the bed. It may be mounted to the bed or freestanding. People in bed can grasp the trapeze with their hands, which enables them to lift themselves. The trapeze assists with repositioning and exercise activities.

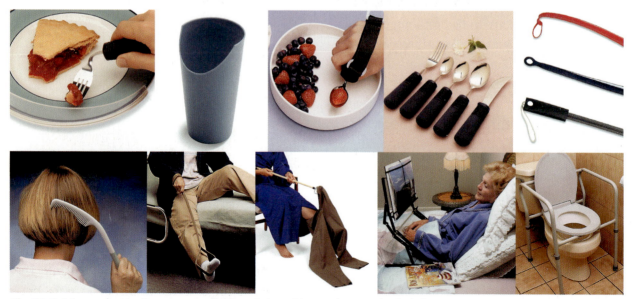

Fig. 21-2. *Many adaptive items are available to help residents adapt to physical changes.* (Photos courtesy of North Coast Medical, Inc. 800-821-9319)

Rehabilitation and Restorative Care

4. Explain guidelines for maintaining proper body alignment

Residents who are confined to bed need to maintain proper body alignment. This aids recovery and prevents injury to muscles and joints. Chapter 10 gives specific instructions for positioning residents. The following guidelines help residents maintain good alignment and make progress when they can get out of bed.

Guidelines:
Alignment and Positioning

G   Observe principles of alignment. Remember that proper alignment is based on straight lines. The spine should be in a straight line. Pillows or rolled or folded blankets can support the small of the back and raise the knees or head in the supine position. They can support the head and one leg in the lateral position (Fig. 21-3).

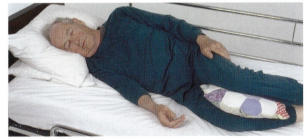

Fig. 21-3. Pillows or rolled or folded blankets help provide extra support.

G   Keep body parts in natural positions. In a natural hand position, the fingers are slightly curled. Use a rolled washcloth, gauze bandage, or rubber ball inside the palm to support the fingers in this position (Fig. 21-4). Use footboards to keep covers from resting on feet in the supine position.

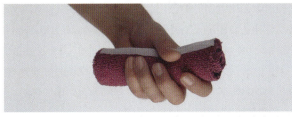

Fig. 21-4. Handrolls keep fingers from curling tightly.

G   Prevent external rotation of hips. When legs and hips turn outward during bedrest, hip contractures can result. A contracture is the permanent and often very painful stiffening of a joint and muscle. A rolled blanket or towel tucked alongside the hip and thigh can keep the leg from turning outward.

G   Change positions often to prevent muscle stiffness and pressure sores. This should be done at least every two hours. The position used will depend on the resident's condition and preference. Check the skin every time you reposition the resident.

5. Explain care guidelines for prosthetic devices

A prosthesis is a device that replaces a body part that is missing or deformed because of an accident, injury, illness, or birth defect. It is used to improve a person's ability to function and/or to improve appearance. Examples of prostheses include the following:

*   Artificial limbs, such as for the hands, arms, feet, and legs, are made to resemble the body part that they are replacing (Fig. 21-5). Many advances have been made and continue to be made in the field of prosthetic limbs. Today's artificial limbs are usually made of strong and lightweight plastics and other materials, such as carbon fiber. Most artificial limbs are attached by belts, cuffs, or suction. Direct bone attachment is a newer method of attaching the limb to the body.

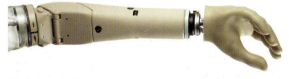

Fig. 21-5. One type of prosthetic arm. (MOTION CONTROL UTAH ARM. PHOTO BY KEVIN TWOMEY.)

*   An artificial breast is made of a lightweight, soft, spongy material. It usually fits into a regular bra or in the pocket of a special bra called a mastectomy bra.

- A hearing aid is a small, battery-operated device that amplifies sound for persons with hearing loss. Many elderly residents have hearing aids.

- Eyeglasses are an optical instrument worn in front of the eyes for correcting vision. They consist of frames that hold a pair of lenses. Many people wear eyeglasses.

- An artificial eye, or ocular prosthetic, replaces an eye that has been lost to disease or injury. It is usually made of plastic, although some are made of glass. It is held in place by suction. An ocular prosthetic does not provide vision. It can, however, improve appearance.

- Dentures are artificial teeth. They may be necessary when a tooth or teeth have been damaged, lost, or must be removed. Many elderly residents have dentures.

See Chapter 4 for more information on eyeglasses and hearing aids and Chapter 13 for more information on denture care.

Guidelines:
Amputation and Prosthesis Care

G   If residents have had a body part amputated, they must make many physical, psychological, social, and occupational adjustments to their disability. Be supportive.

G   Because prostheses are specially-fitted, expensive pieces of equipment (some cost tens of thousands of dollars), only care for them as assigned. Handle them carefully. Follow the care plan.

G   A nurse or therapist will demonstrate application of a prosthesis. Follow instructions to apply and remove the prosthesis. Follow the manufacturer's care directions.

G   Keep a prosthesis and the skin under it dry and clean. The socket of the prosthesis must be cleaned daily when the prosthesis is removed. It may be cleaned more often, if needed. Follow the care plan and the nurse's instructions.

G   If ordered, apply a stump sock before putting on the prosthesis.

G   Observe the skin on stump. Watch for signs of skin breakdown caused by pressure and abrasion. Report any redness or open areas. Never try to fix a prosthesis. Report any problems to the nurse.

G   Do not show negative feelings about the stump during care.

G   If the person has a hearing aid, make sure he or she is wearing it and that it is working properly.

G   If the resident has eyeglasses, make sure they are clean and that he or she wears them.

G   If instructed to care for an artificial eye, first wash your hands. Provide privacy for the resident. Put on gloves before beginning care. Artificial eyes are held in by suction. They will come out quickly when pressure is applied below the lower eyelid. Wash eye with solution and rinse in warm water. Never clean or soak the eye in alcohol. It will crack the plastic and destroy it. Moisten the artificial eye and place it far under upper eyelid. Pull down on lower eyelid and the eye should slide into place.

G   If the artificial eye is to be removed and not reinserted, line an eye cup or basin with a soft cloth or a piece of 4x4 gauze. This prevents scratches and damage. Fill with water or saline solution. Place the eye in the container and close the container. Make sure the container is labeled with the resident's name and room number.

G   If the artificial eye is removed, wash the eye socket with warm water or saline. Use a clean gauze square to clean it. Clean the eyelid with a clean cotton ball. Wipe gently from inner corner (canthus) outward.

6. Describe how to assist with range of motion exercises

Range of motion (ROM) exercises are exercises that put a joint through its full arc of motion. The goal of ROM exercises is to decrease or prevent contractures, improve strength, and increase circulation. **Passive range of motion (PROM) exercises** are used when residents cannot move on their own; a staff member performs these exercises without the resident's help. When helping with PROM exercises, support the resident's joints and move them through the range of motion. **Active range of motion (AROM) exercises** are performed by a resident himself. Your role in AROM exercises is to encourage the resident. **Active assisted range of motion (AAROM) exercises** are done by the resident with some assistance and support from a staff member.

You will not do ROM exercises without an order from a doctor, nurse, or physical therapist. Follow the care plan. You will repeat each exercise three to five times, once or twice a day. You will work on both sides of the body. During ROM exercises, begin at the resident's head and work down the body. Exercise the upper extremities (arms) before the lower extremities (legs). Give support above and below the joint. Move the joints gently, slowly, and smoothly through the range of motion to the point of resistance. Stop the exercises if the resident complains of pain. Report pain to the nurse.

Range of motion exercises are specific for each body area. They include the following movements (Fig. 21-6):

- **Abduction**: moving a body part away from the midline of the body

- **Adduction**: moving a body part toward the midline of the body

- **Dorsiflexion**: bending backward

- **Rotation**: turning a joint

- **Extension**: straightening a body part

- **Flexion**: bending a body part

- **Pronation**: turning downward

- **Supination**: turning upward

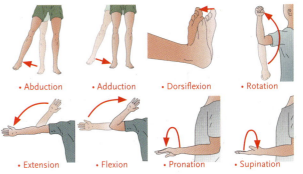

- Abduction   - Adduction   - Dorsiflexion   - Rotation
- Extension   - Flexion   - Pronation   - Supination

Fig. 21-6. *Different range of motion body movements.*

Assisting with passive range of motion exercises

1. Wash your hands.

2. Identify yourself by name. Identify the resident by name.

3. Explain procedure to resident. Speak clearly, slowly, and directly. Maintain face-to-face contact whenever possible.

4. Provide for resident's privacy with curtain, screen, or door.

5. Adjust bed to a safe level, usually waist high. Lock bed wheels.

6. Position the resident lying supine—flat on his or her back—on the bed. Use proper alignment.

7. Repeat each exercise at least 3 times. While supporting the limbs, move all joints gently, slowly, and smoothly through the range of motion to the point of resistance. Stop if any pain occurs.

8. **Shoulder**. Support the resident's arm at the elbow and wrist during ROM for the shoulder. Place one hand under the elbow and

the other hand under the wrist. Raise the straightened arm from the side position forward to above the head and return arm to side of the body (flexion/extension) (Fig. 21-7).

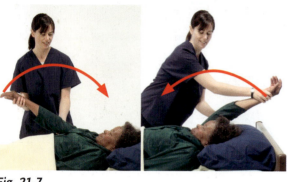

Fig. 21-7.

Raise the arm to side position above head and return arm to side of the body (abduction/adduction) (Fig. 21-8).

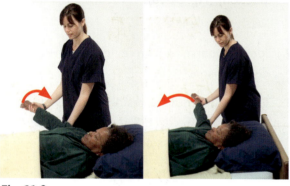

Fig. 21-8.

9. **Elbow**. Hold the resident's wrist with one hand, the elbow with the other hand. Bend the elbow so that the hand touches the shoulder on that same side (flexion). Straighten the arm (extension) (Fig. 21-9).

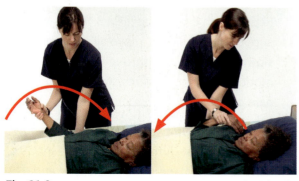

Fig. 21-9.

Exercise the forearm by moving it so the palm is facing downward (pronation) and then the palm is facing upward (supination) (Fig. 21-10).

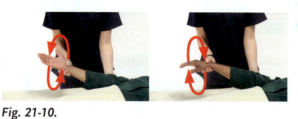

Fig. 21-10.

10. **Wrist**. Hold the wrist with one hand and use the fingers of the other hand to help the joint through the motions. Bend the hand down (flexion); bend the hand backwards (extension) (Fig. 21-11).

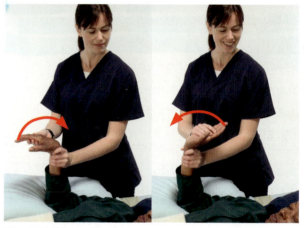

Fig. 21-11.

Turn the hand in the direction of the thumb (radial flexion). Then turn it in the direction of the little finger (ulnar flexion) (Fig. 21-12).

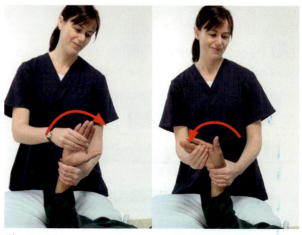

Fig. 21-12.

Rehabilitation and Restorative Care

11. **Thumb**. Move the thumb away from the index finger (abduction). Move the thumb back next to the index finger (adduction) (Fig. 21-13).

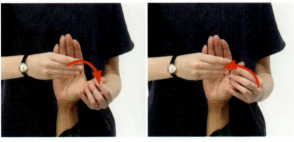

Fig. 21-13.

Touch each fingertip with the thumb (opposition) (Fig. 21-14).

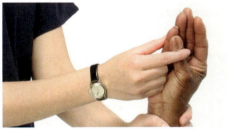

Fig. 21-14.

Bend thumb into the palm (flexion) and out to the side (extension) (Fig. 21-15).

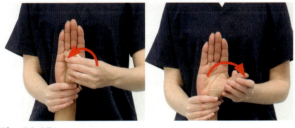

Fig. 21-15.

12. **Fingers**. Make the hand into a fist (flexion). Gently straighten out the fist (extension) (Fig. 21-16).

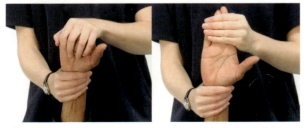

Fig. 21-16.

Spread the fingers and the thumb far apart from each other (abduction). Bring the fingers back next to each other (adduction) (Fig. 21-17).

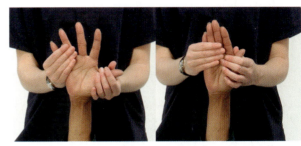

Fig. 21-17.

13. **Hip**. Support the leg by placing one hand under the knee and one under the ankle. Straighten the leg and raise it gently upward.

Move the leg away from the other leg (abduction). Move the leg toward the other leg (adduction) (Fig. 21-18).

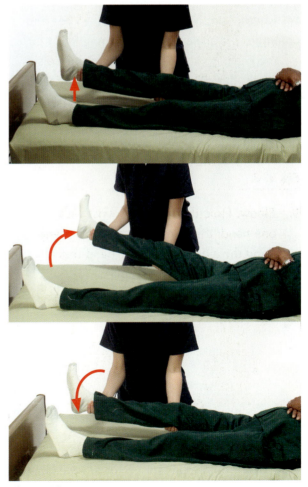

Fig. 21-18.

Gently turn the leg inward (internal rotation), then turn the leg outward (external rotation) (Fig. 21-19).

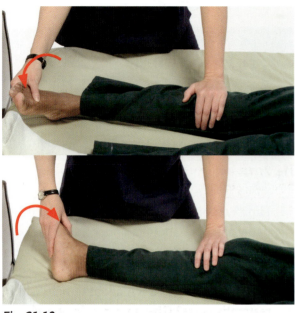

Fig. 21-19.

14. **Knees**. Support the leg under the knee and under the ankle while performing ROM for the knee. Bend the leg to the point of resistance (flexion). Return leg to resident's normal position (extension) (Fig. 21-20).

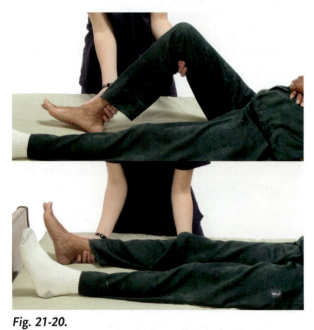

Fig. 21-20.

15. **Ankles**. Push/pull foot up toward the head (dorsiflexion). Push/pull foot down, with the

toes pointed down (plantar flexion) (Fig. 21-21).

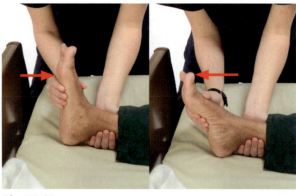

Fig. 21-21.

Turn the inside of the foot inward toward the body (supination). Bend the sole of the foot so that it faces away from the body (pronation) (Fig. 21-22).

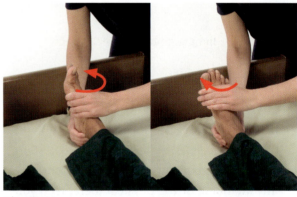

Fig. 21-22.

16. **Toes**. Curl and straighten the toes (flexion and extension) (Fig. 21-23).

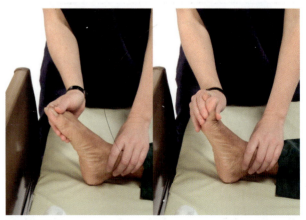

Fig. 21-23.

Gently spread the toes apart (abduction) (Fig. 21-24).

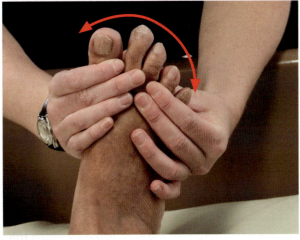

Fig. 21-24.

17. Return resident to comfortable position. Return bed to lowest position. Remove privacy measures.

18. Place call light within resident's reach.

19. Wash your hands.

20. Report any changes in resident to nurse.

21. Document procedure using facility guidelines. Note any decrease in range of motion or any pain experienced by the resident. Notify the nurse or the physical therapist if you find increased stiffness or physical resistance. Resistance may be a sign that a contracture is developing.

7. Describe the benefits of deep breathing exercises

Deep breathing exercises help expand the lungs, clearing them of mucus and preventing infections (such as pneumonia). Residents who are paralyzed or who have had surgery are often told to do deep breathing exercises regularly to expand the lungs.

The care plan may include using a deep breathing device called an incentive spirometer (Fig. 21-25). Do not assist with these exercises if

you have not been trained. Ask the nurse for instructions.

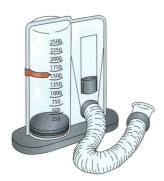

Fig. 21-25. *Incentive spirometers are used for deep breathing exercises.*

Chapter Review

1. What does rehabilitation involve?

2. What attitudes can a NA adopt to help with restorative care? Give an example of each.

3. List 10 problems that a lack of mobility can cause.

4. What are some benefits of regular exercise?

5. Look at the adaptive devices in Figure 21-2. Choose one and briefly describe how it might help a resident recovering from or adapting to a physical condition.

6. List three guidelines to follow to help residents maintain good alignment.

7. List and describe four prosthetic devices.

8. What should be observed about the skin on the stump of an amputated body part?

9. Why should alcohol not be used to clean an artificial eye?

10. What is the goal of ROM exercises?

11. When performing ROM exercises, where should the NA begin? Which parts of the body should be exercised first?

12. Describe the difference between passive, active, and active assisted range of motion exercises.

13. Why are deep breathing exercises performed?

22
Special Care Skills

1. Understand the types of residents who are in a subacute setting

Subacute care is a kind of specialized care that falls between acute care and long-term care. This type of care can take place in hospitals and in skilled nursing facilities. People in subacute settings require more treatment, monitoring, and services than regular long-term care provides. Subacute care may be necessary due to recent surgery, injuries, or chronic illnesses, such as AIDS (Fig. 22-1). Complex wound care, specialized infusion therapy, dialysis, and mechanical ventilation may also require subacute care. Dialysis cleanses the body of waste that the kidneys cannot remove due to chronic kidney failure. A mechanical ventilator is a machine that assists with or replaces breathing when a person cannot breathe on his own.

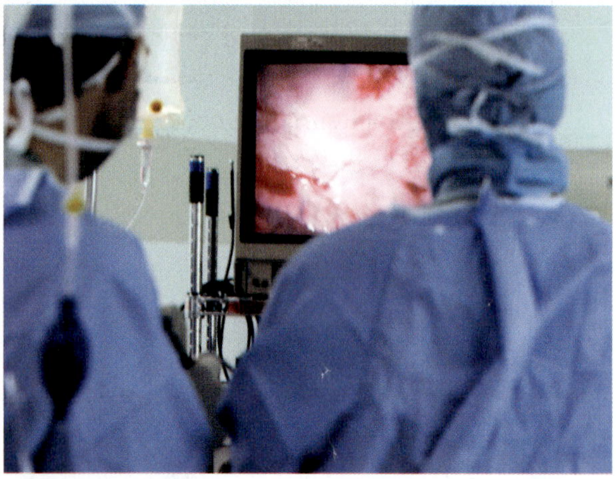

Fig. 22-1. Subacute care provides a higher level of care; it may be necessary due to surgery, illness, serious wounds, dialysis or mechanical ventilation.

2. Discuss reasons for and types of surgery

There are many reasons why surgery is performed, including the following:

- To relieve symptoms of a disease
- To repair or remove problem tissues and structures
- To improve appearance or correct function of damaged tissues
- To diagnose disease
- To cure a disease

Surgeries generally fall into three categories: elective, urgent, and emergency. Elective surgery is surgery that is chosen by the patient and is planned in advance. Generally, the surgery is not absolutely necessary. Plastic surgery, such as having a facelift, is an example of an elective surgery.

Urgent surgery is surgery that must be performed for health reasons, but is not an emergency. Urgent surgery may even be planned and scheduled in advance, as with heart surgery, such as coronary artery bypass surgery.

Emergency surgery is unexpected and unscheduled surgery that is performed immediately to save a patient's life or a limb. A gunshot wound, car accident, or ruptured appendix are examples of situations that can require emergency surgery.

When a person has surgery, anesthesia will usually be given. **Anesthesia** involves the use of medication to block pain during surgery and other medical procedures. Local anesthesia involves the injection of an anesthetic directly into the surgical site or area to block pain. It is used for minor surgical procedures, and the person may remain awake during the surgery. Regional anesthesia involves injection of an anesthetic into a nerve or group of nerves to block sensation in a particular region of the body. It is limited to an area, but to a larger area than for a local anesthetic. One example of a regional anesthetic is an epidural, which is used during childbirth to block pain in the body in the lower half of the body, from the waist down. General anesthesia is inhaled or injected directly into a vein and affects the brain and the entire body. The person is unaware of his surroundings and does not feel any pain. It blocks any memory of the procedure. This type of anesthesia is stopped when the surgery has been completed.

3. Discuss preoperative care

Depending on where you work, your duties may include giving **preoperative**, or before surgery, care. Preoperative care includes both physical and psychological preparation. Before a person has surgery, a doctor will explain the procedure, the risks and benefits, and what to expect after surgery. The person will be encouraged to ask questions and give opinions. This is part of informed consent (Chapter 3), a process in which a person, with the help of a doctor, makes informed decisions about his or her health care. The person must sign a written consent form for surgery, or have one signed by a guardian or someone with medical power of attorney.

People who are going to have surgery often experience anxiety, fear, worry, and sadness, and other emotions (Fig. 22-2). It is often helpful to express these concerns to members of the healthcare team. Being prepared psychologically may help the resident cope better after surgery. As a nursing assistant, part of your role in assisting with this preparation means listening to

a resident's concerns. Report any concerns or questions to the nurse. Also report to the nurse if the person requests a visit from clergy.

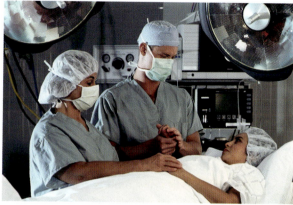

Fig. 22-2. *Patients often have many worries before surgery. A compassionate response by staff may help alleviate concerns.*

A person who is having surgery will require preoperative physical preparation, as well. Follow these general guidelines to assist with physically preparing a resident for surgery:

Guidelines:
Preoperative Care

G   Before surgery, there will be an order for the resident to receive NPO (nothing by mouth). This time usually ranges anywhere from two to eight hours. Having this medical order means that nothing is allowed by mouth, including water, ice chips, food, etc. Remove the water pitcher, glass, and any other food and fluids from the immediate area. Explain to the resident why you are doing this. Report any concerns to the nurse.

G   Assist the resident with urinating before surgery.

G   For some residents having surgery of the gastrointestinal tract, the bowels may need to be cleared. An enema or suppository may be ordered. Assist as trained, ordered, and allowed. Be ready to bring the bedpan or portable commode when needed. Provide plenty of privacy.

G   Assist with bathing as needed. Dressing the person in loose-fitting clothes may make it easier to change into a gown later.

G   Make sure call light is within reach every time before you leave the room.

G   Measure and record vital signs as ordered.

G   Remove dentures, glasses, contact lenses, hearing aids, jewelry, hairpieces, hairpins, and any other personal items. Store these safely according to facility policy. For local or regional anesthetic, the doctor may want the person to wear hearing aids and dentures, so that communication will be easier.

G   Assist person to change into gown, if required.

G   Transfer to a stretcher/gurney if necessary.

G   Make sure the resident's identification bracelet is accurate and on the wrist or ankle prior to transport. You may need to verify if the resident has any known allergies by asking this question or verifying what is written on an allergy bracelet.

4. Describe postoperative care

Postoperative, or after surgery, care begins immediately following surgery. The goal of postoperative care is to prevent infections, promote healing, and return the person to a state of health. Immediate postoperative concerns are problems with breathing, mental status, pain, and wound healing. Complications of surgery can also include urinary retention or infections, constipation, blood pressure variances, and blood clots. Careful postoperative monitoring is critical.

After surgery, the resident is taken to the recovery room and may remain there for some time. This depends on the type of surgery the resident had, as well as how long the surgery was, what type and how much anesthetic was used, and the resident's level of consciousness.

While the resident is in recovery, your duties will include changing bed linens and gathering equipment. Equipment needed may include the following:

*   Bed protector

*   Towels and washcloths

*   Vital signs equipment

*   Emesis basin

*   Pillows and other positioning devices

*   Warming blankets

*   IV pole

*   Oxygen and suction equipment

When the resident returns to the room, use the following guidelines to assist with postoperative care:

Guidelines:
Postoperative Care

G   Move furniture as needed to allow for the transfer back into bed from the stretcher.

G   Assist with transferring the resident back into bed. (Chapter 10 has information on stretcher transfers.)

G   Return dentures, glasses, contact lenses, and hearing aids to the resident. Remember that without these items, residents may not be able to talk, eat, see, or hear.

G   Measure and record vital signs often after surgery as directed. The schedule may look like this: every 15 minutes for the first hour, every 30 minutes for the next hour to two hours, every hour for the next four hours, and then every four hours. Report any changes immediately.

G   Reposition the resident every hour to two hours, or as ordered. Elevate the extremities as ordered.

G   Assist with deep breathing and coughing exercises (Chapter 21).

G Apply anti-embolic hose to reduce the risk of blood clots, if ordered. Assist with leg exercises as instructed.

G Apply binders as ordered. Binders are stretchable pieces of fabric that can be fastened. They hold dressings in place and give support to surgical wounds. Binders can also reduce swelling and ease discomfort.

G Encourage proper nutrition and fluid intake. Proper food and fluid intake can speed the recovery process. The resident may be on a high-protein diet to promote wound healing.

G Assist with elimination. Always provide plenty of privacy for elimination.

G Help with bathing and grooming as requested and as ordered.

G Assist with ambulation as needed and as ordered. Be encouraging and positive.

Observing and Reporting:
Postoperative Care

Report the following signs and symptoms of complications to the nurse immediately:

O/R Changes in vital signs

O/R Difficulty breathing

O/R Mental changes, such as confusion or disorientation

O/R Changes in consciousness

O/R Pale or bluish skin

O/R Skin that is cold or clammy

O/R Increase in amount of drainage

O/R Swelling at IV site

O/R IV that is not dripping

O/R Nausea or vomiting

O/R Numbness or tingling

O/R Resident complaints of pain

5. List care guidelines for pulse oximetry

When residents have had surgery, are on oxygen, are in intensive care, or have cardiac or respiratory problems, a pulse oximeter may be used. A **pulse oximeter** is a noninvasive device that uses a light to determine the amount of oxygen in the blood (also called oxygen saturation). A pulse oximeter also measures a person's pulse rate.

A sensor is clipped on a person's finger, earlobe, or toe (Fig. 22-3). A light passes through the skin, and the percentage of oxygen in the blood and the pulse rate are displayed. An alarm will sound if the oxygen level becomes less than optimal.

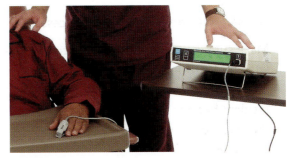

Fig. 22-3. A pulse oximeter.

Normal blood oxygen level usually measures between 95% and 100%. However, what is normal may differ from person to person. Report any increase or decrease in oxygen levels to the nurse.

Guidelines:
Pulse Oximeter

G Report to the nurse immediately if the alarm on the pulse oximeter sounds.

G Tell the nurse if the pulse oximeter falls off or if the resident requests you remove it.

G Check the skin around the device often. Report any of the following:

Swelling

Bluish, or cyanotic, skin

Shiny, tight skin

Skin that is cold to the touch

Sores, redness, or irritation

Numbness or tingling

Pain or discomfort

G Check vital signs as ordered. Report changes to the nurse.

6. Describe telemetry and list care guidelines

Telemetry is used to measure the heart rhythm and rate on a continuous basis. Wires are attached to the chest with sticky pads or patches. The wires are connected to a battery-powered portable unit, which sends data to computer screens at a monitoring station. This data is monitored and assessed at all times by specially trained staff.

Telemetry may be necessary due to chest pain, heart or lung disease, heart or lung surgery, irregular heartbeats, or certain medications that affect heart rhythm or rate.

Guidelines:
Telemetry

G Report to the nurse if the pads become wet or soiled. Report if pads appear loose or fall off.

G Report if the alarm sounds. The alarm may sound if the pads disconnect, or if the battery is low.

G Check the skin around the pads often. Report any of the following:

Swelling

Sores, redness, or irritation

Fluid or blood draining from skin

Broken skin

G Report resident complaints of chest pain or discomfort, as well as any difficulty breathing.

G Check vital signs as ordered. Report changes to the nurse.

7. Explain artificial airways and list care guidelines

An **artificial airway** is any plastic, metal, or rubber device inserted into the respiratory tract to maintain or promote breathing. Artificial airways keep the airway open. This is necessary when the airway is obstructed due to illness, injury, secretions, or aspiration. Some residents who are unconscious will need an artificial airway.

The artificial airway is inserted using a method called intubation. **Intubation** involves the passage of a plastic tube through the mouth, nose, or an opening in the neck and into the trachea (windpipe). There are different types of artificial airways (Fig. 22-4). One common type is a **tracheostomy**, which is a surgically-created opening through the neck into the trachea. A hollow tube, called a tracheostomy tube, is inserted through this opening into the trachea. It is also called a "trach tube." More information on this type of artificial airway may be found in the next Learning Objective.

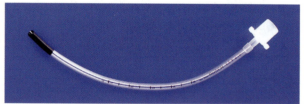

Fig. 22-4. *An endotracheal tube is a type of artificial airway that is inserted through the mouth and then into the trachea.* (PHOTO COURTESY OF RUSCH - A TELEFLEX COMPANY.)

Guidelines:
Artificial Airways

G Observe the resident closely. If the tubing falls out, tell the nurse immediately.

G Check vital signs as ordered. Report changes to the nurse.

G Perform oral care often, as directed.

G Watch for biting and tugging on tube. If a resident is doing this, tell the nurse.

G Use other methods of communication if the person cannot speak. Try writing notes, drawing pictures, and using communication boards. Watch for hand and eye signals.

G Be supportive and reassuring. It can be frightening and uncomfortable to have an artificial airway. Some residents may choke or gag. Be empathetic. Imagine how it might feel to have a tube in your nose, mouth, or throat.

8. Discuss care for a resident with a tracheostomy

A tracheostomy is a type of artificial airway commonly seen in long-term care (Fig. 22-5). Tracheostomies may be necessary for many reasons, including the following:

- Tumors/cancer
- Infection
- Severe neck or mouth injuries
- Facial surgery and facial burns
- Long-term unconsciousness or coma
- Obstruction in the airway
- Paralysis of muscles related to breathing
- Aspiration as a result of muscle or sensory problems in the throat
- Severe allergic reaction
- Gunshot wound

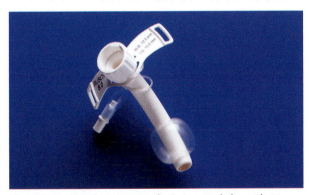

Fig. 22-5. *A tracheostomy tube is inserted through a surgically-created opening in the neck into the trachea.*
(PHOTO COURTESY OF RUSCH - A TELEFLEX COMPANY)

This procedure is usually temporary, but it can be permanent. It is easier to suction and attach respiratory equipment with a tracheostomy than with other artificial airways.

When the tracheostomy is first placed, it may be difficult for the resident to adapt to breathing through the tube. This can cause anxiety and frustration. It may be difficult for the resident to talk at first, which also causes fear. During this time, be especially supportive and encouraging. Use other methods of communication, such as writing notes, drawing pictures, using communication boards, and using hand and eye signals. Check on the resident often, and answer call lights immediately. People can usually learn to talk through a trach tube.

Care of the tracheostomy may include skin care around the opening, helping with dressing changes, and cleaning the device. Suctioning may be required. Nursing assistants do not perform suctioning or trach care. Your responsibilities will mostly include observing and reporting.

Observing and Reporting:
Tracheostomies

Report any of the following to the nurse:

O/R Shortness of breath

O/R Trouble breathing

O/R Gurgling sounds

O/R Any signs of skin breakdown around the opening, such as irritation, rash, cracks, breaks, sores, or bleeding on the skin

O/R The type and amount of discharge the resident coughs up through the tracheostomy (normal discharge looks like white mucus or saliva)

O/R Any increase in the amount of discharge

O/R Discharge that is thick, yellow, green, bloody, or has an odor (this may indicate an infection or other problem in the lungs)

O/R Mouth sores or discomfort

It is very important to prevent infection when caring for residents with tracheostomies. They are prone to respiratory infections. Wash your hands often and wear gloves when indicated. Keep equipment clean. Anything that is dropped on the floor must be sterilized before it can be used in contact with the tubes. Great care must be taken so that nothing gets into the tube which can cause an infection in the lungs.

9. List care guidelines for residents requiring mechanical ventilation

Residents in a subacute unit may be on a mechanical ventilator (Fig. 22-6). **Mechanical ventilation** is using a machine to assist with or replace breathing (inflate and deflate the lungs) when a person is unable to do this on his own. A person may require mechanical ventilation due to cardiac or respiratory arrest, lung injuries and diseases, or head and spinal cord injuries.

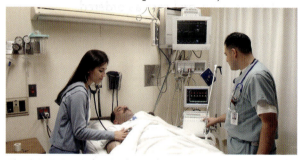

Fig. 22-6. *A mechanical ventilator.* (PHOTO COURTESY OF PULMONETIC SYSTEMS)

Residents will not be able to speak while on the mechanical ventilator. This is because air will no longer reach the larynx (vocal cords). Not being able to speak may increase anxiety. The resident may think that no one will know if he or she is having trouble breathing. Being on a ventilator has been compared to breathing through a straw. Think about how that might feel. Residents will need a lot of support while connected to the ventilator. Enter the room often so that the resident can see you. This reassures residents that they are being carefully observed. Clipboards, notepads, and communication boards will help with communication.

Residents on a ventilator are often heavily sedated. A **sedative** is an agent or drug that helps calm and soothe a person and may cause sleep. Being sedated helps prevent people on ventilators from feeling discomfort and anxiety. Even if a resident seems unaware of what is happening, continue to speak to him or her and explain what you are doing.

Guidelines:
Mechanical Ventilator

G   Ventilators cause an increased risk for a special type of pneumonia. Wash your hands often when working with residents on mechanical ventilators.

G   Report to the nurse if the alarm sounds.

G   If you notice tubing that is disconnected or loose, report it immediately.

G   Answer the call light promptly.

G   Follow the care plan for repositioning instructions. Give regular, careful skin care to prevent pressure sores. Check the skin around the intubation site often, as well as on the rest of the body. Report any of the following:

Swelling

Sores, redness, irritation

Fluid or blood draining from skin

Broken skin

G   Report if the resident is pulling on or biting the tube. Report if the resident is anxious, fearful, or upset.

G   Be patient during communication. Observe body language. Watch for hand or eye signals.

G   Check on the resident often, so that the resident can see you are there. Be supportive, kind, and empathetic.

10. Describe suctioning and list signs of respiratory distress

Subacute care units include residents who require suctioning by nurses or respiratory therapists. Suctioning removes mucus and secretions from the lungs when a person cannot do this on his own. A person who has a tracheostomy may require suctioning. Suctioning can be performed through the nose, mouth, or throat.

Suctioning is normally a sterile procedure. Nursing assistants do not perform suctioning; nurses or respiratory therapists will perform the suctioning. A portable pump, operated on battery power or electrical power, may be used to suction the resident (Fig. 22-7). A canister or bottle on the pump collects the mucus and secretions.

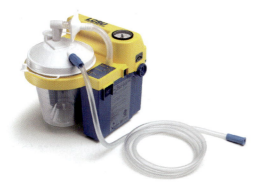

Fig. 22-7. This is one type of suctioning pump. Nursing assistants do not perform suctioning. They help by reporting signs of respiratory distress and monitoring vital signs. (PHOTO COURTESY OF LAERDAL MEDICAL CORPORATION)

A person who needs frequent suctioning may show signs of respiratory distress. Signs of respiratory distress include the following:

- Gurgling sound of secretions

- Difficulty breathing

- Elevated respiratory rate

- Pale, bluish, or gray skin around the eyes, mouth, fingernails or toenails

- Nostrils flaring (nostrils opening wider when breathing in may show that a person is having to work harder to breathe)

- Retracting (chest appears to sink in below the neck with each breath)

- Sweating

- Wheezing

Guidelines:
Suctioning

G   Report signs of respiratory distress to the nurse immediately.

G   Monitor vital signs closely, especially respiratory rate. Report changes.

G   Follow Standard Precautions. Don gloves, gown, mask, or goggles as directed.

G   Assist the nurse with suctioning as needed. You may be asked to have a towel or washcloth ready to clean the resident after suctioning. Give oral care as ordered.

G   Report resident complaints of pain or difficulty breathing.

11. Describe chest tubes and explain related care

Chest tubes are hollow drainage tubes that are inserted into the chest during a sterile procedure. They can be inserted at the bedside or during surgery. Chest tubes drain air, blood, or fluid that has collected inside the pleural cavity or space. The pleural cavity is the space between the layers of the pleura, the thin membrane that covers and protects the lungs. Chest tubes are also inserted to allow a full expansion of the lungs. Some conditions that require chest tube insertion include the following:

- Pneumothorax: air or gas in the pleural space

- Hemothorax: blood in the pleural space

- Empyema: pus in the pleural space
- Certain types of surgery
- Chest trauma or injuries

A doctor normally inserts chest tubes. The chest tube is connected to a bottle of sterile water. Suction is sometimes attached to the system to encourage drainage. This system must be sealed so that air cannot enter the pleural cavity. The system must be airtight.

When X-rays show that the air, blood, or fluid has been drained, the tube is removed. Medications may be used to prevent or treat infection.

Guidelines:
Chest Tubes

G   Be aware of the number and location of chest tubes. Tubes may be in the front, back, or side of the body.

G   Check vital signs as directed. Report any changes immediately to the nurse.

G   Report signs of respiratory distress to the nurse immediately. Report complaints of pain.

G   Keep the drainage system below the level of the resident's chest.

G   Make sure drainage containers remain upright and level at all times.

G   Make sure that tubing is not kinked. If tubing becomes kinked, report to the nurse right away.

G   Watch for disconnected tubing. If this happens, report it immediately.

G   Certain equipment is kept nearby in case tubes are pulled out. Do not remove these items from the area.

G   Observe chest drainage for color and amount. Report any changes in color or amount immediately.

G   Report if there is an increase or decrease in bubbling in the drainage system. Report if there are clots in the tubing.

G   Follow the repositioning schedule. Be very gentle with turning and repositioning. You must move the resident and the tubes at the same time to prevent tubes from coming out. Always get enough help.

G   Report odor in the chest tube area.

G   Provide rest periods as needed.

G   Follow fluid intake orders. Measure intake and output carefully as ordered.

G   If asked to help with coughing and deep breathing exercises, be encouraging and patient.

Other residents who require more direct care and close observation by staff include residents with IVs (Chapter 14) and residents with tube feedings (Chapter 15).

Chapter Review

1. What is different about the type of care provided in a subacute setting as compared to the type of care provided in regular long-term care?

2. Briefly describe three types of surgeries.

3. Which type of anesthesia is inhaled or injected directly into a vein and affects the brain and entire body?

4. List eight guidelines for assisting with pre-operative care.

5. List eight guidelines for assisting with post-operative care.

6. List 10 signs and symptoms to report about a resident after surgery.

7. List two reasons why a resident may need a pulse oximeter.

8. What is important to report about the skin when a resident is using a telemetry unit?

9. What are alternate methods of communication nursing assistants can use with residents who have artificial airways?

10. What are a nursing assistant's responsibilities with tracheostomy care?

11. In what ways can a nursing assistant show support for a resident who is on a ventilator?

12. Why might a resident be anxious while on a ventilator?

13. List five signs of respiratory distress.

14. What types of fluids are drained by chest tubes?

15. List 12 guidelines for caring for residents with chest tubes.

23

Death and Dying

1. Discuss the stages of grief

Death can occur suddenly without warning, or it can be expected. Older people, or those with terminal illnesses, may have time to prepare for death. A **terminal illness** is a disease or condition that will eventually cause death. Preparing for death is a process. It affects the dying person's emotions and behavior.

Dr. Elisabeth Kubler-Ross researched and wrote about the grief process. Her book, *On Death and Dying*, describes five stages that dying people and their families or friends may experience before death. These five stages are described below. Not all residents go through all the stages. Some may stay in one stage until death. Residents may move back and forth between stages during the process.

Denial. People in this stage may refuse to believe they are dying. They often think that a mistake has been made. They may demand lab work be repeated. They may talk about the future and avoid discussion about their illnesses. They may simply act like it is not happening. This is the "No, not me" stage.

Anger. Once they start to face the possibility of their death, people become angry. They may be angry because they think they are too young or that they have always taken care of themselves. Anger may be directed at staff, visitors, roommates, family, or friends. Anger is a normal, healthy reaction. The caregiver must learn not to not take it personally. This is the "Why me?" stage.

Bargaining. Once people have begun to believe that they really are dying, they may make promises to God. They may somehow try to bargain for recovery. This is the "Yes me, but..." stage.

Depression. As dying people become physically weaker and their symptoms get worse, they may become deeply sad or depressed (Fig. 23-1). They may cry or withdraw or be unable to do even simple things. They need physical and emotional support. Listen to residents and be understanding.

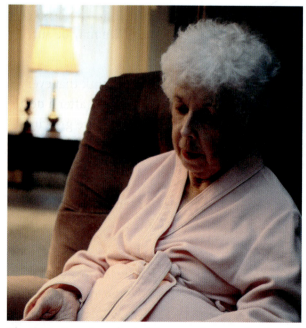

Fig. 23-1. A person who is dying may become depressed and withdrawn. Give emotional support to these residents. Listen closely and be kind and compassionate.

Acceptance. Most people who are dying are eventually able to accept death and prepare for it. They may ask to see an attorney or accountant. They may arrange with loved ones for the care of important people or things. They may plan for their last days or for the ceremonies to follow. At this stage, people who are dying may seem detached.

These stages of dying may not be possible for someone who dies suddenly, unexpectedly, or quickly. You cannot force anyone to move from stage to stage. You can only listen, and be ready to offer your help.

2. Describe the grief process

Dealing with grief after the death of a loved one is a process as well. Grieving is an individual process. No two people will grieve in exactly the same way. Clergy, counselors, or social workers can help people who are grieving. Family members or friends may have any of the following reactions to the death of a loved one:

Shock. Even when death is expected, family members and friends may still be shocked after it occurs. Many of us do not know what to expect after the death of a loved one. We may be surprised by our feelings.

Denial. Sometimes we want to think that everything will quickly return to normal after a death. Denying or refusing to believe we are grieving can help people deal with the hours or days after a death. But eventually we must face our feelings. Grief can be overwhelming. Some people may take years to face their feelings. Professional help can be very valuable.

Anger. Although it is hard to admit it, many of us feel angry after a death. We may be angry with ourselves, at God, at the doctors, or even at the person who died. There is nothing wrong with feeling anger as a part of grief.

Guilt. It is very common for families, friends, and caregivers to feel guilty after a death. We may wish we had done more for the dying person. We may simply feel that he or she did not deserve to die. We may feel guilty that we are still living.

Regret. Often we regret what we did or did not do for the dying person. We may regret things we said or did not say. Many people carry regrets with them for years.

Sadness. Feeling depressed is very common after a death. We may cry or feel emotionally unstable. We may have headaches or insomnia when we cannot express our sadness.

Loneliness. Missing someone who has died is very normal. It can bring up other feelings, such as sadness or regret. Many things may remind us of the person who died. The memories may be painful at first. With time, we usually feel less lonely and memories are less painful.

3. Discuss how feelings and attitudes about death differ

Death is a very sensitive topic; many people find it hard to discuss. Feelings and attitudes about death can be formed by many factors.

Experience with death. Someone who has been through other deaths may have a different understanding of death than someone who has not.

Personality type. Open, expressive people may have an easier time talking about and coping with death than those who are very reserved or quiet. Sharing feelings is one way of working through fears and concerns.

Religious beliefs. Religious practices and beliefs affect a person's experience with death (Fig. 23-2). This includes the dying process, rituals at the time of death, burial or cremation, services after death, and mourning customs. For example, some Catholics do not believe in cremation. Orthodox Jews may not believe in viewing the body after death. Beliefs about what happens after death can also influence grieving. Those who believe in an afterlife, such as heaven, may be comforted by this.

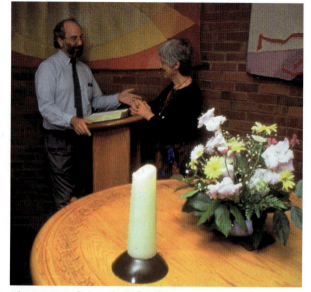

Fig. 23-2. *Religious beliefs influence a person's feelings about death.*

Cultural background. The practices we grow up with will affect how we deal with death. Cultural groups may have different practices to deal with death and grieving. Some groups have meals and other services but say very little about a person's death. In other groups, talking about and remembering the person who has died may be a comfort to family and friends (Fig. 23-3).

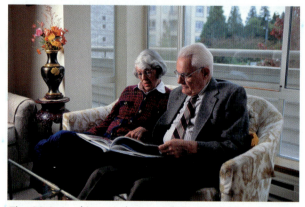

Fig. 23-3. *Looking at photos and sharing stories about a person who is dying or who has died is one way family and friends may grieve.*

4. Discuss how to care for a dying resident

Follow the care plan when caring for a dying resident. However, keep these guidelines in mind to help make the resident as comfortable as possible:

Guidelines:
Dying Resident

G **Diminished senses**. Reduce glare and keep room lighting low (Fig. 23-4). Hearing is usually the last sense to leave the body. Speak in a normal tone. Tell resident about any procedures that are being done. Describe what is happening in the room. Do not expect an answer. Ask few questions. Encourage family to speak to the resident, but to avoid subjects that are disturbing. Observe body language to anticipate a resident's needs.

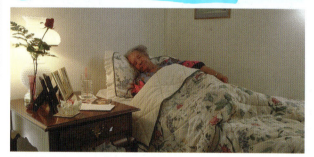

Fig. 23-4. *Keep a dying resident's room softly lit without glare.*

G **Care of the mouth and nose**. Give mouth care often. If the resident is unconscious, give mouth care every two hours. The lips and nostrils may be dry and cracked. Apply lubricant, such as lip balm, to lips and nose.

G **Skin care**. Give bed baths and incontinence care as needed. Bathe perspiring residents often. Skin should be kept clean and dry. Change sheets and clothes for comfort. Keep sheets wrinkle-free. Skin care to prevent pressure sores is important.

G **Comfort**. Pain relief is critical. Residents may not be able to tell you that they are in pain. Observe for signs of pain. Report them. Frequent changes of position, back massage, skin care, mouth care, and proper body alignment may help.

Body temperature usually rises. Many residents are more comfortable with light covers. However, fever may cause chills. Use extra blankets if residents need more warmth.

To control pain, residents may be connected to a patient-controlled analgesia (PCA) device (Fig. 23-5). A PCA is a method of pain control that allows patients to administer pain medication to themselves. They press a button to give themselves a dose of pain medication. Report any complaints of pain or discomfort to the nurse immediately.

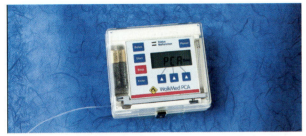

Fig. 23-5. *A patient-controlled analgesia (PCA) device.*
(PHOTO COURTESY OF MCKINLEY MEDICAL WWW.MCKINLEYMED.COM)

G   Environment. Put favorite objects and photographs where the resident can easily see them. They may give comfort. Make sure the room is comfortable, appropriately lit, and well ventilated. When leaving the room, place the call light within reach, even if the resident is unaware of his or her surroundings.

G   Emotional and spiritual support. Residents who are dying may be afraid of what is happening and of death. Listening may be one of the most important things you can do for a dying resident. Pay attention to these conversations. Report any comments about fear to the nurse.

People who are dying may also need the quiet, reassuring, and loving presence of another person. Touch can be very important. Holding your resident's hand can be comforting.

Do not avoid the dying person or his or her family. Do not deny that death is approaching, and do not tell the resident that anyone knows how or when it will happen. Do give accurate information in a reassuring way. No one can take away another's fear of death. However, your supportive and reassuring presence can help.

Some dying residents may seek spiritual comfort from clergy. Tell the nurse immediately if resident requests a clergy person. Give privacy for visits from clergy, family, and friends. Do not discuss your religious or spiritual beliefs with residents or their families or make recommendations.

Take the time to sort out your own feelings about death. If you are not comfortable with the topic, dying residents will feel it. Speak to the nurse if you need resources to help you deal with your feelings.

Advance Directives

You first learned about advance directives and DNR orders in Chapter 3. Advance directives allow people to choose what medical care they want or do not want if they cannot make those decisions themselves. A DNR order tells medical professionals not to perform CPR. DNR orders may be written for a person who has a terminal illness, someone who almost certainly will not be saved by CPR, a person not expected to live long, and/or a person who simply wants to let nature take its course.

If a resident has an advance directive in place, you may be asked to continue to monitor vital signs, such as temperature, pulse, respirations, and blood pressure, and report the readings to the nurse. Comfort measures, such as pain medication, will continue to be used. However, depending on what the advance directive states, performing CPR or any extraordinary measures may be prohibited, no matter how the vital signs have changed or declined. Extraordinary measures are measures used to prolong life when there is no reasonable expectation of recovery. When a person with a DNR order stops breathing or the heart stops, he or she will die unless the heart or breathing restarts on its own. This is not likely to happen. By law, advance directives and DNR orders must be honored. Respect each resident's decisions about advance directives.

5. Describe ways to treat dying residents and their families with dignity and honor their rights

Working in a long-term care facility with elderly and ill residents will probably expose you to death more often than other people are exposed to it. You can treat residents with dignity when they are approaching death by respecting their rights and their preferences. There are some legal rights to remember when caring for the terminally ill:

The right to refuse treatment. Remember that whether you agree or disagree with a resident's decisions, the choice is not yours. It belongs to the person involved. Sometimes, when a resident is not able to make a decision, he has told family members how he wishes things to be done. Be supportive of family members. Do not judge them. They are most likely following the resident's wishes.

The right to have visitors. When death is close, it is an emotional time for all those involved. Saying goodbye can be a very important part of dealing with a loved one's death. It may also be very reassuring to the dying person to have someone in the room, even if they do not seem to be aware of their surroundings.

The right to privacy. Privacy is a basic right, but privacy for visiting, or even when the person is alone, may be even more important now.

Other rights of a dying person are listed below in "The Dying Person's Bill of Rights." This was created at a workshop on "The Terminally Ill Patient and the Helping Person," sponsored by Southwestern Michigan In-Service Education Council, and appeared in the *American Journal of Nursing*, Vol. 75, January 1975, p. 99.

I have the right to:

- Be treated as a living human being until I die.

- Maintain a sense of hopefulness, however changing its focus may be.

- Be cared for by those who can maintain a sense of hopefulness, however changing this might be.

- Express my feelings and emotions about my approaching death in my own way.

- Participate in decisions concerning my care.

- Expect continuing medical and nursing attentions even though "cure" goals must be changed to "comfort" goals.

- Not die alone.

- Be free from pain.

- Have my questions answered honestly.

- Not be deceived.

- Have help from and for my family in accepting my death.

- Die in peace and dignity.

- Retain my individuality and not be judged for my decisions, which may be contrary to the beliefs of others.

- Discuss and enlarge my religious and/or spiritual experiences, whatever these may mean to others.

- Expect that the sanctity of the human body will be respected after death.

- Be cared for by caring, sensitive, knowledgeable people who will attempt to understand my needs and will be able to gain some satisfaction in helping me face my death.

Ways to treat dying residents and their families with dignity include the following:

- Respect their wishes in all possible ways. Communication between staff is extremely important at this time so that everyone understands what the resident's wishes are. Listen carefully for ideas on how to provide simple gestures that may be special and appreciated.

- Do not isolate or avoid a resident who is dying. Enter his or her room regularly.

- Be careful not to make promises that cannot or should not be kept.

- Continue to involve the dying person in facility activities. Be resident-centered. Do not talk with other staff members about your personal life when caring for a resident.

- Listen if a dying resident wants to talk but do not offer advice. Do not make judgmental comments.

- Do not babble or be especially cheerful or sad. Sometimes you may be nervous when you know that a resident is dying. That nervousness may lead to giggling or talking too much. If you let your emotions get out of hand, you may be so sad and upset that you cannot be any help to the resident who needs you. Remain professional.

- Keep the resident as comfortable as possible. The nurse needs to know immediately if pain medication is requested. Keep the resident clean and dry.

- Assure privacy when it is desired.

- Respect the privacy of the family and other visitors. They may be upset and not want to be social at this time. They may welcome a friendly smile, however, and should not be isolated, either.

- Help with the family's physical comfort. If requested, get them coffee, water, chairs, blankets, etc.

Residents' Rights

Life Support Measures

Life support measures are used when vital body systems are not working well enough to support life on their own. These measures include feeding tubes, mechanical ventilation, dialysis, etc. The decision to remain on life support or to discontinue life support is often part of a person's advance directives. When the decision is made to discontinue life support and the body is not able to function without these supports, the person will die. This may happen immediately or the resident may live for a short time. As with any advance directive and personal decision regarding treatment, do not judge a resident's (or a family member's) choice to remain on or discontinue life support. This is a private and personal decision. Respect the resident's wishes. Do not make comments about his or her choices to anyone, including family members, other residents, or staff.

6. Define the goals of a hospice program

Hospice is the term for the special care that a dying person needs. It is a compassionate way to care for dying people and their families. Hospice care uses a holistic approach. It treats the person's physical, emotional, spiritual, and social needs.

Hospice care can be given seven days a week, 24 hours a day. There is always a nurse on call to answer questions, make a visit, or solve a problem. Hospice care may be given in a hospital, at a care facility, or in the home. A hospice can be any location where a person who is dying is treated with dignity by caregivers. Hospice care is available with a doctor's order.

Any caregiver may give hospice care, but often specially-trained nurses, social workers, and volunteers provide hospice care. The hospice team may include doctors, nurses, social workers, counselors, nursing assistants, home health aides, therapists, clergy, dietitians, and volunteers.

Hospice care helps to meet all needs of the dying resident. Family and friends, as well as the resident, are directly involved in care decisions. The resident is encouraged to participate in family life and decision-making as long as possible.

In long-term care, goals focus on recovery, or on the resident's ability to care for him- or herself as much as possible. However, in hospice care, the goals are the comfort and dignity of the resident. This type of care is called **palliative care**. This is an important difference. You will need to change your mindset when caring for hospice residents. Focus on pain relief and comfort, rather than on teaching them to care for themselves. Report complaints or signs of pain to the nurse immediately. Residents who are dying need to feel independent for as long as possible. Caregivers should allow residents to have as much control over their lives as possible. Eventually, caregivers may have to meet all basic needs.

Other attitudes and skills useful in hospice care include the following:

Be a good listener. It is hard to know what to say to someone who is dying or to his or her loved ones. Most often, people need someone to listen to them (Fig. 23-6). Review the listening skills in Chapter 4. A good listener can be a great comfort. Some people, however, will not want to confide in you. Never push someone to talk.

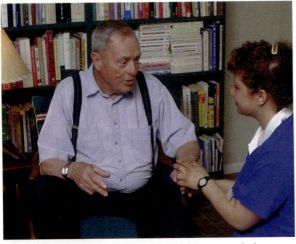

Fig. 23-6. Being a good listener can be a great help to a dying resident and his or her family.

Respect privacy and independence. Relatives, friends, clergy, or others may visit a dying resident. Make it easy for these difficult visits to take place. Stay out of the way when you can. Do not join in the conversation unless you are asked to do so. Understand that some people wish to be alone with their dying loved ones. Dying residents can have some independence even when they need total care. Let the resident make choices when possible, such as when to bathe or what to eat or drink.

Be sensitive to individual needs. Different residents and families will have different needs. The more you know what is needed, the more you can help. Some residents need a quiet and calm atmosphere. Others like a cheery presence. They might like you to talk or stay close by. Ask family members or friends how you can help.

Be aware of your own feelings. Caring for people who are dying can be draining. Know your lim-

its. Respect them. Discuss your feelings of frustration or grief with another care team member.

Recognize the stress. Just realizing how stressful it is to work with people who are dying is a first step toward caring for yourself. Talking with a counselor about your experiences at work can help you understand and work through your feelings. Remember, however, that you must keep specific information confidential. Your supervisor may be able to refer you to a counselor or support group.

Take good care of yourself. Eating right, exercising, and getting enough rest are ways of taking care of yourself (Fig. 23-7). Remember to care for your emotional and spiritual health, too. Talk about and acknowledge your feelings. Take time out to do things for yourself, such as reading a book, taking a bubble bath, or whatever you enjoy. Spiritual needs may be met by attending religious services, reading, praying, meditating, or just taking a quiet walk. Meeting your needs allows you to best meet other people's needs.

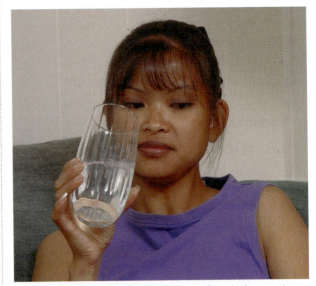

Fig. 23-7. Taking good care of yourself, including eating right, drinking plenty of water, and relaxing, is a way to help you tend to your own needs when caring for people who are dying.

Take a break when you need to. Find ten minutes to sit down and relax or stand up and stretch. These ideas may be enough of a break in some situations.

7. Explain common signs of approaching death

Death can be sudden or gradual. Physical changes occur that can be signs of approaching death. Vital signs and skin color are often affected. Disorientation, confusion, and reduced responsiveness may occur. Vision, taste, and touch usually diminish. However, hearing is often present until death occurs.

Common signs of approaching death include the following:

- Blurred and failing vision
- Unfocused eyes
- Impaired speech
- Diminished sense of touch
- Loss of movement, muscle tone, and feeling
- A rising or below-normal body temperature
- Decreasing blood pressure
- Weak pulse that is abnormally slow or rapid
- Slow, irregular respirations or rapid, shallow respirations, called **Cheyne-Stokes** respirations
- A "rattling" or "gurgling" sound as the person breathes
- Cold, pale skin
- Mottling (bruised appearance), spotting, or blotching of the skin caused by poor circulation

- Perspiration
- Incontinence (both urine and stool)
- Disorientation or confusion

8. List changes that may occur in the human body after death

When death occurs, the body will not have heartbeat, pulse, respiration, or blood pressure. The muscles in the body become stiff and rigid. This is a temporary condition called "**rigor mortis**" which is Latin for "stiffness of death." The eyelids may remain open or partially open with the eyes in a fixed stare. The mouth may remain open. The body may be incontinent of both urine and stool.

Though these things are a normal part of death, they can be frightening. Tell the nurse immediately to help confirm the death.

9. Describe postmortem care

Postmortem care is care of the body after death. Be sensitive to the needs of the family and friends after death. They may wish to sit by the bed to say goodbye. They may wish to stay with the body for a while. Allow them to do so. Be aware of religious and cultural practices that the family wants to observe. Facilities will have different policies on postmortem care. Always follow your facility's policies and procedures. Perform assigned tasks.

Guidelines:
Postmortem Care

- G   Rigor mortis may make the body difficult to move. Talk to the nurse if you need help performing postmortem care.
- G   Bathe the body. Be very gentle to avoid bruising.
- G   Place drainage pads where needed. This is most often under the head and/or under the

perineum (the genital and anal area). Be sure to follow standard precautions.

G   Do not remove any tubes or other equipment. A nurse or the funeral home will do this.

G   Put dentures back in the mouth if instructed by the nurse. Close the mouth. You may need to place a rolled towel under the chin to support the closed mouth position. If this is not possible, place dentures in a denture cup near the head.

G   Close the eyes carefully.

G   Position the body on the back with legs straight. Fold arms across the abdomen. Put a small pillow under the head.

G   Follow facility policy on personal items. Check to see if you should remove jewelry. Always have a witness if personal items are removed or given to a family member. Document what was given and to whom.

G   Strip the bed after the body has been removed.

G   Open windows to air the room, as needed. Straighten up.

G   Respect the wishes of family and friends. Be sensitive to their needs. Only perform assigned tasks.

G   Document according to your facility's policy.

Residents' Rights

Comforting Others

After a loved one has died, show family and friends to a comfortable place to sit and talk privately. Ask if you can contact anyone for them. Provide water or another beverage. If family members want to be left alone with the deceased, provide privacy by leaving the room and closing the door. Family and friends should not feel they are being rushed out of the facility.

It is natural to feel upset and not know what to say when someone has died. Many people talk a lot when feeling stressed. Show your support without

talking very much. Listen patiently and do not interrupt (Fig. 23-8). The family may want to repeat what happened and how it occurred. It is helpful for them to repeat this story.

What you say is not as important as is being sincere. Simply saying "I am so sorry," is fine. Avoid clichés such as, "It is for the better." If you can say it honestly, saying something like "your mother will be missed here," is supportive and kind. Ask your supervisor before sending a sympathy card to a family or attending the funeral service. It is important to respect professional boundaries.

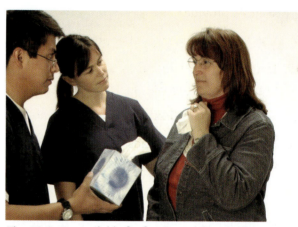

Fig. 23-8. *Be available for family and friends if they want to talk. Allow them to express their feelings.*

Home Care Focus

After a client has died, ask family members or friends how you can be of help. If you are working with a hospice program, you may be asked to answer the phone, make coffee or a meal, supervise children, or keep family members company. Do not leave the home until the client's body has been removed or until your supervisor says you may leave.

Chapter Review

1. Describe one behavior a nursing assistant might see at each stage of dying.

2. Describe five possible feelings/emotions in the grief process.

3. How would you describe your personality type? What helps you work through difficult feelings like those associated with grief?

4. Which sense is usually present until death occurs?

5. What are some of the ways to give emotional and spiritual support for a dying resident?

6. What measures may help a dying resident who is in pain?

7. List three legal rights to remember when caring for the terminally ill.

8. What is the focus in palliative care? How does it differ from the usual care nursing assistants provide?

9. List 10 common signs of approaching death.

10. List five changes that may occur in the human body after death.

11. What is postmortem care?

12. Where are drainage pads most often needed during postmortem care?

24
Introduction to Home Care

1. Explain the purpose of and need for home health care

Institutional health care delivered in hospitals and long-term care facilities is expensive. To reduce costs, hospitals have begun to discharge patients earlier. Many people who are discharged have not fully recovered their strength and stamina. Many require skilled assistance or monitoring. Others need only short-term assistance at home. Most insurance companies are willing to pay for a part of this care because it is less expensive than a long hospital or facility stay.

The growing numbers of older people and chronically ill people are also creating a demand for home care services. Family members who in the past would care for aging or ill relatives frequently leave home towns to live and work in distant areas. In addition, they often have other responsibilities or problems that interfere with their ability to provide care. For example, family members who work or who care for young children may be unable to look after aging relatives as they become frail and less functional.

Most people who need some medical care prefer the familiar surroundings of home to an institution. They choose to live alone or receive care from a relative or friend. Home health aides can provide assistance to the chronically ill, the elderly, and family caregivers who need relief from the physical and emotional stress of caregiving. Many home health aides also work in assisted living facilities. Assisted living facilities allow independent living in a home-like environment, with professional care available as needed. Home health aides may be former nursing assistants who decided to make a change from working in facilities or hospitals to working in the home.

As advances in medicine and technology extend the lives of people with chronic illnesses, the number of people needing health care will increase. Home services will be needed to provide continued care and assistance as chronic illnesses progress. For example, people with acquired immunodeficiency syndrome (AIDS), a chronic illness that is infecting more and more people throughout the world, will require in-home assistance. They will also require disease-specific health care as their illnesses progress. Improvements in medications and better management of the disease have already shown that people with AIDS can live longer, with an improved quality of life.

One of the most important reasons for health care in the home is that most people who are ill or disabled feel more comfortable at home (Fig. 24-1). Health care in familiar surroundings improves mental and physical well-being. It has proven to be a major factor in the healing process.

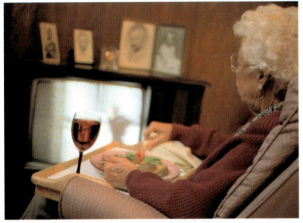

Fig. 24-1. People who are ill or disabled often feel more comfortable being cared for in their own homes, where everything is familiar.

2. Describe a typical home health agency

Many home health aides are employed by home health agencies. **Home health agencies** are businesses that provide health care and personal services in the home. Healthcare services provided by home health agencies may include nursing care, specialized therapy, specific medical equipment, pharmacy and intravenous (IV) products, and personal care. Personal care services may include housekeeping, shopping, help with activities of daily living, and cooking.

Clients who need home care are referred to a home health agency by their doctors. They can also be referred by a hospital discharge planner, a social services agency, the state or local department of public health, the welfare office, a local agency on aging, or a senior center. Clients and family members can also choose an agency that meets their needs.

Once an agency is chosen and the doctor has made a referral, a staff member performs an assessment of the client. This determines how the care needs can best be met. The home environment will also be evaluated to determine whether it is safe for the client. The services home health agencies provide depend on the size of the agency. Small agencies may provide

basic nursing care, personal care, and housekeeping services. Larger agencies may provide speech, physical, and occupational therapies, and medical social work. Some common services include the following:

- Physical, occupational, and speech therapy

- Medical-surgical nursing care, including medication management, wound care, care of different types of tubes, catheterization, and management of clients with AIDS, diabetes, chronic obstructive pulmonary disease (COPD), and congestive heart failure (CHF)

- Intravenous infusion therapy

- Maternal, pediatric, and newborn nursing care

- Nutrition therapy/dietary counseling

- Medical social work

- Personal care, including bathing; taking vital signs; skin, nail and hair care; meal preparation; light housekeeping; ambulation; and range of motion exercises

- Homemaker/companion services

- Medical equipment rental and service

- Pharmacy services

- Hospice services

All home health agencies have professional staff who make decisions about what services are needed. These professionals, who may be doctors, nurses, or other licensed professionals, also reassess clients' needs for service, write care plans, and schedule services.

Once staff determine the amount and types of care needed, assignments are given. A home health aide may be assigned to spend a certain number of hours each day or week with a client providing care and services. While the care plan and the assignments are developed by the supervisor or case manager, input from all members of the care team is needed. All HHAs are under the supervision of a skilled professional: either a nurse, a physical therapist, a speech language pathologist or therapist, or an occupational therapist. Figure 24-2 shows a typical home health agency organization chart.

3. Explain how working for a home health agency is different from working in other types of facilities

In some ways, working as a home health aide is similar to working as a nursing assistant. Most of the basic medical procedures and many of the personal care procedures you perform will be the same. However, some aspects of working in the home are very different from working in other care facilities.

Housekeeping: You may have housekeeping responsibilities, including cooking, cleaning, laundry, and grocery shopping, for at least some of your clients.

Family contact: You may have a lot more contact with clients' families in the home than you would in a facility.

Independence: You will work independently as a home health aide. Your supervisor will monitor your work, but you will spend most of your hours working with clients without direct supervision. Thus, you must be a responsible and independent worker.

Communication: Good written and verbal communication skills are important. Keep informed of changes in the client care plan. You must keep others informed of changes you observe in the client and the client's environment.

Transportation: You will have to get yourself from one client's home to another. You will need

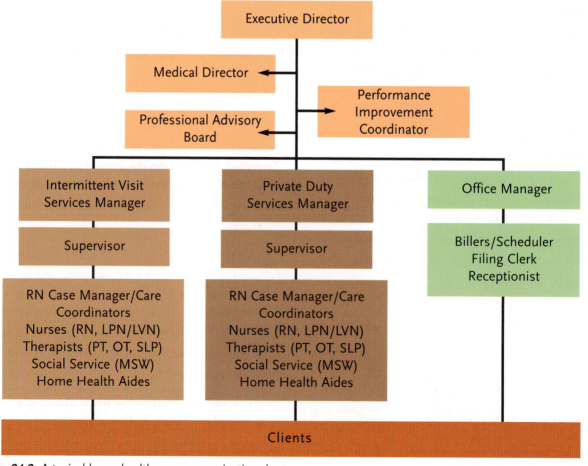

Fig. 24-2. *A typical home health agency organization chart.*

to have a dependable car or know how to use public transportation. You may also face bad weather conditions. Clients need your care—rain, snow, or sleet.

Safety: You need to be aware of personal safety when you are traveling alone to visit clients. You may be visiting clients in high-crime areas. Be aware of your surroundings, walk confidently, and avoid dangerous situations, such as visits after dark.

Flexibility: Each client's home will be different. You will need to adapt to the changes in environment. In a care facility, you know what supplies will be available and what kind of cleanliness and organization to expect at work. In home care, you may not know until you get there.

Working environment: Long-term care facilities are built to make caregiving easier and safer. They have wide doors, large bathing facilities, and special equipment for transferring residents. If needed, other caregivers are close by and can help move a resident or answer questions you may have. In home care, the layout of rooms, stairs, lack of equipment, cramped bathrooms, rugs, clutter, and even pets can complicate caregiving.

Client's home: In a client's home, you are a guest (Fig. 24-3). You need to be respectful of the client's property and customs. The client is in control most of the time. If there are any customs that seem unsafe, talk to your supervisor.

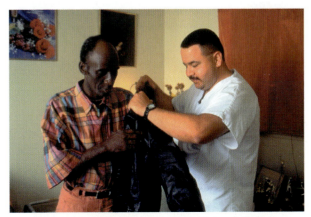

Fig. 24-3. *In a client's home, the HHA is a guest and must respect customs and property.*

Clients' comfort: One of the best things about home care is that it allows clients to stay in the familiar and comfortable surroundings of their own homes. This can help most clients recover or adapt to their condition more quickly.

4. Discuss the client care plan and explain how team members contribute to the care plan

Just as residents in long-term care have a personal care plan, so does the client in home health care. The care plan is individualized for each client. It is developed to help achieve the goals of care. It lists tasks that team members, including home health aides, must perform. It states how often these tasks should be done and how they should be carried out. For example, the care plan for a client who has had a stroke may list the following HHA responsibilities:

- Range of motion exercises to be performed daily

- Vital signs, such as temperature, pulse, and blood pressure, to be taken once a day or more

- Diet and fluid requirements

The care plan is a guide to help the client attain and maintain the best level of health possible. **Activities not listed on the care plan should not be performed**. The HHA care plan is part of this overall plan of care. It must be followed very carefully.

Care planning should involve input from the client and/or the family, as well as from health professionals. Professionals will assess the client's physical, financial, social, and psychological needs. After the doctor prescribes treatment, the supervisor, nurses, and other care team members create the care plan.

Many factors are considered when creating a care plan. These include the following:

- The client's health and physical condition

- The client's diagnosis and treatment

- The client's goals or expectations

- Whether additional services and resources, including transportation, equipment, or supplementary income, are needed (for example, a social worker may arrange transportation for the client to and from appointments with his or her doctor)

The psychological (mental and emotional) and socio-economic (social and economic) status of the client and the family are other important considerations. The agency will assess how the client and family are reacting to the medical problems. Family members may be absent or unavailable for some clients. For example, a client may have only elderly and ailing relatives to help with care. Family members may have jobs to go to or children to care for. Some families may have relatives who are unwilling to assist in care. For some families, problems like alcoholism and substance abuse can make it difficult to provide care. Housing and financial resources may also be lacking. A medical social worker may be sent to the home to assess the situation and make referrals. The medical social worker can assist with long-term care planning.

Input from all members of the care team is needed to develop the client care plan. For instance, a 250-pound, elderly client requests a tub bath. The supervisor assigns it. The home health aide finds that the client has no adaptive equipment and is unable to move to the tub. The assignment puts the home health aide and the client at risk of injury. The home health aide must communicate this. The assignment needs to be changed to a sponge bath or shower, or the client needs to get adaptive equipment. The supervisor is responsible for reassessing the assignment and making changes to the care plan.

Multiple care plans may be necessary for some clients. In these situations, the supervisor will coordinate the client's overall care. There will be one care plan for the home health aide to follow. There will be separate care plans for other providers, such as the physical therapist.

Care plans must be updated as the client's condition changes. Reporting changes and problems to the supervisor is a very important role of the home health aide. That is how the care team revises care plans to meet the client's changing needs (Fig. 24-4).

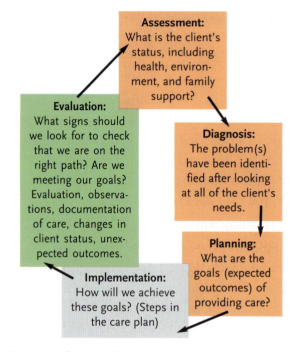

Fig. 24-4. *The care planning process.*

5. Describe the role of the home health aide and explain typical tasks performed

The role of home health aides is to improve or maintain the independence, health, and well-being of clients. This is done by providing or assisting with personal care, assisting with ADLs (activities of daily living), and performing assigned tasks. It is also accomplished by promoting self-care. HHAs can reinforce the teachings of other team members and promote behavior that improves health, such as diet and exercise.

Home health aides provide services directly to their clients in several ways:

HHAs provide care or assist with self-care, depending on the care plan. A care plan may include the following, depending on your state's regulations:

- Bathing
- Dressing
- Grooming
- Toileting
- Assisting with range of motion (ROM) exercises and ambulation (walking)
- Transferring from bed to chair or wheelchair
- Measuring vital signs (temperature, pulse rate, respiratory rate, blood pressure, and pain level)
- Feeding
- Reminding the client about medications
- Giving skin care
- Using medical supplies and equipment, such as walkers and wheelchairs
- Changing of simple dressings
- Making and changing beds
- Light cleaning, including dusting, vacuuming, washing dishes
- Teaching home management

HHAs maintain a safe, secure, and comfortable home life for clients and their families. This may include light housekeeping, food shopping, meal preparation, and doing laundry.

Home health aides are also role models. They promote clients' independence by practicing good housekeeping, nutrition, and healthcare skills. For example, encouraging clients to do tasks for themselves helps ensure that health will be maintained between visits.

In addition, home health aides teach by example. By performing procedures and giving help efficiently and cheerfully, they provide the family with a model for caregiving. Home health aides are not intended to replace a family member. Rather, HHAs support and strengthen the family.

In Chapter 2 you learned about scope of practice. A scope of practice defines the things you are allowed to do and how to do them correctly. Laws and regulations on what aides can and cannot do vary from state to state. However, some procedures are not performed by home health aides under any circumstances. Tasks that are said to be outside the scope of practice of a home health aide include the following:

- HHAs do not administer medications unless trained and assigned to do so. Only a few states allow home health aides to do this. However, it always requires additional training. Home health aides may assist the clients with self-administered medications in certain situations.

- HHAs do not insert or remove tubes or objects (other than a thermometer) in a client's body. These procedures are called "invasive," and are performed only by licensed professionals.

- HHAs do not honor a request to do something outside the scope of practice, not listed in the job description, or not on the assignment sheet. In this situation an HHA should explain that he or she cannot do the task requested. The request should then be reported to a supervisor. This is true even if a nurse or doctor asks the HHA to perform the task. The HHA should refuse to perform the task and explain why. Refusing to do something that the HHA cannot legally do is the HHA's right and responsibility.

- HHAs do not perform procedures that require sterile technique. For example, changing a sterile dressing on a deep, open wound requires sterile technique.

- HHAs do not diagnose or prescribe treatments or medications.

- HHAs do not tell the client or the family the diagnosis or the medical treatment plan. This is the responsibility of the doctor or nurse.

Know which tasks are outside your scope of practice and do not perform them. Many of these specialized tasks require more training. It is important to learn how to refuse a task for which you have not been trained, or which is outside your scope of practice.

Tip

Setting Boundaries

In professional relationships, boundaries must be set. Boundaries are the limits to or within the relationships. Home health aides, like other professionals, are guided by ethics and laws which set limits for their relationships with clients. These boundaries help support a healthy client-worker relationship. Working in clients' homes may make it more difficult to honor the boundaries of professional relationships. Clients may feel that you are their friend because you are in their homes. If the worker and client become personally involved with each other, it makes it more difficult to enforce rules. You may want to give your client extra help or let her skip the exercise she dislikes. The client may expect you to break the rules because she thinks you are friends. Emotional attachments to clients weaken your judgment and are unprofessional. Be friendly, warm, and caring with clients. But behave professionally and stay within the limits of set boundaries. Follow your agency rules and the care plan's instructions. They are in place for everyone's protection. Ask your supervisor for help if your client asks you to do things you are not allowed to do.

---

6. Explain common policies and procedures for home health aides

You will be told where to locate a list of policies and procedures that all staff members are expected to follow. Common policies at home health agencies include the following:

- Keep all information confidential. Keeping information confidential means not telling anyone about it. This is not only an agency rule, it is also the law. See Chapter 3 for more information on confidentiality, including the Health Insurance Portability and Accountability Act (HIPAA). The agency and all its employees must keep all information about clients and their families confidential. Be careful where you keep your notes and assignment sheets. Keeping your paperwork in the open where someone could read it, or losing your notes or assignments, is a breach of confidentiality. Confidentiality also extends to the agency's personnel files and clinical records. This means your employer cannot give out information about you from your job application or other records.

- Follow the client's care plan. Home health aides should perform all tasks assigned by the care plan. They should not do any tasks that are not included or approved by the case manager or supervisor. If the client or family requests changes, they should be told to speak to the supervisor.

- Report to the supervisor at regular arranged times, and more frequently if necessary. For example, home health aides must report the following to their supervisors: important events or changes in clients and their families; an accident on the job; and anything that delays or prevents them from going to or completing an assignment.

- Do not discuss personal problems with the client or the client's family. Discussing your personal problems is unprofessional. You must act in a professional manner. Clients should see you as someone whose job is to provide care, rather than as a friend.

- Be punctual and dependable. Employers expect this of all employees.

- Follow deadlines for documentation and paperwork. Timely and accurate documentation is very important.

- Provide all client care in a pleasant, professional manner.

- Do not give or accept gifts. Gift giving and receiving is not allowed because it is unprofessional. Gift giving can cause other problems as well. For example, a client may forget giving an object as a gift and report it as stolen. Some clients who give gifts may believe they deserve special treatment.

Your employer will have policies and procedures for every client care situation. These have been developed to give quality care and protect client safety. You must always follow your employer's policies and procedures. For more on professionalism and professional behavior, including proper grooming, see Chapter 2.

7. Demonstrate how to organize care assignments

To finish all your assignments each day, you have to work efficiently. To be efficient, you need to decide the order in which to do your tasks. For example, you are assigned to work with an elderly client from 2:00 to 4:00 p.m. on Monday. Your supervisor has told you that this client needs some housekeeping, dinner preparation, and personal care. When you arrive at the client's home, you see what tasks need to be done. It is a good idea to make a list of the tasks you will do and the order in which you will do them (Fig. 24-5).

Two hours is not a lot of time to do all those tasks. You will have to work quickly. You will not have any extra time to turn on the television or sit down and have coffee. If you had not planned the tasks before you started, you might have spent too long cleaning the kitchen and never have made dinner. Making a list of tasks

helps you be most efficient. It is also helpful to include the client in your planning. A client may not cooperate with your schedule if he or she has different priorities. It takes good communication, and sometimes negotiation, to arrange a schedule that works.

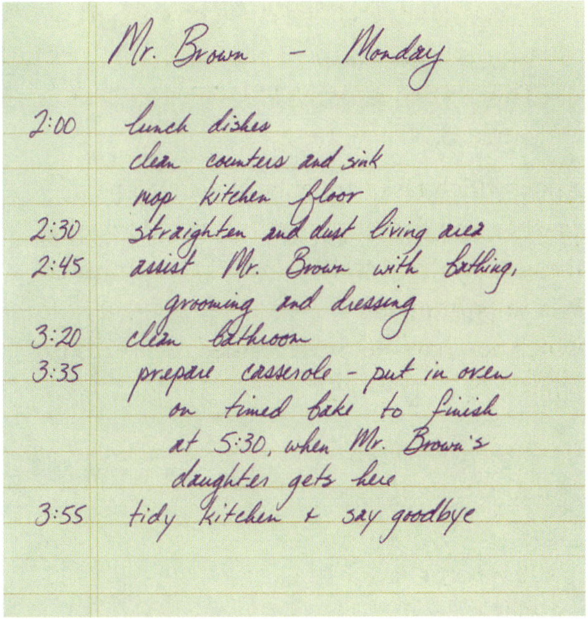

Fig. 24-5. *Making a list of tasks to be done will help you organize to perform them efficiently.*

If you run out of time with a client, you have to stay late to finish all your tasks. That makes you late to your next assignment. You then do not have enough time to do everything the next client needs. Completing assignments efficiently means you are not always running late. It means you will do a better job.

8. Identify an employer's responsibilities

Agencies should teach home health aides about their policies and procedures. Agencies must make sure that HHAs are educated and are able to perform all assigned tasks. Your employer's responsibilities include the following:

- Provide a written job description. The job description tells what you are expected to do during your working hours (Fig. 24-6).

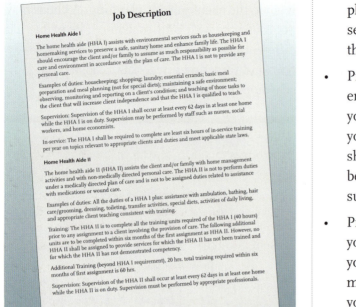

Fig. 24-6. *Your employer should provide you with a job description.*

- Provide testing and skills evaluation before you are sent to care for clients.

- Provide initial training and continuing in-service training. Initial training includes an explanation of the policies and procedures of the agency. You should also be trained in the agency's documentation system. In-service training is a federal requirement. It keeps your skills fresh and helps you do an even better job. OSHA regulations require employers to offer AIDS and Hepatitis B education as well.

- Provide appropriate preparation for each assignment. The agency should teach you to properly care for each client's special needs and conditions. You should be told why the client needs service and what the goals of care are. If other team members are involved, their responsibilities should also be explained to you.

- Provide supervision. Supervisors support and teach you how to do new tasks. They help you find solutions to problems and adjust to new situations. Supervisors check with clients to assure the goals of the care plan are being met. They will also check to see that clients are satisfied with the care they are receiving.

- Provide information about supervision. Your employer should tell you when and where you will meet with your supervisor and what you will discuss in these meetings. You should also be told how the supervisor can be reached for help, and when and why the supervisor will visit your clients' homes.

- Provide proper equipment and supplies for you to safely do your work. For example, your agency should provide the gloves you must sometimes wear to protect you and your client from infection.

9. Identify the client's rights in home health care

Clients in home care have legal rights, just as residents in long-term care do. These rights relate to how clients must be treated. They provide an ethical code of conduct for healthcare workers. Home health agencies give clients a list of these rights and review each right with them. Review Chapter 3 for more on legal rights.

The first right listed in the box below states that clients have the right to receive considerate, dignified, and respectful care. Remember that reporting abuse or suspected abuse is not an option—it is the law. Two other basic clients' rights are the right to be fully informed of the goals of care and of the care itself, and the right to participate in care planning. Your employer should develop an agreement with each client about the goals of care before service is provided. Your employer should also make every effort to involve clients and their families in care planning (Fig. 24-7). Each of us knows how our bodies work best and what makes us comfortable. People who feel in control of their bodies, lives, and health have greater self-esteem. They are more likely to continue a treatment plan and to cooperate with caregivers. Clients also have a right to know what the agency expects to happen as a result of their care. These expected outcomes are sometimes called the goals of the care plan. Clients should be informed of barriers to their care. For example, a client's failure to eat enough healthy food can be an obstacle to getting well.

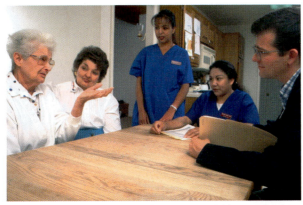

Fig. 24-7. *Clients and their families should be involved in care planning.*

Client's Bill of Rights

Home health clients and their formal caregivers have a right to not be discriminated against based on race, color, religion, national origin, age, gender, sexual orientation, or disability. Furthermore, clients and caregivers have a right to mutual respect and dignity, including respect for property. Caregivers are prohibited from accepting personal gifts and borrowing from clients.

Clients have the right:

- to have relationships with home health providers that are based on honesty and ethical standards of conduct;

- to be informed of the procedure they can follow to lodge complaints with the home health provider about the care that is, or fails to be, furnished and about a lack of respect for property;

- to know about the disposition of such complaints;

- to voice their grievances without fear of discrimination or reprisal for having done so; and

- to be advised of the telephone number and hours of operation of the state's home care hotline, which receives questions and complaints about local home health agencies, including complaints about implementation of advance directive requirements.

Clients have the right:

- to be notified in advance about the care that is to be furnished, the disciplines of the caregivers who will furnish the care, and the frequency of the proposed visits;

- to be advised of any change in the plan of care before the change is made;

- to participate in planning care and planning changes in care, and to be advised that they have the right to do so;

- to be informed in writing of rights under state law to make decisions concerning medical care, including the right to accept or refuse treatment and the right to formulate advance directives;

- to be notified of the expected outcomes of care and any obstacles or barriers to treatment;*

- to be informed in writing of policies and procedures for implementing advance directives, including any limitations if the provider cannot implement an advance directive on the basis of conscience;

- to have healthcare providers comply with advance directives in accordance with state law;

- to receive care without condition or discrimination based on the execution of advance directives; and

- to refuse services without fear of reprisal or discrimination.

* The home health provider or the client's physician may be forced to refer the client to another source of care if the client's refusal to comply with the plan of care threatens to compromise the provider's commitment to quality care.

Clients have the right:

- to confidentiality of their medical record as well as information about their health, social, and financial circumstances and about what takes place in the home; and

- to expect the home health provider to release information only as required by law or authorized by the client, and to be informed of procedures for disclosure.

Clients have the right:

- to be informed of the extent to which payment may be expected from Medicare, Medicaid, or any other payer known to the home health provider;

- to be informed of the charges that will not be covered by Medicare;

- to be informed of the charges for which the client may be liable;

- to receive this information orally and in writing before care is initiated and within 30 calendar days of the date the home health provider becomes aware of any changes; and

- to have access, upon request, to all bills for service the client has received regardless of whether the bills are paid out-of-pocket or by another party.

Clients have the right:

- to receive care of the highest quality;

- in general, to be admitted by a home health provider only if it has the resources needed to provide the care safely and at the required level of intensity, as determined by a professional assessment; a provider with less than optimal resources may nevertheless admit the client if a more appropriate provider is not available, but only after fully informing the client of the provider's limitations and the lack of suitable alternative arrangements; and

- to be told what to do in the case of an emergency.

The home health provider shall assure that:

- all medically-related home care is provided in accordance with physicians' orders and that a plan of care specifies the services and their frequency and duration; and

- all medically-related personal care is provided by an appropriately trained home health aide who is supervised by a nurse or other qualified home health care professional.

Clients have the responsibility:

- to notify the provider of changes in their condition (e.g., hospitalization, changes in the plan of care, symptoms to be reported);

- to follow the plan of care;

- to notify the provider if the visit schedule needs to be changed;

- to inform providers of the existence of any changes made to advance directives;

- to advise the provider of any problems or dissatisfaction with the services provided;

- to provide a safe environment for care to be provided; and

- to carry out mutually-agreed-upon responsibilities.

To satisfy Medicare certification requirements, the Centers for Medicare & Medicaid Services (CMS) requires that agencies:

1. Give a copy of the Bill of Rights to each client during the admission process.

2. Explain the Bill of Rights to the client and document that this has been done.

Agencies may have clients sign a copy of the Client's Bill of Rights to acknowledge receipt.

Chapter Review

1. Name three reasons for the increase in demand for home health care.

2. List ten common services provided by a typical home health agency.

3. Which one of the many differences between working as an aide for a home health agency and working for a facility is most important to you?

4. What are the factors considered when forming a client care plan?

5. How can home health aides be good role models for clients and their families?

6. What does the phrase "home health aides teach by example" mean?

7. List five tasks said to be outside the scope of practice for a home health aide.

8. List five common policies home health agencies have.

9. Create a sample schedule for a two-hour morning visit to Mrs. Smith. Use tasks different from those listed in Figure 24-5.

10. What type of preparation should an employer provide before sending HHAs to care for clients?

11. How do supervisors help HHAs and clients?

12. If a home health aide sees or suspects that a client is being abused, what is her responsibility?

13. What is one important reason that clients should be involved in their care planning?

14. Pick five rights from the Client's Bill of Rights that are most important to you and explain why you chose those particular rights.

25

Infection Prevention and Safety in the Home

Chapter 5 contains most of the important infection prevention and control material. It includes information on standard precautions, isolation precautions, hand hygiene, PPE, infectious diseases, handling spills, equipment and linen, and much more. This chapter contains information on how infection prevention may need to be modified in the home.

Chapter 6 contains most of the information on general safety guidelines. In this chapter you will find additional safety information for the home.

If possible, review both Chapters 5 and 6 before reading this chapter.

1. Discuss disinfection in the home

Measures like sterilization and disinfection are used to decrease the spread of pathogens and disease. An object can only be called "clean" if it has not been contaminated with pathogens. An object that is "dirty" has been contaminated with pathogens. Here is a list of just some of the objects that are considered "dirty" in the home:

- The floor
- Saliva and other discharges from the mouth and nose; this includes any objects that come into contact with these discharges, such as hands, toothbrushes, sinks, napkins, pillowcases, cigarettes, eating utensils, handkerchiefs, etc.

- Body wastes, such as stool (feces) and urine; this includes anything that comes into contact with these wastes, such as toilet paper, underwear, bed linens, and toilets
- Drainage from wounds; this includes objects that come in contact with drainage, such as dressings, tissues, cloths, clothing, and bed linens
- Spoiled food; this includes objects that come into contact with this food, such as other food, dishes, cooking utensils, kitchen working areas, and surfaces

Sterilization is a measure that destroys all microorganisms, including pathogens. Disinfection is a process that kills some pathogens, but not all microorganisms. Disinfection does not destroy all pathogens.

In home care, you may disinfect items used by the client. You will also disinfect some areas while doing housekeeping tasks. The care plan and your assignments will specify what disinfection you need to do.

General methods of disinfection are by wet and dry heat and by chemicals. Wet heat disinfection uses boiling water to disinfect. Dry heat disinfection means baking in the oven. See Chapter 29 for information on household chemical disinfecting solutions. The method used depends on the type of item that needs to be disinfected. Your agency will have policies and procedures for disinfection in the home.

Disinfecting using wet heat

Equipment: items to be disinfected, clean pot with enough room to hold items, clean lid for pot, cold water, timer or clock, stove, potholders

1. Wash your hands.

2. Place items in the pot and fill it with water. Make sure water covers all items, leaving enough room at the top for steam to escape.

3. Place lid on pot and place covered pot on burner on stove.

4. Turn on heat and bring water to a boil. Do not open the lid at any time during boiling.

5. Boil for 20 minutes. You should see steam escaping from the sides of the pot.

6. Turn off heat. Allow items and water to cool.

7. After items have cooled, remove the cover with the potholders.

8. Remove the items. Place on a rack or a clean towel to air dry.

9. Wash and dry the disinfecting equipment. Return to proper storage.

10. Wash your hands.

11. Document the procedure.

Disinfecting using dry heat

Equipment: items to be disinfected, clean metal pan (cookie sheet, cake pan, etc.), timer or clock, oven, potholders

1. Wash your hands.

2. Place items in the pan.

3. Place sheet or cake pan in the oven.

4. Turn on oven to 350° F. Bake for one hour. Keep oven door closed while items are baking.

5. Turn off heat. Allow items to cool.

6. After items have cooled, remove with the potholders.

7. Store the items.

8. Wash and dry the disinfecting equipment. Return to proper storage.

9. Wash your hands.

10. Document the procedure.

2. Describe guidelines for assisting a client when isolation precautions have been ordered

Transmission-based, or isolation precautions are used when caring for persons who are infected or suspected of being infected with a disease. When ordered, these precautions are used in addition to standard precautions. Follow these guidelines for assisting with isolation procedures in the home:

Guidelines:
Isolation Procedures

G Serve food using disposable dishes and utensils that are discarded in specially marked bags and stored in covered garbage containers. When items cannot be discarded, they must be washed thoroughly in very hot water with detergent and bleach. Family members should use separate dishes and utensils.

G Wear disposable gloves when handling soiled laundry. Bag laundry in the client's room and carry it to the laundry area in the bag. Wash the client's laundry separately. Use hot water and detergent.

G A solution of bleach and water (one part bleach to nine parts water) should be mixed in a clearly labeled, plastic spray bottle and stored in a safe place. The bleach solution can be used to clean up spills of blood or body fluids and to disinfect surfaces that may have been contaminated.

G A client in contact or airborne isolation should use a separate bathroom if possible. If the client uses the same bathroom as others, disinfect it after each use by the client.

Remember that clients in isolation may be fearful or concerned about what is happening. Listen to what the client is telling you and allow time to talk with your client about his concerns. Reassure clients that it is the disease, not the person, that is being isolated. Explain why these steps are being taken. Relay any requests outside your scope of practice to your supervisor. Review Chapter 5 for more on standard and isolation precautions.

Spills

In addition to guidelines for cleaning spills found in Chapter 5, follow these tips:

- When blood or body fluids are spilled, put on gloves before starting to clean up the spill. In some cases, industrial-strength gloves are best.

- If blood or body fluids are spilled on a hard surface such as a linoleum floor or countertop, remove the spill first. First put on gloves, then wipe up the spill with rags or paper towels. Then clean immediately using a solution of one part household bleach to nine parts water. You can mix the solution in a bucket and wipe the area with rags or paper towels dipped in the solution. Or, mix the solution in a plastic spray bottle and spray the area before wiping. Be careful not to spill bleach or bleach solution on clothes, carpets, or bedding. It can discolor and damage fabrics. Your employer may provide commercial sprays for cleaning spills.

- If blood or body fluids are spilled on fabrics such as carpets, bedding, or clothes, do not use bleach to clean the spill. Commercial disinfectants that do not contain bleach are available. If you have no disinfectant, wear gloves and wipe up spills. Then use soap and water to clean the area. Clean carpet with regular carpet cleaner. Use gloves to load soiled bedding or clothes into the washing machine and add color-safe bleach to the washer with the laundry detergent.

3. List ways to adapt the home to principles of good body mechanics

Chapters 6 and 10 contain more in-depth information on body mechanics. Following are several strategies that can help you apply good body mechanics in the home:

Have the right tools for a job. For example, if you cannot reach an object on a high shelf, use a step stool rather than climbing on a counter or straining to reach.

Have footrests and pillows available. You can make any position safer and more comfortable by using footrests and pillows to keep the body in alignment. For example, tasks that require standing for long periods can be more comfortable if you rest one foot on a footrest. This position flexes the muscles in the lower back and keeps the spine in alignment. When sitting, using a footrest allows for a more comfortable leg position. Crossing the legs disrupts alignment. It should be avoided. Using pillows can make any chair more comfortable. Use pillows behind the back to keep the back straight.

Keep tools, supplies, and clutter off the floor. Keep frequently-used items on shelves or counters where they can be easily reached without lifting. Keeping things organized will also help you find what you need without straining.

Sit when you can. Whenever you can sit to do a job, do so. Chopping vegetables, folding clothes, and other tasks can be done easily while sitting. For jobs like scouring the bathtub, kneel or use a low stool. Avoid bending at the waist.

Use gait or transfer belts when assisting clients with ambulation or transfers. In Chapter 10 you learned correct procedures for safely assisting clients with ambulation and transfers.

Make sure the homes you work in are safe for your clients, their family members, and yourself. Working in a home that is neglected puts you at risk of injury. Do remember, however, that you are a visitor in the client's home. Unless an immediate danger exists, check with your supervisor and the client before making any significant changes.

A nurse or case manager will assess the safety of the homes in which you work. However, you will spend more time in the home than any other member of the care team. Look for safety hazards. Immediately report to your supervisor any hazards you observe.

4. Identify common types of accidents in the home and describe prevention guidelines

You learned about these common types of accidents—falls, burns/scalds, poisoning, cuts, and choking—in Chapter 6. The HHA needs to be able to identify hazards and take action to remove them. This will include working with the client, the client's family, and/or other members of the care team. Prevention is the key to safety. As you work, watch for safety hazards, and report unsafe conditions to your supervisor promptly.

Below you will find guidelines for how to prevent common types of accidents in the home:

Falls: Falls can be caused by an unsafe environment or by loss of abilities. Falls are particularly common among the elderly. Older people are often more seriously injured by falls because their bones are more fragile. Be especially alert to the risk of falls with your elderly clients.

Follow these tips to guard against falls in the home:

- Clear all walkways of clutter, throw rugs, and cords (Figs. 25-1 and 25-2).

- Avoid waxing floors, and use non-skid mats or carpeting where appropriate.

- Have clients wear non-skid shoes. Make sure shoelaces are tied.

- Have clients wear clothing that fits properly, e.g. is not too long.

- Keep frequently-used personal items close to the client.

- Immediately clean up spills on the floor.

- Mark uneven flooring or stairs with colored tape to indicate a hazard.

- Improve lighting where necessary.

- Lock wheels before helping a client into or out of a wheelchair.

- Return adjustable beds to their lowest positions when you have finished with care.

- Offer trips to the bathroom often. Respond to clients' requests for bathroom assistance promptly.

- Leave furniture in the same place as you found it.

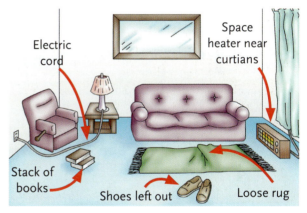

Fig. 25-1. *Be aware of unsafe conditions in your clients' homes. This living room contains many tripping and fire hazards.*

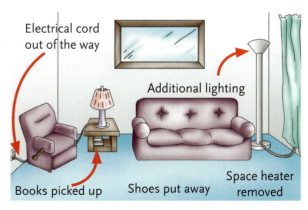

Fig. 25-2. *You can help prevent accidents. The hazards shown in Figure 25-1 have been removed. Talk with your client about changes that need to be made to avoid hazards.*

Burns/Scalds: Burns can be caused by dry heat (e.g. hot iron, stove, other electrical appliances), wet heat (e.g. hot water or other liquids, steam), or chemicals (e.g. lye, acids). Small children, older adults, or people with loss of sensation due to paralysis are at the greatest risk of burns. Scalds are burns caused by hot liquids. It takes five seconds or less for a serious burn to occur when the temperature of a liquid is 140°F. Cof-

fee, tea, and other hot drinks are usually served at 160°F to 180°F. These temperatures can cause almost instant burns that require surgery.

Follow these tips to guard against burns and scalds:

- Roll up sleeves and avoid loose clothing when working at or near the stove (Figs. 25-3 and 25-4).

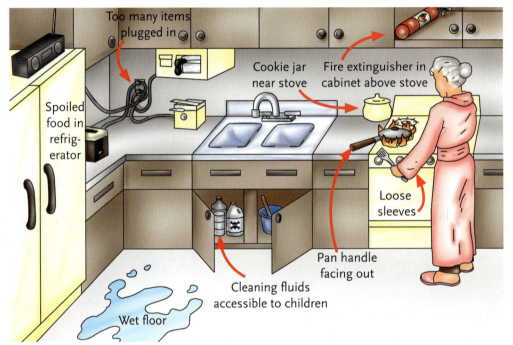

Fig. 25-3. *Unsafe working conditions in the kitchen can lead to burns and other injuries.*

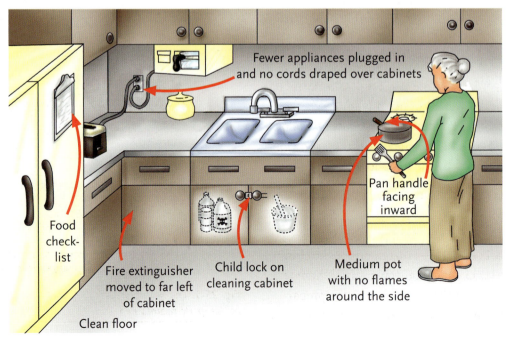

Fig. 25-4. *Prevent burns, other injuries, and fires by following safe practices in the kitchen.*

- Check that the stove and appliances are off when you leave.

- Suggest that the hot water heater be set lower than normal. It should be set at 120°F to 130°F to avoid burns from scalding tap water.

- Always check water temperature with a thermometer or your wrist before using.

- Keep space heaters away from clients' beds, chairs, and draperies. Never allow space heaters to be used in the bathroom.

- Report frayed electrical cords or unsafe-looking appliances immediately. Do not use these appliances.

- Let clients know when you are about to pour or set down a hot liquid.

- Pour hot drinks away from clients. Keep hot drinks and liquids away from edges of tables. Put a lid on them.

- Make sure clients are sitting down before serving hot drinks.

Poisoning: Homes contain many harmful substances that should not be swallowed. These include cleaning products, paints, medicines, toiletries, and glues. Lock these products away from confused clients, clients with limited vision, and children. Clients who have a diminished sense of taste or smell due to stroke or head injury might eat spoiled food. Check the refrigerator and cabinets frequently for foods that are moldy, sour, or spoiled. Investigate any odors you notice. Have the number for the Poison Control Center posted by the telephone.

Cuts: Cuts typically occur in the kitchen or bathroom. Keep any sharp objects, including knives, peelers, graters, food processor blades, scissors, nail clippers, or razors out of the reach of children. Lock sharp objects away if there is a confused client in the home. If you are preparing food, cut away from yourself, use a cutting board, and keep your fingers out of the way. Know proper first aid for cuts (see Chapter 7).

Choking: Choking can occur when eating, drinking, or swallowing medication. Babies and young children who put objects in their mouths are at great risk of choking. People who are weak, ill, or unconscious may choke on their own saliva. A person's tongue can also become swollen and obstruct the airway. To guard against choking, keep small objects out of the reach of babies and small children. Cut food into bite-sized pieces for clients who have trouble with utensils and for children.

Position infants on their backs for sleeping after feeding. Infants should sleep on their backs to prevent sudden infant death syndrome (SIDS). Never put pillows, small toys, or other objects in a crib. Clients should eat in as upright a position as possible to avoid choking. Elderly clients with swallowing difficulties may have a special diet with liquids thickened to the consistency of honey or syrup.

Household Tips for Preventing Accidents

Bathroom

Falls: Use non-skid bathmats in tubs and showers. Request grab bars for the tub, shower, and toilet if the client is weak and unsteady (Figs. 25-5 and 25-6).

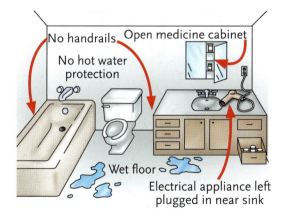

Fig. 25-5. *The bathroom is full of safety hazards if it is not properly maintained.*

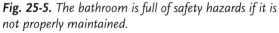

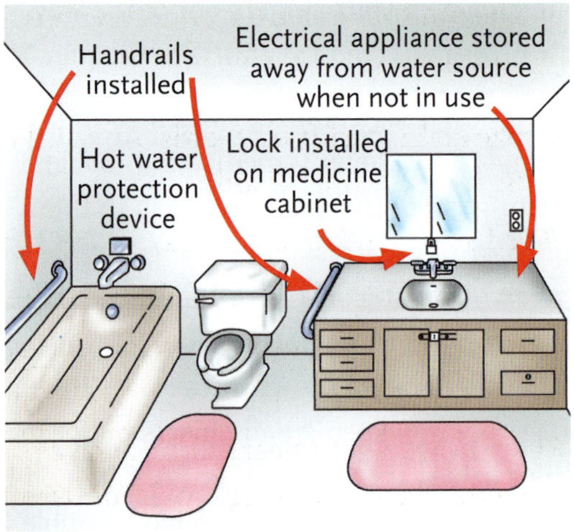

Fig. 25-6. This bathroom has been made safer by using special devices and by cleaning and straightening.

Burns: Check water temperature with a bath thermometer or on your wrist. Put away electrical appliances when they are not in use. Do not use electrical appliances near a water source.

Drowning: Do not leave young children unattended near any water. This includes bathtubs, swimming pools, buckets or basins of water, puddles, ponds, drainage ditches, toilets, or sinks. Do not leave anyone who is ill and weak alone in a tub. Do not leave clients who are dizzy or confused alone in the tub or shower.

Poisoning: Suggest that all medications be stored in containers with childproof caps and in locked cabinets. Never tell children that medication is candy. Be sure all medicines are labeled and your client reads medicine labels with his or her eyeglasses if reading glasses are necessary. Store client's medications separately from medications taken by other members of the family.

Cuts: Put away razors and other sharp objects (such as nail scissors) when they are not in use.

Kitchen

Falls: Fasten high chair safety belt.

Burns: Turn pot handles out of sight and toward the back of the stove. Stir food, especially if cooked in a microwave. This ensures that it is uniformly warm and not too hot before serving. Cool hot liquids with an ice cube before serving, as appropriate.

Poisoning: Keep emergency numbers, including the Poison Control Center, near the phone. Suggest that all household cleaning products and other chemicals be locked away.

Cuts: Keep cutlery put away. If you are using a knife and put it down for a moment, place it away from the edge of the counter or table. Make sure the blade is pointed away from the counter or table edge. Keep other sharp kitchen tools in safe places, out of the reach of children.

Choking: Do not give infants and toddlers popcorn, peanuts, hard candy, gum, or foods such as hot dogs or grapes. These items are easily inhaled, causing choking. Cut all foods into small, bite-size pieces suitable for the age of the child. For elderly clients who have difficulty swallowing, serve softer foods and foods cut into small pieces. Encourage clients to take small bites of food, chew thoroughly, and eat slowly. Keep plastic storage bags out of reach. Discard plastic bags from dry cleaners or other vendors.

Bedroom

Falls: If available, keep a nightlight on to illuminate pathways. Do not leave children unattended on high surfaces. This includes cribs, beds, changing tables, high chairs, and playpens. Do not turn your back when you are changing a child on a high surface. Be sure crib side rails are raised before you leave the room.

Burns: Do not allow clients to smoke in bed or when unattended. Be especially not to allow smoking around oxygen equipment. When a client is unattended, place a call signal nearby.

Cuts: Be sure sharp objects are put away.

Choking: Report any cribs that have wide spaces between the slats. The infant's head could become wedged between them. Keep crib away from drapes and blinds. Infants and toddlers can strangle on the cords. Do not prop up bottles for infants and toddlers. Keep pillows out of cribs to avoid suffocation. Examine all toys for loose or removable parts.

Living Area

Falls: Request walkers or canes for clients who need support when walking. Talk to your supervisor about having handrails installed where necessary. Keep the floors clear. Keep electrical and extension cords out of the way. Be sure shoes are sturdy and shoelaces are tied. For small children, place safety gates, if available, at the tops and bottoms of stairs. Be certain the gates are secure and closed. Use hardware-mounted gates at the top of stairs.

Burns: Suggest that electrical outlets be covered with baby-proof plugs. Keep lighters and matches out of reach and out of sight. Never smoke around children.

Poisoning: Keep plants out of children's reach. Many common plants are poisonous.

Cuts: Keep sharp objects out of children's reach. Do not allow children to run, jump, or play roughly with any toy or object that could stab.

Choking: Do not permit young children to play with balloons or rubber bands. These objects are easily inhaled. Do not allow children to run and jump with food in their mouths.

Garage and Outdoors

Never leave children at home alone or alone in a vehicle. Make sure all children are fastened into an approved car seat. Child car seats should be placed in the back seat of the automobile. Children should never sit in the front seat of a car equipped with dual airbags. Supervise children at play. Keep walkways clear of toys and other obstructions, as well as snow and ice.

For more information on safety in the home for clients with dementia, see Chapter 19.

5. List home fire hazards and describe fire safety guidelines

Recognize and report fire hazards. Any of the following can be a fire hazard:

- Wood stoves and kerosene, gas, or electric heaters that appear old, damaged, or faulty

- Unvented heaters used in small, enclosed areas or sleeping areas

- Space heaters used near fabrics such as draperies, bedspreads, or towels, or used to dry clothing or towels

- Flammable materials such as gasoline, kerosene, or paint thinner stored near stoves, heaters, furnaces, hot water heaters, or other appliances

- Frayed or exposed electrical wires

- Matches or lighters left within reach of children or incapacitated adults

- Careless smoking, smoking in bed, cigarettes left burning, or confused clients smoking

Guidelines:
Reducing Fire Hazards

G Never work wearing loose or flowing clothing, especially around the stove. Roll up clients' sleeves and avoid loose clothing when client may be cooking or around the stove.

G Store potholders, dish towels, and other flammable kitchen items away from the stove.

G Never store cookies, candy, or other items that may attract children above or near the stove.

G Discourage careless smoking and smoking in bed. If clients must smoke, check to be sure that cigarettes are extinguished. Empty ashtrays frequently. Before emptying ashtrays, make sure there are no hot ashes or hot matches in them.

G Stay in or near the kitchen when anything is cooking or baking.

G Do not leave the clothes dryer on when you leave the house. Lint can catch fire.

G Turn off space heaters when no one is home or everyone is asleep.

G Be sure there are working smoke alarms in the home. Check monthly to see that alarms are working. Replace batteries when needed.

G Have fire extinguishers on hand. Every home should have a fire extinguisher in the kitchen. Do not store the kitchen fire extinguisher near or above the stove, because you need to be able to get to it if the stove is on fire. Check that the homes you work in have fire extinguishers that have not expired. Know where the extinguisher is stored and how to operate it.

See Chapter 6 for more information on fire safety.

6. Identify ways to reduce the risk of automobile accidents

Since you may be driving to and from clients' homes, you will need to protect your safety on the road.

Plan your route. Trying to read a map or directions while driving can be very dangerous. When you must drive to a new location, study the map or directions before you start your car. Plan the route you will take.

Minimize distractions. Paying attention to the road can help you avoid accidents. Keep your eyes on the road and your hands on the wheel. If music is distracting, do not listen in the car. Do not talk on your cell phone while driving.

Use turn signals. Using your turn signals lets other drivers know what you are planning to do. Always use turn signals when preparing to turn or change lanes.

Use caution when backing up. Many accidents occur when drivers back up. When you back up, look around carefully. Turn your head to both sides and look behind your car. It is safest to turn your head and look behind you while backing up rather than relying on your rear view mirror.

Drive at a safe speed. Follow speed limits to be sure you are not driving too fast. Road conditions such as ice or heavy rain may mean you have to drive at a slower speed.

Always wear your seat belt. Although it may not help you avoid an accident, it will certainly help protect you if an accident occurs. Always buckle up, no matter how short the distance you must drive. Require your passengers to wear their seat belts as well.

7. Identify guidelines for using your car on the job

Keep the following in mind when using your car on the job:

- Park in safe, well-lit areas.

- Lock doors, both when driving and when you leave your car.

- Do not leave valuables in the car. If you must leave something in the car, put it out of sight.

- Have valid car insurance and carry the insurance card with you.

- Keep your proof of registration or registration card with you, not in the car. If your car is stolen, you do not want the thief to have this important document.

- Keep track of the miles you drive for work. Document them accurately. Lying about your mileage is the same as stealing from your employer.

- Keep your car in good working order. Get your car serviced at the appropriate times.

- Make sure you have good tires. Keep the gas tank full.

8. Identify guidelines for working in high-crime areas

If an assignment takes you to an area where crime is a problem, use caution. If you are using public transportation, be alert at all times. The following tips can help you avoid trouble:

- Park in well-lit areas as close as possible to the home you are visiting.

- Try to leave valuables at home when you must work in a dangerous area.

- If possible, do not take your purse with you. If you must take it, hold your purse or bag tightly, close to your body.

- Lock your car and do not leave any valuables in it.

- Walk confidently. Look as though you know where you are going (Fig. 25-7).

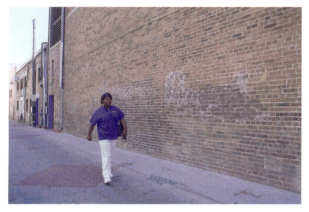

Fig. 25-7. Be cautious but look confident if you enter a high-crime area.

- Carry a whistle so you can make a loud noise to startle an attacker and get help.

- Carry your keys in your hand to unlock your car as soon as you arrive. If necessary, you can also use them as a weapon.

- Do not sit in your car, even with the doors locked. Drive away as soon as you reach your car.

- Try to avoid unsafe areas after dark.

- If you are concerned about your safety in a particular area, leave the area immediately. Contact your supervisor.

- Do not approach a home where strangers are hanging around. Go to your car and drive to a safe area. Use your cell phone or the nearest phone in a safe area, and call your supervisor.

- Call your client before you visit so they know approximately when to expect you.

- Never enter a vacant home.

- If necessary, ask your supervisor to arrange for an escort or another care provider to go with you.

- Be sure someone knows your schedule. Call the office at the end of your work day.

Chapter Review

1. How would an HHA disinfect using wet heat? How would an HHA disinfect using dry heat?

2. List two items that are considered "dirty" in the home. Can you think of two examples of dirty items that are not listed in Learning Objective 1?

3. When serving food to an infectious client using dishes and utensils that cannot be discarded, what should the HHA do?

4. List five strategies of applying good body mechanics in the home.

5. List eight tips to guard against falls in the home.

6. List eight tips to guard against burns in the home.

7. For each of the following rooms in a house, list one way to prevent accidents: bathroom, kitchen, bedroom, living area, garage, and outdoors.

8. List seven guidelines for reducing fire hazards.

9. Why is it a good idea not to use a cell phone when driving?

10. Why is it a bad idea to leave car registration or insurance documents in the car?

11. Is it okay for an HHA to guess the number of miles he drove to a client's house and back? Why or why not?

12. If an HHA approaches a house where strangers are hanging around, what should he do?

13. Why is it a good idea for an HHA to carry his keys in his hand before reaching his car?

26

Medications in Home Care

1. List four guidelines for safe and proper use of medications

People who need home care often need medications. Clients who have problems such as coronary artery disease, high blood pressure, and diabetes may take many drugs, all with different effects. Home health aides do not usually handle or give medications. However, you need to understand the kinds of medicine your clients may be taking. You also need to know what to do if a client experiences side effects or refuses to take medication.

Guidelines:
Safe and Proper Use of Medications

G Never handle or give medications unless you are specifically trained and assigned to do so. Do not touch the inside of a medicine bottle or the pills or other medicines themselves. Do not put any medication in a client's mouth. Handling or giving medication can have serious consequences. You are not trained to give medications.

G Observe clients taking their medication. Although you cannot handle or give medication, you can remind clients to take their medications. You can also bring medication containers to clients, and provide water or food as needed to take with the medication. Always observe, report, and document as appropriate.

G Know the difference between prescription drugs and over-the-counter drugs. Antibiotics (such as penicillin), heart drugs (such as nitroglycerin), and potent pain medications (such as codeine) are examples of prescription drugs. Aspirin or cold medications, such as decongestants, are over-the-counter drugs (Fig. 26-1).

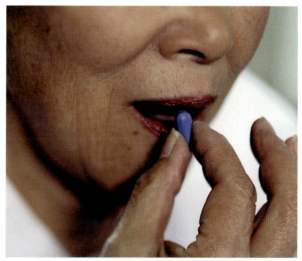

Fig. 26-1. *Be aware of all medications a client is taking. Know the difference between prescription and over-the-counter medications.*

G Be aware of all medications a client is taking. There are many possible side effects and interactions among medications. Watch for symptoms such as itching, trembling or shaking, anxiety, stomachache, diarrhea, confusion, vomiting, rash, hives, or headache. Any of these symptoms could indicate a side effect or interaction. Report any of these symptoms to your supervisor.

2. Identify the five "rights" of medications

Knowing and remembering the five "rights" of medications will help prevent mistakes.

1. **The Right Client**: Always check the label on the medication container to make sure the client's name is on it.

2. **The Right Medication**: Check the expiration date and the name of the medication before giving the container to the client. Make sure the medication name on the container matches the name listed in the care plan.

3. **The Right Time**: Make sure the instructions on the container label for what time or how often to take the medication match the instructions in the care plan.

4. **The Right Route**: Check the label for instructions on how the medication is to be taken. Make sure the instructions on the label match those in the care plan.

5. **The Right Amount**: Make sure the instructions on the container label for how much medication to take match the instructions in the care plan.

If the medication label and the care plan do not agree on any of the five "rights," call your supervisor. Also, if there is not enough information, or if you have noticed another problem with the medication (for example, the client's name is not on the container), call your supervisor.

Dosages

Medications come from the pharmacy with the instructions printed on the label (Fig. 26-2). When assisting a client to self-administer medication, read the directions on the bottle before handing the bottle to the client. Dosage means how much medication should be taken each time it is taken (the right amount). A capsule, tablet or pill will be ordered with both the strength of one pill, and how many are to be taken each time. For example, the bottle may read "Zolpidem 10 mg tablets, take one tablet."

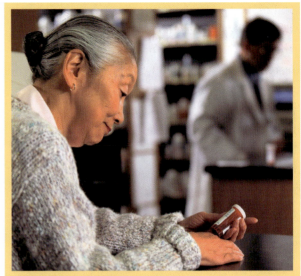

Fig. 26-2. *Medications come with instructions from the pharmacist. Instructions include the dosage and when and how to take the medication.*

The label will state how the medication should be taken (the right route). For example, the Zolpidem should be "taken by mouth at bedtime." Sometimes the prescription states to "take as needed." This means it is not required to take the drug; it should be taken when the client has symptoms. The Zolpidem is to be taken as needed for sleep.

Liquid oral medications may be ordered in teaspoons, tablespoons, or portions of either. For example, the dose may be one-fourth of a teaspoon or one-half tablespoon. Provide the client a measuring spoon—not a spoon used at the table—to measure the dose. Medications which are to be put into the eyes or ears will be labeled with the number of drops per dose. A nasal spray label will state how many sprays are in one dose. Medications for inhalers may be pre-measured into dose-size packages.

Learn the abbreviations that are approved by your agency. If abbreviations are unclear or confusing, call your supervisor. Always call your supervisor if you have a concern or question.

3. Explain how to assist a client with self-administered medications

Some elderly people have a hard time remembering to take all their medications. In addition, there may be instructions to remember. Examples of instructions include taking pills with food or on an empty stomach, or drinking plenty of fluids. Pay close attention to the medication schedule. The nurse usually sets this schedule. Become familiar with all doctors' instructions on how and when to take medications. Use forms as ordered to assist (Fig. 26-3). If the specified time for a dose passes, remind the client to take the medicine. Report to your supervisor if the client does not take a medication that has been ordered.

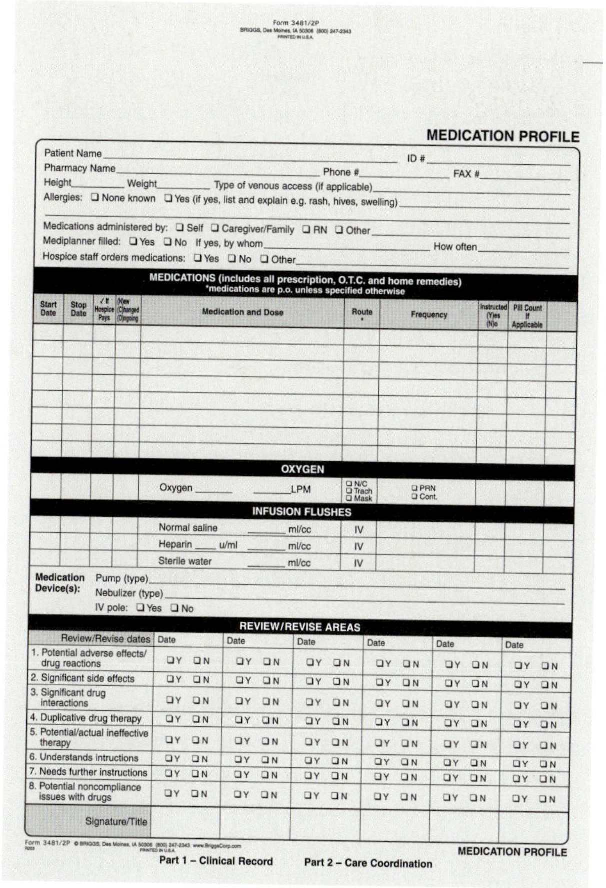
Form 3481/2P
BRIGGS, Des Moines, IA 50306 (800) 247-2343
PRINTED IN U.S.A.

MEDICATION PROFILE

Patient Name ______ ID # ______
Pharmacy Name ______ Phone # ______ FAX # ______
Height ______ Weight ______ Type of venous access (if applicable) ______
Allergies: ❑ None known ❑ Yes (if yes, list and explain e.g. rash, hives, swelling) ______

Medications administered by: ❑ Self ❑ Caregiver/Family ❑ RN ❑ Other ______
Mediplanner filled: ❑ Yes ❑ No If yes, by whom ______ How often ______
Hospice staff orders medications: ❑ Yes ❑ No ❑ Other ______

MEDICATIONS (includes all prescription, O.T.C. and home remedies)
*medications are p.o. unless specified otherwise

Start Date	Stop Date	✓ If Hospice Pays	(N)ew (C)hanged (O)ngoing	Medication and Dose	Route *	Frequency	Instructed (Y)es (N)o	Pill Count If Applicable	

OXYGEN

				Oxygen ______ ______ LPM	❑ N/C ❑ Trach ❑ Mask	❑ PRN ❑ Cont.			

INFUSION FLUSHES

				Normal saline ______ ml/cc	IV				
				Heparin ____ u/ml ______ ml/cc	IV				
				Sterile water ______ ml/cc	IV				

Medication Device(s): Pump (type) ______
Nebulizer (type) ______
IV pole: ❑ Yes ❑ No

REVIEW/REVISE AREAS

Review/Revise dates	Date	Date	Date	Date	Date	Date
1. Potential adverse effects/ drug reactions	❑Y ❑N	❑Y ❑N	❑Y ❑N	❑Y ❑N	❑Y ❑N	❑Y ❑N
2. Significant side effects	❑Y ❑N	❑Y ❑N	❑Y ❑N	❑Y ❑N	❑Y ❑N	❑Y ❑N
3. Significant drug interactions	❑Y ❑N	❑Y ❑N	❑Y ❑N	❑Y ❑N	❑Y ❑N	❑Y ❑N
4. Duplicative drug therapy	❑Y ❑N	❑Y ❑N	❑Y ❑N	❑Y ❑N	❑Y ❑N	❑Y ❑N
5. Potential/actual ineffective therapy	❑Y ❑N	❑Y ❑N	❑Y ❑N	❑Y ❑N	❑Y ❑N	❑Y ❑N
6. Understands intructions	❑Y ❑N	❑Y ❑N	❑Y ❑N	❑Y ❑N	❑Y ❑N	❑Y ❑N
7. Needs further instructions	❑Y ❑N	❑Y ❑N	❑Y ❑N	❑Y ❑N	❑Y ❑N	❑Y ❑N
8. Potential noncompliance issues with drugs	❑Y ❑N	❑Y ❑N	❑Y ❑N	❑Y ❑N	❑Y ❑N	❑Y ❑N
Signature/Title						

Form 3481/2P © BRIGGS, Des Moines, IA 50306 (800) 247-2343 www.BriggsCorp.com
PRINTED IN U.S.A.
MEDICATION PROFILE
Part 1 – Clinical Record **Part 2 – Care Coordination**

Fig. 26-3. *Many home health agencies use medication forms to help the client or aide document the client's self-medication.* (REPRINTED WITH PERMISSION OF BRIGGS CORPORATION, 800-247-2343, WWW.BRIGGSCORP.COM)

If specified, you may be instructed to help the client with self-medication by doing any of the following:

- Remind the client when it is time for medication.
- Check for right person, medication, time, expiration date, route, and amount.
- Read the medication label for the client.
- Identify the container and bring the bottle or container of medication to the client.
- Bring client equipment needed to prepare and self-administer medication.
- Provide food or water to take with the medication, as directed.
- Shake liquid medications if ordered by the care plan.
- Open and close containers.
- Position client for taking medication.
- Observe the client taking the medication.
- Document that the client took the medication, the time, and any other medications or food taken at the same time.
- Report any possible reactions to your supervisor. Call your supervisor if there are any problems or questions.
- Clean and store or dispose of special medication equipment after use.
- Return medication to storage.

Home health aides are <u>NOT</u> allowed to do any of the following:

- Break apart or crush capsules or tablets
- Mix medication with food or drink
- Pour or mix medication from one bottle into another, even if both contain the same medicine
- Touch medication directly with your hands
- Assist with self-administration of medicine if the client's name is different from that on the label
- Assist with medication whose label has been removed or changed
- Assist with medicine if medication name does not match the name on the care plan
- Use appearance alone to identify a medication

- Assist client in taking more or less of a medication than is ordered
- Remove or change a medication label
- Assist client with medicine at a time when it is not ordered
- Provide the wrong liquid for swallowing medications
- Put medication into the client's mouth
- Draw up solution for injections
- Give the client an injection
- Dispose of used injection needles/syringes
- Insert suppositories or other medication into the rectum
- Insert or apply vaginal medication
- Do special cleaning of the client's eyelids or eyelashes to prepare for eye medications
- Put drops into the eye, ear, or nose
- Apply prescription medications to the skin

Some clients have reactions to certain medications, or some medications will interact with others, causing problems. To avoid these problems, document all medication that is taken. Report drugs, prescription or nonprescription, that the client takes that are not part of the care plan. Even a pill as innocent as aspirin should be noted. It is very important to report to your supervisor and document any reactions the client may have to medications.

Avoiding certain foods or substances can be important when taking certain medications. For example, drugs that have sedative or calming effects should never be mixed with alcohol. If the client does not follow these restrictions, notify your supervisor immediately. The doctor and pharmacist will inform the client and the family of any possible side effects from the medication. Be aware of what side effects to watch for. Common side effects include dizziness, drowsiness, headache, nausea and vomiting, or confusion. More serious side effects occur when there is an allergic reaction to the medication. Allergic reactions with symptoms like hives, fever, rash, or difficulty breathing can be life-threatening. They may require emergency help.

Medication Nebulizer

A medication nebulizer is a small device that turns liquid medication into a fine mist so that it can be inhaled. It is also known as an atomizer. This device helps clients who have lung problems to bring medication deep into the lungs. The medication loosens mucus in the lungs and helps the client cough it up.

Depending on your agency's and state's rules, you may be allowed to assist the client with the use of the medication nebulizer. You should not perform any activity that is not listed in the care plan. If allowed to assist, your duties may include the following:

- Gathering the necessary equipment and supplies
- Properly positioning the client
- Putting normal saline in the nebulizer
- Turning on the equipment
- Timing the treatment
- Checking to make sure the client is using the equipment properly
- Turning off the equipment
- Cleaning and storing the equipment properly
- Documenting your observations and reporting to your supervisor

You must be very careful to prevent infection when assisting with a nebulizer. If microorganisms get into the medicine or on the mouthpiece, they can go deep into the client's lungs when he uses the nebulizer. Always wash your hands before and after touching the air hose, medication container, or medication bottle.

If your client is using oxygen, it should be left on while using the medication nebulizer. Observe all oxygen safety precautions. Do not try to repair the equipment if it is not working properly. Contact your supervisor.

If you notice any of the following signs, it may mean that the client is not getting enough oxygen while using the nebulizer:

- Rapid pulse and respirations
- Difficulty breathing
- Cold, clammy skin

- Blue or darkened lips, fingernails, or eyelids
- Inability to sit still
- Lack of response when you call his name

If your client shows any of these signs, stop the procedure and immediately notify your supervisor.

4. Identify observations about medications that should be reported right away

If a client shows signs of a reaction to a medication, or complains of side effects, report it right away. Your supervisor can assess whether the symptom is caused by the medication. Your responsibility is to report your observations.

Observing and Reporting:
Medications

- ^O/_R Dizziness, fainting
- ^O/_R Nausea, vomiting
- ^O/_R Rash, hives, itching
- ^O/_R Difficulty breathing, swelling of the throat or eyes
- ^O/_R Drowsiness
- ^O/_R Headache, blurred vision
- ^O/_R Abdominal pain
- ^O/_R Diarrhea
- ^O/_R Any other unusual sign

In addition, report any of the following problems immediately:

- ^O/_R Client refuses to take medication as directed.
- ^O/_R Client takes the wrong dose (amount) of medication.
- ^O/_R Client takes medication at the wrong time.
- ^O/_R Client takes the wrong medication.
- ^O/_R A medication container is missing or empty.

5. Describe what to do in an emergency involving medications

If a client has a severe allergic reaction to a medication, takes the wrong dose, or takes medications together that cause complications, emergency medical treatment is necessary. Treat an overdose, whether it was accidental or intentional, as a poisoning. Call the local poison control number immediately. Follow their instructions. Poison control will send paramedics or an ambulance if needed.

For severe drug reactions or interactions, call 911 or 0 for emergency help. Stay with the client. Do not give any liquids, food, or other medications unless instructed to do so by emergency personnel. Notify your supervisor as soon as possible.

6. Identify methods of medication storage

You may be required to assist with the proper storage of medications. Keep the following in mind:

- Keep the client's medications in one place, separate from medicine used by other members of the household.

- If there are young children or a disoriented elderly person in the home, recommend to the family that medications be locked away.

- All medications should be kept in childproof containers if children are in the home. To avoid an accidental overdose, keep medications out of the reach of children.

- If medicine requires refrigeration, make sure the bottle is toward the back on an upper shelf, out of a child's reach (Fig. 26-4).

- All medications should be stored away from heat and light, as appropriate.

- The client or a family member should discard medications that have expired, are not labeled, or are discolored. Make sure these medications are not discarded in the trash. Children or animals may have access to them. Ask your supervisor for specific disposal instructions. If the client or family will not dispose of expired medications, inform your supervisor. Do not dispose of them yourself.

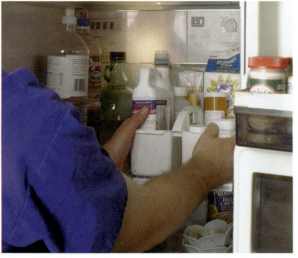

Fig. 26-4. Store medication properly. Keep medications out of the reach of children.

7. Identify signs of drug misuse and abuse and know how to report these

Drug misuse and abuse may be accidental or deliberate. It includes the following:

- Refusing to take medications
- Taking the wrong dose or taking it at the wrong time
- Mixing medication with alcohol
- Taking drugs that have not been prescribed
- Taking illegal drugs

Misuse and abuse of drugs is extremely dangerous. It can even be fatal.

If your client refuses to take certain medications, explain that recovery often depends on taking the right medication. If the client still refuses, notify your supervisor. Do not push the client to take the medication. However, try to find out what is making him or her reluctant to take it.

Getting the client to express uncertainties may help you get information to the care team. A doctor or nurse can then persuade the client to take the medication or adjust the treatment.

People may avoid taking prescribed medication because they cannot afford it or because they have difficulty getting it. Sometimes the client is confused about which drugs to take, at what hour, and in what quantities. You can help. If the client wants to know why he needs to be taking certain medications, ask the nurse or doctor to provide an explanation. People who have conditions that affect mental function, such as Alzheimer's disease, will greatly benefit from your friendly reminders. Other reasons people do not take medicine are the dislike of side effects and difficulty swallowing the pills. These problems can be overcome once you have informed your supervisor.

Be alert to the signs of misuse or abuse and report them to your supervisor immediately.

Observing and Reporting:
Drug Misuse and Abuse

- ^O/R Depression
- ^O/R Anorexia
- ^O/R Change in sleep patterns
- ^O/R Withdrawn behavior or moodiness
- ^O/R Secrecy
- ^O/R Verbal abusiveness
- ^O/R Poor relationships with family members

The drugs that pose the highest risk for causing drug dependency are pain medications, tranquilizers, muscle relaxers, and sleeping pills.

Chapter Review

1. What are the four guidelines for promoting safe and proper use of medications? Briefly describe why each guideline is important.

2. List the five "rights" of medications and explain what they mean.

3. What should an HHA do if she has noticed any problem with a client's medication?

4. List ten tasks an HHA may perform if she is instructed to help a client with self-medication.

5. List 18 tasks an HHA may NOT do with regard to medications.

6. What are four signs of an allergic reaction to a medication?

7. Name five side effects of medications.

8. List seven signs an HHA should report immediately to her supervisor that might indicate a reaction to medication.

9. How should an HHA treat an overdose? Whom should she call?

10. What is the best place to keep medications if there are young children in the home?

11. List five signs of drug abuse and misuse.

12. What are two common reasons people avoid taking prescribed medications?

27
New Mothers, Infants, and Children

1. Explain the growth of home care for new mothers and infants

New mothers and their babies used to stay in the hospital for several days after delivery. Today, new restrictions by insurers and the popularity of natural childbirth techniques have changed that. Many new mothers and their babies are sent home as early as 24 hours after an uncomplicated delivery. Thus, new mothers today return home more tired and uncomfortable. They are less confident feeding and handling their babies than women were in the past.

Home care helps ease the transition from hospital to home. It allows the mother to rest and recover. Home health aides also assist with household management when an expectant mother is put on **bed rest** by her doctor. Bed rest is ordered if a woman shows signs of early labor, has a history of miscarriage or premature deliveries, or is extremely ill. Stopping all activity and staying in bed helps prevent labor from starting before the baby is ready to be born. An expectant mother may have to stay mostly in bed for a period of a few weeks up to a few months.

2. Identify common neonatal disorders

Neonatal is the medical term for newborn. Doctors who specialize in caring for newborn babies are called **neonatologists**. A newborn baby is sometimes called a **neonate**. While most babies are born healthy, some babies are born with diseases or disorders that require special care. Babies born prematurely or at low birth weight, or who are injured during birth, will also need special care.

The most common neonatal disorders include the following:

- Prematurity (birth more than three weeks before due date)
- Low birth weight
- Cerebral palsy
- Cystic fibrosis
- Down syndrome
- Viral or bacterial infections
- Susceptibility to sudden infant death syndrome (SIDS)

3. Explain how to provide postpartum care

Care for a new mother will be spelled out in the care plan. Each situation will be different. The care needed will depend on the mother's condition, the baby's condition, and the situation in the home. Care will depend on how much support the mother has from her husband or partner, family, friends, or others.

A new mother may need the following types of assistance:

- Basic care for the baby, such as feeding, diapering, bathing

- Basic care for herself, such as rest, meal preparation, monitoring vital signs, and comfort measures such as heat, ice, or sitz baths

- Light housekeeping and laundry

- Care of older children

- Meal planning and shopping for the family

The birth of a baby is a tremendous physical feat. Monitoring vital signs is important for checking the stability of a mother during her initial recovery period. Temperature, pulse, respirations, blood pressure and changes in pain level, if any, are vital measurements that track the successful physical transition from pregnancy to motherhood. After a woman has given birth, vital signs are usually taken often. You may be asked to monitor vital signs every 15 minutes, every 30 minutes, or every hour. Follow the care plan's instructions. Check with your supervisor if you have any questions.

You may be required to monitor the amount and color of the new mother's lochia. The lochia is the vaginal flow that occurs after giving birth. This flow comes from the uterine wall where the placenta was attached. Similar to a monthly menses, the discharge is at first bright red in color. Over the next number of days the flow changes color to a duller red and then to pink. During the second week, the flow continues to change color from pink to a yellowish white and then finally disappears. The lochia may be quite heavy for a couple of days after birthing. It usually lessens gradually over the next 7 to 10 days. However, it can also last much longer, depending upon the person. Report the number of sanitary pads a new mother uses, and report any changes in flow or color to your supervisor. Increased amounts of lochia or a brightening in color are signs that should not be ignored.

In some cases, special care for the mother or baby may be needed. You may be asked to assist the mother in caring for a cesarean section incision or an episiotomy. A **Cesarean section**, or C-section, is a surgical procedure in which the baby is delivered through an incision in the mother's abdomen. An **episiotomy** is an incision made in the perineal area during vaginal delivery that enlarges the vaginal opening for the baby's head. Generally self-dissolving stitches are used to repair this incision. Your job duties regarding an episiotomy include careful observation and reporting. Observe for signs of infection, including swelling at the site, redness, radiating heat, increased pain and any wound changes such as discharge that is foul-smelling, or yellow or green in color. You may also assist with complete cleansing of the perineal area after voiding and bowel movements. It is common to use a squeeze bottle of warmed water to rinse the perineum followed by drying from front to back. Other comfort measures you may assist with are sitz baths and frequent sanitary pad changes. Follow all care guidelines.

If the baby is on a monitor (for pulse and respiration) or receiving oxygen, you may be asked to monitor the equipment. Sometimes a new mother needs help with breastfeeding. Report to your supervisor if she is having difficulties. She may need the assistance of a breastfeeding expert, called a lactation consultant.

Observing and Reporting:
Postpartum Care

O/R Fever

O/R Change in amount of vaginal flow

O/R Odor in vaginal flow

O/R Changes in color of vaginal flow (e.g. bright red after it had been pink)

O/R Pain in the pelvic region

O/R Swelling, redness or pain in the legs

O/R Changes in vital signs

O/R Swelling, redness, heat, pain, or discharge at surgical site or site of episiotomy

4. List important observations to report and document

Your supervisor should instruct you about observations to make. You may be documenting the baby's or the mother's vital signs regularly. You may also be documenting how much and how often the baby eats, how long the baby nurses, the baby's sleeping patterns, and how many diapers are changed. Document and/or report any observations that seem important to you. In addition, pay attention to the following:

The home: Is it clean, healthy, and safe?

The family: Are older children maintaining their regular routines? Do the husband or partner and other family members know how they can help?

The mother: Is she able to rest? Does she seem to be handling everything? Is she depressed, crying, or moody? Watch for signs of **postpartum** (after birth) **depression**, similar to signs of depression described in Chapter 20.

The baby: Is the baby eating regularly, wetting and soiling diapers, and sleeping well? Does the baby have good color?

The baby's room or space: Is there a safe place for the baby to sleep? Is the crib, bassinet, or bed free of pillows, toys, or excess bedding that could cause suffocation? Is the room temperature comfortably warm?

5. Explain guidelines for safely handling a baby

Wash your hands thoroughly before touching a baby or any baby supplies. Preventing the spread of germs is extremely important around a newborn baby. See that all visitors and family members wash their hands frequently, especially before touching or holding the baby. People with colds or signs of illness should stay away from a newborn, or wear a mask to prevent transmission of disease.

Always lift and hold a baby safely, according to the procedure below. Newborn babies cannot hold their heads up without assistance. Leaving the head unsupported can cause injury. Be sure all visitors and family members hold the baby safely.

Never leave a baby in an unsafe location or position. **The only safe place to leave a baby is in a crib with the side rails up or in an adult's arms.** Do not leave babies in swings, carriers, seats, or on blankets on the floor unless you can see them at all times. Never put seats, swings, or carriers on tables, chairs, or countertops. Even when changing a baby's diaper, never leave the baby on a table or countertop without keeping at least one hand on the baby at all times. Letting go, even for one second, can be dangerous. Never leave a baby or any child alone in a bath.

Never put a baby down on his or her abdomen. Babies should be placed on their backs. Crib mattresses should be firm. Infants should not be placed on a blanket, comforter, pillow, or sheepskin to sleep. These items can cause suffocation and may contribute to SIDS, which occurs when a baby stops breathing and dies.

Supervise older children and pets around babies. Jealousy can cause even well-behaved children and pets to harm babies. Older children may not mean to hurt a baby, but may not know how to touch or handle a baby.

Picking up and holding a baby

1. Wash your hands.

2. Reach one hand under the baby and behind his head and neck. Cradle the head and neck in your hand. Support the head at all times when lifting or holding a newborn.

3. With the other hand, support the baby's back and bottom.

4. There are several ways to hold a baby safely: the cradle hold; the football hold; and upright against your chest (Figs. 27-1 through 27-3). Always be sure the baby's head and neck are supported.

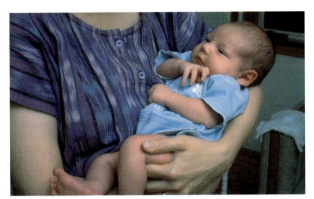

Fig. 27-1. The cradle hold has the baby's head and neck resting in the crook of one elbow and the legs in the other arm. You must support the back with one or both hands.

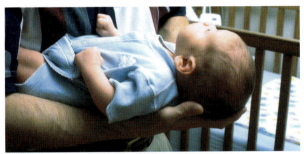

Fig. 27-2. The football hold is accomplished by holding the baby's head in one hand and supporting the baby's back with the arm on the same side of your body. The baby's body will lie along the side of your body.

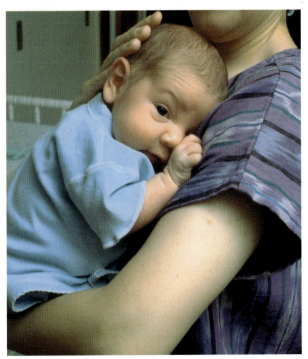

Fig. 27-3. When holding a baby upright against your chest, you must support the baby's head, neck, and back with one hand while keeping the other arm under the baby's bottom to support his or her weight.

Keep in mind that most infants love to be held. They are very sensitive to touch. You should also talk to them while performing personal care; they respond well to stimulation. Although babies are helpless, they are sensitive to their environment. They can see, taste, hear, and smell.

6. Describe guidelines for assisting with feeding a baby

Assisting with Breastfeeding

Many pediatricians encourage mothers to breastfeed, or nurse, their babies. Breastfeeding provides the perfect nutrition for infants. The decision to breast- or bottle-feed is a personal one that each mother must make for herself. If a mother chooses breastfeeding, she may need support while learning how to breastfeed. Many professionals recommend that women try breastfeeding for at least two weeks before deciding whether to continue. The first two weeks may be challenging for the mother. Your support can help her get off to a good start.

Discuss with the mother how much help she wants or needs. Ask her questions to determine her experience with and knowledge of breastfeeding: Did you breastfeed your other children? If yes, for how long? If no, what made you decide to do so now? Did the nurses in the hospital teach you about breastfeeding? Did you take any newborn classes before delivery? The mother may only want you to help her get into position. Or, she may need your coaching throughout the process. Make sure she knows that lactation consultants can help solve breastfeeding problems. Report any problems you observe or the client shares with you.

Mothers nursing for the first time may experience embarrassment, fear of pain, and/or lack of self-confidence. You can help the new mother by remaining calm, being supportive and confident in her ability to nurse, and creating an atmosphere in which she can comfortably nurse without interruption. Help for nursing mothers is available from the La Leche League International, listed in the phone book and also found online at lalecheleague.net.

Women have different breastfeeding styles. Some are very comfortable and will nurse anytime, including in the presence of others. Others may want more privacy while nursing. Be sensitive to individual preferences. A calm setting where the mother can relax will help her body provide the most milk for the baby.

Guidelines:
Helping a Mother with Breastfeeding

G Remind the mother to wash her hands. Help her get in position for breastfeeding, usually sitting upright in a comfortable chair or in bed supported by pillows. Provide a low footrest if possible and a pillow for the mother's lap (Fig. 27-4). Some mothers are able to breastfeed while lying down. Others, however, find this more difficult, especially with a newborn baby.

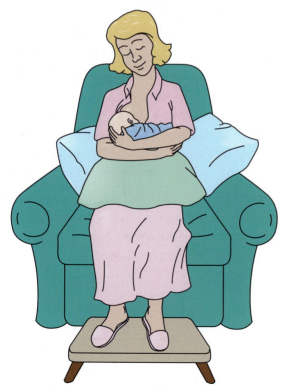

Fig. 27-4. A new mother usually prefers to nurse in an upright sitting position. Provide support with pillows and a footrest.

G Provide privacy. Close the door and occupy older children if necessary.

G Change the baby's diaper if necessary before bringing him to the mother. If desired, use a towel or blanket to cover the mother's breast and baby's head after baby has latched on.

G If necessary, remind the mother how to hold the nipple and areola between thumb and forefinger to allow baby to latch on. If baby does not latch on right away, have the mother stroke his cheek with her nipple.

G Good nutrition and plenty of fluids are important for nursing mothers. Offer snacks and frequent drinks of water, juice, or milk.

G Observe the baby nursing to be sure he stays latched on properly (Fig. 27-5). If needed, the mother can use one hand to hold the breast tissue away from the baby's nose.

There is no need to move the baby from one breast to the other until the baby stops nursing on his own. The longer the baby nurses on one side, the more of the denser, fattier "hindmilk" he receives.

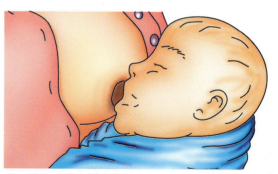

Fig. 27-5. When the baby is properly latched on to the mother's nipple, his mouth covers much of the areola. The nipple is sucked straight out rather than at an angle. This ensures the best milk flow and prevents the nipples from becoming sore.

G If the mother needs to reposition the baby or wishes to try for a better latch, she can break the suction by pressing down on the breast above the nipple or by gently putting her finger in the baby's mouth.

G Help the mother burp the baby when switching breasts and when finishing the feeding.

G   Change the baby's diaper after the feeding. Help the mother lay the baby down safely.

G   Many women find it helpful to tie a ribbon or place a pin on the side the baby last fed on. This helps them remember to start the baby's feeding on that side next time, so the breasts will be emptied more evenly.

Assisting with Bottle Feeding

Many women choose to bottle feed their babies some or all of the time. Bottle-fed newborns require special formula. Infant formula is commercially prepared and provides the nutrition babies need. Regular whole milk does not supply the proper nourishment for babies and would upset their digestive systems.

There are many brands and types of formula. If you are doing the shopping, know exactly which type you need to buy. The three most common types are ready-to-feed formula, concentrated liquid formula, and powdered formula (Fig. 27-6).

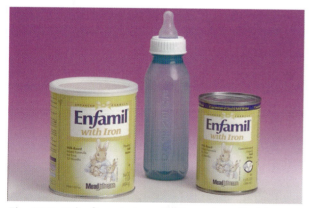

Fig. 27-6. Baby formula is available ready-to-feed in cans or bottles, concentrated in cans, or powdered in cans.

Ready-to-feed or **prepared formula** is sold in bottles or cans. This formula is ready to use. Do not dilute it or mix it with water. If the formula comes in a bottle, simply shake, unscrew the cap, and screw on a standard nipple and ring. Discard any formula remaining in the bottle after feeding. If the ready-to-feed formula comes in a can, shake the can before opening it with a sterilized can opener. Pour into sterile bottles. Store remaining formula in a sterile container, and keep covered and refrigerated, for no more than two days. Ready-to-feed formula is the most convenient to use. It is also the most expensive.

Concentrated formula is sold in small cans. It must be mixed with sterile water before using. Shake the can and open it with a sterile can opener. Measure an amount into a marked bottle and add an equal amount of sterile water. Screw on the nipple and ring, and shake to mix. Sterile water can be purchased in small bottles or in gallon jugs. You can also make sterile water by bringing water to a boil and then cooling. Store unused concentrate in a sterile container, covered and refrigerated, for no more than two days.

Powdered formula is sold in one- or two-pound cans. It is carefully measured and mixed with sterile water. A scoop is included in the can for measuring. Mix the powder and sterile water in sterile bottles or a sterilized pitcher or covered container. Follow the directions on the package carefully. Once mixed, the formula can be stored for two days in the refrigerator. Shake before feeding. Powdered formula is the most difficult to use, but is usually the cheapest to buy.

Before feeding, bottles should be warmed. To heat, immerse the bottle in warm tap water for several minutes. Bottles of formula just out of the refrigerator will take longer to warm. Never use the microwave to warm bottles. This can create hot spots in the liquid that can burn the baby (Fig. 27-7). Always shake the bottle after warming and shake a few drops of formula onto the inside of your wrist. It should feel warm, not hot or cold.

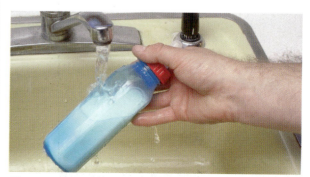

Fig. 27-7. Warm bottles in warm tap water—not in the microwave!

Sterilizing bottles

Equipment: clean bottles, nipples, and rings to be sterilized (these should be washed in hot, soapy water using a bottle brush, and allowed to drain), large kettle filled halfway with water, tongs, clean dish or paper towels to set sterile bottles on

1. Wash your hands.

2. Bring water to a boil and put bottles, nipples, and rings in. Use tongs to push bottles under water.

3. Bring water to a boil again and boil for five minutes.

4. Using tongs, remove bottles, nipples, and rings, draining the water into the pot. Set everything on the clean towels. When dry, store in a clean, dry cabinet.

5. Discard water.

Assisting with bottle feeding

1. Wash your hands.

2. Prepare bottle and formula as directed.

3. Sit in a comfortable chair and hold the baby safely in either the cradle hold or football hold.

4. Stroke the baby's lips with the bottle nipple until he opens his mouth. Put the bottle nipple in the baby's mouth.

5. Be sure the baby's head is higher than his body during feeding. Also make sure the nipple stays full of milk so the baby does not swallow air (Fig. 27-8).

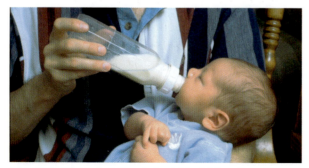

Fig. 27-8. *The baby's head should be higher than his body during feeding.*

6. Talk or sing to the baby while feeding. Feedings are the high points of his days and should be special times.

7. When the baby is through or has stopped sucking, burp him (see procedure below). Resume feeding or, if finished, change the diaper (see procedure later in chapter). Put the baby down safely.

8. Wash your hands and document the feeding, how much was consumed, and any other observations.

9. Throw out unused formula left in bottle. Wash the bottle, nipple, and ring in hot soapy water with a bottle brush, and allow to dry. Sterilize before using again.

Babies must be burped after each feeding to release air swallowed during feeding. Burping prevents babies from developing gas. Gas can be very uncomfortable for them. Burping in the middle of a feeding may allow a baby to eat more.

Burping a baby

1. Wash your hands.

2. Assemble equipment: a clean towel, cloth diaper, or burp pad.

3. Pick up the baby safely. There are two different positions to use for burping. Most people like to hold the baby against the shoulder to burp (Fig. 27-9). However, babies who are very small, who have breathing problems, or who tend to choke or spit up should be held on the lap with the head supported by holding the baby's chin with the thumb and forefinger (Fig. 27-10). This position allows you to watch the baby for signs of respiratory distress, especially color changes, and spit-up. Whichever position you use, put the burp pad under the baby's chin to catch any spit-up.

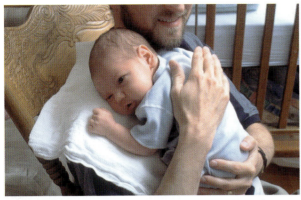

Fig. 27-9. Holding a baby against the shoulder to burp is common.

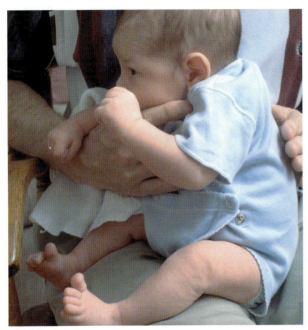

Fig. 27-10. Babies who have breathing problems or who choke or spit up will be held on the lap with the head supported to burp.

4. With the baby in a safe and comfortable position, pat the baby's back gently with your flat hand. Concentrate on the area between the shoulder blades. Some people like to pat up and down the baby's back. Others like to massage the back using an upward motion with the flat hand. Use any technique that works for you. The more relaxed and comfortable the baby is, the sooner the burp will come.

5. After the baby has burped, return him or her to a safe position or resume feeding.

Schedule and Feeding

The mother has the right to determine how to handle her new baby's schedule. For example, if a mother wants her baby to be fed whenever he cries, whether she is present or not, the HHA should respect her wishes. It is also the mother's decision what to feed her baby. Do not make judgments or express your opinion on whether the mother should be breastfeeding or using formula to feed her baby. If any behavior causes you to be concerned, report it to your supervisor.

7. Explain guidelines for bathing and changing a baby

Keeping a baby clean is important to his health. Follow the guidelines for safely handling a baby. In addition, remember the following guidelines:

Guidelines:
Bathing and Changing a Baby

G Because you could come into contact with body fluids, wear disposable gloves when bathing or changing a baby. Remember, however, that gloves can make a wet baby slippery! Be very careful when handling a baby during a bath.

G Whether bathing or changing a baby, keep one hand on the infant at all times. Have all supplies ready so you **never** have to take both hands off the baby.

G Give baths in a warm place. Close doors and windows to prevent drafts. Dry the baby's head immediately after washing hair.

G Be very careful about bath temperature. Always test the temperature of the water (either on the inside of your wrist or with a bath thermometer).

G Keep the baby's bottom dry. Be sure the area is thoroughly dried after a bath. Moisture contributes to diaper rash. Dry the bottom after changing a diaper. Leaving the diaper off for a few moments when changing the baby allows air to circulate and helps prevent diaper rash.

G Do not use powder unless directed to do so. Babies who are very small, premature, or who have breathing problems can be harmed by inhaling baby powder.

Giving an infant sponge bath

Equipment: disposable gloves, clean basin, blanket or towel to pad surface, washcloth and towel, baby cleanser or mild soap, baby shampoo or mild shampoo, cotton hat, lotion or oil, cotton ball or cotton-tipped swabs and alcohol, diaper ointment if used, clean diaper, clean clothes or sleeper, clean receiving blanket

1. Wash your hands.

2. Put on gloves. Be careful—gloves make the baby slippery!

3. Give the bath in a warm place. Use a blanket or towel to pad the surface the baby will lie on. Have all your supplies within reach. You will need to keep one hand on the baby during the entire bath. Remove caps from shampoo and cleanser to make it easier.

4. Fill the basin with warm water. Test the temperature on the inside of your wrist. Put the bottle of lotion or oil in the warm water to warm it.

5. With the baby still dressed, hold him or her in the football hold. Wet the washcloth and gently wipe the eyes, from the inner corner to the outer (Fig. 27-11). Then clean the rest of the face. Use only warm water—no soap.

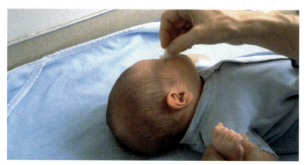

Fig. 27-11. *Wipe with eyes from the inner area to the outer area only using warm water.*

6. To wash hair, hold the baby in the football hold with the head over the basin. Use the washcloth to wet the hair. Using a small amount of shampoo, lather the baby's hair (Fig. 27-12). Rinse with the washcloth. Pat the head dry immediately with the towel. Put a cotton hat over the baby's head. Much heat is lost through the head. Be careful to keep the head warm.

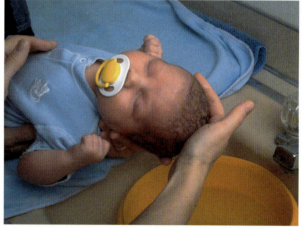

Fig. 27-12. *Lather the hair with a small amount of shampoo and, after rinsing, immediately dry the head.*

7. Lay the baby down on the padded surface. Always keep at least one hand on the baby.

8. Undress the upper body. Wash the neck, chest, back, arms, and hands using the washcloth and small amounts of soap. Rinse using the washcloth and water from the basin (Fig. 27-13). Pat dry. Cover the upper body with a towel.

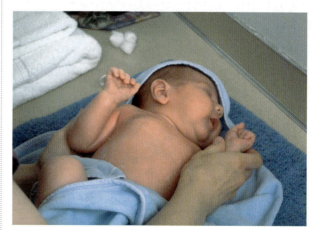

Fig. 27-13. *Uncover only the area that you are washing. Keep one hand on the baby at all times.*

9. Undress the lower body, removing the diaper. Wash the baby's abdomen and legs. Rinse. Pat dry.

10. Wash the perineal area last. For a girl, wipe the perineal area from front to back. For a boy who has recently been circumcised, do not wash the area of the circumcision. Follow special instructions to care for the circumcision.

11. Wash the baby's bottom thoroughly and dry the entire area completely with the towel. Moisture can contribute to diaper rash.

12. As gently and quickly as possible, rub lotion over the baby's body. Avoid the umbilical cord stump if it has not yet healed. Use lotion on the face only if skin is very dry. Be extremely careful not to get any lotion near the eyes. Keep the baby covered except for the part you are rubbing.

13. Diaper and dress the baby. Wrap baby in blanket and put him or her down safely.

14. Put used towels and washcloth in the laundry. Discard water. Clean basin and store. Store other supplies. Discard gloves.

15. Wash your hands.

16. Document the bath, including any observations.

Giving an infant tub bath

In addition to the supplies listed in the procedure above for a sponge bath, you will need a large basin or baby bath tub. You may also bathe a baby in a clean sink. Follow the first six steps in the procedure for a sponge bath for preparing the bath and washing the baby's face and hair.

1. Lay the baby down on the padded surface and undress him or her completely. Immerse baby in the basin. Support the head and neck above water with one hand at all times (Fig. 27-14).

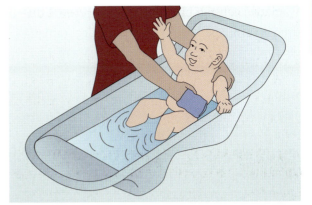

Fig. 27-14. The baby's head and neck must be supported at all times.

2. Using the washcloth and small amounts of soap, wash the baby from the neck down.

3. Remove the baby from the bath and lay him or her down on the padded surface. Keep one hand on the baby at all times. Cover baby with a towel and pat dry (Fig. 27-15).

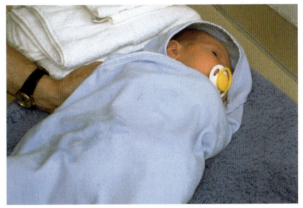

Fig. 27-15. Immediately dry and cover the baby after the bath.

4. Apply lotion, keeping the baby covered as much as possible.

5. Diaper, dress, and wrap the baby in a receiving blanket. Put him or her down safely.

6. Put used linens in the laundry. Discard bath water. Clean and store basin. Store all supplies. Discard gloves.

7. Wash your hands.

8. Document the bath, including any observations.

Diapers catch the baby's urine and feces. Children wear diapers until they are toilet trained—generally between two and three years of age. Diapers are either cloth or disposable, made of paper and plastic. Cloth diapers are used with special waterproof diaper covers or with diaper pins or other fasteners and waterproof pants.

A newborn will need between eight and twelve diaper changes in 24 hours. As babies get older, they use fewer diapers each day. The appearance, consistency, and smell of a baby's feces will depend on what he or she is fed. Some newborn babies have loose bowel movements with every feeding, as many as eight a day. Others have different schedules. Babies must be changed frequently to avoid diaper rash or irritation.

Changing cloth or disposable diapers

Equipment: clean disposable diaper or clean cloth diaper, diaper cover or pins or other fasteners and waterproof pants, wipes or a washcloth wet with warm water, diaper ointment or oil if used, clean clothes if clothes are soiled or wet

1. Wash your hands.

2. Put on gloves.

3. Change the diaper in a warm place. You need a padded surface, which may be a special changing table or a countertop. Never turn your back on the baby. Keep one hand on baby at all times, and stand so as to leave no space between your body and the changing surface. Have supplies within reach.

4. Undress the baby to remove wet or soiled diaper. Set it aside for handling later.

5. Clean the perineal area with wipes or washcloth. Remove all traces of feces. Spread the legs to clean thoroughly. For girls, wipe from front to back and spread the labia to clean as needed.

6. Let air circulate on the bottom for a moment. Exposure to air prevents diaper rash. Apply ointment or oil as directed.

7. **For disposable diapers**: Unfold the diaper and expose tapes. Place the diaper flat under the baby's bottom with the tapes in back. Bring the front of the diaper up between the baby's legs and bring the back sides around and over the front (Fig. 27-16). Peel tapes open and tape the side of the diaper securely to the front.

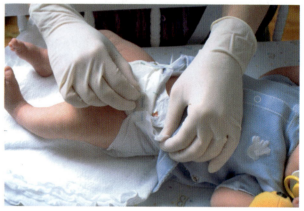

Fig. 27-16. *A disposable diaper is fastened with adhesive or Velcro tape attached to the back sides of the diaper.*

For cloth diapers with a diaper cover: Fold the diaper in thirds lengthwise. Then open out the back corners about three inches (Fig. 27-17). Lay the back of the diaper inside the back of the diaper cover (the back of the diaper cover has the tabs extending from it). Place the diaper and cover underneath the baby's bottom. Bring the front of the diaper and cover up through the baby's legs. Bring the tabs around from the sides to the front of the diaper cover and use them to close the cover securely over the diaper. Check that all the edges of the diaper are tucked under the cover.

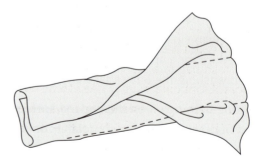

Fig. 27-17. *After folding the diaper in thirds, open out the back corners about three inches.*

For cloth diapers with pins or other fasteners and waterproof pants: Fold the diaper lengthwise in thirds, then open out the back corners about three inches. Place the diaper under the baby's bottom and bring the front of the diaper up between the baby's legs. Fold down the front of the diaper to the inside (next to baby's skin) so that the diaper covers the genitals and lower abdomen. Bring the corners of the diaper around the baby's sides and pin or fasten them to the front of the diaper. Hold your fingers inside the diaper next to baby's skin when pinning to avoid sticking the baby (Fig. 27-18). You do not need to pin through all layers. Just pin enough to fasten the back of the diaper to the front. When diaper is securely fastened, put waterproof pants over the diaper to keep urine from leaking.

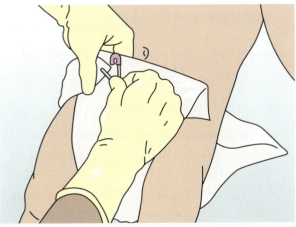

Fig. 27-18. Keep your fingers between the baby's skin and the diaper to avoid sticking the baby.

8. Dress the baby in clean clothes and put him down safely.

9. Dispose of diaper properly. Disposable diapers can be rolled into a ball (dirty side in), sealed with tapes, and disposed of in a special trash bag in a sealed container to prevent odors. Cloth diapers may need to be soaked before washing or removal by a diaper service. Check with the baby's mother or your supervisor for instructions.

10. Remove gloves.

11. Wash your hands.

12. Clean changing area and store supplies.

13. Wash hands again as needed.

14. Document any observations, including unusual color, consistency, or odor.

8. Identify how to measure weight and length of a baby

As part of your duties, you may be asked to measure a new baby's weight and length. Measurement of a newborn is not normally difficult, but they do tend to squirm and wiggle when naked and on a hard, flat surface. Always keep one hand on the baby at all times.

The infant may need to be naked for an accurate weight. Follow instructions. Use an infant scale when measuring the baby's weight.

Measuring a baby's weight

Equipment: infant scale, clean paper or pad, pen

1. Wash your hands.

2. Place an infant scale on a firm surface.

3. Place a clean paper or pad on the scale.

4. Start with scale balanced at zero before weighing baby.

5. Undress the baby.

6. Place the baby on the scale protecting the sides so he or she does not roll. Keep at least one hand on the baby at all times.

7. Read and remember the weight. If possible, lock the weight into place.

8. Remove the baby and dress him or her. Put baby in crib.

9. Wash your hands.

10. Document the weight, including any observations.

A baby's length measurement can be obtained with the baby dressed.

Measuring a baby's length

Equipment: paper with inch markings on it or plain paper, tape measure, pencil

1. Wash your hands.

2. Prepare a firm surface with a clean sheet of paper that has inch markings on it.

3. Place the baby on the firm surface. Keep at least one hand on the baby at all times.

4. Place the baby's head at the beginning of the measured markings.

5. Straighten the baby's knee.

6. Make a pencil mark on the paper at the baby's heel.

7. Determine and remember length.

8. Remove the baby and put him in his crib.

9. Wash your hands.

10. Document the length, including any observations.

When a paper with inch markings is not available, follow these steps:

1. Wash your hands.

2. Prepare a firm clean surface with a plain sheet of paper on it. The paper must be longer than the baby.

3. Place the baby on the firm surface. Keep at least one hand on the baby at all times.

4. Make a pencil mark on the paper at the top of the baby's head.

5. Straighten the baby's knee.

6. Make another mark at the baby's heel.

7. Remove the baby and put him in his crib.

8. With the tape measure, measure the distance between the marks. Remember length.

9. Wash your hands.

10. Document the length, including any observations.

9. Explain guidelines for special care

At birth the **umbilical cord** that connected the baby to the placenta inside the mother's uterus is cut. The stump of the cord remains attached to a newborn's navel for up to three weeks. Proper care of the cord stump is necessary to prevent infection and allow healing.

- With every diaper change, moisten the cord with rubbing alcohol. Use a cotton ball or cotton-tipped swabs soaked in rubbing alcohol to swab the area around the navel and cord. This helps the stump dry up and fall off.

- Never pull on or handle the cord. It will fall off by itself. The baby will feel no pain when the cord falls off.

- Keep diapers folded down away from the cord to allow air to circulate and prevent irritation (Fig. 27-19).

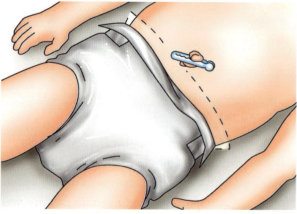

Fig. 27-19. *Keep diapers folded down, away from the cord, to allow air to circulate and to prevent irritation.*

- Do not give an infant a tub bath until the cord has fallen off.

Taking an infant's axillary or tympanic temperature

An infant's temperature is typically taken by the axillary or tympanic methods. Rectal temperatures are no longer recommended due to the chance of damaging rectal tissue. Oral temperatures are never taken for infants because the method is too difficult and dangerous.

Equipment: mercury-free thermometer, digital thermometer, or tympanic thermometer, disposable probe cover, if needed

1. Wash your hands.

2. Be sure thermometer is clean. Put on disposable probe cover, if used. For mercury-free thermometer, shake thermometer down to below the lowest number.

3. **For axillary temperature**: Undress the upper body on one side. Lay the baby on a padded surface. Place the tip of the thermometer under the arm and hold the baby's arm close to his body, so the thermometer tip touches skin on all sides (Fig. 27-20). Keep thermometer in place for 3 to 5 minutes for a mercury-free glass thermometer, or until the signal sounds for a digital thermometer.

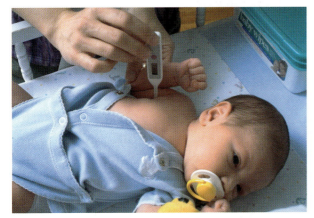

Fig. 27-20. *Leave the thermometer in place for three to five minutes or until it beeps.*

For tympanic temperature: Lay the baby on his side. Pull the outside of the ear gently toward the back of the head. Insert the thermometer tip into the ear, pointing toward the opposite eye (Fig. 27-21). Be sure the ear is sealed by the thermometer. Press the button and hold for one second.

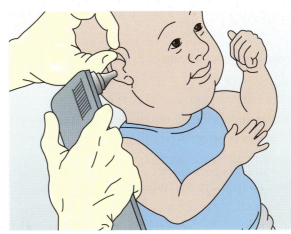

Fig. 27-21. *After gently pulling the outside of the ear back, insert the thermometer tip into the ear.*

4. For all methods, remove the thermometer and read the temperature. Keep one hand on the baby at all times.

5. Dress the baby and put him down safely.

6. Clean and store thermometer and supplies.

7. Wash your hands.

8. Document temperature.

Circumcision is the removal of part of the foreskin of the penis. It is commonly performed on male babies. Some religions require circumcision. Other parents choose to have their baby circumcised for hygienic or social reasons.

The circumcision is usually performed in the hospital or at the doctor's office when the baby is only days old. Afterwards, the circumcision site needs special care to heal. This usually includes covering the tip of the penis with a gauze pad rubbed with petroleum jelly to prevent the diaper from irritating the site. However, some types of circumcision require different care. Follow your supervisor's instructions and the care plan carefully.

Some babies who need special care will have medical equipment in the home. You will probably not be responsible for operating or handling the equipment. However, it is helpful to be familiar with various items. Always follow your supervisor's instructions before touching any medical equipment.

Apnea monitor: Apnea is the state of not breathing. Some babies may stop breathing for periods of time due to immaturity of the lungs or other reasons. The apnea monitor alerts parents or caregivers if breathing has stopped. Many apnea monitors also monitor heart rate.

Ventilator or oxygen equipment: Some babies with breathing problems need to be given oxygen. Oxygen is considered a medication. In most states it cannot be given by a home health aide. In addition, HHAs are not allowed to change the amount of oxygen being given. As always, be careful when working around oxygen, as it is flammable. Follow your supervisor's instructions carefully when working in a home where oxygen is in use. See Chapter 14 for more information on oxygen and related care.

10. Identify special needs of children and describe how children respond to stress

You may have contact with children in several ways. You may be assigned to care for a client's children when the client is unable to care for them. The client may be absent, or unable to care for them due to illness, injury, or disability. In this case you are a substitute for the parent. In other cases, the child may be the client and is suffering from a disease or disability that requires home care. In either case, it is important to understand some basic principles of caring for and working with children.

Children have the same basic physical and emotional needs as adults (see Chapter 8). They also have some special physical, mental, and emotional needs. Children's growing bodies need adequate and nutritious food and fluids, exercise, fresh air, and plenty of sleep. Their developing minds need to be stimulated by age-appropriate activities, opportunities for learning, and chances for increasing independence. Emotionally, children need love and affection, reassurance, encouragement, security and guidance. They also need consistent and constructive discipline. In addition, children need protection from injury and illness. Chapter 8 describes child development in more detail.

Children with disabilities have the same physical and emotional needs as other children (Fig. 27-22). Remember to treat these children as children first. Disabilities may make normal social contact with other children difficult. However, it is important for children with disabilities to interact with others their own age.

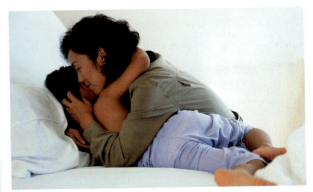

Fig. 27-22. *Children with disabilities have the same emotional needs as other children. They need love and acceptance, reassurance, encouragement, security and guidance, and consistent and constructive discipline.*

Children may experience stress due to a variety of reasons, including unmet needs, problems at school or at home, unstable families, disability, illness, and unfamiliar caregivers in the home. Many factors influence how children respond to stress, such as how old the child is, what is causing the stress, how severe the stress is, how long it lasts, and how often it occurs.

School-age children may react to stress by rebelling, skipping school, daydreaming, lying, cheating, or stealing. They may also feel guilty and feel that they are to blame for the family's problems. Adolescents may also react to stress in negative ways, such as staying out all night, dropping out of school, and abusing drugs or alcohol.

11. List symptoms of common childhood illnesses and the required care

Most childhood illnesses are caused by bacterial or viral infections. These include colds, flu, and various infections causing fever, diarrhea, vomiting, or coughs. You can help prevent illness by preventing the spread of infection in the home. Handwashing, cleaning, and disinfection are the best ways to control infection (see Chapter 5). Treatment for some of the most common symptoms of childhood illnesses is described below.

Fever: Fever may indicate serious illness. It should always be reported to your supervisor. Rest and fluids are recommended for fevers. Treatment for a fever may also include acetaminophen, or a lukewarm bath or sponging. Home health aides never give any medication, including over-the-counter medications. You can assist by making sure the family caregiver follows a doctor's dosage instructions for all medications. The strength of over-the-counter drugs varies in infant, children, and adult formulas. It is especially important to follow dosage instructions. Giving too much acetaminophen, for example, can cause liver damage or failure. In general, children should not be given aspirin, as it has been associated with some serious disorders.

Diarrhea: Diarrhea, or frequent loose or watery bowel movements, can have many causes. In children, it is often caused by a virus. Cramps and abdominal pain may accompany diarrhea. Children with diarrhea should rest and drink plenty of clear liquids, including water, broth, and diluted juices. Doctors may recommend electrolyte-replacement drinks to prevent dehydration. Usually, children with diarrhea should avoid solid foods until the problem subsides. Then they may follow the BRAT diet: bananas, rice, applesauce, and toast. Other starchy foods, such as pasta or crackers, are also allowed. Milk products, fruits, vegetables, and fatty foods should be avoided until the bowels return to normal.

Vomiting: The treatment for vomiting is similar to the treatment for diarrhea, including rest and clear liquids, and later the BRAT diet. Always call your supervisor if symptoms continue. Follow instructions in the care plan or your assignment sheet carefully.

12. Identify guidelines for working with children

The following suggestions may help you establish a trusting and honest relationship with the children in your care.

Introduce yourself. Treat children as important members of the family, and worthy of your notice. Be friendly, tell the children your name, and explain why you are there.

Maintain routine. As much as possible, stick with the family's regular schedule. The comfort of a routine can help ease the stress children may feel if someone in their household needs home care.

Give comfort. Children who are hurt, angry, or sad may need a hug, a pat, or soothing words to make them feel more secure (Fig. 27-23).

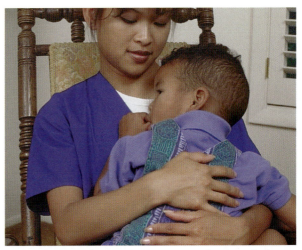

Fig. 27-23. Comforting children can make them feel more secure.

Offer encouragement and praise. Praise and encouragement contribute to the child's sense of self-worth and self-confidence. Word your praise so that it does not belittle other children.

Do not make comparisons. Children should not be compared to each other.

Use positive phrases. Children often respond better to guidance such as, "Let's try it this way..." rather than "no" or "don't."

Listen. Pay attention when children attempt to communicate. Do not interrupt them or deny their feelings. Help them to express what they are feeling by using your communication skills.

Answer. Respond to children's questions immediately, willingly, and clearly. If you do not know the answer or are not sure you are the right person to answer it, tell the child. Take the child's question to the appropriate person.

Do not force children to eat. Like adults, children do not always feel like eating. Do not allow a meal to become a power struggle. Children are usually motivated to eat when meals are simple but attractive and contain their favorite foods.

Involve children in household activities. Children feel capable and responsible when they are given household tasks to perform (Fig. 27-24). Like all people, they like to feel they are making a contribution to the family.

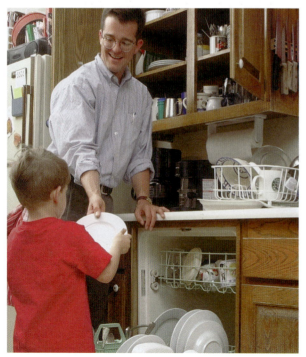

Fig. 27-24. Help children contribute.

Encourage children to play. Children need to exercise and socialize with other children (Fig. 27-25). Playing helps children express themselves and be creative. Exercise is important for their growth and health. Socialization is especially important for children who are learning social skills.

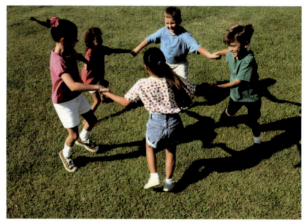

Fig. 27-25. Encourage children to play with others.

Recognize individual needs. Not all children are the same. They have different needs for sleep, food, and exercise. They grow and develop at different paces.

Be nonjudgmental. As with any client, you must accept a child regardless of disabilities or problems.

13. List the signs of child abuse and neglect and know how to report them

Child abuse is the physical, sexual, or psychological mistreatment of a child. Children who are abused can range in age from infant to adolescent. Sexual abuse of children includes inappropriate touching of a child's body, sexual contact, penetration, or sharing sexual stories or material with children. Psychological abuse includes verbal abuse, such as name-calling, social isolation, and seclusion. **Child neglect** is the purposeful or unintentional failure to provide for the needs of a child. Children who are neglected may not receive adequate food, water, medications, supervision, or shelter.

Children should never be harmed, threatened, or teased. They must be treated with respect and concern. Adults must talk to children calmly and quietly and give them positive comments, praise, and encouragement.

Child abuse or neglect can come from any-one who is responsible for a child's care. This includes parents, guardians, paid caregivers, teachers, friends, or relatives. The law requires that health professionals must report suspected child abuse. **If you observe or suspect abuse or neglect, or if a child reports that someone has abused or neglected him or her, you must imme-diately report this to your supervisor.** It not only is the right thing to do, but you and your agency can get into trouble for not reporting suspected abuse or neglect. Follow your employer's proce-dures for reporting abuse or suspected abuse.

Observing and Reporting:
Child Abuse

If you observe any of these signs of child abuse or neglect, or if you suspect abuse or neglect, speak to your supervisor immediately.

- Child has burns, cuts, bruises, abrasions, or fractured bones.
- Child stares vacantly or watches intently.
- Child is extremely quiet.
- Child avoids eye contact. In some cultures, however, it is the norm to avoid eye contact.
- Child is afraid of adults.
- Child behaves aggressively.
- Child exhibits excessive activity or hyperac-tivity. Some hyperactive children, however, have a chemical imbalance that produces this behavior.
- Child tells you that someone is abusing him or her.

Chapter Review

1. Why are new mothers often more tired and uncomfortable when they get home than women were in the past?
2. What kind of doctor specializes in working with newborns?
3. List five tasks an HHA may do to assist a new mother.
4. What might an HHA be asked to routinely document in caring for a newborn and mother?
5. What should an HHA always do before touching or picking up a baby?
6. Where are the only safe places to leave a baby?
7. Why must a baby's head be supported when he is being held?
8. Why should a baby NOT be put to sleep on his stomach or on a blanket or comforter?
9. Why are women encouraged to breastfeed?
10. How should a bottle be warmed?
11. How is concentrated formula mixed?
12. For what length of time can ready-to-feed formula be refrigerated?
13. How does burping help a baby?
14. Why should an HHA have all supplies ready before bathing or changing a baby?
15. How can an HHA test the temperature of a baby's bath water?
16. How many diaper changes will a newborn typically need in 24 hours?
17. What should an HHA do to care for the um-bilical cord stump every time a baby's diaper is changed?
18. What does circumcision care generally require?

19. What is important to report about a new mother's lochia?

20. Why may an HHA be assigned to care for a client's children?

21. Why is it important to treat children with disabilities as children first?

22. List five factors that influence how children respond to stress.

23. Name each of the three symptoms of illness outlined in Learning Objective 11 and describe one common treatment for each.

24. If a child asks an HHA a question and she does not know the answer, what should she do?

25. Why is maintaining routine important for children?

26. List six common signs of child abuse.

28

Meal Planning, Shopping, Preparation, and Storage

1. Explain how to prepare a basic food plan and list food shopping guidelines

It is very important to plan meals for a week or at least several days before shopping. When planning, take into account the client's dietary restrictions and food preferences, the number of family members present at meals, and the client's budget.

On a large sheet of paper, write out the days for which you will shop. Leave space under each day for meals and snacks. You may end up serving the meals in a different order. However, by planning for each day, you will plan the right number of meals and buy the right amount of food (Fig. 28-1).

Fill in breakfasts, lunches, dinners, and snacks for each day. Ask the client or family for ideas or look in cookbooks. Plan to have leftovers that can be easily reheated on days you will not be in the home. Plan plenty of nutritious snacks; clients may need as many as three snacks a day. Remember to list beverages as well.

When your meal plan is completed, make your shopping list. On another large sheet of paper,

	MONDAY	TUESDAY	WEDNESDAY	THURSDAY	FRIDAY
BREAKFAST	Oatmeal w/Raisins Toast Juice	Scrambled eggs Orange Coffee	WAFFLES BANANAS JUICE	POACHED EGG ½ GRAPEFRUIT COFFEE	CORN FLAKES STRAWBERRIES OJ
SNACK	PEARS CHEESE	BRAN MUFFIN MILK	SLICED PEACH TOAST MILK	BRAN MUFFIN MILK	PEARS CHEESE
LUNCH	TOSSED SALAD W/ TURKEY, TOMATO, + CUCUMBER	CHICKEN SOUP SOURDOUGH BREAD ICED TEA	ROAST BEEF SANDWICH APPLESAUCE	TOMATO SOUP HAM SANDWICH	CHICKEN SALAD SANDWICH TOMATO SLICES
SNACK	BRAN MUFFIN MILK	APPLE SLICES CHEDDAR CHEESE	ENGLISH MUFFIN HOT TEA	APPLE SLICES CHEDDAR CHEESE	BANANA BREAD MILK
DINNER	ROAST BEEF POTATOES CARROTS APPLESAUCE	SMOKED HAM MASHED POTATOES GRAVY GREEN BEANS	BAKED POTATO W/ BROCCOLI AND CHEESE SOURDOUGH BREAD	BAKED CHICKEN PEAS + CARROTS CANTALOUPE	TUNA CASSEROLE SOURDOUGH BREAD PEACHES + YOGURT
SNACK	HOT COCOA ENGLISH MUFFIN	GRAHAM CRACKERS MILK	CORN MUFFIN MILK	BANANA BREAD ~~BLUEBERRY FOAM~~ MILK	CORN MUFFIN MILK

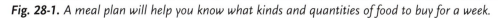

Fig. 28-1. *A meal plan will help you know what kinds and quantities of food to buy for a week.*

write down categories including produce, meats, canned goods, frozen foods, dairy, and other. Leave space under each category to list the foods you need to buy. Listing items by category will save you time in the grocery store. Go through your plan meal by meal. Write down all of the ingredients you will need for each meal. Remember to include beverages. Check the refrigerator, cabinets, and pantry for ingredients. Many ingredients you need may already be in the home.

Keep a shopping list going all the time so family members, clients, and you can write down things you run out of during the week.

Nutritious Snacks

Take into account the client's dietary needs when planning snacks.

- Low-salt pretzels and tomato juice or vegetable juice
- Celery with peanut butter or cream cheese and milk
- Graham crackers and milk
- Rice cakes with peanut butter and milk
- Cereal and milk
- Yogurt
- Baked tortilla chips with salsa
- Carrot or celery sticks with salsa
- Crackers and cheese
- Gelatin with fruit
- Bran muffin and milk
- Raisins, dates, figs, prunes, or dried apricots
- Trail mix
- Smoothies made with yogurt, milk, and fruit blended together
- Fresh fruit
- Apple with peanut butter
- Apple with cheese

Meals that Make Good Leftovers

- Beef stew
- Chili
- Spaghetti with sauce
- Casseroles
- Red beans and rice
- Split pea soup
- Lentil soup
- Chicken soup
- Macaroni and cheese
- Lasagna
- Meat loaf
- Pot roast

Guidelines:
Shopping for Clients

G Use coupons. If your client receives a newspaper, scan it for coupons from stores or manufacturers. Clip and use only those coupons for items you have already planned to buy.

G Check store circulars for advertised specials. Compare foods by reading the unit price tags that are on the shelves in front of the products (Fig. 28-2). Store brands are usually cheaper than advertised brands.

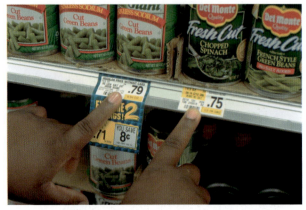

Fig. 28-2. *Compare foods by reading the unit price tags.*

G Buy fresh foods that are in season, when they are at peak flavor and inexpensive. You may also want to buy seasonal foods for canning, freezing, or preserving. Newspaper ads usually tell you which foods are plentiful. Follow your client's preferences when buying in-season foods.

G Buy in quantity. Large amounts or larger sizes are usually more economical, but do not buy more than you can store.

G Shop from your list. Do not be tempted by items that are not on your list.

G Avoid processed, already-mixed, or ready-made foods. They are usually more expensive and less nutritious. When time allows, buy staples, or basic items.

G Loaves of bread are generally a better buy than rolls or crackers. Day-old bread is usually sold at reduced prices. Buy enriched and whole-grain breads, if the client agrees. Get different varieties from time to time.

G Milk can be bought in many forms. Choose the type that the client prefers. Skim, one percent, or two percent milk contains lower fat and is usually cheaper than whole milk. Evaporated milk is usually cheaper than whole milk; it is useful in cooking.

G Buy a cheaper brand when appearance is not important. For example, store-brand mushroom bits are fine to use in a casserole and cheaper than name-brand mushroom pieces.

G Read labels to be sure you are getting the kind of product and the quantity you want. Read labels for ingredients that may be harmful to your client, such as excessive salt or sodium or sugar.

G Estimate the cost per serving before buying. Divide the total cost by the number of servings to determine the cost per serving.

G Consider the amount of waste in bones and fat when buying cheaper cuts of meat. Some

cuts of less expensive meats yield only half of what leaner cuts yield per pound. For clients on low-fat/low-cholesterol diets, pick lean meats and take the skin off chicken and turkey parts. The skin holds much of the fat.

Inexpensive Meals

- Pasta dishes
- Baked stuffed potatoes
- Rice and beans
- Tuna casserole
- Chicken thighs or legs
- Hamburger casserole
- Pot roast
- Stews
- Lentil soup
- Split pea soup

When deciding what to buy, keep these four factors in mind:

1. **Nutritional value**: Does this food contain essential nutrients, vitamins, and minerals? Is it unprocessed, without added salt or sugar?

2. **Quality**: Is this food fresh and in good condition? Fruits, vegetables, and meats should look fresh. Canned goods should not be dented, rusted, or bulging (bulging cans may be a sign of bacterial growth). Milk and dairy products should not have passed their expiration dates.

3. **Price**: Is this the most economical choice? If it costs more, is it worth it?

4. **Preference**: Will my client like this food? Can I make an appealing meal using this food?

2. List and define common health claims on food labels

Food packages often make claims about the health benefits of the food they contain. Remember that food labels are advertising designed to convince you to buy a product. Although some regulations exist about what labels can claim, read health claims carefully before making a decision to buy.

Key Claims in Food Label Advertising

Low-fat, nonfat, fat-free, reduced fat, or light: If a product is labeled low-fat or nonfat, it usually does not contain much fat. Always read the label anyway to determine the fat content of the food.

Products labeled "reduced fat" or "light" contain less fat than other versions of the same product. For example, salad dressing labeled "reduced fat" should contain 25 percent less fat than regular salad dressing. But it may still be high in fat. Salad dressing labeled "light" should contain 50 percent less fat than regular. Read the label to determine fat content. Some foods labeled low-fat, nonfat, or reduced fat may contain fat substitutes. In general, the best food and dollar value is found in products that do not contain these substitutes.

Cookies, cakes, and other treats labeled "fat-free" or "reduced fat" usually contain a lot of sugar and calories. Remember that all sweets should be used sparingly, as they provide little or no food value. Also remember that extra calories, especially sugars, are quickly converted to fat by the body.

Low-sodium, sodium-free, or no salt added: For clients who must reduce their sodium or salt intake, foods labeled "low-sodium" or "sodium-free" are important. Most foods naturally contain some sodium. Avoid foods that list salt or sodium as added ingredients. In general, canned foods and prepared foods like soups and frozen dinners usually have a lot of added salt and should be avoided.

Cholesterol-free: Cholesterol-free foods may be useful for those clients who must restrict their cholesterol intake. However, the best way to limit cholesterol is to avoid foods containing animal fats, such as butter, cheese, whole milk, eggs, red meats, and organ meats.

Sugar-free or no sugar added: Clients who must restrict their weight or who are diabetic must be very careful about consuming any sugar. Sugar-free products can be helpful, but you must read the labels carefully. Sugar-free products may contain artificial sweeteners, such as saccharin or aspartame. These have no food value and should be used sparingly. Foods sweetened with fruit juice may still contain a lot of calories. Diabetics may need to avoid fruit-juice-sweetened products as well as sugar-sweetened ones.

Organic: Organic food is produced without using most conventional pesticides, fertilizers made with synthetic ingredients or sewage sludge, bioengineering, or ionizing radiation. Organic meat, poultry, eggs, and dairy products come from animals that are given no antibiotics or growth hormones. Before a product can be labeled "organic," a government-approved certifier inspects the farm where the food is grown to make sure the farmer is following all the rules to meet USDA organic standards. Companies that handle or process organic food before it gets to the supermarket or restaurant must be certified, too. Organic food differs from conventionally produced food in the way it is grown, handled, and processed (Fig. 28-3).

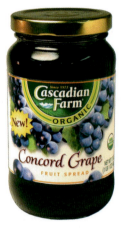

Fig. 28-3. Organic fruit spreads are one type of organic food.

Natural, healthy, or good for you: These claims may have little or no meaning. Buy whole, unprocessed grains, fresh fruits and vegetables, and lean meats, poultry, and fish, and you will

Meal Planning, Shopping, Preparation, and Storage

know you are buying food that is healthful and nutritious. Do not be swayed by the advertising you see on labels; check the facts before you buy.

3. Explain the information on the FDA-required Nutrition Facts label

The Food and Drug Administration (FDA) requires that all packaged foods contain a standardized nutrition label, called "Nutrition Facts." This label contains information about the nutritional content of food. Because the label is in the same format on all foods, it is easy to compare different products (Fig. 28-4).

Regular Frozen Lasagna

Nutrition Facts
Serving size 1 Package (10.75 oz.)

Amount Per Serving

Calories 360   **Calories from Fat** 120

	% Daily Value
Total Fat 13g	20%
Saturated Fat 7g	35%
Cholesterol 35mg	11%
Sodium 960mg	40%
Total Carbohydrate 40g	14%
Dietary Fiber 6g	23%
Sugars 10g	
Protein 21g	

Calcium	35%
Vitamin A	10%
Vitamin C	10%
Iron	6%

Fig. 28-4. The FDA-required Nutrition Facts label contains standard nutritional information that makes it easier to compare different products.

The Nutrition Facts label gives you the following information:

Serving size and number of servings per container: Check the size of the serving. Remember that a serving may be a different amount than what a client actually eats.

Calories per serving and calories from fat per serving: The number of calories per serving tells you how much food energy a serving contains. It does not tell you how much nutritional value the food has. A candy bar is high in calories, providing quick energy, but has very few nutrients and lots of fat and sugar.

The number of calories from fat tells you a lot about the fat content of a food. In general, no more than one-third, or roughly 30 percent, of the total calories should come from fat. Thus, potato chips containing 110 calories per ounce and 80 calories from fat per ounce are not a good food choice. With more than two-thirds of their calories from fat, they are a high-fat food.

Amounts and percent daily values: For each of the following items, the label tells you two things. First, how much a serving contains, and second, what percent of the recommended daily total a serving contains. For example, crackers that contain three grams of fat per serving contain 5 percent of the recommended daily total of fat. These recommended daily totals are based on a 2,000-calorie diet. Someone who eats fewer than 2,000 calories per day should have less fat each day. Someone who eats more than 2,000 calories per day can have more fat. The label provides information on total fat and saturated fat, cholesterol, sodium, total carbohydrates, dietary fiber, sugars, and protein. The FDA-required label gives amounts and daily totals for the percentage of the daily recommended amount one serving of the food provides.

Vitamins and minerals: The label lists the percentages of the recommended daily total for certain vitamins and minerals. If the label says one serving contains 50 percent of the vitamin C needed each day, you know this food is a good source of vitamin C.

4. List guidelines for safe food preparation

Food-borne illnesses affect up to 100 million people each year. Elderly people are at increased risk partly because they may not see, smell, or taste that food is spoiled. They also may not have the energy to prepare and store food safely. For people who have weakened immune systems because of AIDS or cancer, a food-borne illness can be deadly.

Guidelines:
Safe Food Preparation

G   Wash hands frequently. Wash your hands thoroughly before beginning any food preparation.

G   Wash your hands after touching nonfood items, and after handling raw meat, poultry, or fish.

G   Keep your hair tied back or covered.

G   Wear clean clothes or a clean apron.

G   Wear gloves when you have a cut on your hands.

G   Avoid coughing or sneezing around food. If you cough or sneeze, wash your hands immediately.

G   Keep everything clean. Clean and disinfect countertops and other surfaces before, during (as necessary), and after food preparation.

G   Handle raw meat, poultry, and fish carefully. Use an antibacterial kitchen cleaner or a dilute bleach solution to clean any countertops on which meat juices were spilled. Wrap paper or packaging containing meat juices in plastic and discard immediately.

G   Once you have used a knife or cutting board to cut fresh meat, do not use it for anything else until it has been washed in hot soapy water, rinsed in clear water, and allowed to

air dry. Cutting boards made of plastic, glass, nonporous acrylic, and solid wood can also be washed in the dishwasher. Use one cutting board for fresh produce and bread, and a separate cutting board for raw meat, poultry, and seafood (Fig. 28-5). This helps prevent contamination of food.

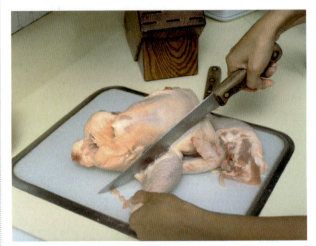

Fig. 28-5. *Carefully wash areas used to cut raw meat.*

G   Use hot, soapy water to wash utensils.

G   Use clean dishcloths, sponges, and towels. Change them frequently. Sponges may be washed in the dishwasher to disinfect them.

G   Defrost frozen foods in the refrigerator, not on the countertop. Do not remove meats or dairy products from the refrigerator until just before use.

G   Wash fruits and vegetables thoroughly in running water to remove pesticides and bacteria.

G   Cook meats, poultry, and fish thoroughly to kill any harmful microorganisms they may contain. Heat leftovers thoroughly. Never leave food out for more than two hours. Put warm foods in the refrigerator before they are cool, so that bacteria does not have a chance to grow. Keep cold foods cold and hot foods hot. Use cooked meat, poultry, fish, and baked dishes within three to four days.

G   Do not use cracked eggs. Do not consume or serve raw eggs.

G   Never taste and stir with the same utensil.

5. Identify methods of food preparation

The following basic methods of food preparation will allow you to prepare a variety of healthy meals:

Boiling: Food is cooked in boiling water until tender or done. This is the best method for cooking pasta, noodles, rice, and hard- or soft-boiled eggs (Fig. 28-6).

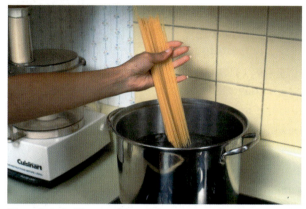

Fig. 28-6. Boiling works well for pasta and other grains.

Steaming: Steaming is a healthy way to prepare vegetables. A small amount of water is boiled in the bottom of a saucepan and food is set over it on a rack (Fig. 28-7). The pan is tightly covered to keep the steam in.

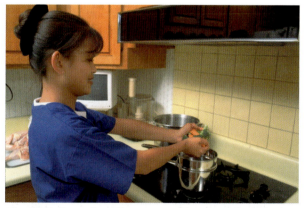

Fig. 28-7. Steaming allows vegetables to retain their vitamins and flavor.

Poaching: Fish or eggs may be cooked by poaching in barely boiling water or other liquid. Eggs are cracked and shells discarded before poaching. Fish may be poached in milk or broth, on top of the stove or in the oven in a baking dish (Fig. 28-8).

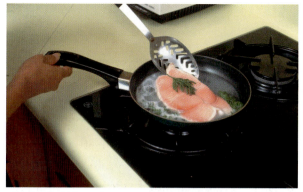

Fig. 28-8. Fish and eggs can both be poached.

Roasting: Used for meats and poultry or some vegetables, roasting is a simple way to cook. Dry heat roasting means food is roasted in an open pan in the oven (Fig. 28-9). Meats and poultry are **basted**, or coated with juices or other liquid, during roasting.

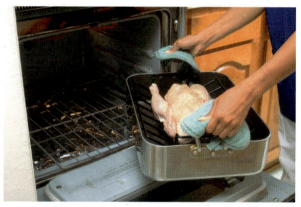

Fig. 28-9. Meats roast well at high temperatures (450°) but may need to be basted. Vegetables can also be roasted.

Braising: Braising is a slow-cooking method that uses moist heat. Liquid such as broth, wine, or tomato sauce is poured over and around meat or vegetables, and the pot is covered. The meat or vegetables are then slowly cooked at a temperature just below boiling. Braising is a good way to tenderize tough meats and vegetables, since the long cooking breaks down their fibers. Braising may be done in the oven or on the stove top.

Baking: Baking is used for many foods, including breads, poultry, fish, and vegetables. Baking is done at moderate heat, 350°F to 400°F. Foods such as potatoes and winter squash bake very well (Fig. 28-10).

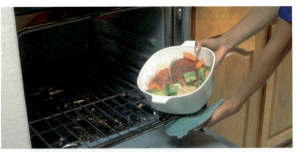

Fig. 28-10. *Many vegetables and meats can be baked together.*

Broiling: Used primarily for meats, broiling involves cooking food close to the source of heat at a high temperature for a short time (Fig. 28-11). Meat must be tender to be broiled successfully; inexpensive and lean cuts are often better cooked using moist heat. The "broil" setting on the oven can also be used to melt cheese or brown the top of a casserole. Leave the oven door ajar when broiling and never leave the kitchen; things can burn very fast.

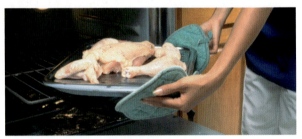

Fig. 28-11. *Broiling involves cooking at a very high temperature.*

Sautéing or stir-frying: These are quick cooking methods for vegetables and meats. Use a small amount of oil in a frying pan or wok over high heat (Fig. 28-12).

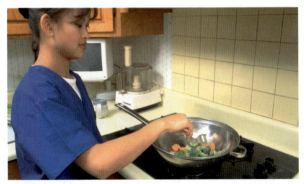

Fig. 28-12. *Stir frying is quick and uses very little fat. Food must be stirred constantly to prevent it from sticking.*

Microwaving: Microwave ovens are safe to use for defrosting, reheating, and cooking. However "cold spots" can occur in microwaved foods because of the irregular way the microwaves enter the oven and are absorbed by the food. If food does not cook evenly, bacteria may survive and cause food-borne illness.

To minimize cold spots, stir and rotate the food once or twice during cooking. Arranging foods uniformly in a covered dish and turning large foods upside down during cooking also help. When defrosting food in the microwave, remove food from store wrap first. Foam trays and plastic wraps may melt and cause chemicals to migrate into the food. Place food in a microwave-safe bowl instead. Foods being reheated in the microwave should be steaming and hot to the touch, or at least 165°F. Cover foods. Stir them from the outside in to encourage safe, even heating.

To insure that meat is properly cooked, use a meat thermometer or the oven's temperature probe. This verifies that the food has reached a safe temperature. Check in several places to be sure red meat is 160°F and poultry 180°F. Check for visual signs of doneness. Juices should run clear and meat should not be pink.

Never place metal thermometers or any metal object in the microwave oven. Be aware that some clients cannot be near a microwave during operation.

Frying: Frying uses a lot of fat and is the least healthy way to cook. Avoid frying foods for clients (Fig. 28-13).

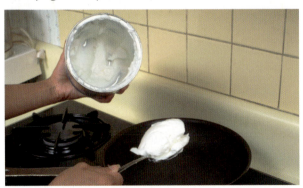

Fig. 28-13. *Avoid frying foods because it is one of the least healthy ways to cook.*

Fresh, uncooked foods: Many fruits and vegetables have the most nutrients when eaten fresh, as in salads (Fig. 28-14). However, fresh fruits and vegetables may be difficult for some clients to chew or digest. Wash fruits and vegetables well to remove any chemicals or pesticides.

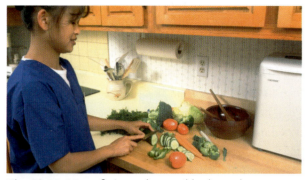

Fig. 28-14. Many fruits and vegetables have the most nutrients when eaten uncooked and fresh.

Preparing Mechanically Altered Diets

You learned about special diets in Chapter 15. If a client has chewing or swallowing difficulties, weakness, paralysis, dental problems, or is recovering from surgery, the doctor may order a liquid, soft or mechanical soft, or pureed diet for a short time.

For soft, mechanical soft, or pureed diets, foods are prepared with blenders, food processors, or cutting utensils. Chopped foods are foods that have been cut up into very small pieces. When chopping food, use a sharp knife and a clean cutting board (separate boards for raw meat and for vegetables and other foods). Grinding breaks the foods up into even smaller pieces. Pureed foods are cooked and then ground very fine or strained. A little liquid is added to give them the consistency of baby food. Grinding and pureeing can be done in a blender or food processor. However, fruits and vegetables can be also be pureed by pushing them through a colander with the back of a spoon.

All equipment used must be kept very clean to help prevent infection and illness. Take the blender or food processor apart after every use. Wash each piece that has come in contact with food in warm soapy water, and rinse thoroughly. Wash the cutting board after each use. This is especially important after chopping raw meat, poultry, and fish. Wash it with soap, or in the dishwasher, before using it again. Allow cutting board to air dry.

Changing the texture of food may make it lose its appeal. Season it according to the client's preferences to make it more appealing. Talk about the food being served using positive words. Pureeing also causes nutrients to be lost, so vitamin supplements may be ordered. Constipation and dehydration are complications of a pureed diet. It is very important to follow directions exactly.

Preparing Nutritional Supplements

Illness and injury may call for nutritional supplements to be added into the client's diet. Certain medications also change the need for nutrients. For example, some medication prescribed for high blood pressure increases the need for potassium.

Nutritional supplements may come in a powdered form or liquid form. Powdered supplements need to be mixed with a liquid before being taken; the care plan will include instructions on how much liquid to add.

When preparing supplements, make sure the supplement is mixed thoroughly. Make sure the client takes it at the ordered time. Clients who are ill, tired, or in pain may not have much of an appetite. It may take a long time for him to drink a large glass of a thick liquid. Be patient and encouraging. If a client does not want to drink the supplement, do not insist that he do so. However, do report this to your supervisor.

6. Identify four methods of low-fat food preparation

1. **Cook lean**. Boiling, steaming, broiling, roasting, and braising are all methods of cooking that require little or no added fat. Broiling also allows fats in meat to drip out before food is consumed. This lowers the fat content even more.

2. **Drain fat**. When using ground meat, brown it first. Then drain it on paper towels to remove excess fat.

3. **Plan lean**. Choosing foods with lower fat content to begin with will make low-fat cooking easier. Planning meals around grains will help cut the fat content. Low-fat meals based on grains include pasta dishes, rice and beans, baked or stuffed potatoes, and soups.

4. **Substitute or cut down**. Sometimes high-fat ingredients can be left out or replaced to lower the fat content of a recipe. Leave out or cut down the amount of cheese used on sandwiches or to top casseroles. Substitute plain nonfat yogurt for mayonnaise or sour cream. Nonfat cottage cheese can also be used. Try it on a baked potato instead of sour cream.

Food Appearance, Texture, and Portion Size

Keep the color and texture of foods in mind when planning meals. For example, do not serve two types of green vegetables at the same meal. Rather than green beans and spinach, try green beans and carrots instead. Serving food that is similar in texture may make the meal less interesting. For example, mashed potatoes and mashed rutabagas are similar. Try a boiled or baked potato instead. To promote appetites, make sure that food is attractively arranged on the plate. It should look appealing. Avoid putting large portions on the plate, unless the client normally eats larger amounts of food. Plan on smaller portions, but have enough food available in case the client requests seconds. Small, frequent meals may be ordered for some clients. For more information on how to make mealtime appealing, see Chapter 15.

7. List four guidelines for safe food storage

1. **Buy cold food last; get it home fast**. After shopping, put away refrigerated foods first.

2. **Keep it safe; refrigerate**. Maintain refrigerator temperature between 36°F and 40°F. Maintain freezer temperature at 0°F. Refrigerated items that spoil easily should be kept in the rear of the refrigerator, not the door. Look on the jar or package to determine if food requires refrigeration once it has been opened (Fig. 28-15). Do not refreeze items after they have been thawed.

3. **Use small containers that seal tightly**. Foods cool more quickly when stored in smaller containers. Store with enough room around them for air circulation. Never leave foods out for more than two hours. Tightly cover all foods. To prevent dry foods, such as cornmeal and flour, from becoming infested with insects, store these items in tightly-sealed containers. If you find items that are already infested, discard them. Use a clean container to store a fresh supply. Check dry storage areas periodically for signs of insects and rodents.

4. **When in doubt, throw it out!** If you are not sure whether food is spoiled, do not take any chances. Discard it. Check the expiration dates on foods, especially perishables.

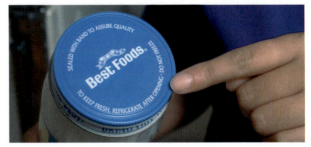

Fig. 28-15. *Look for refrigeration guidelines on food labels.*

Check the refrigerator often for spoiled foods. Discard any you find. Throw out foods that have become moldy (mold cannot just be scraped off).

Chapter Review

1. When planning a meal for a client, what are factors that the HHA should take into account?

2. List ten examples of nutritious snacks.

3. What are two reasons that an HHA should buy fresh foods that are in season?

4. Why is more expensive meat sometimes a better deal?

5. Why are processed or ready-made foods not as desirable as food made from scratch?

6. What does it mean if a food is labeled "organic?"

7. What information can be learned by looking at the number of calories from fat in a food?

8. What is the longest period of time that it is safe to leave cooked food unrefrigerated?

9. What needs to happen after an HHA has used a cutting board to cut fresh meat?

10. How can pesticides be removed from fresh fruits and vegetables?

11. How can a sponge be disinfected?

12. Briefly describe each of the following food preparation methods: boiling; steaming; poaching; roasting; braising; baking; broiling; sauteing; microwaving; and frying.

13. What equipment is used to prepare soft, mechanical soft, or pureed diets?

14. An HHA has browned ground beef to make soft tacos for her client. What should be done before adding the seasoning to make it lower in fat?

15. Give an example of one low-fat substitution in addition to those listed in the text.

16. When is it acceptable to refreeze an item?

17. What does the phrase, "When in doubt, throw it out" mean?

18. If an HHA finds insects in the flour, what should he do?

Conversion Tables

Liquid Measures				
1 gal=	4 qt=	8 pt=	16 cups=	128 fl oz
1/2 gal=	2 qt=	4 pt=	8 cups=	64 fl oz
1/4 gal=	1 qt=	2 pt=	4 cups=	32 fl oz
	1/2 qt=	1 pt=	2 cups=	16 fl oz
	1/4 qt=	1/2 pt=	1 cup=	8 fl oz

Dry Measures			
1 cup=	8 fl oz=	16 tbsp=	48 tsp
3/4 cup=	6 fl oz=	12 tbsp=	36 tsp
2/3 cup=	5 1/3 fl oz=	10 2/3 tbsp=	32 tsp
1/2 cup=	4 fl oz=	8 tbsp=	24 tsp
1/3 cup=	2 2/3 fl oz=	5 1/3 tbsp=	16 tsp
1/4 cup=	2 fl oz=	4 tbsp=	12 tsp
1/8 cup=	1 fl oz=	2 tbsp=	6 tsp
		1 tbsp=	3 tsp

Emergency Substitutions

Emergency substitutions can sometimes be made, although it is best to use the ingredients called for in recipes.

Vegetables	
Ingredient	Substitute
1 cup canned tomatoes	1 1/3 cups cut-up fresh tomatoes, simmered 10 minutes
1/2 lb. fresh mushrooms	4-oz can mushrooms
Legumes	With the exception of lentils, dry beans can be used interchangeably to suit personal preference.

Herbs, Spices, Seasonings	
Ingredient	Substitute
1 tbsp snipped fresh herbs	1 tsp. same herb, dried, or 1/4 tsp powdered or ground
1 tsp dry mustard	2 tsp prepared mustard
1 tsp pumpkin pie spice	1/2 tsp cinnamon, 1/2 tsp ginger, 1/8 tsp ground allspice, 1/8 tsp nutmeg

Baking	
Ingredient	Substitute
1 tsp baking powder	1/4 tsp baking soda plus 1/2 tsp cream of tartar
1 pkg active dry yeast	1 tbsp dry yeast
1 cup oil	1/2 lb. butter or margarine
1 cup brown sugar	1 cup granulated sugar

Thickeners	
Ingredient	Substitute
1 tbsp cornstarch	2 tbsp flour, or 1 1/3 tbsp quick-cooking tapioca
1 tbsp flour	1/2 tbsp cornstarch, or 2 tsp quick-cooking tapioca, or two egg yolks
1 tbsp tapioca	1 1/2 tbsp flour

29

The Clean, Safe, and Healthy Home Environment

1. Describe how housekeeping affects physical and psychological well-being

Providing a safe, clean, and orderly environment has always been an essential part of home health care. Illness and disability cause great stress. Clients feel better physically and psychologically and recover more quickly when their homes and families receive care and support. Infection and accidents are prevented. In addition, families who lack some knowledge to manage their homes can be taught valuable household management skills. These skills include sanitation, safety, personal hygiene, nutrition, meal planning, shopping, child care, food preparation, communication skills, and specific healthcare techniques. You can be a role model for your clients and their families by performing tasks efficiently and cheerfully.

2. List qualities needed to manage a home and describe general housekeeping guidelines

It takes efficiency, planning, knowledge, and skills to manage a household. You will need to know how to use your time and energy well. This is so that you do not neglect your primary responsibility—the personal care of the client.

Sensitivity is another important quality when caring for your clients' homes. You must respect the customs, beliefs, and feelings of your cli-

ents and their families. How would you feel if a stranger were handling your personal items and possessions? How would you feel if you could no longer care for your home yourself?

Be sensitive when you ask members of the household for help with housekeeping as well. Know when it is appropriate to ask for assistance and how to ask for it in an appropriate way. Some family members may be experiencing such stress that they are unable to help at all.

Your assignments will vary. They may include simple cleaning and organizing of the client's room or general cleaning throughout the house. Some clients require management of all household functions, including finances. You may be required to dust, straighten, vacuum, sweep, wash dishes, clean the bathroom and kitchen, and do laundry. Your assignments will outline the specific duties to be performed (Fig. 29-1).

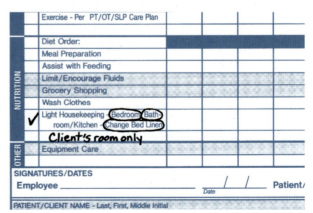

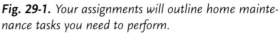

Fig. 29-1. Your assignments will outline home maintenance tasks you need to perform.

Your assignments may list specific days on which tasks should be performed or you may be allowed to make your own schedule. Flexibility is important and allows you to meet the client's and family's needs. If you receive requests for services not listed in your assignments or complaints about how tasks are done, contact your supervisor.

Most agencies require that aides perform light housekeeping. This usually involves dusting, straightening, vacuuming or sweeping floors and floor coverings, cleaning bathrooms and the kitchen, and disposing of trash. Light housekeeping does not involve moving heavy furniture, washing windows, taking down drapes, cleaning the attic and basement, or mowing the lawn.

Guidelines:
Housekeeping

G   Invite family participation. Depending on their abilities and availability, clients and family members may be asked to participate in housekeeping tasks.

G   Invite family and client input when you determine the tasks that need to be done and the methods used.

G   Use cleaning materials and methods that are acceptable to and approved by clients and their families. Any efforts you make toward improving the home environment should coincide with the client's choices, lifestyle, and values.

G   Be organized when performing tasks. Write out detailed daily and weekly schedules. Seek feedback from your supervisor and the client and family.

G   Build some flexibility into the schedule to allow for changes in the client's condition, needs, appointments, or social activities.

G   Organize cleaning materials and equipment by placing them in one closet. Place cleaning materials in a pail, a carrying bin that has a handle, a laundry basket, or a shopping bag (Fig. 29-2). Do not leave cleaning equipment around the home.

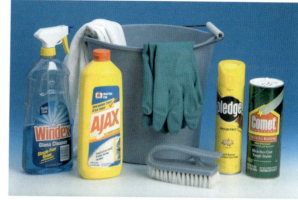

Fig. 29-2. *Keep cleaning materials and equipment organized.*

G   Familiarize yourself with the cleaning materials and equipment. Read the labels and instruction booklets. Ask the client, family members, or your supervisor how the equipment works if you are unfamiliar with it.

G   Maintain a safe environment as well as a clean and healthy one. Do not wax floors if your client is unsteady. Mop up spills immediately.

G   Use housekeeping procedures and methods that promote good health. Many diseases may be transmitted through improper food handling, dishwashing, handwashing, and unclean bathrooms and kitchens.

G   Observe the home environment for signs of infestation by roaches, rats, mice, lice, and fleas. These insects and animals are common carriers of disease. Controlling them is vital to family health and cleanliness.

G   Use good body mechanics in performing home maintenance activities to prevent injury. Housecleaning can require a great deal of bending, standing, stooping, and lifting.

Watch your posture. Kneel instead of stooping for long periods.

G   Clean up and straighten up after every activity. Spills that have dried are difficult to remove later.

G   Carry paper and a small pencil to make note of items that must be purchased or replaced. Maintain a shopping list on a bulletin board, refrigerator door, or other convenient location, and encourage family members to use the list.

G   Use your time wisely and efficiently. For example, prepare food while a load of wash is being done.

3. Describe cleaning products and equipment

Five basic types of home cleaning products are available in the market:

1. All-purpose cleaning agents can be used for many purposes and on several types of surfaces. These include countertops, walls, floors, and baseboards.

2. Soaps and detergents are used for bathing, laundering, and dishwashing.

3. Abrasive cleansers are used mostly to scour hard-to-clean surfaces.

4. Specialty cleaners are used to clean special surfaces, such as glass, metal, or ovens.

5. Non-toxic, environmentally safe cleaning products are made without toxic chemicals. They may be vegetable-based. Some of these products are even made at home with basic ingredients, such as baking soda, vinegar, castile soap, and water.

All cleaning products must be used properly. Many cleaning products are chemicals which can be irritating and can even cause burns. Some chemicals are poisonous when swallowed.

Guidelines:
Using Household Cleaning Products

G   Read and follow the directions on the label of every product you use. Cleaning products can harm the materials you are trying to clean.

G   Do not mix cleaning products. This can cause a dangerous chemical reaction that may harm you or others. In particular, **never mix bleach or products containing bleach with ammonia. The fumes are toxic and can be fatal**.

G   Open windows when cleaning to provide fresh air. Some cleaning products have fumes that are unpleasant or even harmful if you are exposed to them for a long time.

G   Do not leave cleaning products on surfaces longer than the recommended time. Do not scrub too hard on soft surfaces.

A basic set of cleaning tools generally includes two types:

1. Wet mops, pails, toilet brushes, and sponges are tools for softening and removing soil that has dried and hardened on washable surfaces.

2. A vacuum cleaner and attachments, carpet sweeper, dust mop, dust cloths, broom, and brush and dustpan are tools for removing dry dirt and dust.

Remember to be careful with equipment. Replacements can be expensive. Be familiar with the purpose and use of each piece of equipment. Keep it clean and in its proper place. Check the brushes and bags of vacuum cleaners frequently.

4. Describe proper cleaning methods for living areas, kitchens, bathrooms, and storage areas

Not all housekeeping tasks must be performed daily. Some tasks may be done weekly. Others only need to be done once a month or seasonally.

Space out the special tasks. Do each cleaning job properly and efficiently. Do not take a lot of steps and do not reach, bend, and stoop unnecessarily. Experiment a little to find the most comfortable and effective way to do a job. Cleaning can be done when your client is resting, sleeping, or doing another activity. Care of the client is your primary responsibility. However, do not neglect housekeeping.

Guidelines:
Straightening and Cleaning Living Areas

G   Clear up clutter and put objects in their correct places.

G   Pick up newspapers, magazines, and toys as needed.

G   Empty wastebaskets and ashtrays daily.

G   Make the beds each day.

G   Keep essential and frequently-used items, such as eyeglasses, tissues, a wastebasket, telephone, newspaper, magazines, and books, within reach. Organize them on an accessible table, magazine rack, or hanging organizer (Fig. 29-3).

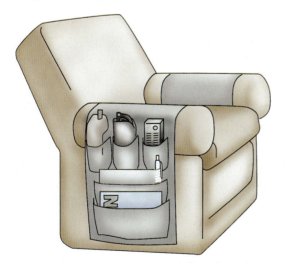

Fig. 29-3. A hanging organizer can help reduce clutter while keeping important items handy.

G   Dust once a week or when necessary. If your client has allergies, you may need to dust daily.

G   Vacuum floors and rugs once a week or more often if indicated. When vacuuming rugs, use long strokes and go over each area repeatedly. If the home does not have a vacuum, use a broom to sweep the floors and rugs. Take care not to raise much dust.

G   Floors covered with vinyl, ceramic tile, and linoleum may be washed. Some wood floors may not. Some floor coverings should be cleaned with water only. Check with the client or family before you begin. After removing loose dirt or crumbs with a vacuum or broom, wash floors with a cloth or mop dipped in warm, sudsy water. Dry the floor after you have washed it or close off the area for the time it takes for the floor to dry (Fig. 29-4). Wet or waxed floors are slippery and are frequent causes of falls in the home.

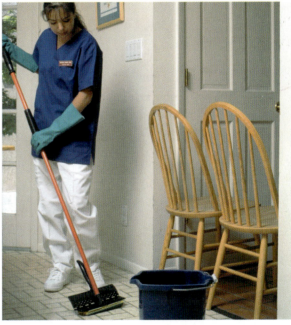

Fig. 29-4. Close off the area for the time it takes the floor to dry.

Handling food on contaminated surfaces, improper dishwashing, and contaminated food storage areas may transmit many diseases. Roaches, rats, and mice may cause disease and allergy by contaminating food with their saliva or through their droppings. Pest control is vital to health and cleanliness. Always report pest control problems to your supervisor.

Guidelines:
Cleaning the Kitchen

G   Clean the kitchen after every use. Ask family members to do the same. Do not wait until the end of the day to clean up. Daily kitchen cleaning tasks include washing dishes, wiping surfaces, taking out garbage, and storing leftover food. Weekly tasks include cleaning the refrigerator and washing the floor. Cleaning cabinets, drawers, and other storage areas is usually done a few times a year.

G   Wash dishes in hot, soapy water using liquid dish detergent. Rinse them in hot water. When working with clients who have an infectious disease or a cold, use boiling water for rinsing and add a tablespoon of chlorine bleach to the soapy water. The combination of heat and chlorine will kill pathogens, or harmful microorganisms.

G   Wash glasses and cups first, then silverware, plates, and bowls. Pots and pans are washed last. Rinse with hot water and dry on a rack. Air drying dishes is more sanitary than drying with a dish towel.

G   If the house has a dishwasher, learn how to correctly load and start it. Dishwashers save time. They may also sterilize dishes because of the high temperature used in washing and drying. Ask the client if you should scrape food from plates before placing in the dishwasher. Empty cups and glasses. Do not place dishes, cups, and flatware too close together. This keeps them from being washed thoroughly. Place dishes, cups, and glasses so that their eating or drinking surfaces are facing the water source.

G   Do not wash the following items in the dishwasher: electrical appliances, certain plastic materials, wooden pieces or utensils, hand-painted or antique dishes, delicate china, crystal, cast iron, most pots and pans, and sharp or carbon steel knives. Use only a dishwasher detergent. Fill the well with only the amount recommended on the label.

G   Clean the outside of the stove, the trays, and burners with hot, sudsy water or an all-purpose cleaner, and rinse. Ovens should be cleaned according to manufacturer's recommendations. Be sure to follow the directions. Do not spray the light bulb inside the oven with cleanser, or it may break. Soak the broiler pan immediately after use.

G   The refrigerator should be totally cleaned once a week. However, you should wipe it out more frequently (Fig. 29-5). If the refrigerator is not a self-defrosting one, the freezer should be defrosted whenever necessary. One-half inch of frost usually means it should be defrosted. To defrost a freezer, turn the dial to the "off" position. Remove all food. Wrap frozen foods in a cooler or newspapers to keep them from defrosting. Defrosting the freezer may take less time if you place pans of hot water in it. Do not use a knife to chip off the frost. This could damage the cooling unit.

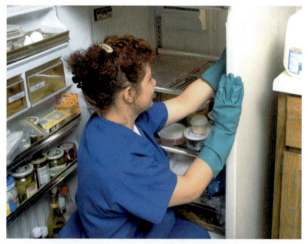

Fig. 29-5. The refrigerator should be totally cleaned once a week, but you should wipe it out more frequently.

G   Mix two tablespoons of baking soda in one quart of warm water. Wipe the inside walls of the refrigerator and freezer. Baking soda will remove odors. Wash the shelves and trays with warm, soapy water.

The Clean, Safe, and Healthy Home Environment

G Clean countertops, tables, and the stove each time they are used. Clean cabinet and drawer fronts and the refrigerator once a week. If a cutting board or other surface has been used to cut fresh meat, scrub the surface thoroughly with soapy water. Rinse well.

G An all-purpose cleaner may be needed to remove grease and cooked foods that have spilled or splashed on surfaces. Clean the sink with a cleanser such as scouring powder or cream.

G Never place food on soiled work or storage areas or in unclean containers. Keep food covered. Close lids of cartons and cover food storage containers to prevent contamination or infestation by insects and rodents. Place leftovers in covered containers and store them in the refrigerator immediately. Use them in two to three days.

G Vacuum, sweep, or dry mop the floor daily. Damp mop uncarpeted floors at least once a week, using hot water and a floor cleaner. Rinse the floor if the label recommends doing so. Dry the floor or close off the area until the floor dries to prevent accidents.

G Dispose of garbage daily. To prevent odor and discourage insects and rodents, rinse out tin cans and bottles before placing them in the garbage pail or recycling bin. Follow the recycling procedures for your client's community. Periodically wash wastebaskets and trash cans with hot, soapy water.

G Store all cleaning materials away from food, food preparation utensils, and food preparation areas. Keep them out of reach of children and confused clients.

A clean, organized, and odor-free bathroom is an important part of improving a family's hygiene and safety. Because it is moist and warm, the bathroom is a reservoir for the growth of microorganisms, mold, and mildew.

Guidelines:
Cleaning the Bathroom

G Involve the entire family in keeping the bathroom clean (Fig. 29-6). Always wash from clean areas to dirty areas, so you do not spread dirt into areas that have already been washed.

G Flush the toilet each time it is used.

G Clean toothbrushes and toothbrush holders.

G Scrub the tub and shower after use.

G Remove hair from drain strainers.

G Hang up all used towels to dry.

G Put away toiletries.

G Rinse the sink after brushing teeth, shaving, and washing.

G Place soiled towels in the laundry hamper after they are dry.

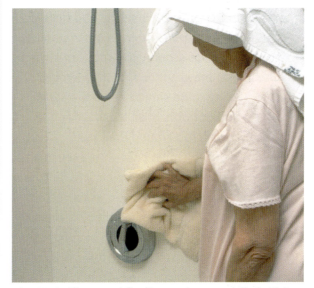

Fig. 29-6. Clients and family members can help by doing such things as wiping out the shower after each use.

The bathroom is the location of many home accidents. Make sure that all bathroom rugs are nonskid. Wipe up puddles of water immediately. If grab bars are not present and your client has difficulty moving about in the bathroom safely, report this to your supervisor.

Cleaning a bathroom

Equipment: approved disinfectant (a cleaning product that kills germs), scouring powder or scouring cream with bleach, sponge, toilet brush, glass cleaner, paper towels, disposable or rubber gloves

1. Put on gloves.

2. Using the disinfectant and sponge, wipe all surfaces and rinse as needed. Be sure to clean the sides, walls, and curtain or door of the shower or tub; the towel racks; holders for toilet paper, toothbrushes, and soap; and window sills.

3. Rinse sponge well or use a different sponge to wipe the outside of the toilet bowl, seat, and lid. As a general cleaning rule, start with the cleanest surface first, then move to dirtier areas.

4. Use a different sponge to clean the bathtub, shower stall, and sink. Use scouring powder or cream for tile and porcelain, and disinfectant or all-purpose cleaner on other surfaces. Remember that scouring powder can scratch. Check with the client or a family member before using it. Be sure to scrub the sides, edges, and bottoms of all these areas. Clean faucets and scrub around their bases. Scrub the inside of the toilet bowl with a brush and scouring powder containing bleach. Be sure to scrub under the rim. If you use a second, stronger toilet cleaner, flush the first cleaning product down the drain first to avoid possible chemical reactions. Wash the toilet brush with a disinfectant solution. Store it in a plastic bag or holder after letting it air dry.

5. Vacuum or dry mop the floor first, then wash if the floor is tile or linoleum. Use an all-purpose floor cleaner in hot water. Wash the floor with a cloth or mop, taking special care to clean the areas at the base of the toilet and sink. Do not leave the floor wet. Dry it carefully to avoid accidents.

6. Clean the mirror and any glass or chrome surfaces using glass cleaner and paper towels or clean rags.

7. Place dry, soiled towels in the laundry hamper. Empty the waste can into a plastic or paper garbage bag and dispose of it. Replace toilet tissue and facial tissue when needed. Open the bathroom window for a short time, if possible, to air the room out. Once a week, wash out the waste can and laundry hamper, and launder the bath mats and rugs.

8. Store supplies.

9. Remove and discard gloves.

10. Wash your hands.

11. Document the cleaning.

Cleaning and organizing storage areas will contribute to the order and organization of the home.

Guidelines:
Cleaning and Organizing Storage Areas

G Every item in the home should have a storage place that is convenient for use. That means storage places should be as close as possible to where they are used (Fig. 29-7). For example, bath towels should be stored in or near the bathroom. Frequently used pots and pans and cooking utensils should be near the stove. Less frequently used items, such as popcorn poppers, should be stored in the less accessible storage places.

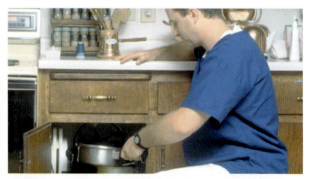

Fig. 29-7. *Store items near where they will be used.*

G Items that are frequently used should be easily seen and reached. When they are used, they should be immediately replaced. Items that are used together should be stored near each other. Arrange food on shelves according to category to save time in searching for items. Dangerous materials such as cleaning products should be stored out of reach of children and confused adults.

G Some storage areas only need to be cleaned occasionally. Remove the stored items and any shelf or drawer liners. Wipe the shelves and drawers with a damp cloth and all-purpose cleaner. Replace the liners or wipe them if they can be cleaned. Food storage areas and other storage areas that are used frequently should be cleaned more often.

G Do not change the client's or the family's storage arrangements without talking to them. If you think changes are needed, discuss your ideas with the family.

Cleaning Solution Ideas

Several types of cleaning solutions can be prepared from common household items when supplies are not available or when the family budget is restricted. Some of these are environmentally safe and non-toxic.

- Baking soda can be used instead of scouring powder. Baking soda can also be diluted with warm water to make a solution that will eliminate odors when used to clean surfaces.

- White vinegar can be used to remove lime or other mineral deposits on sinks, toilets, or chrome fixtures. White vinegar diluted with water can be used instead of glass cleaner and as a general cleaner. Mix solution using one part white vinegar to three parts water (1:3).

- Household bleach, diluted with four parts water, makes a strong disinfectant solution to clean bathroom surfaces. Diluted with nine parts water and stored in a spray bottle, bleach makes a milder disinfectant to use on kitchen counters. Do not spill or splash undiluted bleach or bleach solutions on carpets, clothing, or other surfaces that might be discolored.

5. Describe how to prepare a cleaning schedule

Most house-cleaning tasks should be done either immediately, daily, weekly, monthly, or less often. Take into account the care plan, your assignments, how much help is needed, and how much time you have in a particular home to prepare a cleaning schedule. You may not always stick to the schedule exactly. However, it will guide your work and help you get essential cleaning done. Establishing a schedule for cleaning can also help the family keep a housekeeping routine after your care has ended. Below is a sample cleaning schedule. The client can do almost nothing around the house. Her daughter comes in several times a week, but no family members live with the client.

Cleaning Schedule for Mrs. Hedman

Immediately: Wipe counters, wash dishes, store food, clean spills, put away supplies.

Daily: Straighten up: make bed, sort mail, remove clutter, empty trash, etc. Clean bathroom. (One hour)

Weekly: Wash kitchen floors, wipe refrigerator, scrub sink, vacuum other floors, dust all surfaces, scrub bathtub. (Two to three hours)

Monthly: Clean out refrigerator, defrost freezer. (One hour)

Less often: Clean oven when needed. (One hour)

Cleaning schedules will be different for each client. Be flexible. You will need to adapt your schedule after you make it. Remember that client care is your first priority.

6. List special housekeeping procedures to use when infection is present

You must follow standard precautions with every client. This is true because you cannot know when infection is present (see Chapter 5). However, when a client has a known infectious disease such as influenza, or one that weakens the immune system, such as AIDS or cancer, you need to take special precautions in housecleaning:

- Use disinfectant when cleaning countertops and surfaces in the kitchen and bathroom.

- Clean the client's bathroom daily. Have other family members use a different bathroom if possible.

- Use separate dishes and utensils for the infected client. In some cases, disposable dishes and utensils will be ordered.

- Wash dishes and utensils in the dishwasher or wash dishes in hot soapy water with bleach. Rinse in boiling water, and allow to air dry.

- Disinfect any surfaces that contact body fluids, such as bedpans, urinals, and toilets.

- Frequently remove trash containing used tissues.

- Keep any specimens of urine, stool, or sputum in double bags and away from food or food preparation areas.

7. Explain how to do laundry and care for clothes

You may be expected to do hand or machine washing as part of an assignment. Clean clothes, bed linens, and towels are important for hygiene and comfort.

Laundry Products and Equipment: To do the laundry you will need laundry detergent, a washing machine or a basin for hand washing clothes, and a dryer or a clothesline and pins. The instructions for using washing machines are usually located on the inside of the machine lid.

In general, you will use all-purpose detergent. Some delicate fabrics, underwear, or stockings may require a special detergent. Some clients may prefer a non-detergent soap for use on baby clothes. Bleach, color brighteners, stain removers, and fabric softeners may also be used. Ask the client and family about their preferences for laundry products.

Pretreating: Pretreating means giving special treatment to items that have heavy soil, spots, and stains before washing them. Spots and stains should be treated immediately. The sooner they are treated, the easier they are to remove. Some oily stains harden with age and cannot be removed. Washing and ironing may set some stains, making them difficult or impossible to remove. If you can, identify the source of the stain and treat it according to a stain guide on the pretreating solution.

Bleach: Bleach is used with detergent. However, bleach cannot be used on all fabrics. Be familiar with the type of bleach and the fabric that is being washed. Three types of bleach are used in laundry: liquid chlorine, powdered chlorine, and oxygen or all-fabric bleach. Each type of bleach should be used with caution. Read the instructions on the container carefully.

Liquid chlorine bleaches are excellent stain removers. They whiten clothing. However, they can be very damaging. Bleach should always be diluted in water. Fill the washer, then add liquid bleach and stir the water before adding clothing. Never use liquid chlorine bleach on silk, spandex, wool, or any item that contains these fibers. Be careful not to spray or splash liquid chlorine bleach. It will remove color or damage fabric. Powdered chlorine bleach is more gentle than liquid, but it can also damage clothing. Either type of chlorine bleach is also an excellent disinfectant. Oxygen or all-fabric bleach is used on washable fabrics, but it is most effective in hot water.

Water Temperature: Read the washing instructions for all materials and garments (Fig. 29-8). Warm water is safest for most garments. However, some must be washed in cold to prevent shrinking or colors fading. Hot water is generally used for towels, bed linens, and white or colorfast cottons. Warm is usually used for permanent press, knit, synthetic, sheer, lace, acetate, fabric blends, washable rayons, and plastic. Cold water is used for brightly-colored fabrics or fabrics that are not colorfast.

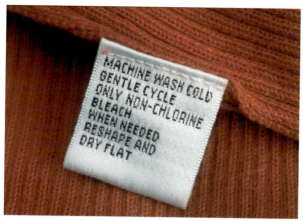

Fig. 29-8. *A care tag gives washing and drying instructions. It can be found on most clothing.*

Washing Action or Cycle: Use the normal setting on the washer for cottons, linens, rayons, sturdy permanent press, knits, synthetics, blends, and most other items. Set the washer on the slow or gentle setting for washable woolens, old quilts, curtains, and delicate or fragile items.

Drying Clothes: Settings on the dryer vary according to the model. Most dryers have a permanent press setting and a delicate setting. The more delicate a fabric, the lower the drying temperature and the shorter the time in the dryer. Heavy items such as towels need higher temperature settings and a longer time in the dryer. Clean the lint filter each time you use the dryer. If your client does not have a clothes dryer, hang clothes on a clothesline using clothespins.

Folding: To reduce the amount of wrinkling, remove all clothes from the dryer immediately. Fold them neatly or place them on hangers. Set aside those that need to be ironed. Return other items to their drawers or closet.

Ironing: Before you begin to iron, check the label of the item for the recommended tempera-

ture. If the label does not recommend a particular setting or the fabric is a blend, use the lowest temperature on the iron. Take special care with pile fabrics, such as velvets and corduroy. They will keep their texture better if ironed on the wrong side over a towel. Dark fabrics, silks, acetates, rayons, linens, and some wools must be pressed on the wrong side to prevent them from becoming shiny. Use a pressing cloth to protect the fabric.

To prevent stretching, iron all fabrics lengthwise. Iron collars, cuffs, and garment facings first. Next, iron the sleeves, then the front and back. Hang or fold clothes immediately. Fasten all hooks and buttons and close zippers. Be sure clothes are completely dry before putting them away.

Maintaining Clothing: You may need to do basic mending or sewing occasionally. This is especially true if you are taking care of a family, an older person with impaired vision, or people who may not have the time or the ability to keep clothing and linens repaired. Some clients who can do their own mending may just need you to thread the needle.

Doing the laundry

1. Sort clothes carefully. Make separate piles of whites, colors, and bright colors. Check clothing labels for special washing instructions. Do not wash anything labeled "Dry Clean Only." If hand washing is recommended, do not wash in the machine.

2. As you sort laundry, check pockets and remove tissues, money, pens, and other items. Remove belts with buckles, trims, and non-washable ornaments. Close zippers, buttons, and other fasteners. Check garments for stains and areas of heavy soil. If appropriate, mend or repair any holes, snags, rips, tears, pulled seams, and weak spots in garments and other items.

3. Pretreat spots and stains before washing. A small amount of liquid detergent or dry detergent dissolved in water can be worked in with an old toothbrush (Fig. 29-9). Pretreat or soak clothing as soon as possible for best results. If you know something is spotted, do not let it sit in the laundry hamper all week until you do the laundry.

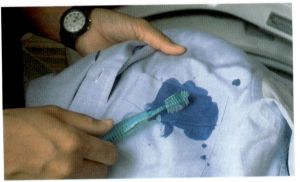

Fig. 29-9. Pretreating helps remove spots, stains, and areas that are heavily soiled.

4. Use the correct water temperature: hot for whites, warm for colors, cold for bright colors.

5. Use the appropriate laundry product(s). Follow the washing instructions on the container.

6. Follow written instructions or client or family instructions for using the washer. Use the correct washing cycle for the load you are laundering.

7. Dry clothes completely either in a dryer or on a clothesline. If using an automatic dryer, follow the drying instructions on clothing labels or the client's preferences. Some fabrics require cooler temperatures.

8. Hand-wash items in warm or cool water, depending on the fabric and instructions. Use a mild detergent or special hand-washing liquid. Line dry or lay items flat on towels to preserve the shape of the garment.

9. Fold or hang clean laundry and sort into categories. Store in drawers or closets.

8. List special laundry precautions to use when infection is present

When a client has a known infectious disease, you must take special precautions when handling laundry:

- Keep client's laundry separate from other family members'.

- Handle dirty laundry as little as possible. Do not shake it. Sort it and put it in plastic bags in the client's room or bathroom. Take it immediately to the laundry area.

- Wear gloves and hold laundry away from your clothes and body when you are handling it.

- Use liquid bleach when fabrics allow.

- Use agency-approved disinfectants in all loads.

- Use hot water.

9. List guidelines for teaching housekeeping skills to clients' family members

In some assignments, you will be asked to teach housekeeping skills to family members. This prepares them to take over housekeeping and care when home care is discontinued. By teaching household management skills, you help families meet their daily needs and become more self-reliant.

Guidelines:
Teaching Family Members

G Get to know the family before starting to teach them. Understand their needs or problems before beginning.

G Be patient. Give people time to learn new skills. Praise their efforts.

G Keep teaching sessions brief.

G Break down tasks into simple steps. Explain each step and demonstrate it.

G Answer all questions.

G Assist the person as necessary. Do not do the task for him or her.

G Remember that each person is an individual and will learn in different ways. Customize your teaching to allow for these differences.

Using Good Body Mechanics in the Home

Review the principles of body mechanics you learned in Chapters 6 and 10. Remember the following additional tips when working in a home:

- Bend the knees, not the back, when lifting things from the floor or when kneeling to pick up objects.

- Carry heavy objects close to the body and distribute the weight evenly. For example, when carrying a basket of clothes, hold it directly in front of the body (Fig. 29-10). Stand close to the work area. When possible, raise the work area to a comfortable level so you do not have to bend your back and neck to do the work.

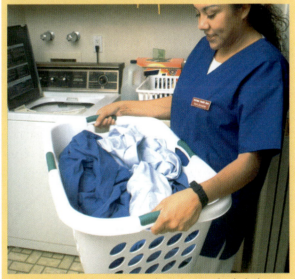

Fig. 29-10. *Holding objects close to your body helps prevent back strain and injury.*

- Try not to lift heavy objects. If you must move heavy objects such as furniture, try pushing, pulling, or rolling, using the entire body.

- Stand erect when doing tasks like washing dishes. Your knees may be slightly bent.

- Avoid lifting heavy objects from the floor. For example, put the clothes basket on a chair before filling it (Fig. 29-11).

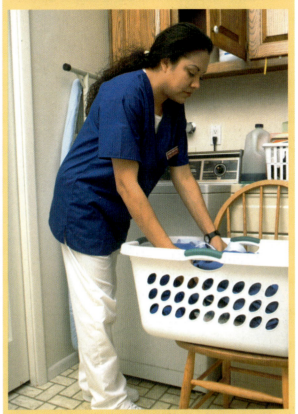

Fig. 29-11. *By placing the basket on a chair close to her, this HHA avoids excessive bending and reaching.*

10. Identify hazardous household materials

Any of the following household materials can have harmful effects:

- Household bleach

- Cleaning products

- Aerosol or spray cans

- Paint

- Chemicals such as turpentine or paint thinner

- Medicines, both prescription and over-the-counter

- Hair spray

- Nail polish remover

These products should be kept in separate cabinets with childproof latches or locks, or up out of the reach of children. If a client is confused, mark these cabinets with signs that indicate danger.

Chapter Review

1. What skills are important in household management?

2. What housekeeping assignments might an HHA be asked to do?

3. What are some housekeeping tasks an HHA should NOT be asked to perform?

4. List ten housekeeping guidelines.

5. Why is it important to read the instructions for cleaning products?

6. Why should cleaning products not be mixed?

7. What two parts of a vacuum cleaner should an HHA check often?

8. How often should wastebaskets and ashtrays be emptied?

9. How should an HHA clean the floors if the home does not have a vacuum?

10. What should an HHA do when washing dishes for clients who have an infectious disease or cold?

11. How frequently should the refrigerator be cleaned?

12. In what time frame should leftover food be eaten?

13. What items should not be washed in the dishwasher?

14. Ideally, where should storage places be located?

15. Describe why it is helpful to make a cleaning schedule.

16. How frequently should an HHA clean the bathroom of a client who has an infectious disease?

17. List two guidelines for dealing with the dishes and utensils of a client with an infectious disease.

18. What is pretreating?

19. List three types of bleach.

20. List the safest temperature for most garments.

21. How can an HHA reduce the amount of wrinkling after clothes have been dried in the dryer?

22. List six guidelines that an HHA should follow when handling laundry of a client with an infectious disease.

23. List five guidelines to follow when teaching family members housekeeping skills.

24. Where should hazardous household materials be kept?

30

Managing Time, Energy, and Money in the Home

1. Explain three ways to work more efficiently

Taking care of the client and other family members who need assistance and support is your most important responsibility. For this to be accomplished, you must maintain an orderly and clean environment. To balance these responsibilities, you must manage your time and energy efficiently. The following are ways to be sure your work schedule is as efficient as possible:

Distribute tasks. Look at the client care plan and your assignments. Note the assigned housekeeping tasks. Divide the tasks and schedule them for the week and the month. Make sure all your assignments can be completed in the time you have. Some tasks are best accomplished together. For example, it is most efficient to do all the laundry on one day. Then you are able to do larger loads and fold and iron all at once. Plan one morning or afternoon to do the laundry. For more efficiency, plan other tasks to do while loads are in the washer or dryer.

Prioritize tasks. Prioritizing your tasks is an important time and energy management skill. Think about the jobs you want to complete throughout the day. Which ones must be done immediately? Which ones must be done at a certain time? Which activities are not absolutely essential and could be put off? Spend time on activities that are most important first.

Simplify tasks. Learn to simplify your tasks. Take time to think about how you will go about doing a task. Try to eliminate a few steps but still get the same result. For example, when baking a cake, can you mix everything in one bowl? When you clean up, can you stack everything on a tray and take it all to the sink at one time?

Be realistic. You may not be able to get everything done even if you plan carefully. Reassess your schedule during the day. Have you finished what you planned or are you behind? When tasks take longer than you expected, or unexpected tasks need to be done, be realistic about what you can do. Do not be afraid to change your plan. It is better to accomplish the highest-priority tasks and let others go unfinished than to do everything half-way. The key to success is to be flexible.

Simple Ways to Conserve Time and Energy

Energize. Use good body mechanics. Take occasional breaks to restore your energy. Alternate longer tasks with shorter tasks, and high-energy tasks with low-energy ones. Take care of yourself—eat right, exercise, and get plenty of rest.

Organize. At the beginning of the day, do a mental rundown of the tasks that must be done and rearrange your schedule if necessary. Plan what must be done and do it. Store frequently-used items in convenient places near the work area. Assemble your equipment and materials before you begin a task. Keep clutter in control and work in good light. Think about how to organize activities and equipment to avoid unnecessary work. Make and use shopping lists.

Economize. Save time and energy by doing a little extra ahead of time. Use trays, baskets, or carts to carry several things at once. Prepare often-used food items ahead of time and freeze them. Cook in quantity and freeze meal-size portions. Cook more than one item in the oven at a time.

Minimize. Look for ways to make tasks shorter and easier. Modify your workspace to make your work more comfortable and easier.

Specialize. Use the right tool for each task. For example, a vegetable peeler is more efficient than a knife for peeling carrots. Take pride in what you are doing. Finally, be sure to thank family members who have picked up, cleaned up, or participated in household chores.

2. Describe how to follow an established work plan with the client and family

The client care plan and your assignments will tell you what tasks are required. You can develop your own work plan. This will allow you to finish all your assigned tasks as quickly and efficiently as possible. For each day or block of time you will spend in a home, list all the tasks you must complete. Then, prioritize them. Mark the most important as "1," the next most important as "2," and so on. Finally, write out a schedule for the day, filling in the highest priority tasks first. If there are tasks that must be done at a certain time, put those tasks on the schedule at the appropriate time.

Remember to distribute tasks so that you are not trying to do all the house cleaning on one afternoon and end up with no time to bathe or care for a client. Simplify tasks whenever possible to allow you to accomplish more.

Following an established work plan will allow you to get more done in less time. It will also allow your clients and families to know what to expect of you. You may even want to discuss the plan with a client or family member as you are making it up or when it is finished. Some people

appreciate knowing what will be happening in their homes at any given time.

3. Discuss ways to handle inappropriate requests

Occasionally, you may be asked to do something that is not in the care plan or your assignments. Because each client's situation is unique, you will not be assigned to the same tasks for every client. For example, the care plan may specify grocery shopping for Mrs. Singer, who lives alone and cannot drive. But if another client who lives with family members asks you to run to the store, you have to say no if it is not in the care plan or your assignments.

Several things will help you handle requests that you must refuse. First, explain that you are only allowed to do tasks assigned in the care plan. Explain that nurses familiar with the client's condition give you your assignments. Emphasize that you would like to help, but that you are limited to the tasks outlined in the care plan and your assignments. After explaining this to the client, contact your supervisor and discuss the request. Your supervisor may add the task requested by the client to your assignments. It is possible it was left out of your assignments by mistake. Be sure to document the client's request and the actions you took to address it.

Establishing a work schedule will also help you handle inappropriate requests. If a client and family know what to expect of you, they may not be tempted to ask you to do other tasks.

Sharing a schedule of everything you must accomplish in a visit may help the client understand your job. If inappropriate requests continue, refer clients or family members to your supervisor.

4. List five money-saving homemaking tips

1. Check store circulars for advertised specials. Plan your menus around foods that are a good

value; for example, raw foods are less expensive than prepared ones. Chapter 28 discusses more ways to plan economical meals.

2. Use coupons. If your client receives a newspaper, scan it for coupons from stores or manufacturers (Fig. 30-1).

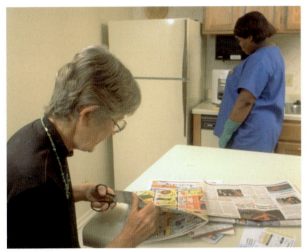

Fig. 30-1. Clipping coupons can save your client money. Some clients may enjoy doing this task themselves.

3. Shop from your list. Do not be tempted by items that are not on your list, even if they are on sale.

4. Avoid convenience stores. Shopping at large supermarkets or discount stores usually guarantees you will get the best prices.

5. Plan ahead. Knowing what you need before you run out will save money. Planning will also save time and energy. For example, you will not have to make a special trip when you discover you are out of laundry detergent.

5. List guidelines for handling a client's money

Different states and employers have different regulations and policies regarding healthcare employees handling clients' money. Find out from your employer whether you will be expected to handle clients' money. If you are not allowed to handle money, never agree to do so, even occasionally. You could get yourself and your employer into serious trouble.

If your state and your employer permit you to handle clients' money, there are several guidelines you must follow in doing so.

Guidelines:
Handling a Client's Money

G Never use a client's money for your own needs, even if you plan to pay it back. This is considered stealing. You could lose your job and/or be arrested.

G Estimate the amount of money you will need before requesting it. If you are making a trip to the grocery store, show the client your list and ask how much he or she is willing to spend on groceries, or how much is budgeted. You may need to take things off your list or estimate the total bill as you go along in the store to stay within the money allotted (Fig. 30-2).

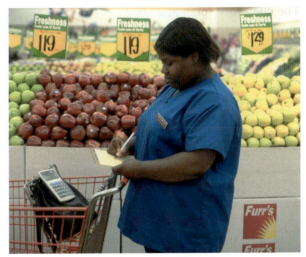

Fig. 30-2. Taking a calculator to the grocery store helps you to stay within the client's budget.

G Take checks rather than cash, when possible. Have the client or family member fill out the name of the store. A signed check that is not made out is as good as cash. If you lose cash or a signed bank check, you may be responsible for paying back the amount.

G Get a receipt for every purchase. This proves how much you spent and provides a record for you and the client.

G Return receipts and change to the client or family member immediately. Do not wait until the end of the day or week to settle up. Do it right away while everything is fresh in your mind. Forgetting to return change could be viewed by the client or a family member as stealing.

G Keep a record of money you have spent. Follow your agency's policies and procedures for documenting money issues. Write down how much you spent and where. Note any change returned to the client. The better record you have, the smaller the chance of any misunderstanding.

G Keep a client's cash separate from yours. If you must use the client's cash, do not put it in your own wallet. Keep it in a separate, safe place. Do the same with change. This will prevent confusion.

G Never offer money advice to clients. You should not even refer clients to others regarding their financial matters.

G Remember, your clients' financial matters are private. Never discuss your clients' money matters with anyone.

Chapter Review

1. List three ways to work more efficiently.

2. What does it mean to "prioritize" tasks?

3. How should the HHA handle requests that she must refuse?

4. How might an HHA help a client and his/her family understand her job? How could this help reduce inappropriate requests?

5. List five money-saving homemaking tips.

6. List six guidelines for handling a client's money.

7. Why is it important to get a receipt for anything purchased with a client's money?

8. How can taking a calculator to the store when shopping for clients be useful?

31

Caring for Your Career and Yourself

1. Discuss different types of careers in the healthcare field

There are many different types of careers in the healthcare field. Some of these are considered direct service. These are the positions that serve the resident, client, or patient directly. Nursing assistants, home health aides, patient care technicians, nurses, physician assistants and doctors all provide direct service. Professionals in therapeutic services, such as occupational, speech, and physical therapists, also offer direct care.

Some specialized technicians work in diagnostic services, such as x-ray technicians, lab technicians, and ultrasound technicians (Fig. 31-1). Diagnostic services are procedures performed to determine a condition and/or its cause.

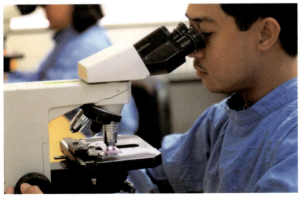

Fig. 31-1. *Lab technicians may conduct tests to help diagnose a condition.*

Medical social workers and substance abuse counselors are part of psychology, counseling, and social work fields. Activities directors and assistants also work in health care. Administra-

tive and support staff, including directors or other executive staff, medical records personnel, receptionists, office managers, and billing staff are part of the healthcare field.

Career opportunities in health care also include the fields of dentistry, nutrition, and pharmacy. Complementary or alternative healthcare fields include chiropracty, massage therapy and homeopathic medicine (Fig. 31-2).

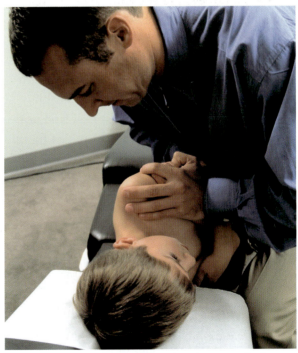

Fig. 31-2. *Chiropractors perform hands-on manipulations, or adjustments, of the spine or other joints.*

There are many opportunities for teachers within health care. Most of the career paths require classes before working in the field, as well as continuing education. Health educators and prevention professionals teach the general population or specific populations, such as diabetics or pregnant women.

There are many opportunities available to you in the healthcare field, depending upon your interest, education, and abilities. The careers listed above are only a fraction of jobs offered in health care. You are reading this textbook most likely because you want to become a nursing assistant and/or home health aide. Those positions may be the best fit for you, or at some point, you may want to try something different. Speak with your supervisor, instructor, or a career counselor if you want more information about other careers in the healthcare field. Review Chapters 1 and 2 for information on the different healthcare settings and educational requirements for care team members.

2. Explain how to find a job and how to write a résumé

You may soon be looking for a job. Nursing assistants may be able to work in long-term care facilities, in assisted living facilities, in hospitals, in the home, and in other places. Home health aides usually look for jobs with home health agencies. To find a job, you must first find potential employers. Then you must contact them to find out about job opportunities. To find employers, use the Internet, newspaper, telephone book, or personal contacts. Try these resources:

- Classified or employment sections of the newspaper list jobs currently available. Circle ads for the positions for which you are qualified. Make a list of names and phone numbers to contact.

- Call the state or local Department of Social Services or Department of Aging. Many states hire or place nursing assistants or home health aides.

- Ask your instructor for potential employers. Some schools maintain a list of employers seeking nursing assistants or home health aides.

- Check the Internet (Fig. 31-3). One good web site is carecareers.net. Other good ones are jobbankinfo.org and monster.com. You can also visit a search engine, such as google.com or yahoo.com. Type in "nursing assistant" or "home health aide" and your city. See what employment opportunities are there.

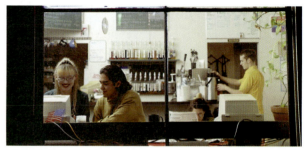

Fig. 31-3. *Searching the Internet is one good way to find a job.*

Once you have a list of potential employers, you need to contact them about job opportunities. Phoning first, unless they mention not to do so, is a good way to find out what opportunities are available. Ask how to apply for a job with each potential employer.

When making an appointment, ask what information to bring with you. Make sure you have it when you go. Some of these documents include the following:

- Identification, including driver's license, social security card, birth certificate, passport, or other official form of identification

- Proof of your legal status in this country and proof that you are legally able to work, even if you are a U.S citizen. Employers must have files showing that employees are legally allowed to work in this country. Do not be offended by this request.

- High school diploma or equivalency, school transcripts, and diploma or certificate from your nursing assistant or home health aide training course. Take the name and phone number of your instructor with you as well.

- References are people who can be called to recommend you as an employee. They can include former employers or former teachers. Do not use relatives or friends as references. You can ask your references beforehand to write letters of recommendation for you, addressed "To whom it may concern," explaining how they know you and describing your skills, qualities, and habits. Take copies of these with you.

Some potential employers will ask you for a résumé and a cover letter. A **résumé** is a summary or listing of relevant job experience and education. It is also called also "curriculum vitae" or "CV." When creating your résumé, include the following:

- Your contact details: name, address, telephone number, e-mail address

- A list of your educational experience, starting with the most current first (for example, nursing assistant training course, college degree, high school diploma or G.E.D. courses)

- A list of your work experience, starting with the most current first (include name of company or organization, your title, dates worked, and a brief summary of duties)

- Any special skills, such as knowledge of computer software, typing skills, or speaking other languages

- Any memberships in professional organizations

- Volunteer work

State at the end of your résumé that references are available upon request. Try to keep your résumé brief (one page is best) and clear. Use nice white or cream-colored paper for printing your résumé.

The cover letter is a letter included with your résumé. It should be no longer than one page in length. This letter briefly states the position you are seeking and why you would be the best person for the job. Emphasize skills you have that would be a good match. Include the following in a cover letter:

- Date

- Sender's name, address, and other contact information

- Recipient's name and address

- Salutation (e.g. "Dear Human Resources Director")

- Introduction (position you are seeking)

- Body (skills/experience that fit job being offered)

- Closing and signature (e.g. "I look forward to hearing from you. Sincerely, Josie Hartman")

3. Identify information that may be required when filling out a job application

On one sheet of paper, write down the general information you will need. Take it with you, along with your résumé, if you have one. This will save time and avoid mistakes.

Include the following general information:

- Your address and phone number

- Your birth date

- Your social security number

- Name and address of the school or program where you were trained and the date you completed it, as well as certification numbers and expiration dates from a certification card, if you have one

- Names, titles, addresses, and phone numbers of former employers, and the dates you worked there

- Salary information from your former jobs

- Reasons why you left each of your former jobs

- Names, addresses, and phone numbers of your references

- Days and hours you can work

- A brief statement of why you are changing jobs or why you want to work as a nursing assistant or home health aide

Fill out the application carefully and neatly (Fig. 31-4). Never lie on a job application. Before you write anything, read the application all the way through once. If you do not understand what is being asked, find out before filling in that space. Fill in all of the blanks. Write "N/A" (not applicable) if the question does not apply to you.

Employment Application

Personal Information

Name: Rosie Ferguson

Date: 12/15/09

Social Security Number: 555-99-9999

Home Address: 8529 Indian School Rd. NE

City, State, Zip: Albuquerque, NM 87112

Home Phone: 505-291-1274

Business Phone: N/A

US Citizen? Yes

If Not, Give Visa No. & Expiration:

Position Applying For

Title: Nursing Assistant

Salary Desired: $10.00/hr

Referred By: Ms. McClain, Instructor, NA Training Center

Date Available: 12/15/09

Education

High School (Name, City, State): Laguna High School, Albuquerque, NM

Graduation Date: December 2009

Technical or Undergraduate School: NA Training Center, Albuquerque, NM

Dates Attended: July – Dec. 2009

Degree Major: N/A

References

Mr. Robert Castro, Instructor, NA Training Center, 505-291-1284

Ms. Scott, Health Occupations, Laguna HS, 505-555-6255

Kate Crawford, Instructor, NA Training Center, 505-291-1294

Fig. 31-4. A sample job application.

By law, your employer must perform a criminal background check on all new aides hired. You may be asked to sign a form granting permission to do this. Do not take it personally; it is a law intended to protect patients, clients, and residents.

4. Discuss proper job interview techniques

Use these tips to make the best impression at a job interview:

- Shower or bathe, and use deodorant.
- Brush your teeth.
- Apply makeup lightly.
- Trim and clean your nails.
- Style clean hair simply.
- Shave or trim facial hair before the interview (men).
- Dress neatly and appropriately. Make sure clothing is clean, ironed, and has no holes in it. Avoid wearing jeans, shorts, or short dresses or skirts. Shoes should be clean and polished.
- Wear little or no jewelry.
- Arrive 10 or 15 minutes early.
- Introduce yourself. Smile and shake hands (Fig. 31-5). Your handshake should be firm and confident.

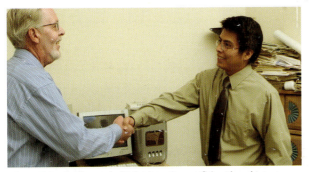

Fig. 31-5. Smile and shake hands confidently when you arrive at a job interview.

- Answer questions clearly and completely.
- Make eye contact to show you are sincere (Fig. 31-6).

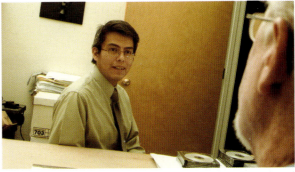

Fig. 31-6. Be polite and make eye contact while interviewing.

- Avoid slang words or expressions.
- Never eat, drink, chew gum, or smoke in an interview.
- Sit up or stand up straight. Look happy to be there.
- Do not bring friends or children with you.
- Relax. You have worked hard to get this far. You understand the work and what is expected of you. Be confident!

Be positive when answering questions. Emphasize what you enjoy or think you will enjoy about the job. Do not complain about previous jobs. Make it clear that you are hardworking and willing to work with all kinds of residents, clients, and patients.

The following are some questions you can expect to be asked:

- Why did you become a nursing assistant?
- What do you like about working as an aide?
- What do you not like? (If this is your first job, you may be asked what you expect to like or dislike.)
- What are your best qualities? What are your weaknesses?
- Why did you leave your last job?
- What kinds of residents or clients do you prefer to work with?

Usually interviewers will ask if you have any questions. Have some prepared. Write them down so you do not forget things you really want to know. Questions you may want to ask include the following:

- What hours would I work?

- What benefits does the job include? Is health insurance available? Would I get paid sick days or holidays?

- What orientation or training will be provided?

- Will my supervisor be available when needed?

- How soon will you be making a decision about this position?

Later in the interview, you may want to ask about salary or wages if you have not already been given this information.

Listen carefully to the answers to your questions. Take notes if needed. You will probably be told when you can expect to hear from the employer. Do not expect to be offered a job at the interview. When the interview is over, stand up and shake hands again. Say something like, "Thank you for taking the time to meet with me today. I look forward to hearing from you."

Send a thank-you letter after every job interview. This states your continued interest in a job. If you have not heard from the employer within the time frame you discussed with your interviewer, call and ask if the job was filled.

5. Describe a standard job description

A job description is an agreement between the employer and the employee. It states the responsibilities and tasks of the job. It also includes the skill required for the job, to whom the employee must report, and the salary range.

The job description is protection for both parties. It protects the employee from the facility or agency changing duties without notifying the employee. It protects the employee from being fired based on something not related to his or her job description. The employer is protected from the employee saying he or she did not

know certain duties were part of the job. The job description reduces misunderstandings and can be used to document what was agreed upon if misunderstandings or legal issues arise.

6. Discuss how to manage and resolve conflict

Everyone experiences conflict at some point in their lives. Families may argue at home; co-workers may disagree on the job, and so on. When conflict at work is not managed or resolved, it may affect the ability to function well. Productivity and the workplace environment may suffer. When conflict occurs, there is a proper time and place to address it. You may need to talk to your supervisor for assistance. In general, follow these guidelines for managing conflict:

Guidelines:
Resolving Conflict

G Plan to discuss the issue at the right time. Do not start a conversation while you are helping residents or patients. Wait until the supervisor has decided on an appropriate time and place. Privacy is important. Shut the door. Limit distractions, such as TV, conversations, radio, etc.

G Agree not to interrupt the person. Do not be rude or sarcastic, or name-call. Use active listening. Take turns speaking.

G   Do not get emotional. Some situations may be very upsetting. However, you will be more effective in communicating and problem-solving if you can keep your emotions out of it.

G   Check your body language to make sure it is not tense, unwelcoming, or threatening. Maintain eye contact and use a posture that says you are listening and interested. Lean forward slightly and do not slouch.

G   Keep the focus on the issue at hand. When discussing conflict, state how you feel when a behavior occurs. Use "I" statements. First describe the actual behavior. Then use "feeling" words to describe how you feel. Let the person know how the problem has affected you. For example, "When you are late to work, I feel upset because I end up doing your work along with my own."

G   People involved in the conflict may need to brainstorm possible solutions. Think of ways that the conflict can be resolved. A solution may be chosen by a supervisor or mediator that does not satisfy everyone. In order to resolve conflict, you may have to compromise. Be prepared to do this.

For more assistance with conflict resolution, speak to your supervisor.

7. Describe employee evaluations and discuss appropriate responses to criticism

Handling criticism is hard for most people. Being able to accept and learn from criticism is important in all relationships, including employment. From time to time you will receive evaluations from your employer. They contain ideas to help you improve your job performance. Here are some tips for handling criticism and using it to your benefit:

•   Listen to the message that is being sent. Do not get so upset that you cannot understand the message.

•   Hostile criticism and constructive criticism are not the same. Hostile criticism is angry and negative. Examples are, "You are useless!" or "You are lazy and slow." Hostile criticism should not come from your employer or supervisor. You may hear hostile criticism from residents, family members, or others. The best response is something like, "I'm sorry you are so disappointed," and nothing more. Give the person a chance to calm down before trying to discuss their comments.

•   Constructive criticism may come from your employer, supervisor, or others. Constructive criticism is meant to help you improve. Examples are, "You really need to be more accurate in your charting," or "You are late too often. You'll have to make more of an effort to be on time." Listening and acting on constructive criticism can help you be more successful in your job. Pay attention to it (Fig. 31-7).

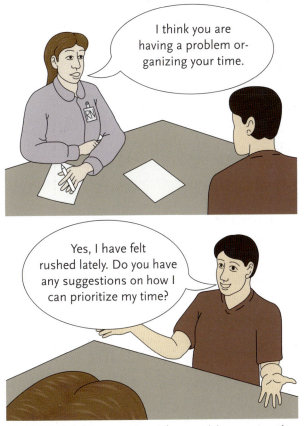

Fig. 31-7. Ask for suggestions when receiving constructive criticism.

- If you are not sure how to avoid a mistake you have made, always ask for suggestions. Avoiding making mistakes will help you improve your performance.

- Apologize and move on. If you have made a mistake, apologize as needed (Fig. 31-8). This may be to your supervisor, a resident, or others. Learn from the incident and put it behind you. Do not dwell on it or hold a grudge. Responding professionally to criticism is important for success in any job.

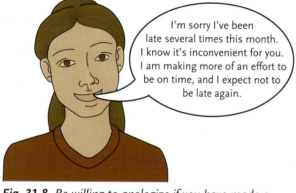

I'm sorry I've been late several times this month. I know it's inconvenient for you. I am making more of an effort to be on time, and I expect not to be late again.

Fig. 31-8. Be willing to apologize if you have made a mistake.

Your evaluation will also cover overall knowledge, conflict resolution, and team effort. Flexibility, friendliness, trustworthiness, and customer service are other things considered. Evaluations are often the basis for salary increases. A good evaluation can help you advance within the facility. Being open to criticism and suggestions for improvement will help you be more successful.

8. Explain how to make job changes

If you decide to change jobs, be responsible. Always give your employer at least two weeks' written notice that you will be leaving. Otherwise, your facility may be understaffed. Both the residents and other staff will suffer. In addition, future employers may talk with past supervisors. People who change jobs too often or who do not give notice before leaving are less likely to be hired.

9. Discuss certification and explain the state's registry

To satisfy the requirements set forth in the Omnibus Budget Reconciliation Act (OBRA), states must regulate nursing assistant training, evaluation, and certification. OBRA mandates 75 hours as the minimum level of initial training and a 12-hour minimum for annual continuing education (called "in-services"). Many states' requirements exceed the minimum hours for the basic training programs and annual in-services. It is a good idea to know your state's rules.

After a nursing assistant has completed an approved training program in his or her state, he or she is given a competency evaluation (a certification exam or test) in order to be certified to work in that state. This exam usually consists of both a written evaluation and a skills evaluation. You must pass both parts in order to be certified to work as a nursing assistant.

OBRA also requires that each state keep a registry of nursing assistants. This registry is maintained by a state department, often by the state's Department of Health. The registry contains nursing assistants' training information, results of certification exams, and any findings of abuse, neglect or theft by nursing assistants. Employers are able to access this list to verify that you have passed the certification exam, as well as to check if your certification is current. They are also able to see if you have been investigated or found guilty of any abuse or neglect.

Nursing assistant registries are also a good source of information for nursing assistants. By contacting the department that oversees the registry, you can find out how you may be able to move your certification from one state to another state. This is called reciprocity.

Each state has different requirements for maintaining certification. Learn your state's requirements. Follow them exactly or you will not be able to keep working. Once you are certified, you can lose your certification if you fail to follow your state's rules. Usually this occurs if you do not work in long-term care for a period of time or fail to get the required number of continuing education hours. You can also lose certification due to criminal activities, including abuse and neglect.

For your state, make sure you know the following:

- How quickly after completing a training program you must take and pass the certification exam

- How many days per year you must work in long-term care to maintain your certification

- How many hours of continuing education you must take each year

Some states do not have a registry for home health aides like the ones they maintain for nursing assistants. If you are a home health aide, ask your employer how best to maintain your certification. Know who is responsible for reporting your work hours and in-service hours to the state.

10. Describe continuing education

The federal government requires that nursing assistants and home health aides have 12 hours of continuing education each year. Some states may require more. "In-service" continuing education courses help you keep your knowledge and skills fresh. Classes also give new information about conditions, challenges you face in working with residents/clients, or regulation changes. You need to be up-to-date on the latest that is expected of you.

If you need more instruction in a particular area, speak to your supervisor. Perhaps he or she can arrange for an in-service continuing education class to be offered on that topic. Your employer may be responsible for offering continuing education courses. However, you are responsible for attending and completing them. Specifically, you must do the following:

- Sign up for the course or find out where it is offered (Fig. 31-9).

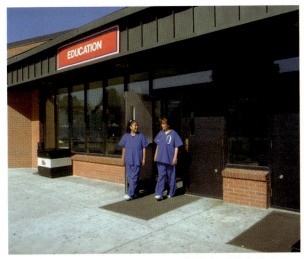

Fig. 31-9. You may want to go outside the in-service programs offered by your employer to take some continuing education courses.

- Attend all class sessions.

- Pay attention and complete all the class requirements.

- Make the most of your in-service programs. Participate! (Fig. 31-10)

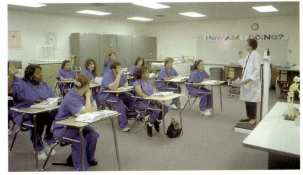

Fig. 31-10. Pay attention and participate during continuing education courses.

- Keep original copies of all certificates and records of your successful attendance so you can prove you took the class.

11. Define "stress" and "stressors"

Stress is the state of being frightened, excited, confused, in danger, or irritated. We may think only bad things cause stress. However, positive situations cause stress, too. For example, getting married or having a baby are usually positive situations. But both can bring enormous stress from the changes they bring to our lives (Fig. 31-11).

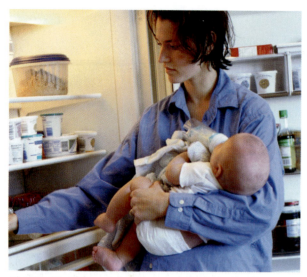

Fig. 31-11. *Although having a new baby is usually a happy time, it can also cause stress.*

You may be thrilled when you get your new job. But starting work may also cause you stress. You may be afraid of making mistakes, excited about earning money or helping people, or confused about your new duties. Learning how to recognize stress and its causes is helpful. Then you can master a few simple methods for relaxing and learn to manage stress.

Defense mechanisms are unconscious behaviors used to cope with stress. See Chapter 20 for more information on defense mechanisms.

A **stressor** is something that causes stress. Anything can be a stressor if it causes you stress. Some examples include the following:

- Divorce
- Marriage
- New baby
- Children growing up
- Children leaving home
- Feeling unprepared for a task
- Starting a new job

- Losing a job
- New responsibilities at work
- Problems at work
- Supervisors
- Co-workers
- Residents/clients
- Illness
- Finances

12. Explain ways to manage stress

Stress is not only an emotional response. It is also a physical response. When we experience stress, changes occur in our bodies. The endocrine system may make more of the hormone adrenaline. This can increase nervous system response, heart rate, respiratory rate, and blood pressure. This is why, in stressful situations, your heart beats fast, you breathe hard, and you feel warm or perspire.

Each of us has a different tolerance level for stress. What one person would find overwhelming may not bother another person. Your tolerance for stress depends on your personality, life experiences, and physical health.

Guidelines:
Managing Stress

To manage the stress in your life, develop healthy habits of diet, exercise, and lifestyle:

G   Eat nutritious foods.

G   Exercise regularly (Fig. 31-12). You can exercise alone or with a partner.

G   Get enough sleep.

G   Drink only in moderation.

G   Do not smoke.

G   Find time at least a few times a week to do something relaxing, such as taking a walk, reading a book, or sewing.

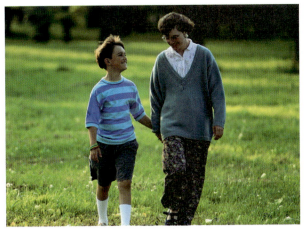

Fig. 31-12. *Exercising regularly is one healthy way to decrease stress.*

Not managing stress can cause many problems. Some of these problems affect how well you do your job. Signs that you are not managing stress include the following:

- Showing anger or being abusive to residents/clients

- Arguing with your supervisor about assignments

- Having poor relationships with co-workers and residents/clients

- Complaining about your job and your responsibilities

- Feeling work-related burnout (burnout is a state of mental or physical exhaustion caused by stress)

- Feeling tired even when you are rested

- Having a difficult time focusing on residents/clients and procedures

Stress can seem overwhelming when you try to handle it yourself. Often just talking about stress can help you manage it better. Sometimes another person can offer helpful suggestions. You may think of new ways to handle stress just by talking it through. Get help from one or more of these resources when managing stress (Fig. 31-13):

- Your supervisor or another member of the care team for work-related stress

- Your family

- Your friends

- Your place of worship

- Your doctor

- A local mental health agency

- Any phone hotline that deals with related problems (check your local yellow pages or the Internet)

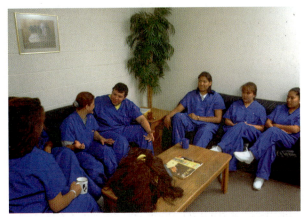

Fig. 31-13. *Support groups can help you deal with different types of stress.*

It is not appropriate to talk to your residents/clients or their family members about your personal or job-related stress.

One of the best ways of managing stress is to develop a plan for managing stress. The plan can include nice things you will do for yourself every day and things to do in stressful situations. When you think about a plan, you first need to answer the following questions:

- What are the sources of stress in my life?

- When do I most often feel stress?

- What effects of stress do I see in my life?

- What can I change to decrease my stress?

- What do I have to learn to cope with because I cannot change it?

When you have answered these questions, you will have a clearer picture of the challenges you face. Then you can come up with strategies for managing stress.

13. Describe a relaxation technique

Sometimes a relaxation exercise can help you feel refreshed and relaxed in only a short time. Below is a simple relaxation exercise. Try it out. See if it helps you feel more relaxed.

The body scan. Close your eyes. Focus on your breathing and posture. Be sure you are comfortable. Starting at the balls of your feet, concentrate on your feet. Find any tension hidden in the feet. Try to relax and release the tension. Continue very slowly. Take a breath between each body part. Move up from the feet, focusing on and relaxing the legs, knees, thighs, hips, stomach, back, shoulders, neck, jaw, eyes, forehead, and scalp. Take a few very deep breaths. Open your eyes.

This exercise takes only about two minutes. If it is helpful for you, try it the next time you need a break, at work or at home.

14. List ways to remind yourself of the importance of the work you have chosen to do

Look back over all you have learned in this program. Your work as a caregiver is very important. Every day may be different and challenging. In a hundred ways every week you will offer help that only a caring person like you can give.

Do not forget to value the work you have chosen to do. It is important. Your work can mean the difference between living with independence and dignity and living without. The difference you make is sometimes life versus death. Look in the face of each of your residents and clients. Know that you are doing important work. Look in a mirror when you get home and be proud of how you make your living (Fig. 31-14).

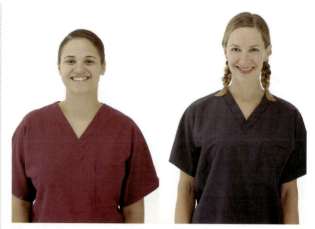

Fig. 31-14. *Be proud of the work you have chosen to do. It is important.*

An important life skill is reflecting on how you spend your time. Learn ways to fully appreciate that what you do has great meaning. Few jobs have the challenges and rewards of working with the elderly, ill, or disabled. Congratulate yourself for choosing a path that includes helping others along the way.

Chapter Review

1. What are direct service positions?

2. What are two good ways to find out about job opportunities with potential employers?

3. List three documents you may need to take with you when applying for a job.

4. What should be done before writing anything on a job application?

5. List 10 things that show potential employers professionalism during an interview.

6. How can you follow up on a job interview?

7. What is contained in a job description?

8. List four guidelines to follow while working on resolving conflicts.

9. What is the difference between hostile and constructive criticism?

10. Why might an employer not hire a person who has changed jobs often?

11. What information does a registry for certified nursing assistants keep?

12. How many hours of continuing education does the federal government require for NAs and HHAs each year?

13. What is stress? Give three examples of stressors you have experienced in the last year. How did you respond to them?

14. List five guidelines for managing stress.

15. What are five resources that are appropriate for an NA or HHA to turn to when trying to manage stress?

16. Before developing a stress management plan, what are four questions that a person should ask herself?

17. What do you think you will like best about being a nursing assistant or home health aide?

Abbreviations

ABCD	airway, breathing, circulation, defibrillation
abd	abdomen
ABR	absolute bedrest
ac, a.c.	before meals
ad lib	as desired
adm.	admission
ADLs	activities of daily living
AIDS	acquired immune deficiency syndrome
amb	ambulate, ambulatory
amt	amount
ap	apical
AROM	active range of motion
ASAP	as soon as possible
as tol	as tolerated
ax.	axillary (armpit)
BID, b.i.d.	two times a day
BM	bowel movement
BP, B/P	blood pressure
BPM	beats per minute
BR	bedrest
BRP	bathroom privileges
BSC	bedside commode
c̄	with
C	Centigrade
CA	cancer
cath.	catheter
CBC	complete blood count
CBR	complete bedrest
CCU	cardiac care unit, cardiovascular care unit
CDC	Centers for Disease Control
C. diff	*clostridium difficile*
CHF	congestive heart failure
ck ✔	check
cl liq	clear liquid
CMS	Centers for Medicare and Medicaid Services
c/o	complains of, in care of
CNA	certified nursing assistant
CNS	central nervous system
COPD	chronic obstructive pulmonary disease
CPR	cardiopulmonary resuscitation
CS	Central Supply
CVA	cerebrovascular accident, stroke
CVP	central venous pressure
CVS	cardiovascular system
CXR	chest X-ray
DAT	diet as tolerated
DM	diabetes mellitus
DNR	do not resuscitate
DOA	dead on arrival
DOB	date of birth
DON	director of nursing
Dr., DR	doctor
drsg	dressing
DVT	deep vein thrombosis
Dx, dx	diagnosis
ECG, EKG	electrocardiogram
EMS	emergency medical services
ER	emergency room
exam	examination
F	Fahrenheit
FBS	fasting blood sugar
FF	force fluids
ft	foot
F/U, f/u	follow-up
FWB	full weight bearing
FYI	for your information
geri chair	geriatric chair
GI	gastrointestinal
h, hr, hr.	hour
H_2O	water
H/A, HA	headache
HBV	hepatitis B virus
HHA	home health aide
HIPAA	Health Insurance Portability and Accountability Act
HIV	human immunodeficiency virus
HOB	head of bed
HS/hs	hours of sleep

ht	height	MSDS	material safety data sheet	post-op	after surgery
HTN	hypertension	NA	nursing assistant	PPE	personal protective equipment
hyper	above normal, too fast, rapid	N/A	not applicable	pre-op	before surgery
hypo	low, less than normal	N/C	no complaints, no call	p.r.n., prn	when necessary
ICU	intensive care unit	NG, ng	nasogastric	PROM	passive range of motion
inc	incontinent	NKA	no known allergies	PT	physical therapist/ therapy
I&O	intake and output	NPO	nothing by mouth	PVD	peripheral vascular disease
IV, I.V.	intravenous (within a vein)	NVD	nausea, vomiting and diarrhea	PWB	partial weight bearing
isol	isolation	NWB	non-weight bearing	$\bar{q}$	every
L, lt	left	OBRA	Omnibus Budget Reconciliation Act	qh, qhr	every hour
lab	laboratory	OOB	out of bed	q2h	every two hours
lb.	pound	OR	operating room	q3h	every three hours
lg	large	OSHA	Occupational Safety and Health Administration	q4h	every four hours
LOC	level of consciousness			R, rt.	right
LPN	licensed practical nurse	OT	occupational therapist/therapy	R	respirations, rectal
LTC	long-term care	oz	ounce	RBC	red blood cell/count
LTCF	long-term care facility	$\bar{p}$	after	rehab	rehabilitation
LVN	licensed vocational nurse	pc, p.c.	after meals	res.	resident
M.D.	medical doctor	PCA	patient-controlled anesthesia	resp.	respiration
MDS	minimum data set	PEG	percutaneous endoscopic gastrostomy	RF	restrict fluids
meds	medications			R.I.C.E.	rest, ice, compression, elevation
MI	myocardial infarction	per os	by mouth	RN	registered nurse
min	minute	peri care	perineal care	R/O	rule out
mm Hg	millimeters of mercury	PHI	Protected Health Information	ROM	range of motion
mL	milliliter	PNS	peripheral nervous system	RR	respiratory rate
mod	moderate			$\bar{s}$	without
MRSA	methicillin-resistant *staphylococcus aureus*	PO	by mouth	SNF	skilled nursing facility
				SOB	shortness of breath

SP	standard precautions
spec.	specimen
S&S, S/S	signs and symptoms
SSE	soapsuds enema
staph	*staphylococcus*
stat, STAT	immediately
STD	sexually transmitted disease
std. prec.	standard precautions
STI	sexually transmitted infection
strep	*streptococcus*
T., temp	temperature
TB	tuberculosis
TIA	transient ischemic attack
t.i.d., tid	three times a day
TLC	tender loving care
TPN	total parenteral nutrition
TPR	temperature, pulse and respiration
TWE	tap water enema
U/A, u/a	urinalysis
URI	upper respiratory infection
UTI	urinary tract infection
VRE	vancomycin resistant *enterococcus*
VS, vs	vital signs
WBC	white blood cell/ count

w/c, W/C	wheelchair
WNL	within normal limits
wt.	weight

Symbols

©	copyright
☣	biohazard
△	change, heat
°	degree
♀	female
♂	male
%	percent
☢	radiation

Appendix

Basic Math Skills

Nursing assistants need math skills when doing certain tasks, such as calculating intake and output. A basic math review is listed below:

Addition

```
      2,905              53,138
  +     174          +    3,008
  ─────────          ──────────
      3,079              56,146
```

Subtraction

```
     32,542             549,233
  −    8,710          −   26,903
  ─────────          ──────────
     23,832             522,330
```

Multiplication

```
      4,962                  79
  ×      13          ×        41
  ─────────          ──────────
     14,886                  79
  +  49,620          +     3,160
  ─────────          ──────────
     64,506               3,239
```

Division

```
        34                    39
    ┌─────             ┌─────
  22│  748           14│  546
    − 660               − 420
    ─────               ─────
       88                 126
     − 88               − 126
     ─────             ──────
        0                    0
```

Converting Decimals, Fractions, and Percentages

Decimals, fractions and percentages are different ways of showing the same value. For example, a half can be written in the following ways:

As a decimal: 0.5
As a fraction: 1/2
As a percentage: 50%

Here are common values shown in decimal, fraction, and percentage forms:

Decimal	Fraction	Percentage
0.01	1/100	1%
0.1	1/10	10%
0.2	1/5	20%
0.25	1/4	25%
0.333	1/3	33 1/3%
0.5	1/2	50%
0.75	3/4	75%
1	1/1	100%

Follow these rules for converting decimals, fractions, and percentages:

To convert **from decimal to a percentage**, you will multiply by 100, and add a percent sign (%).

.25 x 100 = 25%

To convert **from a percentage to decimal**, you will divide by 100, and delete the percent sign (%).

80% ÷ 100 = 0.8

To convert a **fraction to a decimal**, you will divide the top number by the bottom number.

$$\frac{2}{3} = 2 \div 3 = 0.67$$

To convert a **decimal to a fraction**, write the decimal over the number 1.

Step 1 $\dfrac{0.5}{1}$

Then multiply top and bottom by 10 for every number after the decimal point (10 for 1 number, 100 for 2 numbers, and so on.)

Step 2 $\dfrac{0.5}{1} \cdot \dfrac{\times 10}{\times 10} = \dfrac{5}{10}$

The resulting fraction is 5/10 (or 1/2 if you simplify the fraction).

To convert a **fraction to a percentage**, you will divide the top number by the bottom number. Then you multiply the result by 100, and add a percent sign (%).

Step 1 $\frac{3}{5} = 3 \div 5 = 0.6$

Step 2 $0.6 \times 100 = 60\%$

To convert a **percentage to a fraction**, first convert to a decimal by dividing by 100. Then use the steps for converting decimal to fractions.

Step 1 $15\% \div 100 = 0.15$

Step 2 $\frac{0.15}{1}$

Step 3 $\frac{0.15}{1} \cdot \frac{\times 100}{\times 100} = \frac{15}{100}$

The resulting fraction is 15/100 (or 3/20 if you simplify the fraction).

Other Useful Information

Multiplication Table

1	2	3	4	5	6	7	8	9	10	11	12
2	4	6	8	10	12	14	16	18	20	22	24
3	6	9	12	15	18	21	24	27	30	33	36
4	8	12	16	20	24	28	32	36	40	44	48
5	10	15	20	25	30	35	40	45	50	55	60
6	12	18	24	30	36	42	48	54	60	66	72
7	14	21	28	35	42	49	56	63	70	77	84
8	16	24	32	40	48	56	64	72	80	88	96
9	18	27	36	45	54	63	72	81	90	99	108
10	20	30	40	50	60	70	80	90	100	110	120
11	22	33	44	55	66	77	88	99	110	121	132
12	24	36	48	60	72	84	96	108	120	132	144

Conversions: Volume

1 milliliter (mL) = 1 cubic centimeter (cc)

1 ounce (oz.) = 30 mL (cc)

¼ cup = 2 oz. = 60 mL (cc)

½ cup = 4 oz. = 120 mL (cc)

1 cup = 8 oz. = 240 mL (cc)

1 Liter = 1000 mL (cc)

Conversions: Weight

2 pints = 1 quart (qt.) = 960 mL (cc)

2 quarts = ½ gallon (gal.) = 1920 cc = 2 liters (L)

4 quarts = 1 gallon (gal.)

2.2 pounds (lbs.) = 1 kilogram (kg)

1 gram (g) = 1000 milligrams (mg)

Conversions: Length

1 inch (in) = 2.54 centimeters (cm) (or round off to 2.5)

12 inches = 1 foot

3 feet = 1 yard

10 millimeters (mm) = 1 centimeter (cm)

100 centimeters (cm) = 1 meter

Glossary

24-hour urine specimen: a urine specimen consisting of all urine voided in a 24-hour period.

abdominal thrusts: method of attempting to remove an object from the airway of someone who is choking.

abduction: moving a body part away from the midline of the body.

abrasion: an injury which rubs off the surface of the skin.

abuse: purposely causing physical, mental, or emotional pain or injury to someone.

acquired immune deficiency syndrome (AIDS): disease caused by the human immunodeficiency virus (HIV) in which the body's immune system is weakened and unable to fight infection.

active assisted range of motion (AAROM) exercises: range of motion exercises performed by a person with some assistance and support.

active neglect: purposely harming a person by failing to provide needed care.

active range of motion (AROM) exercises: range of motion exercises performed by a person by himself.

active TB: type of tuberculosis in which the person shows symptoms of the disease and can spread TB to others; also known as TB disease.

activities of daily living (ADLs): personal daily care tasks, such as bathing, dressing, caring for teeth and hair, toileting, eating and drinking, walking, and transferring.

acute care: care given in hospitals and ambulatory surgical centers for people who have an immediate illness.

adaptive devices: special equipment that helps a person who is ill or disabled to perform ADLs; also called assistive devices.

additive: a substance added to another substance, changing its effect.

adduction: moving a body part toward the midline of the body.

adult daycare: care given at a facility during daytime working hours for people who need some help but are not seriously ill or disabled.

advance directives: legal documents that allow people to choose what medical care they wish to have if they cannot make those decisions themselves.

affected side: a weakened side from a stroke or injury; also called the weaker or involved side.

ageism: prejudice toward, stereotyping of, and/or discrimination against older persons or the elderly.

agitated: the state of being excited, restless, or troubled.

agnostics: persons who claim that they do not know or cannot know if God exists.

AIDS dementia complex: term for a group of symptoms including memory loss, poor coordination, paralysis, and confusion that occur during the late stages of AIDS.

alternative medicine: practices and treatments used instead of conventional healthcare methods.

Alzheimer's disease: a progressive, incurable disease that causes tangled nerve fibers and protein deposits to form in the brain, which eventually cause dementia.

ambulation: walking.

ambulatory: capable of walking.

amputation: the removal of some or all of a body part, usually a foot, hand, arm or leg; may be the result of an injury or disease.

anal incontinence: the inability to control the bowels, leading to involuntary passage of stool; also called fecal incontinence.

anesthesia: the use of medication to block pain during surgery and other medical procedures.

angina pectoris: the medical term for chest pain, pressure, or discomfort due to coronary artery disease.

anorexia: an eating disorder in which a person does not eat or exercises excessively to lose weight.

antimicrobial: destroying or resisting pathogens.

anxiety: uneasiness or fear, often about a situation or condition.

apathy: a lack of interest.

apical pulse: the pulse located on the left side of the chest, just below the nipple.

apnea: the state of not breathing.

arm lock: position in which the caregiver places his arm under the resident's armpit, grasping the resident's shoulder, while the resident grasps the caregiver's shoulder; also called lock arm.

arthritis: a general term that refers to inflammation of the joints; causes stiffness, pain, and decreased mobility.

artificial airway: any plastic, metal, or rubber device inserted into the respiratory tract to maintain or promote breathing.

aspiration: the inhalation of food, drink, or foreign material into the lungs.

assault: the act of threatening to touch a person without his or her permission.

assisted living : living facilities for people who do not need skilled, 24-hour care, although they do require some help with daily care.

assistive devices: special equipment that helps a person who is ill or disabled to perform ADLs; also called adaptive devices.

asthma: a chronic inflammatory disease that causes difficulty with breathing and coughing and wheezing.

atheist: person who claims there is no God and actively denies God's existence.

atherosclerosis: a hardening and narrowing of the blood vessels.

atrophy: the wasting away, decreasing in size, and weakening of muscles from lack of use.

autoimmune illness: an illness in which the body's immune system attacks normal tissue in the body.

axillae: underarms.

baseline: initial values that can then be compared to future measurements.

basted: coated with juices or other liquid during roasting.

battery: touching a person without his or her permission.

bed rest: stopping all activity and staying in bed in order to prevent labor from starting before a baby is ready to be born.

benign prostatic hypertrophy: a disorder that occurs in men as they age, in which the prostate becomes enlarged and causes pressure on the urethra, leading to frequent urination, dribbling of urine, difficulty in starting the flow of urine, and urinary retention.

benign tumors: tumors that are considered non-cancerous.

bias: prejudice.

bloodborne pathogens: microorganisms found in human blood, body fluid, draining wounds, and mucous membranes that can cause infection and disease in humans.

Bloodborne Pathogens Standard: federal law that requires that healthcare facilities protect employees from bloodborne health hazards.

body mechanics: the way the parts of the body work together whenever a person moves.

bone: rigid tissue that protects organs and works together to allow the body to move.

bony prominences: areas of the body where bone is close to the skin.

brachial pulse: the pulse inside the elbow, about 1-1 1/2 inches above the elbow.

bronchiectasis: condition in which the bronchial tubes are permanently enlarged, causing chronic coughing and thick sputum; may be result of chronic infections and inflammation.

bronchitis: an irritation and inflammation of the lining of the bronchi.

bulimia: an eating disorder in which a person binges, eating huge amounts of foods or very fattening foods, and then purges, or eliminates the food by vomiting, using laxatives, or exercising excessively.

calculi: kidney stones that form when urine crystallizes in the kidneys.

cardiopulmonary resuscitation (CPR): medical procedures used when a person's heart or lungs have stopped working.

cataracts: a condition in which milky or cloudy spots develop in the eye, causing vision loss.

catastrophic reaction: overreacting to something in an unreasonable way.

catheter: a thin tube inserted into the body that is used to drain or inject fluids.

causative agent: a pathogen or microorganism that causes disease.

C cane: a straight cane with a curved handle at the top.

cells: basic units of the body that divide, develop, and die, renewing tissues and organs.

Centers for Disease Control and Prevention (CDC): a government agency under the Department of Health and Human Services (HHS) that issues information to protect the health of individuals and communities.

Centers for Medicare & Medicaid Services (CMS): a federal agency within the U.S. Department of Health and Human Services that is responsible for Medicare and Medicaid, among many other responsibilities.

central nervous system: part of the nervous system that is composed of the brain and spinal cord.

cerebrovascular accident (CVA): a condition that occurs when blood supply to a part of the brain is cut off suddenly by a clot or a ruptured blood vessel; also called a stroke.

Cesarean section: a surgical procedure in which a baby is delivered through an incision in the mother's abdomen.

chain of infection: a way of describing how disease is transmitted from one living being to another.

chancres: open sores.

charting: writing down important information and observations about residents.

chest tubes: hollow drainage tubes that are inserted into the chest to drain air, blood, or fluid that has collected inside the pleural cavity or space.

Cheyne-Stokes: slow, irregular respirations or rapid, shallow respirations.

chickenpox: a highly contagious viral illness that strikes nearly all children.

child abuse: physical, emotional, and sexual mistreatment of children, as well as neglect and maltreatment.

child neglect: the purposeful or unintentional failure to provide for the needs of a child.

chlamydia: sexually transmitted disease that causes yellow or white discharge from the penis or vagina and burning with urination.

chronic illness: a disease or condition that is long-term or long-lasting.

chronic kidney failure: condition that occurs when the kidneys cannot eliminate certain waste products from the body; also called chronic renal failure.

chronic obstructive pulmonary disease (COPD): a chronic lung disease that cannot be cured; causes difficulty breathing.

chronic renal failure: condition that occurs when the kidneys cannot eliminate certain waste products from the body; also called chronic kidney failure.

circadian rhythm: the 24-hour day-night cycle.

circumcision: the removal of part of the foreskin of the penis.

cite: in a long-term care facility, to find a problem through a survey.

claustrophobia: the fear of being in a confined space.

clean: in health care, a condition in which objects are not contaminated with pathogens.

clean catch specimen: a urine specimen that does not have the first and last urine included.

clichés: phrases that are used over and over again and do not really mean anything.

closed bed: a bed completely made with the bedspread and blankets in place.

closed fracture: a broken bone that does not break the skin.

Clostridium difficile (C-diff, C. difficile): bacterial illness that causes diarrhea and can cause colitis.

cognition: the ability to think logically and quickly.

cognitive: related to thinking and learning.

cognitive impairment: loss of ability to think logically; concentration and memory are affected.

colitis: inflammation of the large intestine that causes diarrhea and abdominal pain; also called irritable bowel syndrome.

colorectal cancer: cancer of the gastrointestinal tract; also known as colon cancer.

colostomy: surgically-created diversion of stool or feces to an artificial opening through the abdomen; stool will generally be semi-solid.

combative: violent or hostile behavior.

combustion: the process of burning.

communication: the process of exchanging information with others by sending and receiving messages.

compassionate: caring, concerned, considerate, empathetic, and understanding.

complementary medicine: treatments that are used in addition to the conventional treatments prescribed by a doctor.

complex carbohydrates: carbohydrates that are broken down by the body into simple sugars for energy; found in foods such as bread, cereal, potatoes, rice, pasta, vegetables, and fruits.

concentrated formula: a type of formula for infants that is sold in small cans and must be mixed with sterile water before using.

condom catheter: catheter that has an attachment on the end that fits onto the penis; also called an external or "Texas" catheter.

confidentiality: the legal and ethical principle of keeping information private.

confusion: the inability to think clearly.

congestive heart failure (CHF): a condition in which the heart is no longer able to pump effectively; blood backs up into the heart instead of circulating.

conscientious: guided by a sense of right and wrong; having principles.

conscious: the state of being mentally alert and having awareness of surroundings, sensations, and thoughts.

constipation: the inability to eliminate stool, or the difficult and painful elimination of a hard, dry stool.

constrict: to narrow.

contracture: the permanent and often very painful stiffening of a joint and muscle.

cultural diversity: the variety of people with varied backgrounds and experiences who live and work together in the world.

culture: a system of learned behaviors by a group of people that are considered to be the tradition of that people and are passed on from one generation to the next.

culture change: a term given to the process of transforming services for elders so that they are based on the values and practices of the person receiving care; core values include choice, dignity, respect, self-determination, and purposeful living.

cyanotic: skin that is pale, blue, or gray.

cystitis: inflammation of the bladder that may be caused by bacterial infection.

dandruff: a skin condition that results from an excessive shedding of dead skin cells from the scalp.

dangle: to sit up with the feet over the side of the bed in order to regain balance.

defecation: the act of passing feces from the large intestine out of the body through the anus.

defense mechanisms: unconscious behaviors used to release tension or cope with stress.

degenerative: something that continually gets worse.

dehydration: a condition that results from inadequate fluid in the body.

delirium: a state of severe confusion that occurs suddenly and is usually temporary.

delusions: persistent false beliefs.

dementia: a general term that refers to a serious loss of mental abilities, such as thinking, remembering, reasoning, and communicating.

dental floss: a special kind of string used to clean between teeth.

dentures: artificial teeth.

dermatitis: general term that refers to inflammation of the skin; usually involves swollen, reddened, irritated, and itchy skin.

developmental disabilities: disabilities that are present at birth or emerge during childhood that restrict physical or mental ability.

diabetes: a condition in which the pancreas does not produce enough or does not properly use insulin.

diabetic ketoacidosis (DKA): complication of diabetes that is caused by having too little insulin; also called hyperglycemia or diabetic coma.

diagnosis: physician's determination of an illness.

diarrhea: frequent elimination of liquid or semi-liquid feces.

diastole: phase when the heart relaxes or rests.

diastolic: second measurement of blood pressure; phase when the heart relaxes or rests.

dietary restrictions: rules about what and when individuals can eat.

diet cards: cards that list the resident's name and information about special diets, allergies, likes and dislikes, and other instructions.

digestion: the process of preparing food physically and chemically so that it can be absorbed into the cells.

dilate: to widen.

direct contact: touching an infected person or his secretions.

dirty: in health care, a condition in which objects have been contaminated with pathogens.

disinfection: process that kills pathogens, but not all microorganisms; it reduces the organism count to a level that is generally not considered infectious.

disorientation: confusion about person, place, or time.

disposable: only to be used once and then discarded.

disposable razor: type of razor, usually plastic, that is discarded after one use; requires the use of shaving cream or soap.

diuretics: medications that reduce fluid volume in the body.

domestic violence: physical, sexual, or emotional abuse by spouses, intimate partners, or family members.

do-not-resuscitate (DNR): an order that tells medical professionals not to perform CPR.

dorsal recumbent: position in which a person is flat on her back with her knees flexed and her feet flat on the bed.

dorsiflexion: bending backward.

douche: putting a solution into the vagina in order to cleanse the vagina, introduce medication to treat an infection or condition, or to relieve discomfort.

draw sheet: an extra sheet placed on top of the bottom sheet when the bed is made; also called a turning sheet.

durable power of attorney for health care: a signed, dated, and witnessed paper that appoints someone else to make the medical decisions for a person in the event he or she becomes unable to do so.

dysphagia: difficulty swallowing.

dyspnea: difficulty breathing.

edema: swelling caused by excess fluid in body tissues.

edentulous: having no teeth; toothless.

electric razor: type of razor that runs on electricity; does not require the use of soap or shaving cream.

elimination: the process of expelling solid wastes made up of the waste products of food that are not absorbed into the cells.

elope: in medicine, when a person with Alzheimer's disease wanders away from the protected area and does not return.

emesis: the act of vomiting, or ejecting stomach contents through the mouth.

emotional lability: laughing or crying without any reason, or when it is inappropriate.

empathy: entering into the feelings of others.

emphysema: a chronic disease of the lungs that usually develops as a result of chronic bronchitis and smoking.

enema: a specific amount of water, with or without an additive, that is introduced into the colon to eliminate stool.

epilepsy: an illness of the brain that produces seizures.

episiotomy: an incision made in the perineal area during vaginal delivery of a baby that enlarges the vaginal opening for the baby's head.

ergonomics: the science of designing equipment and work tasks to suit the worker's abilities.

ethics: the knowledge of right and wrong.

exchange lists: lists of similar foods that can be substituted for each other on a meal plan.

expiration: exhaling air out of the lungs.

exposure control plan: plan designed to eliminate or reduce employee exposure to infectious material.

expressive aphasia: inability to speak or speak clearly.

extension: straightening a body part.

facilities: in medicine, places where health care is delivered or administered, including hospitals, long-term care facilities or nursing homes, and treatment centers.

fallacy: a false belief.

farsightedness: the ability to see objects in the distance better than objects nearby.

fasting: not eating food or eating very little food.

fecal impaction: a hard stool that is stuck in the rectum and cannot be expelled; results from unrelieved constipation.

financial abuse: the act of stealing, taking advantage of, or improperly using the money, property, or other assets of another person.

first aid: emergency care given immediately to an injured person.

flammable: easily ignited and capable of burning quickly.

flatulence: air in the intestine that is passed through the rectum, which can result in cramping or abdominal pain; also called flatus or gas.

flexion: bending a body part.

fluid balance: taking in and eliminating equal amounts of fluid.

fluid overload: a condition that occurs when the body is unable to handle the amount of fluid consumed.

foot drop: a weakness of muscles in the feet and ankles that impairs the ability to flex the ankles and walk normally.

force fluids: a medical order for a person to drink more fluids.

Fowler's: position in which a person is in a semi-sitting position (45 to 60 degrees).

fracture: a broken bone.

fracture pan: a bedpan that is flatter than the regular bedpan.

full weight bearing: able to bear 100 percent of the body weight on one or both legs on a step.

functional grip cane: cane that has a straight grip handle.

gait belt: a belt made of canvas or other heavy material used to assist people who are who are weak, unsteady, or uncoordinated; also called a transfer belt.

gastroesophageal reflux disease (GERD): a chronic condition in which the liquid contents of the stomach back up into the esophagus.

gastrostomy: an opening in the stomach and abdomen.

geriatrics: the study of health, wellness, and disease later in life.

gerontology: the study of the aging process in people from mid-life through old age.

gestational diabetes: type of diabetes that appears in pregnant women who have never had diabetes before but who have high glucose levels during pregnancy.

glands: structures that secrete hormones.

glaucoma: a condition in which the fluid inside the eyeball is unable to drain; increased pressure inside the eye causes damage that often leads to blindness.

glucose: natural sugar.

gonads: sex glands.

gonorrhea: sexually transmitted disease that causes greenish or yellowish discharge from the penis and burning with urination in men.

groin: the area from the pubis (area around the penis and scrotum) to the upper thighs.

grooming: practices to care for oneself, such as caring for fingernails and hair.

halitosis: bad breath.

hallucinations: illusions a person sees or hears.

hand antisepsis: washing hands with water and soap or other detergents that contain an antiseptic agent.

hand hygiene: washing hands with either plain or antiseptic soap and water and using alcohol-based hand rubs.

hat: in health care, a collection container that is sometimes inserted into a toilet to collect and measure urine or stool.

healthcare-associated infections (HAIs): infections that patients acquire within healthcare settings that result from treatment for other conditions.

health maintenance organizations (HMOs): a method of health insurance in which a person has to use a particular doctor or group of doctors except in case of emergency.

heartburn: a condition that results from a weakening of the sphincter muscle which joins the esophagus and the stomach; causes a burning sensation in the esophagus.

hemiparesis: weakness on one side of the body.

hemiplegia: paralysis on one side of the body.

hemorrhoids: enlarged veins in the rectum or outside the anus that can cause rectal itching, burning, pain, and bleeding.

hepatitis: inflammation of the liver caused by infection.

Herpes simplex 2: a sexually-transmitted, incurable disease caused by a virus; repeated outbreaks of the disease may occur for the rest of the person's life.

HIV: stands for human immunodeficiency virus, the virus that can cause AIDS.

hoarding: collecting and putting things away in a guarded manner.

holistic: a type of care that involves considering a whole system, such as a whole person, rather than dividing the system into parts.

home health agencies: businesses that provide health care and personal services in the home.

home health care: care that takes place in a person's home.

homeostasis: the condition in which all of the body's systems are working their best.

hormones: chemical substances created by the body that control numerous body functions.

hospice care: holistic, compassionate care given in facilities or homes for people who have six months or less to live.

hygiene: practices used to keep bodies clean and healthy.

hypertension: high blood pressure.

hyperthyroidism: condition in which the thyroid produces too much thyroid hormone, causing the cells to burn too much food.

hypotension: abnormally low blood pressure.

hypothyroidism: condition in which the thyroid produces too little thyroid hormone, causing the body processes to slow down; weight gain and physical and mental sluggishness result.

ileostomy: surgically-created opening into the end of the small intestine to allow feces to be expelled; causes stool to be liquid.

impairment: a loss of function or ability.

incident: an accident or unexpected event during the course of care that is not part of the normal routine in a healthcare facility.

incontinence: the inability to control the bladder or bowels.

indirect contact: touching something contaminated by an infected person.

indwelling catheter: a type of catheter that remains inside the bladder for a period of time; urine drains into a bag.

infection: the state resulting from pathogens invading the body and multiplying.

infection control: the measures practiced in healthcare facilities to prevent and control the spread of disease.

infectious: contagious.

inflammation: swelling.

informed consent: the process in which a person, with the help of a doctor, makes informed decisions about his or her health care.

input: the fluid a person consumes; also called intake.

insomnia: the lack of ability to fall asleep or stay asleep.

inspiration: breathing in.

insulin: a hormone that converts glucose into energy for the body.

insulin reaction: complication of diabetes that can result from either too much insulin or too little food; also known as hypoglycemia.

intake: the fluid a person consumes; also called input.

integument: a natural protective covering, such as the skin.

intervention: a way to change an action or development.

intravenous (IV): into a vein.

intubation: the passage of a plastic tube through the mouth, nose, or opening in the neck and into the trachea.

involuntary seclusion: separating a person from others against the person's will.

involved: term used to refer to the weaker, or affected, side of the body after a stroke or injury.

irreversible: incurable.

isolate: to keep something separate, or by itself.

isolation precautions: method of infection control used when caring for persons who are infected or suspected of being infected with a disease; also called transmission-based precautions.

jaundice: a condition in which the skin, whites of the eyes, and mucous membranes appear yellow.

joint: the place at which two bones meet.

Joint Commission: an independent, not-for-profit organization that evaluates and accredits healthcare organizations.

Kaposi's sarcoma: a rare form of skin cancer that appears as purple or red skin lesions.

karma: the belief that all past and present deeds affect one's future and future lives.

kidney dialysis: an artificial means of removing the body's waste products.

knee-chest: position in which the person is lying on her abdomen with her knees pulled towards the abdomen and her legs separated; arms are pulled up and flexed, and the head is turned to one side.

lactose intolerance: the inability to digest lactose, a type of sugar found in milk and some other dairy products.

latent TB: type of tuberculosis in which the person carries the disease but does not show symptoms and cannot infect others; also known as TB infection.

lateral: position in which a person is lying on either side.

laws: rules set by the government to help people live peacefully together and to ensure order and safety.

length of stay: the number of days a person stays in a healthcare facility.

leukemia: form of cancer in which the body's white blood cells are unable to fight disease.

lever: something that moves an object by resting on a base of support.

liability: a legal term that means someone can be held responsible for harming someone else.

lithotomy: position in which a person lies on her back with her hips at the end of an exam table; legs are flexed, and feet are in padded stirrups.

living will: a document that states the medical care a person wants, or does not want, in case he or she becomes unable to make those decisions for him- or herself.

localized infection: an infection that is confined to a specific location in the body and has local symptoms.

lock arm: position in which the caregiver places his arm under the person's armpit, grasping the person's shoulder, while the person grasps the caregiver's shoulder; also called arm lock.

logrolling: method of moving a person as a unit, without disturbing the alignment of the body.

long-term care (LTC): care given in long-term care facilities (LTCF) for people who need 24-hour, supervised nursing care.

lung cancer: the development of abnormal cells or tumors in the lungs.

lymph: a clear yellowish fluid that carries disease-fighting cells called lymphocytes.

major depression: a type of mental illness that causes many symptoms, including apathy and sadness.

malabsorption: inability to absorb or digest a particular nutrient properly.

malignant tumors: tumors that are considered to be cancerous.

malnutrition: poor nutrition due to improper diet.

malpractice: injury to a person due to professional misconduct through negligence, carelessness, or lack of skill.

managed care: a system or strategy of managing health care in a way that controls costs.

mandated reporters: people who are legally required to report suspected or observed abuse or neglect because they have regular contact with vulnerable populations, such as the elderly in facilities.

mastectomy: the surgical removal of all or part of the breast and sometimes other surrounding tissue.

masturbation: to touch or rub sexual organs in order to give oneself or another person sexual pleasure.

mechanical ventilation: the use of a machine to assist with or replace breathing (inflate and deflate the lungs) when a person is unable to do this on his own.

Medicaid: a medical assistance program for low-income people.

medical asepsis: the process of removing pathogens, or the state of being free of pathogens.

Medicare: a federal health insurance program for people who are 65 or older, are disabled, or are ill and cannot work.

menopause: the end of menstruation.

mental health: a general term that refers to the normal functioning of emotional and intellectual abilities.

mental illness: a disease that affects a person's ability to function at a normal level in the family, home, or community; often produces inappropriate behavior.

metabolism: physical and chemical processes by which substances are produced or broken down into energy or products for use by the body.

microbe: a living thing or organism that is so small that it can be seen only through a microscope; also called microorganism.

microorganism: a living thing or organism that is so small that it can be seen only through a microscope; also called microbe.

Minimum Data Set (MDS): a detailed form with guidelines for assessing residents in long-term care facilities; also details what to do if resident problems are identified.

mode of transmission: method of describing how a pathogen travels from one person to the next person.

modified diets: diets for people who have certain illnesses; also called special or therapeutic diets.

MRSA: stands for methicillin-resistant *Staphylococcus aureus*, an antibiotic-resistant infection often acquired by people in hospitals and other healthcare facilities who have weakened immune systems.

mucous membranes: the membranes that line body cavities, such as the mouth, nose, eyes, rectum, or genitals.

multidrug-resistant organisms (MDROs): microorganisms, mostly bacteria, that are resistant to one or more antimicrobial agents.

multidrug-resistant TB (MDR-TB): type of TB that can develop when a person with active TB does not take all the prescribed medication.

multiple sclerosis (MS): a progressive disease of the nervous system in which the protective covering for the nerves, spinal cord, and white matter of the brain breaks down over time; without this covering, nerves cannot send messages to and from the brain in a normal way.

muscles: groups of tissues that provide movement of body parts, protection of organs, and creation of body heat.

muscular dystrophy: an inherited, progressive disease that causes a gradual wasting of muscle, weakness, and deformity.

myocardial infarction (MI): a condition that occurs when the heart muscle does not receive enough oxygen because blood vessels are blocked; also called a heart attack.

nasal cannula: a device used to deliver oxygen, which consists of a piece of plastic tubing that fits around the face and is secured by a strap that goes over the ears and around the back of the head.

nasogastric tube: a feeding tube that is inserted into the nose and goes to the stomach.

nearsightedness: the ability to see things near but not far.

neglect: harming a person physically, mentally, or emotionally by failing to provide needed care.

negligence: actions, or the failure to act or provide the proper care, that result in unintended injury to a person.

neonatal: pertaining to a newborn infant.

neonate: a newborn baby.

neonatologists: doctors who specialize in caring for newborn babies.

nephritis: an inflammation of the kidneys.

neuropathy: numbness, tingling, and pain in the feet and legs.

nitroglycerin: medication that helps to relax the walls of the coronary arteries, allowing them to open and get more blood to the heart; comes in tablet, patch or spray form.

non-intact skin: skin that is broken by abrasions, cuts, rashes, acne, pimples, or boils.

nonspecific immunity: a type of immunity that protects the body from disease in general.

nonverbal communication: communicating without using words.

non-weight bearing: unable to support any weight on one or both legs.

nutrient: something found in food that provides energy, promotes growth and health, and helps regulate metabolism.

nutrition: how the body uses food to maintain health.

objective information: information based on what a person sees, hears, touches, or smells.

obsessive compulsive disorder: a disorder in which a person uses obsessive behavior to cope with anxiety.

obstructed airway: a condition in which the tube through which air enters the lungs is blocked.

occult: hidden; difficult to see or observe.

Occupational Safety and Health Administration (OSHA): a federal government agency that makes rules to protect workers from hazards on the job.

occupied bed: a bed made while a person is in the bed. An unoccupied bed is a bed made while no resident is in the bed.

ombudsman: the legal advocate for residents; helps resolve disputes and settle conflicts.

Omnibus Budget Reconciliation Act (OBRA): law passed by the federal government that includes minimum standards for nursing assistant training, staffing requirements, resident assessment instructions, and information on rights for residents.

onset: in medicine, the first appearance of the signs or symptoms of an illness.

open bed: a bed made with linen fanfolded down to the foot of the bed.

open fracture: a broken bone that penetrates the skin; also known as a compound fracture.

opportunistic infections: infections that invade the body when the immune system is weak and unable to defend itself.

oral care: care of the mouth, teeth, and gums.

organ: a structural unit in the human body that performs a specific function.

orthotic device: a device that helps support and align a limb and improve its functioning and helps prevent or correct deformities.

osteoarthritis: a common type of arthritis that usually affects the hips, knees, fingers, thumbs, and spine.

osteoporosis: a disease that causes bones to become porous and brittle.

ostomy: a surgically-created opening from an area inside the body to the outside.

outpatient care: care given for less than 24 hours for people who have had treatments or surgery and need short-term skilled care.

output: all fluid that is eliminated from the body; includes fluid in urine, feces, vomitus, perspiration, and moisture in the air that is exhaled.

oxygen concentrator: a box-like device that changes air in the room into air with more oxygen.

oxygen therapy: the administration of oxygen to increase the supply of oxygen to the lungs.

pacing: walking back and forth in the same area.

palliative care: care that focuses on the comfort and dignity of the person rather than on curing him or her.

panic disorder: a disorder in which a person is terrified for no apparent reason.

paralysis: the loss of ability to move all or part of the body, and often includes loss of feeling in the affected area.

paranoid schizophrenia: a brain disorder that centers mainly on hallucinations and delusions.

paraplegia: loss of function of the lower body and legs.

Parkinson's disease: a progressive disease that causes the brain to degenerate; causes stooped posture, shuffling gait, pill-rolling, and tremors.

partial bath: a bath that includes washing the face, hands, underarms, and perineum; is given on days when a complete bed bath, tub bath, or shower is not done.

partial weight bearing: able to support some weight on one or both legs.

passive neglect: unintentionally harming a person physically, mentally, or emotionally by failing to provide needed care.

passive range of motion (PROM) exercises: range of motion exercises performed by another person, without the affected person's help.

pathogens: harmful microorganisms.

payers: people or organizations paying for healthcare services.

pediculosis: an infestation of lice.

peptic ulcers: raw sores in the stomach or the small intestine that cause pain, belching, and vomiting.

percutaneous endoscopic gastrostomy (PEG) tube: a tube placed through the skin directly into the stomach to assist with eating.

perineal care: care of the genitals and anal area.

perineum: the genital and anal area.

peripheral nervous system: part of the nervous system made up of the nerves that extend throughout the body.

peripheral vascular disease (PVD): a disease in which the legs, feet, arms, or hands do not have enough blood circulation due to fatty deposits in the blood vessels that harden over time.

peristalsis: involuntary contractions that move food through the gastrointestinal system.

perseveration: repeating words, phrases, questions, or actions.

personal: relating to life outside one's job, such as family, friends, and home life.

personal protective equipment (PPE): equipment that helps protect employees from serious workplace injuries or illnesses resulting from contact with workplace hazards.

phantom sensation: pain or feeling from a body part that has been amputated; caused by remaining nerve endings.

phlegm: thick mucus from the respiratory passage.

phobia: an intense form of anxiety.

physical abuse: any treatment, intentional or not, that causes harm to a person's body; includes slapping, bruising, cutting, burning, physically restraining, pushing, shoving, or even rough handling.

pillaging: taking things that belong to someone else.

pneumonia: a bacterial, viral, or fungal infection that causes acute inflammation in a portion of lung tissue.

policy: a course of action that should be taken every time a certain situation occurs.

portable commode: a chair with a toilet seat and a removable container underneath; used for elimination.

portal of entry: any body opening on an uninfected person that allows pathogens to enter.

portal of exit: any body opening on an infected person that allows pathogens to leave.

positioning: the act of helping people into positions that will be comfortable and healthy for them.

postmortem care: care of the body after death.

postoperative: after surgery.

postpartum depression: a type of depression that occurs after giving birth.

post traumatic stress disorder: an anxiety-related disorder brought on by a traumatic experience.

posture: the way a person holds and positions his body.

powdered formula: a type of formula for infants that is sold in cans and is measured and mixed with sterile water.

pre-diabetes: a condition that occurs when a person's blood glucose levels are above normal but not high enough for a diagnosis of Type 2 diabetes.

preferred provider organizations (PPOs): a network of providers that contract to provide health services to a group of people.

prehypertension: a condition in which a person has a systolic measurement of 120–139 mm Hg and a diastolic measurement of 80–89 mm Hg; indicator that the person does not have high blood pressure now but is likely to have it in the future.

premature: term for babies who are born before 37 weeks gestation (more than three weeks before the due date).

preoperative: before surgery.

prepared formula: a type of formula for infants that is sold in bottles or cans and is ready to use.

pressure points: areas of the body that bear much of its weight.

pressure sore: a serious wound resulting from skin breakdown; also called bed sore or decubitus ulcer.

procedure: a method, or way, of doing something.

professional: having to do with work or a job.

professionalism: how a person behaves when on the job; it includes how a person dresses, the words he uses, and the things he talks about.

progressive: term used to mean that a disease gets worse, causing greater and greater loss of health and abilities.

pronation: turning downward.

prone: position in which a person is lying on his stomach.

prosthesis: a device that replaces a body part that is missing or deformed because of an accident, injury, illness, or birth defect; used to improve a person's ability to function and/or his appearance.

protected health information (PHI): a person's private health information, which includes name, address, telephone number, social security number, e-mail address, and medical record number.

providers: people or organizations that provide health care, including doctors, nurses, clinics, and agencies.

psychosocial: having to do with social interaction, emotions, intellect, and spirituality.

psychological abuse: any behavior that causes a person to feel threatened, fearful, intimidated, or humiliated in any way; includes verbal abuse, social isolation, and seclusion.

psychotherapy: a method of treating mental illness that involves talking about one's problems with mental health professionals.

pulse oximeter: a device that measures a person's blood oxygen level and pulse rate.

puree: to chop, blend, or grind food into a thick paste of baby food consistency.

quad cane: cane that has four rubber-tipped feet and a rectangular base.

quadriplegia: loss of function of the legs, trunk, and arms.

rabbi: religious leader of the Jewish faith.

radial pulse: the pulse located on the inside of the wrist, where the radial artery runs just beneath the skin.

range of motion (ROM) exercises: exercises that put a joint through its full arc of motion.

ready-to-feed: a type of formula for infants that is sold in bottles or cans and is ready to use.

receptive aphasia: inability to understand spoken or written words.

rehabilitation: care given in facilities or homes by a specialist to restore or improve function after an illness or injury.

reincarnation: a belief that some part of a living being survives death to be reborn in a new body.

renovascular hypertension: a condition in which a blockage of arteries in the kidneys causes high blood pressure.

repetitive phrasing: repeating words, phrases, or questions.

reproduce: to create new life.

reservoir: a place where a pathogen lives and grows.

residents' rights: numerous rights identified in the OBRA law that relate to how residents must be treated while living in a facility; they provide an ethical code of conduct for healthcare workers.

resistant: state in which drugs no longer work to kill specific bacteria.

respiration: the process of breathing air into the lungs and exhaling air out of the lungs.

restraint: a physical or chemical way to restrict voluntary movement or behavior.

restraint alternatives: any intervention used in place of a restraint or that reduces the need for a restraint.

restraint-free: the state of being free of restraints and not using restraints for any reason.

restrict fluids: a medical order that limits the amount of fluids a person takes in.

résumé: a summary or listing of relevant job experience and education; also called also "curriculum vitae" or "CV."

rheumatoid arthritis: a type of arthritis in which joints become red, swollen, and very painful, and movement is restricted.

rigor mortis: the Latin term for the temporary condition after death in which the muscles in the body become stiff and rigid.

rotation: turning a joint.

routine urine specimen: a urine specimen that can be collected any time a person voids.

safety razor: a type of razor that has a sharp blade with a special safety casing to help prevent cuts; requires the use of shaving cream or soap.

scabies: contagious skin condition caused by a tiny mite burrowing into the skin, where it lays eggs; causes intense itching and a skin rash that may look like thin burrow tracks.

scalds: burns caused by hot liquids.

scope of practice: defines the things that healthcare providers are legally allowed to do and how to do them correctly.

sedative: an agent or drug that helps calm and soothe a person and may cause sleep.

sexual abuse: forcing a person to perform or participate in sexual acts against his or her will; includes unwanted touching, exposing oneself, and sharing pornographic material.

sexual harassment: any unwelcome sexual advance or behavior that creates an intimidating, hostile, or offensive working environment; includes requests for sexual favors, unwanted touching, and other acts of a sexual nature.

sexually transmitted diseases (STDs): diseases caused by sexual contact with an infected person; also called venereal diseases.

sexually transmitted infections (STIs): infections caused by sexual contact with an infected person; a person may be infected, and may potentially infect others, without showing signs of the disease.

sharps: needles or other sharp objects.

shearing: rubbing or friction that results from the skin moving one way and the bone underneath it remaining fixed or moving in the opposite direction.

shingles: non-contagious skin rash caused by the varicella-zoster virus (VZV), which is the same virus that causes chickenpox; causes pain, tingling, or itching in an area, which later develops into a rash of fluid-filled blisters.

shock: a condition that occurs when organs and tissues in the body do not receive an adequate blood supply.

shower chair: a sturdy, water- and slip-resistant chair designed to be placed in a tub or shower.

simple carbohydrates: carbohydrates that are found in foods such as sugars, sweets, syrups, and jellies and have little nutritional value.

Sims': position in which a person is in a left side-lying position; lower arm is behind the back and the upper knee is flexed and raised toward the chest.

situation response: a temporary condition that may be caused by a crisis, temporary changes in the brain, side effects from medications, interactions among medications, or severe change in the environment.

sitz bath: a warm soak of the perineal area given to clean perineal wounds and reduce inflammation and pain.

skilled care: medically necessary care given by a skilled nurse or therapist; is available 24 hours a day.

slide board: a wooden board that helps transfer people who are unable to bear weight on their legs; also called a transfer board.

special diets: diets for people who have certain illnesses; also called therapeutic or modified diets.

specific immunity: a type of immunity that protects against a particular disease that is invading the body at a given time.

specimen: a sample that is used for analysis in order to try to make a diagnosis.

sphygmomanometer: a blood pressure cuff.

spiritual: of, or relating to, the spirit or soul.

sputum: the fluid a person coughs up from the lungs.

standard precautions: a method of infection control in which all blood, body fluids, non-intact skin, and mucous membranes are treated as if they were infected with an infectious disease.

sterilization: a measure that destroys all micro-organisms, including pathogens.

stethoscope: an instrument designed to listen to sounds within the body.

stoma: an artificial opening in the body.

straight catheter: a catheter that does not remain inside the person; it is removed immediately after urine is drained.

stress: the state of being frightened, excited, confused, in danger, or irritated.

stressor: something that causes stress.

subacute care: care given in a hospital or in a long-term care facility for people who have had an acute injury or illness or problem resulting from a disease.

subjective information: information that a person cannot or did not observe, but is based on something reported to the person that may or may not be true.

substance abuse: the use of legal or illegal drugs, cigarettes, or alcohol in a way that is harmful to the abuser or to others.

sudden infant death syndrome (SIDS): the sudden and unexpected death of a baby for no known reason, usually during sleep.

suffocation: death from a lack of air or oxygen.

sundowning: becoming restless and agitated in the late afternoon, evening, or night.

supination: turning upward.

supine: position in which a person lies flat on his back.

suppository: a medication given rectally to cause a bowel movement.

surgical asepsis: the state of being free of all microorganisms, not just pathogens; also called sterile technique.

surgical bed: a bed made to easily accept residents who must return to bed on stretchers.

susceptible host: an uninfected person who could get sick.

sympathy: sharing in the feelings and difficulties of others.

syphilis: sexually transmitted disease that can cause chancres on the penis and, if untreated, rash, sore throat, or fever.

systemic infection: an infection that is in the bloodstream and is spread throughout the body, causing general symptoms.

systole: phase where the heart is at work, contracting and pushing blood out of the left ventricle.

systolic: first measurement of blood pressure; phase when the heart is at work, contracting and pushing the blood from the left ventricle of the heart.

tact: the ability to understand what is proper and appropriate when dealing with others; being able to speak and act without offending others.

telemetry: the application of a cardiac monitoring device that sends information about the heart's rhythm and rate to a monitoring station.

terminal illness: a disease or condition that will eventually cause death.

therapeutic diets: diets for people who have certain illnesses; also called special or modified diets.

tissues: groups of cells that perform similar tasks.

total parenteral nutrition (TPN): the intravenous infusion of nutrients administered directly into the bloodstream, bypassing the digestive tract.

tracheostomy: a surgically-created opening through the neck into the trachea.

transfer belt: a belt made of canvas or other heavy material used to assist people who are who are weak, unsteady, or uncoordinated; also called a gait belt.

transfer board: a wooden board that helps transfer people who are unable to bear weight on their legs; also called a slide board.

transient ischemic attack: a warning sign of a CVA/stroke resulting from a temporary lack of oxygen in the brain; symptoms may last up to 24 hours.

transmission: passage or transfer.

transmission-based precautions: method of infection control used when caring for persons who are infected or suspected of being infected with a disease; also called isolation precautions.

trauma: severe injury.

triggers: situations that lead to agitation.

tuberculosis: an airborne disease carried on very small mucous droplets suspended in the air.

tumor: a group of abnormally growing cells.

Type 1 diabetes: type of diabetes in which the body does not produce enough insulin; is usually diagnosed in children and young adults and will continue throughout a person's life.

Type 2 diabetes: common form of diabetes in which either the body does not produce enough insulin or the body fails to properly use insulin; typically develops after age 35 and is the milder form of diabetes.

ulceration: scarring.

ulcerative colitis: a chronic inflammatory disease of the large intestine; causes cramping, diarrhea, pain, rectal bleeding, and loss of appetite.

umbilical cord: the cord that connects a baby to the placenta inside the mother's uterus.

unoccupied bed: a bed made while nobody is in the bed.

upper respiratory infection (URI): a bacterial or viral infection of the nose, sinuses, and throat; commonly called a cold.

ureterostomy: surgically created opening from an ureter to the abdomen for urine to be eliminated.

urinary incontinence: the inability to control the bladder, which leads to an involuntary loss of urine.

urinary tract infection (UTI): inflammation of the bladder and the ureters that results in a painful burning during urination and the frequent feeling of needing to urinate; also called cystitis.

urination: the act of passing urine from the bladder through the urethra to the outside of the body; also known as micturition or voiding.

vaginitis: an infection of the vagina that may be caused by a bacteria, protozoa (one-celled animals), or fungus (yeast).

validating: giving value to or approving.

vegans: people who do not eat or wear any animals or animal products.

vegetarians: people who do not eat meat, fish, or poultry and who may or may not eat eggs and dairy products.

verbal abuse: the use of language—spoken or written—that threatens, embarrasses, or insults a person.

verbal communication: communicating using words or sounds, spoken or written.

vital signs: measurements that show how well the vital organs of the body are working; consist of body temperature, pulse, respirations, blood pressure, and level of pain.

VRE: vancomycin-resistant *enterococcus*, a genetically changed strain of *enterococcus* that originally developed in people who were exposed to the antibiotic vancomycin.

walker: adaptive equipment used for people who are unsteady or who lack balance; usually has four rubber-tipped feet and/or wheels.

wandering: walking around aimlessly.

workplace violence: verbal, physical, or sexual abuse of staff by residents or other staff members.

wound: a type of injury to the skin.

yarmulke: a small skullcap worn by Jewish men as a sign of their faith.

Index